New Technologies for the Treatment of Coronary and Structural Heart Diseases

New Technologies for the Treatment of Coronary and Structural Heart Diseases

Editor

Alberto Polimeni

MDPI • Basel • Beijing • Wuhan • Barcelona • Belgrade • Manchester • Tokyo • Cluj • Tianjin

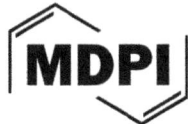

Editor
Alberto Polimeni
Magna Graecia University
of Catanzaro
Italy

Editorial Office
MDPI
St. Alban-Anlage 66
4052 Basel, Switzerland

This is a reprint of articles from the Special Issue published online in the open access journal *Journal of Clinical Medicine* (ISSN 2077-0383) (available at: https://www.mdpi.com/journal/jcm/special_issues/coronary_structural_heart).

For citation purposes, cite each article independently as indicated on the article page online and as indicated below:

LastName, A.A.; LastName, B.B.; LastName, C.C. Article Title. *Journal Name* **Year**, *Article Number*, Page Range.

ISBN 978-3-03943-559-3 (Hbk)
ISBN 978-3-03943-560-9 (PDF)

© 2020 by the authors. Articles in this book are Open Access and distributed under the Creative Commons Attribution (CC BY) license, which allows users to download, copy and build upon published articles, as long as the author and publisher are properly credited, which ensures maximum dissemination and a wider impact of our publications.

The book as a whole is distributed by MDPI under the terms and conditions of the Creative Commons license CC BY-NC-ND.

Contents

About the Editor ix

Preface to "New Technologies for the Treatment of Coronary and Structural Heart Diseases" . xi

Alberto Polimeni, Sabato Sorrentino, Salvatore De Rosa, Carmen Spaccarotella, Annalisa Mongiardo, Jolanda Sabatino and Ciro Indolfi
Transcatheter Versus Surgical Aortic Valve Replacement in Low-Risk Patients for the Treatment of Severe Aortic Stenosis
Reprinted from: *J. Clin. Med.* **2020**, *9*, 439, doi:10.3390/jcm9020439 1

Mirosław Gozdek, Kamil Zieliński, Michał Pasierski, Matteo Matteucci, Dario Fina, Federica Jiritano, Paolo Meani, Giuseppe Maria Raffa, Pietro Giorgio Malvindi, Michele Pilato, Domenico Paparella, Artur Słomka, Jacek Kubica, Dariusz Jagielak, Roberto Lorusso, Piotr Suwalski and Mariusz Kowalewski
Transcatheter Aortic Valve Replacement with Self-Expandable ACURATE neo as Compared to Balloon-Expandable SAPIEN 3 in Patients with Severe Aortic Stenosis: Meta-Analysis of Randomized and Propensity-Matched Studies
Reprinted from: *J. Clin. Med.* **2020**, *9*, 397, doi:10.3390/jcm9020397 13

Martin Geyer, Johannes Wild, Marc Hirschmann, Zisis Dimitriadis, Thomas Münzel, Tommaso Gori and Philip Wenzel
Predictors for Target Vessel Failure after Recanalization of Chronic Total Occlusions in Patients Undergoing Surveillance Coronary Angiography
Reprinted from: *J. Clin. Med.* **2020**, *9*, 178, doi:10.3390/jcm9010178 41

Emilija Miskinyte, Paulius Bucius, Jennifer Erley, Seyedeh Mahsa Zamani, Radu Tanacli, Christian Stehning, Christopher Schneeweis, Tomas Lapinskas, Burkert Pieske, Volkmar Falk, Rolf Gebker, Gianni Pedrizzetti, Natalia Solowjowa and Sebastian Kelle
Assessment of Global Longitudinal and Circumferential Strain Using Computed Tomography Feature Tracking: Intra-Individual Comparison with CMR Feature Tracking and Myocardial Tagging in Patients with Severe Aortic Stenosis
Reprinted from: *J. Clin. Med.* **2019**, *8*, 1423, doi:10.3390/jcm8091423 53

Tak-Wah Wong, Chung-Dann Kan, Wen-Tai Chiu, Kin Lam Fok, Ye Chun Ruan, Xiaohua Jiang, Junjiang Chen, Chiu-Ching Kao, I-Yu Chen, Hui-Chun Lin, Chia-Hsuan Chou, Chou-Wen Lin, Chun-Keung Yu, Stephanie Tsao, Yi-Ping Lee, Hsiao Chang Chan and Jieh-Neng Wang
Progenitor Cells Derived from Drain Waste Product of Open-Heart Surgery in Children
Reprinted from: *J. Clin. Med.* **2019**, *8*, 1028, doi:10.3390/jcm8071028 65

Tommaso Gori, Stephan Achenbach, Thomas Riemer, Julinda Mehilli, Holger M. Nef, Christoph Naber, Gert Richardt, Jochen Wöhrle, Ralf Zahn, Till Neumann, Johannes Kastner, Axel Schmermund, Christian Hamm and Thomas Münzel
Hybrid Coronary Percutaneous Treatment with Metallic Stents and Everolimus-Eluting Bioresorbable Vascular Scaffolds: 2-Years Results from the GABI-R Registry
Reprinted from: *J. Clin. Med.* **2019**, *8*, 767, doi:10.3390/jcm8060767 87

Niklas F. Boeder, Melissa Weissner, Florian Blachutzik, Helen Ullrich, Remzi Anadol, Monique Tröbs, Thomas Münzel, Christian W. Hamm, Jouke Dijkstra, Stephan Achenbach, Holger M. Nef and Tommaso Gori
Incidental Finding of Strut Malapposition Is a Predictor of Late and Very Late Thrombosis in Coronary Bioresorbable Scaffolds
Reprinted from: *J. Clin. Med.* **2019**, *8*, 580, doi:10.3390/jcm8050580 . . . . **101**

Chieh-Jen Wu, Hsin-Hung Chen, Pei-Wen Cheng, Wen-Hsien Lu, Ching-Jiunn Tseng and Chi-Cheng Lai
Outcome of Robot-Assisted Bilateral Internal Mammary Artery Grafting via Left Pleura in Coronary Bypass Surgery
Reprinted from: *J. Clin. Med.* **2019**, *8*, 502, doi:10.3390/jcm8040502 . . . . **113**

Dan Mircea Olinic, Mihail Spinu, Calin Homorodean, Mihai Claudiu Ober and Maria Olinic
Real-Life Benefit of OCT Imaging for Optimizing PCI Indications, Strategy, and Results
Reprinted from: *J. Clin. Med.* **2019**, *8*, 437, doi:10.3390/jcm8040437 . . . . **125**

Lucia Agoston-Coldea, Kunal Bheecarry, Carmen Cionca, Cristian Petra, Lelia Strimbu, Camelia Ober, Silvia Lupu, Daniela Fodor and Teodora Mocan
Incremental Predictive Value of Longitudinal Axis Strain and Late Gadolinium Enhancement Using Standard CMR Imaging in Patients with Aortic Stenosis
Reprinted from: *J. Clin. Med.* **2019**, *8*, 165, doi:10.3390/jcm8020165 . . . . **137**

Ryoi Okano, Yi-Jia Liou, Hsi-Yu Yu, I-Hui Wu, Nai-Kuan Chou, Yih-Sharng Chen and Nai-Hsin Chi
Coronary Artery Bypass in Young Patients—On or Off-Pump?
Reprinted from: *J. Clin. Med.* **2019**, *8*, 128, doi:10.3390/jcm8020128 . . . . **153**

Mateusz P. Jeżewski, Michał J. Kubisa, Ceren Eyileten, Salvatore De Rosa, Günter Christ, Maciej Lesiak, Ciro Indolfi, Aurel Toma, Jolanta M. Siller-Matula and Marek Postuła
Bioresorbable Vascular Scaffolds—Dead End or Still a Rough Diamond?
Reprinted from: *J. Clin. Med.* **2019**, *8*, 2167, doi:10.3390/jcm8122167 . . . . **163**

Alessandro Caracciolo, Paolo Mazzone, Giulia Laterra, Victoria Garcia-Ruiz, Alberto Polimeni, Salvatore Galasso, Francesco Saporito, Scipione Carerj, Fabrizio D'Ascenzo, Guillaume Marquis-Gravel, Gennaro Giustino and Francesco Costa
Antithrombotic Therapy for Percutaneous Cardiovascular Interventions: From Coronary Artery Disease to Structural Heart Interventions
Reprinted from: *J. Clin. Med.* **2019**, *8*, 2016, doi:10.3390/jcm8112016 . . . . **185**

Renato Francesco Maria Scalise, Armando Mariano Salito, Alberto Polimeni, Victoria Garcia-Ruiz, Vittorio Virga, Pierpaolo Frigione, Giuseppe Andò, Carlo Tumscitz and Francesco Costa
Radial Artery Access for Percutaneous Cardiovascular Interventions: Contemporary Insights and Novel Approaches
Reprinted from: *J. Clin. Med.* **2019**, *8*, 1727, doi:10.3390/jcm8101727 . . . . **219**

Grzegorz M. Kubiak, Agnieszka Ciarka, Monika Biniecka and Piotr Ceranowicz
Right Heart Catheterization—Background, Physiological Basics, and Clinical Implications
Reprinted from: *J. Clin. Med.* **2019**, *8*, 1331, doi:10.3390/jcm8091331 . . . . **239**

Rabea Asleh and Jon R. Resar
Utilization of Percutaneous Mechanical Circulatory Support Devices in Cardiogenic
Shock Complicating Acute Myocardial Infarction and High-Risk Percutaneous
Coronary Interventions
Reprinted from: *J. Clin. Med.* **2019**, *8*, 1209, doi:10.3390/jcm8081209 255

Isabella C. Schoepf, Ronny R. Buechel, Helen Kovari, Dima A. Hammoud and Philip E. Tarr
Subclinical Atherosclerosis Imaging in People Living with HIV
Reprinted from: *J. Clin. Med.* **2019**, *8*, 1125, doi:10.3390/jcm8081125 289

Matteo Pirro, Luis E. Simental-Mendía, Vanessa Bianconi, Gerald F. Watts, Maciej Banach and Amirhossein Sahebkar
Effect of Statin Therapy on Arterial Wall Inflammation Based on 18F-FDG PET/CT:
A Systematic Review and Meta-Analysis of Interventional Studies
Reprinted from: *J. Clin. Med.* **2019**, *8*, 118, doi:10.3390/jcm8010118 311

Ramez Morcos, Haider Al Taii, Priya Bansal, Joel Casale, Rupesh Manam, Vikram Patel, Anthony Cioci, Michael Kucharik, Arjun Malhotra and Brijeshwar Maini
Accuracy of Commonly-Used Imaging Modalities in Assessing Left Atrial Appendage for
Interventional Closure: Review Article
Reprinted from: *J. Clin. Med.* **2018**, *7*, 441, doi:10.3390/jcm7110441 325

About the Editor

Alberto Polimeni (MD, PhD) is an Interventional Cardiologist. Currently, he works at Magna Graecia University of Catanzaro as Postdoctoral Fellow in Cardiology. He has authored many research articles in the cardiovascular field and was awarded the "Young Researcher Award" in 2010 and 2013 by the Italian Society of Cardiology. In 2016, his project on the percutaneous treatment of mitral valve regurgitation was granted by the European Association of Percutaneous Cardiovascular Interventions (EAPCI). He has been serving as Chair of the Italian Cardiologists of Tomorrow since 2019 and was elected in the ESC Board Committee for Young Cardiovascular Professionals in 2020.

Preface to "New Technologies for the Treatment of Coronary and Structural Heart Diseases"

There has been significant progress in the field of interventional cardiology, from the development of newer devices to newer applications of technology, resulting in improved cardiovascular outcomes. The goal of this Special Issue is to update practicing clinicians and provide a comprehensive collection of original articles, reviews, and editorials.

To this end, we invited state-of-the-art reviews, including reviews of new technology and therapeutics, as well as original research in this area to be considered for inclusion in this issue. Examples include the history and evolution of interventional techniques, reviews of specific devices and technologies for coronary artery disease (i.e., stent technology, atherectomy devices, coronary physiology, intracoronary imaging, and robotics), structural heart diseases (i.e., ASD: atrial septal defect; LAAC: left atrial appendage closure; MC: MitraClip; PFO: patent foramen ovale; TAVI: transcatheter aortic valve implantation), advances in the management of challenging coronary anatomy, new biomarkers of cardiovascular disease (noncoding RNAs, etc.), and interventional techniques in the management of heart failure, peripheral arterial diseases, and pulmonary embolism.

This Special Issue presents the most recent advances in the field of coronary and structural heart diseases as well as their implications for future patient care.

Alberto Polimeni
Editor

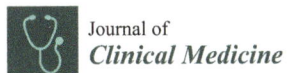

Article

Transcatheter Versus Surgical Aortic Valve Replacement in Low-Risk Patients for the Treatment of Severe Aortic Stenosis

Alberto Polimeni [1], Sabato Sorrentino [1], Salvatore De Rosa [1], Carmen Spaccarotella [1], Annalisa Mongiardo [1], Jolanda Sabatino [1] and Ciro Indolfi [1,2,*]

[1] Division of Cardiology, Department of Medical and Surgical Sciences, "Magna Graecia" University, 88100 Catanzaro, Italy; polimeni@unicz.it (A.P.); sabatosorrentino@hotmail.com (S.S.); saderosa@unicz.it (S.D.R.); spaccarorella@unicz.it (C.S.); mongiardo@unicz.it (A.M.); jolesbt@hotmail.com (J.S.)
[2] URT-CNR, Department of Medicine, Consiglio Nazionale delle Ricerche, 88100 Catanzaro, Italy
* Correspondence: indolfi@unicz.it; Tel.: +39-096-1364-7151; Fax: +39-096-1364-7153

Received: 17 December 2019; Accepted: 4 February 2020; Published: 6 February 2020

Abstract: Recently, two randomized trials, the PARTNER 3 and the Evolut Low Risk Trial, independently demonstrated that transcatheter aortic valve replacement (TAVR) is non-inferior to surgical aortic valve replacement (SAVR) for the treatment of severe aortic stenosis in patients at low surgical risk, paving the way to a progressive extension of clinical indications to TAVR. We designed a meta-analysis to compare TAVR versus SAVR in patients with severe aortic stenosis at low surgical risk. The study protocol was registered in PROSPERO (CRD42019131125). Randomized studies comparing one-year outcomes of TAVR or SAVR were searched for within Medline, Scholar and Scopus electronic databases. A total of three randomized studies were selected, including nearly 3000 patients. After one year, the risk of cardiovascular death was significantly lower with TAVR compared to SAVR (Risk Ratio (RR) = 0.56; 95% CI 0.33–0.95; p = 0.03). Conversely, no differences were observed between the groups for one-year all-cause mortality (RR = 0.67; 95% CI 0.42–1.07; p = 0.10). Among the secondary endpoints, patients undergoing TAVR have lower risk of new-onset of atrial fibrillation compared to SAVR (RR = 0.26; 95% CI 0.17–0.39; p < 0.00001), major bleeding (RR = 0.30; 95% CI 0.14–0.65; p < 0.002) and acute kidney injury stage II or III (RR = 0.28; 95% CI 0.14–0.58; p = 0.0005). Conversely, TAVR was associated to a higher risk of aortic regurgitation (RR = 3.96; 95% CI 1.31–11.99; p = 0.01) and permanent pacemaker implantation (RR = 3.47; 95% CI 1.33–9.07; p = 0.01) compared to SAVR. No differences were observed between the groups in the risks of stroke (RR= 0.71; 95% CI 0.41–1.25; p = 0.24), transient ischemic attack (TIA; RR = 0.98; 95% CI 0.53–1.83; p = 0.96), and MI (RR = 0.75; 95% CI 0.43–1.29; p = 0.29). In conclusion, the present meta-analysis, including three randomized studies and nearly 3000 patients with severe aortic stenosis at low surgical risk, shows that TAVR is associated with lower CV death compared to SAVR at one-year follow-up. Nevertheless, paravalvular aortic regurgitation and pacemaker implantation still represent two weak spots that should be solved.

Keywords: TAVR; TAVI; low risk; STS; aortic stenosis; SAVR

1. Introduction

Transcatheter aortic valve replacement (TAVR) has been established as a standard of care for patients with severe aortic stenosis (AS) deemed at prohibitive or high surgical risk [1]. Of note, over the last years, its use has progressively increased, along with continuous improvements of devices and implantation techniques, to encompass patients at lower surgical risk [2,3]. Indeed, both the balloon-expandable as well as self-expandable devices were non-inferior to the surgical aortic valve replacement (SAVR) for short- and long-term outcomes in intermediate-risk patients [4] and are becoming a feasible alternative in appropriately selected low-risk patients. However, since SAVR has shown a low rate of mortality and stroke in these relatively young and healthy patients [5], some have hypothesized that the benefit of using TAVR may be futile over SAVR. Moreover, peri-procedural TAVR outcomes such as vascular access complications, conduction disturbances, bleeding and post-procedural paravalvular leak (PVL) after TAVR need further investigations in this large portion of patients [6]. Very recently, two randomized trials, the Safety and Effectiveness of the SAPIEN 3 Transcatheter Heart Valve in Low Risk Patients With Aortic Stenosis (PARTNER 3) trial [7], using the balloon-expandable valve, and the Evolut Low Risk Trial [8], using a self-expandable nitinol-frame valve, independently demonstrate that TAVR is non-inferior to SAVR in patients at low surgical risk. However, the non-inferiority design of these trials may be underpowered to detect statistical differences in hard clinical endpoints, as most were powered only for composite endpoints. Given this context, we have undertaken a systematic review and meta-analysis of the available evidence on TAVR to better characterize the safety and efficacy of the currently FDA-approved transfemoral TAVR in comparison with SAVR in patients with symptomatic aortic valve stenosis and at low operatory risk.

2. Methods

2.1. Search Strategy and Study Selection

Published randomized trials comparing transcatheter to surgical aortic valve replacement were searched for within Medline, Scholar and Scopus electronic databases up to March 19th, 2019. The following syntax was used for the search: "transcatheter aortic valve replacement" OR "TAVR" OR "TAVI" AND "surgical aortic valve replacement" OR "SAVR" OR "SAVI" AND "low risk". Time of publication and language were not limiting criteria for our analysis. All reports including the search terms were independently screened by two investigators for relevance and eligibility (A.P., S.S.). Additionally, references from relevant articles were also scanned for eligible studies. The authors discussed their evaluation and any disagreement was resolved through discussion and re-reading. All selected trials were thoroughly checked and classified by the author's institution in order to avoid any effect from duplicity of data. The study protocol was registered in PROSPERO (CRD42019131125).

Studies were considered eligible if the following statements applied: (a) randomized clinical trials; (b) they involved a study population with aortic stenosis; (c) they compared TAVR versus SAVR; (d) they included mostly transfemoral TAVR (>95%); (e) they included patients at low risk (Society of Thoracic Surgeons (STS) score: ≤4); (f) follow-up length of 1 year; (g) they reported the following outcome data (all-cause mortality, cardiovascular death, myocardial infarction, stroke, transient ischemic attack, aortic regurgitation, new-onset atrial fibrillation, permanent pacemaker implantation, major and minor bleedings). Exclusion criteria were (just one was sufficient for study exclusion): duplicate publication, observational data.

2.2. Data Abstraction, Validity Assessment and Analysis

Baseline characteristics, as well as numbers of events, were extracted from the single studies, through careful scanning of the full article by two independent reviewers (A.P., S.S.). Divergences were resolved by consensus. In particular, the following data were abstracted: year of publication, location, number of study patients, study design, clinical outcome data (all-cause mortality, cardiovascular death, myocardial infarction, stroke, transient ischemic attack, aortic regurgitation, new-onset atrial fibrillation, permanent pacemaker implantation, major and minor bleedings) and baseline patients' characteristics. Selection and data abstraction were performed according to the PRISMA statement [9]. The primary endpoint of this analysis was cardiovascular death. Further outcomes were: all-cause mortality, myocardial infarction (MI), stroke, transient ischemic attack (TIA), aortic regurgitation, new-onset atrial fibrillation, permanent pacemaker implantation, life-threatening or disabling bleeding and acute kidney disease (AKI) stage II or III. The quality of randomized trials included in the meta-analysis was appraised by using Cochrane methods (selection bias, performance bias, detection bias, attrition bias, reporting bias and other bias) as previously described [10].

2.3. Statistical Analysis

The summary measure used was the Risk Ratio (RR) with 95% confidence. The random-effects model was used, as previously described, to combine the collected values [11,12]. This model calculates a weighted average of the relative risks by incorporating within-study and between-study variations. Heterogeneity was assessed by means of the Cochrane Q test using a chi-squared function, with $p < 0.10$ considered significant for heterogeneity, as previously described [13]. Additionally, I^2 values were calculated for the estimation of variation in weighted mean differences among studies attributable to heterogeneity. Power calculation of the meta-analysis was performed as described by Valentine et al. [14]. Small study effects were evaluated through graphical inspection of funnel plots, as already previously described [15]. Forest plots were used to graphically display the results of the meta-analysis, as already previously described [16]. Briefly, the measure of effect (RR) for every single study included (represented by a square) is plotted, together with confidence intervals, represented by horizontal lines. The area of each square is proportional to the study's weight in the meta-analysis. The overall measure of effect is reported on the bottom line of the plot as a diamond, whose lateral ends indicate the confidence interval for the summary effect. Analyses were performed by means of RevMan 5.3.

3. Results

3.1. Search Results

Our search retrieved a total of 2660 entries, which were reduced to 2145 studies after an initial pre-screening. A total of 110 studies were then excluded for one of the following reasons: (a) they were not related to our research question; (b) they were not original articles. In the assessment of eligibility, a further seven studies were excluded. Finally, a total of three studies were included [7,8,17]. The study selection procedure was reported in detail in Figure 1.

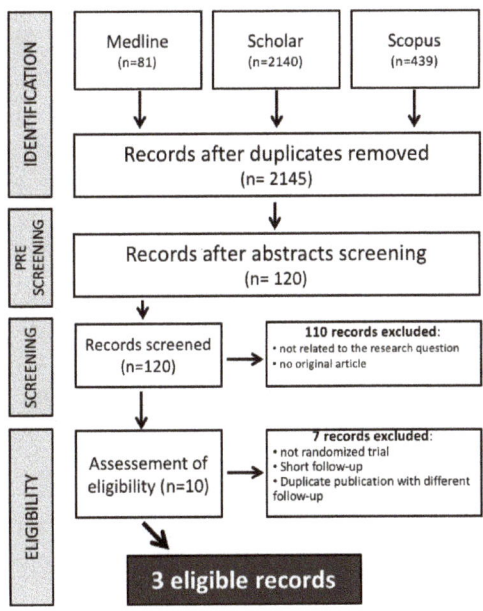

Figure 1. Study selection flow chart.

3.2. Study Characteristics

The main characteristics of the selected studies were reported in Table 1. Quality assessment revealed a high study quality (Supplementary Figure S1). The specific study designs made both patients' and investigators' blinding impossible. Endpoint assessment and data analysis was blinded in all included studies. A total of 2629 patients were included of which 1363 patients were randomized to TAVR and 1266 to SAVR.

Baseline clinical and procedural characteristics across the trials are reported in Table 2. Across the studies, patients were predominantly male, one-fourth of patients had diabetes mellitus and less than 1% had creatinine level >2 mg/dL at presentation. The mean STS score was less than 3% across all the trials. In the TAVR arm, the most frequently implanted valve was a self-expandable valve which included Corevalve, Evolute R and Evolute PRO (Medtronic), whereas the remaining patients ($n = 496$) were treated with a balloon-expandable valve, Sapien 3 (Edwards).

3.3. Study Outcomes

After one year, the risk of cardiovascular death was significantly lower with TAVR compared to SAVR (Risk Ratio (RR) = 0.56; 95% CI 0.33–0.95; $p = 0.03$; $I^2 = 0\%$; Figure 2A). Similarly, a trend risk reduction for one-year all-cause mortality was also observed in favor of TAVR (RR = 0.67; 95% CI 0.42–1.07; $p = 0.10$; $I^2 = 0\%$; Figure 2B). The effect was consistent also in fixed effect and no evidence of publication bias was found for this endpoint. Among the secondary endpoint, patients undergoing TAVR have a lower risk of new-onset of atrial fibrillation compared to SAVR (RR = 0.26; 95% CI 0.17–0.39; $p < 0.00001$; $I^2 = 75\%$; Figure 2C), major bleeding (RR = 0.30; 95% CI 0.14–0.65; $p < 0.002$; $I^2 = 84\%$; Figure 2D) and AKI stage II or III (RR = 0.28; 95% CI 0.14–0.58; $p = 0.0005$; $I^2 = 0\%$; Figure 2E).

Conversely, TAVR was associated to a higher risk of aortic regurgitation (RR = 3.96; 95% CI 1.31–11.99; $p = 0.01$; $I^2 = 41\%$; Figure 3A) and permanent pacemaker implantation (RR = 3.47; 95% CI 1.33–9.07; $p = 0.01$; $I^2 = 89\%$; Figure 3B) compared to SAVR. No differences were observed between the groups in the risks of stroke (RR = 0.71; 95% CI 0.41–1.25; $p = 0.24$; $I^2 = 29\%$; Figure 3C), TIA (RR = 0.98; 95% CI 0.53–1.83; $p = 096$; $I^2 = 0\%$; Figure 3D) and MI (RR = 0.75; 95% CI 0.43–1.29; $p = 0.29$; Figure 3E). The effect was consistent also in fixed effect and no evidence of publication bias was found for this endpoint for all the secondary outcomes.

Table 1. Characteristics and endpoint definitions of included randomized trials.

Study	Year	Location	N	Study Design	Primary Endpoint	Mortality Reported	Valve Type	Randomization	Follow-Up (Years)
NOTION	2015	Multicenter	280	RCT	Death from any cause, stroke, or myocardial infarction	Yes	CoreValve (Medtronic)	TAVR vs. SAVR	1
ELRT	2019	Multicenter	1403	RCT	Death from any cause or disabling stroke	Yes	CoreValve, Evolut R, or Evolut PRO (Medtronic)	TAVR vs. SAVR	1
PARTNER 3	2019	Multicenter	950	RCT	death from any cause, stroke, or rehospitalization	Yes	Sapien 3 (Edwards)	TAVR vs. SAVR	1

Abbreviations: RCT = randomized clinical trials; TAVR = transcatheter aortic valve replacement; SAVR = surgical aortic valve replacement.

Table 2. Patient's characteristics.

	NOTION 2015		ELRT 2019		PARTNER 3 2019	
	TAVR	SAVR	TAVR	SAVR	TAVR	SAVR
N of patients, n	145	135	725	678	496	454
Age, yrs	79.2	79	74.1	73.6	73.3	73.6
Male, %	53.8	52.6	64	66.2	67.5	71.1
Creatinine > 2 mg/dL, %	1.4	0.7	0.4	0.1	0.2	0.2
Peripheral vascular disease, %	4.1	6.7	7.5	8.3	6.9	7.3
Diabetes, %	17.9	20.7	31.4	30.5	31.2	30.2
Chronic lung disease, %	11.7	11.9	15	18	5.1	6.2
Prior Stroke, %	16.6	16.3	10.2	11.8	3.4	5.1
Prior MI, %	5.5	4.4	6.6	4.9	5.7	5.8
Prior AF, %	27.8	25.6	15.4	14.5	15.7	18.8
STS score, %	2.9	3.1	1.9	1.9	1.9	1.9

Yrs = years; MI = myocardial infarction; AF = atrial fibrillation; STS = Society of Thoracic Surgeons.

A

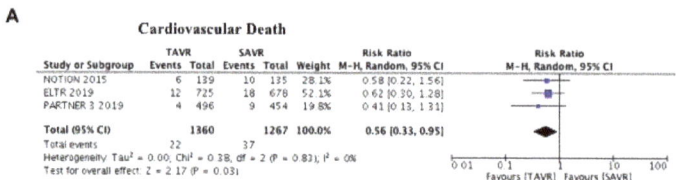

B

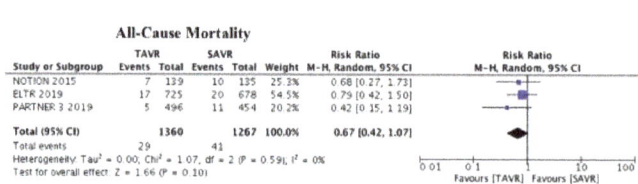

C

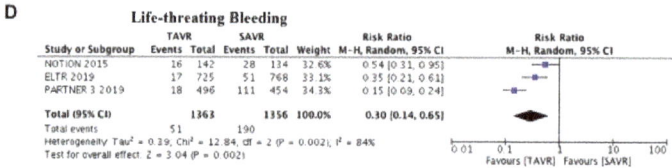

D

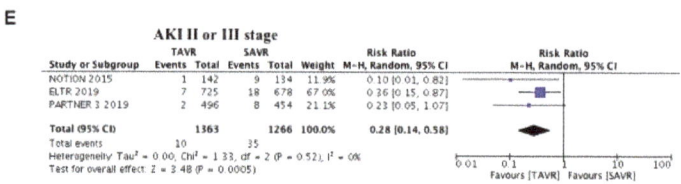

E

Figure 2. Meta-analysis of cardiovascular death, all-cause mortality, new-onset atrial fibrillation, life-threating bleeding, acute kidney injury II or III stage. (**A**) Forest plot and summary effect of the difference in the incidence of cardiovascular death, showing a significantly lower incidence in the TAVR arm ($p = 0.03$). (**B**) Forest plot and summary effect of the difference in the incidence of all-cause mortality showing no difference between transcatheter aortic valve replacement (TAVR) and surgical aortic valve replacement (SAVR; $p = 0.10$). (**C**) Forest plot and summary effect of the difference in the incidence of new-onset atrial fibrillation, showing a significantly lower incidence in the TAVR arm ($p < 0.001$). (**D**) Forest plot and summary effect of the difference in the incidence of life-threating bleeding, showing a significantly lower incidence in the TAVR arm ($p < 0.002$). (**E**) Forest plot and summary effect of the difference in the incidence of acute kidney injury II or III stage, showing a significantly lower incidence in the TAVR arm ($p < 0.0005$).

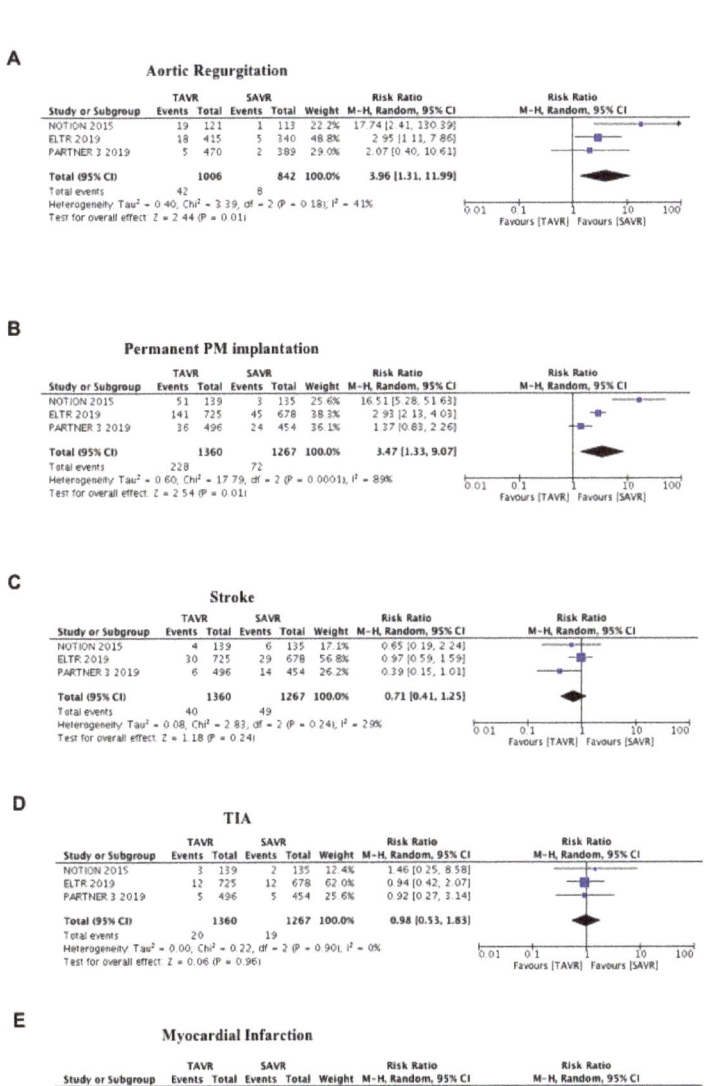

Figure 3. Meta-analysis of aortic regurgitation, permanent PM implantation, stroke, transient ischemic attack (TIA) and myocardial infarction. (**A**) Forest plot and summary effect of the difference in the incidence of aortic regurgitation, showing a significantly lower incidence in the SAVR arm ($p = 0.01$). (**B**) Forest plot and summary effect of the difference in the incidence of permanent PM implantation, showing a significantly lower incidence in the SAVR arm ($p = 0.01$). (**C**) Forest plot and summary effect of the difference in the incidence of stroke, showing no difference between TAVR and SAVR ($p = 0.24$). (**D**) Forest plot and summary effect of the difference in the incidence of TIA, showing no difference between TAVR and SAVR ($p = 0.96$). (**E**) Forest plot and summary effect of the difference in the incidence of myocardial infarction, showing no difference between TAVR and SAVR ($p = 0.29$).

4. Discussion

We performed a meta-analysis with only randomized studies comparing a one-year outcome after treatment of severe aortic stenosis with TAVR or SAVR in patients at low surgical risk.

Recently, several meta-analyses showed promising results of TAVR [18–20]. However, there are some differences with our meta-analysis. Kheiri et al. performed a meta-analysis of patients at low risk, but including transapical TAVR [21] and a post-hoc analysis of the SURTAVI trial [22]. Similarly, Kolte and colleagues also included in their work the post-hoc analysis of the SURTAVI trial finding a significant difference in the rate of all-cause death [20]. Conversely, we found only a nonsignificant difference in such hard clinical end-points. A recently updated meta-analysis [18] of RCTs including all surgical risk categories had reported a reduction in all-cause mortality up to two years of TAVR irrespective of baseline surgical risk. However, in the subgroup at low surgical risk, they had reported only all-cause mortality outcomes with a dishomogenous follow-up. Hence, different TAVR access approaches were performed in most of the studies. In our meta-analysis, we included only studies with >95% of transfemoral access-site since current data and expertise strongly favor the femoral artery as the preferred and most widespread access route for TAVR.

In the present meta-analysis, including three randomized studies and nearly 3000 patients, we found a superiority of TAVR against SAVR for cardiovascular death (primary endpoint) at the one-year follow-up (Figure 2A). Interestingly, results on this hard clinical endpoint were strongly homogeneous across individual studies and could be explained by several factors. Patients undergoing TAVR had less: acute kidney injury (Figure 2E); new-onset atrial fibrillation (Figure 2C); major bleedings (Figure 2D). These factors could have a strong impact on mortality, also in the long-term.

The second key finding of our meta-analysis is a significant reduction in the risk of AKI in patients undergoing TAVI compared with SAVR. Several studies have shown that AKI is a serious complication after both TAVR and SAVR. Adams and colleagues reported a lower incidence with TAVR compared to SAVR (6.0% vs. 15.1%; $p < 0.001$) [23]. Similarly, Bagur et al. showed that 9% suffered from AKI after TAVR, whereas SAVR was associated with an incidence of AKI in 26% [24]. These results could be of impact, in fact, AKI was associated with an increased risk of 30-day and long-term (up to seven years) mortality (42.3% versus 22.7% for seven-year mortality; HR 1.71 (95% CI 1.30–2.25)) [25].

The third key finding of our meta-analysis is a significant reduction in the risk of new-onset atrial fibrillation (NOAF) in patients undergoing TAVI compared with SAVR. New-onset atrial fibrillation (NOAF) has emerged in the last few years as a potential prognostic factor in patients undergoing TAVR [12]. NOAF after TAVR could be detrimental due to atrio-ventricular dyssynchrony resulting in reduced cardiac output and increased filling pressures. In addition, NOAF could be responsible for fatal cerebrovascular events. Recently, Gargiulo et al. performed a meta-analysis of eight studies encompassing 4959 patients to investigate the role of NOAF as a potential prognostic factor in patients undergoing TAVR. Interestingly, they found a borderline increase of 30-day and a significant increase in one-year all-cause death in the NOAF group compared with those in sinus rhythm [26].

The fourth key finding of our meta-analysis is a significant reduction in the risk of NOAF in patients undergoing TAVI compared with SAVR. The impact of bleeding on hard clinical endpoints in patients undergoing TAVR was already discussed by Piccolo et al. [27]. Among patients with severe aortic stenosis undergoing TAVR, both access-site and non-access-site bleeding were independently associated with an increased risk for mortality.

Finally, all these three factors (bleedings, AKI, NOAF) for the reasons mentioned above, could explain, at least in part, the superiority of TAVR against SAVR for cardiovascular death, also in a population at low surgical risk at one-year follow-up.

Cerebral embolization is a common complication leading to stroke after TAVR and SAVR [28]. In this meta-analysis, we found no difference in stroke and TIA rates between the groups. These results are in line with the results of single studies [7,8,17].

However, some concerns should be raised, and some limitations should be mentioned about TAVR: (1) paravalvular aortic regurgitation; (2) major incidence of pacemaker implantation; (3) durability at longer follow-up.

Paravalvular aortic regurgitation and the need for permanent pacemaker implantation have historically been the limit of TAVR compared with SAVR. Nevertheless, advances in TAVR technology, along with operator experience, precise valve sizing and implantation technique, may further reduce the associated pacemaker implantations and paravalvular aortic regurgitation risks. However, in a recent real-world study of TAVR among lower surgical risk patients, promising rates of 30-day moderate-to-severe paravalvular leak (0.5%) and permanent pacemaker implantation (6.5%) were reported [29].

Finally, the question of durability has been an Achilles heel of TAVR. Some recent data seem to suggest similar longevity between transcatheter and surgical tissue valves out to five to seven years. A post-hoc analysis wherein investigators looked for valve dysfunction and failure in the NOTION trial showed that bioprosthetic valve dysfunction was numerically lower in TAVR group over five years (55.4% versus 65.2%, $p = 0.10$) [30] compared to SAVR. However, to date, it is not clear if that is good enough to get TAVR into younger patients.

5. Limitations

As for any meta-analysis, some limitations should be acknowledged that are related to: (1) different definitions in the studies for different endpoints; (2) differences in the baseline characteristics between the studies; (3) not all the outcomes are reported in the studies; (4) short-term follow-up.

6. Conclusions

The present meta-analysis, including three randomized studies and nearly 3000 patients with severe aortic stenosis at low surgical risk, shows that TAVR is associated with lower CV death compared to SAVR at 1-year follow-up. Nevertheless, paravalvular aortic regurgitation and pacemaker implantation still represent two weak spots that should be solved.

Supplementary Materials: The following are available online at http://www.mdpi.com/2077-0383/9/2/439/s1, Figure S1: Quality assessment.

Author Contributions: A.P. and S.S. designed the study and acquired, analyzed and interpreted data. A.P. and J.S. did the literature search and study selection procedures. S.D.R., A.M., C.S. and C.I. drafted the manuscript, with critical revisions for important intellectual content from all authors. All authors have read and agreed to the published version of the manuscript.

Conflicts of Interest: The authors declare no conflict of interest.

References

1. Smith, C.R.; Leon, M.B.; Mack, M.J.; Miller, D.C.; Moses, J.W.; Svensson, L.G.; Tuzcu, E.M.; Webb, J.G.; Fontana, G.P.; Makkar, R.R.; et al. Transcatheter versus surgical aortic-valve replacement in high-risk patients. *N. Engl. J. Med.* **2011**, *364*, 2187–2198. [CrossRef]
2. Indolfi, C.; Bartorelli, A.L.; Berti, S.; Golino, P.; Esposito, G.; Musumeci, G.; Petronio, S.; Tamburino, C.; Tarantini, G.; Ussia, G.; et al. Updated clinical indications for transcatheter aortic valve implantation in patients with severe aortic stenosis: Expert opinion of the Italian Society of Cardiology and GISE. *J. Cardiovasc. Med. (Hagerstown)* **2018**, *19*, 197–210. [CrossRef]
3. Sorrentino, S.; Giustino, G.; Moalem, K.; Indolfi, C.; Mehran, R.; Dangas, G.D. Antithrombotic Treatment after Transcatheter Heart Valves Implant. *Semin. Thromb. Hemost.* **2018**, *44*, 38–45. [CrossRef]
4. Spaccarotella, C.; Mongiardo, A.; De Rosa, S.; Indolfi, C. Transcatheter aortic valve implantation in patients at intermediate surgical risk. *Int. J. Cardiol.* **2017**, *243*, 161–168. [CrossRef]

5. Barbanti, M.; Tamburino, C.; D'Errigo, P.; Biancari, F.; Ranucci, M.; Rosato, S.; Santoro, G.; Fusco, D.; Seccareccia, F.; Group, O.R. Five-Year Outcomes of Transfemoral Transcatheter Aortic Valve Replacement or Surgical Aortic Valve Replacement in a Real World Population. *Circ. Cardiovasc. Interv.* **2019**, *12*, e007825. [CrossRef] [PubMed]
6. Pilgrim, T.; Windecker, S. Newer-Generation Devices for Transcatheter Aortic Valve Replacement: Resolving the Limitations of First-Generation Valves? *JACC Cardiovasc. Interv.* **2016**, *9*, 373–375. [CrossRef] [PubMed]
7. Mack, M.J.; Leon, M.B.; Thourani, V.H.; Makkar, R.; Kodali, S.K.; Russo, M.; Kapadia, S.R.; Malaisrie, S.C.; Cohen, D.J.; Pibarot, P.; et al. Transcatheter Aortic-Valve Replacement with a Balloon-Expandable Valve in Low-Risk Patients. *N. Engl. J. Med.* **2019**, *380*, 1695–1705. [CrossRef] [PubMed]
8. Popma, J.J.; Deeb, G.M.; Yakubov, S.J.; Mumtaz, M.; Gada, H.; O'Hair, D.; Bajwa, T.; Heiser, J.C.; Merhi, W.; Kleiman, N.S.; et al. Transcatheter Aortic-Valve Replacement with a Self-Expanding Valve in Low-Risk Patients. *N. Engl. J. Med.* **2019**, *380*, 1706–1715. [CrossRef] [PubMed]
9. Moher, D.; Liberati, A.; Tetzlaff, J.; Altman, D.G.; Group, P. Preferred reporting items for systematic reviews and meta-analyses: The PRISMA statement. *Int. J. Surg.* **2010**, *8*, 336–341. [CrossRef]
10. Polimeni, A.; Anadol, R.; Munzel, T.; Indolfi, C.; De Rosa, S.; Gori, T. Long-term outcome of bioresorbable vascular scaffolds for the treatment of coronary artery disease: A meta-analysis of RCTs. *BMC Cardiovasc. Disord.* **2017**, *17*, 147. [CrossRef] [PubMed]
11. Polimeni, A.; Passafaro, F.; De Rosa, S.; Sorrentino, S.; Torella, D.; Spaccarotella, C.; Mongiardo, A.; Indolfi, C. Clinical and Procedural Outcomes of 5-French versus 6-French Sheaths in Transradial Coronary Interventions. *Medicine (Baltimore)* **2015**, *94*, e2170. [CrossRef] [PubMed]
12. Sorrentino, S.; Giustino, G.; Mehran, R.; Kini, A.S.; Sharma, S.K.; Faggioni, M.; Farhan, S.; Vogel, B.; Indolfi, C.; Dangas, G.D. Everolimus-Eluting Bioresorbable Scaffolds Versus Everolimus-Eluting Metallic Stents. *J. Am. Coll. Cardiol.* **2017**, *69*, 3055–3066. [CrossRef] [PubMed]
13. De Rosa, S.; Polimeni, A.; Petraco, R.; Davies, J.E.; Indolfi, C. Diagnostic Performance of the Instantaneous Wave-Free Ratio: Comparison With Fractional Flow Reserve. *Circ. Cardiovasc. Interv.* **2018**, *11*, e004613. [CrossRef] [PubMed]
14. Valentine, J.C.; Pigott, T.D.; Rothstein, H.R. How Many Studies Do You Need? *J. Educ. Behav. Stat.* **2010**, *35*, 215–247. [CrossRef]
15. Santarpia, G.; De Rosa, S.; Polimeni, A.; Giampa, S.; Micieli, M.; Curcio, A.; Indolfi, C. Efficacy and Safety of Non-Vitamin K Antagonist Oral Anticoagulants versus Vitamin K Antagonist Oral Anticoagulants in Patients Undergoing Radiofrequency Catheter Ablation of Atrial Fibrillation: A Meta-Analysis. *PLoS ONE* **2015**, *10*, e0126512. [CrossRef] [PubMed]
16. Polimeni, A.; De Rosa, S.; Sabatino, J.; Sorrentino, S.; Indolfi, C. Impact of intracoronary adenosine administration during primary PCI: A meta-analysis. *Int. J. Cardiol.* **2016**, *203*, 1032–1041. [CrossRef]
17. Thyregod, H.G.; Steinbruchel, D.A.; Ihlemann, N.; Nissen, H.; Kjeldsen, B.J.; Petursson, P.; Chang, Y.; Franzen, O.W.; Engstrom, T.; Clemmensen, P.; et al. Transcatheter Versus Surgical Aortic Valve Replacement in Patients With Severe Aortic Valve Stenosis: 1-Year Results From the All-Comers NOTION Randomized Clinical Trial. *J. Am. Coll. Cardiol.* **2015**, *65*, 2184–2194. [CrossRef]
18. Kheiri, B.; Osman, M.; Bakhit, A.; Radaideh, Q.; Barbarawi, M.; Zayed, Y.; Golwala, H.; Zahr, F.; Stone, G.W.; Bhatt, D.L. Meta-Analysis of Transcatheter Aortic Valve Replacement in Low-Risk Patients. *Am. J. Med.* **2020**, *133*, e38–e41. [CrossRef]
19. Ando, T.; Ashraf, S.; Villablanca, P.; Kuno, T.; Pahuja, M.; Shokr, M.; Afonso, L.; Grines, C.; Briasoulis, A.; Takagi, H. Meta-Analysis of Effectiveness and Safety of Transcatheter Aortic Valve Implantation Versus Surgical Aortic Valve Replacement in Low-to-Intermediate Surgical Risk Cohort. *Am. J. Cardiol.* **2019**, *124*, 580–585. [CrossRef]
20. Kolte, D.; Vlahakes, G.J.; Palacios, I.F.; Sakhuja, R.; Passeri, J.J.; Inglessis, I.; Elmariah, S. Transcatheter Versus Surgical Aortic Valve Replacement in Low-Risk Patients. *J. Am. Coll. Cardiol.* **2019**, *74*, 1532–1540. [CrossRef]
21. Nielsen, H.H.; Klaaborg, K.E.; Nissen, H.; Terp, K.; Mortensen, P.E.; Kjeldsen, B.J.; Jakobsen, C.J.; Andersen, H.R.; Egeblad, H.; Krusell, L.R.; et al. A prospective, randomised trial of transapical transcatheter aortic valve implantation vs. surgical aortic valve replacement in operable elderly patients with aortic stenosis: The STACCATO trial. *EuroIntervention* **2012**, *8*, 383–389. [CrossRef] [PubMed]

22. Serruys, P.W.; Modolo, R.; Reardon, M.; Miyazaki, Y.; Windecker, S.; Popma, J.; Chang, Y.; Kleiman, N.S.; Lilly, S.; Amrane, H.; et al. One-year outcomes of patients with severe aortic stenosis and an STS PROM of less than three percent in the SURTAVI trial. *EuroIntervention* **2018**, *14*, 877–883. [CrossRef] [PubMed]
23. Adams, D.H.; Popma, J.J.; Reardon, M.J. Transcatheter aortic-valve replacement with a self-expanding prosthesis. *N. Engl. J. Med.* **2014**, *371*, 967–968. [CrossRef] [PubMed]
24. Bagur, R.; Webb, J.G.; Nietlispach, F.; Dumont, E.; De Larochelliere, R.; Doyle, D.; Masson, J.B.; Gutierrez, M.J.; Clavel, M.A.; Bertrand, O.F.; et al. Acute kidney injury following transcatheter aortic valve implantation: Predictive factors, prognostic value, and comparison with surgical aortic valve replacement. *Eur. Heart J.* **2010**, *31*, 865–874. [CrossRef]
25. Kliuk-Ben Bassat, O.; Finkelstein, A.; Bazan, S.; Halkin, A.; Herz, I.; Salzer Gotler, D.; Ravid, D.; Hakakian, O.; Keren, G.; Banai, S.; et al. Acute kidney injury after transcatheter aortic valve implantation and mortality risk-long-term follow-up. *Nephrol. Dial. Transplant.*. (published online ahead of print, 2018 Aug 28). *Nephrol. Dial. Transplant.* **2018**. [CrossRef]
26. Gargiulo, G.; Capodanno, D.; Sannino, A.; Barbanti, M.; Perrino, C.; Capranzano, P.; Stabile, E.; Indolfi, C.; Trimarco, B.; Tamburino, C.; et al. New-onset atrial fibrillation and increased mortality after transcatheter aortic valve implantation: A causal or spurious association? *Int. J. Cardiol.* **2016**, *203*, 264–266. [CrossRef]
27. Piccolo, R.; Pilgrim, T.; Franzone, A.; Valgimigli, M.; Haynes, A.; Asami, M.; Lanz, J.; Raber, L.; Praz, F.; Langhammer, B.; et al. Frequency, Timing, and Impact of Access-Site and Non-Access-Site Bleeding on Mortality Among Patients Undergoing Transcatheter Aortic Valve Replacement. *JACC Cardiovasc. Interv.* **2017**, *10*, 1436–1446. [CrossRef]
28. Giustino, G.; Sorrentino, S.; Mehran, R.; Faggioni, M.; Dangas, G. Cerebral Embolic Protection During TAVR: A Clinical Event Meta-Analysis. *J. Am. Coll. Cardiol.* **2017**, *69*, 465–466. [CrossRef]
29. Waksman, R.; Rogers, T.; Torguson, R.; Gordon, P.; Ehsan, A.; Wilson, S.R.; Goncalves, J.; Levitt, R.; Hahn, C.; Parikh, P.; et al. Transcatheter Aortic Valve Replacement in Low-Risk Patients With Symptomatic Severe Aortic Stenosis. *J. Am. Coll. Cardiol.* **2018**, *72*, 2095–2105. [CrossRef]
30. Sondergaard, L.; Ihlemann, N.; Capodanno, D.; Jorgensen, T.H.; Nissen, H.; Kjeldsen, B.J.; Chang, Y.; Steinbruchel, D.A.; Olsen, P.S.; Petronio, A.S.; et al. Durability of Transcatheter and Surgical Bioprosthetic Aortic Valves in Patients at Lower Surgical Risk. *J. Am. Coll. Cardiol.* **2019**, *73*, 546–553. [CrossRef]

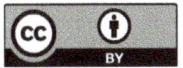 © 2020 by the authors. Licensee MDPI, Basel, Switzerland. This article is an open access article distributed under the terms and conditions of the Creative Commons Attribution (CC BY) license (http://creativecommons.org/licenses/by/4.0/).

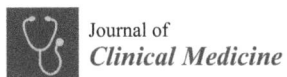

Journal of
Clinical Medicine

Article

Transcatheter Aortic Valve Replacement with Self-Expandable ACURATE neo as Compared to Balloon-Expandable SAPIEN 3 in Patients with Severe Aortic Stenosis: Meta-Analysis of Randomized and Propensity-Matched Studies

Mirosław Gozdek [1,2], Kamil Zieliński [2,3], Michał Pasierski [2,4], Matteo Matteucci [5,6], Dario Fina [5,7], Federica Jiritano [5,8], Paolo Meani [5,9], Giuseppe Maria Raffa [10], Pietro Giorgio Malvindi [11], Michele Pilato [10], Domenico Paparella [12,13], Artur Słomka [2,14], Jacek Kubica [1], Dariusz Jagielak [15], Roberto Lorusso [5], Piotr Suwalski [4] and Mariusz Kowalewski [2,4,5,*] on behalf of Thoracic Research Centre

1 Department of Cardiology and Internal Medicine, Nicolaus Copernicus University, Collegium Medicum, 85067 Bydgoszcz, Poland; gozdekm@wp.pl (M.G.); kubicajw@gmail.com (J.K.)
2 Thoracic Research Centre, Nicolaus Copernicus University, Collegium Medicum in Bydgoszcz, Innovative Medical Forum, 85067 Bydgoszcz, Poland; kamilziel@gmail.com (K.Z.); michalpasierski@gmail.com (M.P.); artur.slomka@cm.umk.pl (A.S.)
3 Department of Cardiology, Warsaw Medical University, 02091 Warsaw, Poland
4 Clinical Department of Cardiac Surgery, Central Clinical Hospital of the Ministry of Interior and Administration, Centre of Postgraduate Medical Education, 02607 Warsa, Poland; suwalski.piotr@gmail.com
5 Department of Cardio-Thoracic Surgery, Heart and Vascular Centre, Maastricht University Medical Centre, 6229 HX Maastricht, The Netherlands; teo.matte@libero.it (M.M.); dario.fina88@gmail.com (D.F.); fede.j@hotmail.it (F.J.); paolo.meani@ospedaleniguarda.it (P.M.); roberto.lorussobs@gmail.com (R.L.)
6 Department of Cardiac Surgery, Circolo Hospital, University of Insubria, 21100 Varese, Italy
7 Department of Cardiology, IRCCS Policlinico San Donato, University of Milan, 20097 Milan, Italy
8 Department of Cardiac Surgery, University Magna Graecia of Catanzaro, 88100 Catanzaro, Italy
9 Department of Intensive Care Unit, Maastricht University Medical Centre (MUMC+), 6229 HX Maastricht, The Netherlands
10 Department for the Treatment and Study of Cardiothoracic Diseases and Cardiothoracic Transplantation, IRCCS-ISMETT (Instituto Mediterraneo per i Trapianti e Terapie ad alta specializzazione), 90127 Palermo, Italy; giuseppe.raffa78@gmail.com (G.M.R.); mpilato@ISMETT.edu (M.P.)
11 Wessex Cardiothoracic Centre, University Hospital Southampton, Southampton SO16 6YD, UK; pg.malvindi@hotmail.com
12 GVM Care & Research, Department of Cardiovascular Surgery, Santa Maria Hospital, 70124 Bari, Italy; domenico.paparella@uniba.it
13 Department of Emergency and Organ Transplant, University of Bari Aldo Moro, 70121 Bari, Italy
14 Chair and Department of Pathophysiology, Nicolaus Copernicus University, Collegium Medicum, 85067 Bydgoszcz, Poland
15 Department of Cardiac Surgery, Gdańsk Medical University, 80210 Gdańsk, Poland; kardchir@gumed.edu.pl
* Correspondence: kowalewskimariusz@gazeta.pl; Tel.: +0048-502-269-240

Received: 30 December 2019; Accepted: 30 January 2020; Published: 1 February 2020

Abstract: Frequent occurrence of paravalvular leak (PVL) after transcatheter aortic valve replacement (TAVR) was the main concern with earlier-generation devices. Current meta-analysis compared outcomes of TAVR with next-generation devices: ACURATE neo and SAPIEN 3. In random-effects meta-analysis, the pooled incidence rates of procedural, clinical and functional outcomes according to VARC-2 definitions were assessed. One randomized controlled trial and five observational studies including 2818 patients (ACURATE neo $n = 1256$ vs. SAPIEN 3 $n = 1562$) met inclusion criteria. ACURATE neo was associated with a 3.7-fold increase of moderate-to-severe PVL (RR (risk ratio): 3.70 (2.04–6.70); $P < 0.0001$), which was indirectly related to higher observed 30-day mortality with

ACURATE valve (RR: 1.77 (1.03–3.04); $P = 0.04$). Major vascular complications, acute kidney injury, periprocedural myocardial infarction, stroke and serious bleeding events were similar between devices. ACURATE neo demonstrated lower transvalvular pressure gradients both at discharge ($P < 0.00001$) and at 30 days ($P < 0.00001$), along with lower risk of patient–prosthesis mismatch (RR: 0.29 (0.10–0.87); $P = 0.03$) and pacemaker implantation (RR: 0.64 (0.50–0.81); $P = 0.0002$), but no differences were observed regarding composite endpoints early safety and device success. In conclusion, ACURATE neo, as compared with SAPIEN 3, was associated with higher rates of moderate-to-severe PVL, which were indirectly linked with increased observed 30-day all-cause mortality.

Keywords: meta-analysis; ACURATE neo; SAPIEN 3; transcatheter aortic valve replacement

1. Introduction

Since first its mention by Cribier in 2002 [1], transcatheter aortic valve replacement (TAVR) has been complementary method to surgical aortic valve replacement (SAVR) in inoperable or high-risk patients with severe symptomatic aortic stenosis. Similar [2] or even lower [3] one-year mortality rate of TAVR, as compared to SAVR, was shown in selected groups of patients. Hence, TAVR is now considered to be an alternative treatment option and is recommended not only in inoperable, high or increased risk surgical patients [2–5] but also in intermediate and lower risk individuals [6–10]. Commercially available earlier-generation transcatheter valves, despite providing good clinical outcomes, were not free from shortcomings; indeed, high rates of conduction abnormalities, permanent pacemaker implantation (PPI) or vascular complications remained important issues to be addressed. More importantly, though, higher incidence of paravalvular leak (PVL), in turn associated with increased late mortality and higher rate of other adverse clinical incidents, as compared to SAVR [11–13], often outweigh the benefits of transcatheter approach.

To minimize these shortcomings, technological innovations were developed in next-generation valves including the following: balloon-expandable SAPIEN 3 (Edwards Lifesciences, Irvine, CA, USA) and self-expandable ACURATE neo (Boston Scientific Corporation, Marlborough, MA, USA). Since direct comparisons of these two devices are few and one recent randomized controlled trial (RCT) [14] did not demonstrate non-inferiority of the ACURATE neo device as compared to SAPIEN 3 as opposed to previous observational studies [15–21] that, however, pointed to comparable or superior results with ACURATE, the debate is ongoing.

The objective of the present investigation was to evaluate and compare short-term results of TAVR with ACURATE neo and SAPIEN 3 in patients presenting with symptomatic severe native aortic valve stenosis.

2. Experimental Section

2.1. Data Sources and Search Strategy

The systematic review and meta-analysis were performed in accordance to MOOSE statement and PRISMA guidelines [22,23]. The MOOSE checklist is available as Table A1. We searched PubMed, ClinicalKey, the Web of Science and Google Scholar all until October 2019. Search terms were as follows: "ACURATE neo" (or "ACCURATE neo"), "Symetic ACURATE", "Boston ACURATE" and/or "SAPIEN 3", "SAPIEN III" and "transcatheter valve" or "aortic". The literature was limited to peer-reviewed articles published in English. References of original articles were reviewed manually and cross-checked.

2.2. Selection Criteria and Quality Assessment

Studies were included if having met all of the following criteria: (1) human study; (2) study or study arms comparing directly strategy of transcatheter aortic valve replacement with ACURATE neo and SAPIEN 3; (3) RCT or propensity score matched observational study. Studies were excluded if they fell into the following categories: (1) in-vitro study; (2) single arm; (3) adjustment not PS or methods not reported; (4) outcomes of interest not reported; and (5) sub-studies or overlapping populations. No restrictions regarding number of patients included or characteristic of the population were imposed. Two reviewers (M.G. and K.Z.) selected the studies for the inclusion, extracted studies and patients' characteristics of interest and relevant outcomes. Two authors (M.G. and K.Z.) independently assessed the trials' eligibility and risk of bias. Any divergences were resolved by consensus.

Quality of RCTs was appraised by using the components recommended by the Cochrane Collaboration [24]; observational studies were, instead, appraised with ROBINS-I (Risk of Bias in Nonrandomised Studies-of Interventions), a tool used for assessment of the bias (the selection of the study groups; the comparability of the groups; and the ascertainment of either the exposure or outcome of interest) in cohort studies included in a systematic review and/or meta-analysis [25].

2.3. Endpoints Selection

Endpoints were established according to the Valve Academic Research Consortium-2 (VARC-2) definitions [26]. Procedural outcomes of interest were predilatation and postdilatation, procedural times and contrast volume. Clinical endpoints assessed included the following: PPI, major vascular complications (MVC), serious bleeding (life-threatening and/or major), acute kidney injury (AKI), stroke, myocardial infarction and 30-day mortality. Functional outcomes were as follows: mean transvalvular gradients, prosthesis-patient mismatch (PPM), and mild and moderate-to-severe paravalvular leak (PVL). Composite endpoints were as per VARC-2: device success (defined as absence of procedural death, correct position of 1 valve in the proper location, mean gradient < 20 mm Hg or peak velocity < 3 m/s, absence of moderate-to-severe PVL and absence of PPM) and early safety (composite of all-cause death, any stroke, life-threatening or disabling bleeding, major vascular complications, coronary artery obstruction requiring intervention, acute kidney injury (stage 2 or higher), rehospitalization for valve-related symptoms or congestive heart failure, valve-related dysfunction requiring repeat procedure, and valve-related dysfunction determined by echocardiography (mean aortic valve gradient ≥ 20 mm Hg and either effective orifice area ≤ 0.9–1.1 cm^2 (depending on body surface area) or Doppler velocity index < 0.35; or moderate or severe prosthetic PVL).

2.4. Statistical Analysis

Data were analyzed according to intention-to-treat principle, wherever applicable. Risks ratios (RR) and 95% confidence intervals (95% CI) served as primary index statistics for dichotomous outcomes. For continuous outcomes, mean difference (MD) and corresponding 95% CI were calculated by using a random effects model. To overcome the low statistical power of Cochran Q test, the statistical inconsistency test $I^2 = [(Qdf)/Q] \times 100\%$, where Q is the chi-square statistic and df is its degrees of freedom, was used to assess heterogeneity [27]. It examines the percentage of inter-study variation, with values ranging from 0% to 100%. An I^2 value of 25% indicates low heterogeneity, 50% are suggestive of moderate heterogeneity and 70% of high heterogeneity. Because of high degree of heterogeneity anticipated among predominantly nonrandomized trials, an inverse variance (DerSimonian–Laird) random-effects model was applied as a more conservative approach for observational data accounting for between- and within-study variability. Whenever a single study reported median values and interquartile ranges instead of mean and standard deviation (SD), the latter were approximated as described by Wan and colleagues [28]. In case there were "0 events" reported in both arms, calculations were repeated, as a sensitivity analysis, using risk difference (RD) and respective 95% CI. Additionally, we performed a set of meta-regression analyses to address potential relationships between 30-day all-cause mortality and other endpoints and baseline characteristics assessed. For the analyses of clinical endpoints, RCTs and PS-matched studies were analyzed separately. Review Manager 5.3 (The Nordic Cochrane Centre, Copenhagen, Denmark) was used for statistical computations. P-values

≤ 0.05 were considered statistically significant and reported as two-sided, without adjustment for multiple comparisons.

3. Results

3.1. Study Selection and Bias

Study selection process and reasons for exclusion of some studies are described in Figure 1.

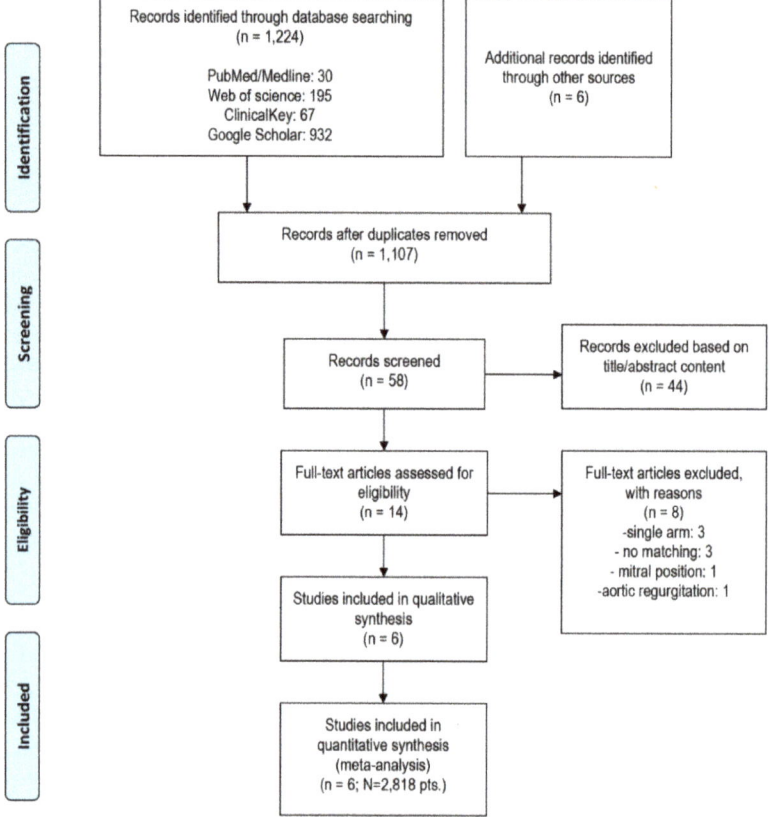

Figure 1. Study selection and inclusion process.

Systematic search of the online databases allowed collection of 58 potentially eligible records that were retrieved for scrutiny. Of those, 52 were further excluded because they were not pertinent to the design of the meta-analysis or did not meet the explicit inclusion criteria. One RCT [14] and five observational studies [15–19] enrolling the total of 2818 patients were eventually included in the analysis. Potential sources of the studies' bias were analyzed with the use of components recommended by the Cochrane Collaboration and ROBINS-I tool, and the results are enclosed as Table A2. Overall, the studies reported moderate risk of bias. Most commonly, biases arose from participants selection for the study by designated heart teams and subjective distribution of the participants within the study arms. All but one study [14] lacked a core lab assessment of PVL and central adjudication of clinical events.

Patients were divided into two groups: those treated with ACURATE neo transcatheter valve (n = 1256) and SAPIEN 3 transcatheter valve (n = 1562). Summary of the valve characteristics is available as Table 1.

Table 1. Valve characteristics and features.

ACURATE neo (Boston Scientific Corporation)	SAPIEN 3 (Edwards Lifesciences)
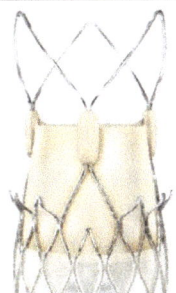	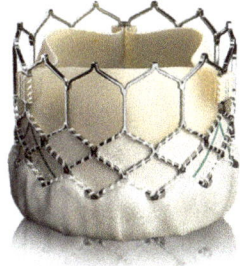
Supra-annular	Intra-annular
Porcine pericardial leaflet tissue	Bovine pericardial leaflet tissue
Self-expanding, deployment in a top-down mechanism of nitinol frame.	Balloon-expandable cobalt-chromium frame
Transfemoral sheath size (valve size)	
18-French for all devices: Small (23 mm), Medium (25 mm), Large (27 mm).	Ready for ultra-low profile: 14 F (20, 23, 26 mm); 16 F (29 mm), 18 F (20, 23, 26 mm), 21 F (29 mm)
Special features	
-Upper and lower crown; -Three stabilization arches; -Outer and inner pericardial skirt.	-Outer sealing and inner skirt at the inflow

Studies' characteristics, as well as definitions or diagnostic criteria for assessed clinical endpoints, are reported in Table 2. Table A3 lists selection criteria for the procedure and valve, as well as inclusion and exclusion criteria within particular studies. Patients' baseline characteristics and detailed procedural characteristics are available as Tables A4 and A5. All studies reported data on 30-day clinical outcomes; three reported Kaplan–Meier estimates of survival at longer-term follow-ups [15,16,18].

Table 2. Baseline characteristics of included studies.

Study	Barth S et al. 2019 [15]		Costa et al. 2019 [16]		Husser O et al. 2017 [17]		Lanz J et al. 2019 [14]		Mauri V et al. 2017 [18]		Schaefer A et al. 2017 [19]	
	ACURATE neo	SAPIEN 3	ACURATE neo	SAPIEN 3	ACURATE neo	SAPIEN 3	ACURATE neo	SAPIEN 3	ACURATE neo	SAPIEN 3	ACURATE neo	SAPIEN 3
Study period	2012–2016		09.2014–02.2018		01.2014–01.2016		02.2017–02.2019		02.2014–08.2016		2012–2016	
Design	MC, RCS, PM		SC, RCS, PM		MC, RCS, PM		MC, RCT		MC, RCS, PM		SC, RCS, PM	
Number of pts.	329	329	48	48	311	622	372	367	92	92	104	104
Age	81.0 ± 5.0	81.0 ± 6.0	82.3 ± 3.8	83.3 ± 2.3	81.0 ± 6.0	81.0 ± 6.0	82.6 ± 4.3	83.0 ± 3.9	82.8 ± 6.5	81.9 ± 5.3	81.7 ± 5.5	81.2 ± 6.2
Female (%)	NR		70.8	68.8	60.8	55.3	59.0	55.0	92.4	92.4	69.2	65.4
BMI (kg/m^2)	28.7 ± 5.5	28.4 ± 5.8	27.8 ± 4.6	27.1 ± 3.9	27.0 ± 5.0	27.0 ± 5.0	27.3 ± 4.4	27.9 ± 4.7	27.3 ± 5.5	26.0 ± 4.7	27.1 ± 5.1	26.8 ± 5.0
STS-PROM (%)	NR		4.0 ± 3.3	3.8 ± 1.7	NR		3.7 ± 1.8	3.7 ± 1.9	NR		5.8 ± 3.8	5.4 ± 3.6
Logistic EuroSCORE (%)	18.8 ± 14.7	19.1 ± 13.6	NR	NR	18.0 ± 10.0	18.0 ± 12.0	NR	NR	16.2 ± 8.8	16.6 ± 8.8	15.9 ± 9.3	13.7 ± 9.0
NYHA III/IV (%)	79.0	78.1	NR		256	489	77.0	73.0	NR		86.5	88.5
EF (%)	53.0 ± 13.0	54.0 ± 15.0	54.5 ± 9.7	56.1 ± 9.7	NR	NR	56.4 ± 11.1	57.1 ± 10.7	59.0 ± 8.0	59.0 ± 10.0	NR	NR
EF < 35% (%)	9.4	10.3	NR		5.8	5.5	NR	NR	NR		26.0*	22.1 [1]
Mean aortic gradient (mmHg)	44.0 ± 15.0	45.0 ± 14.0	51.3 ± 14.5	51.3 ± 17.2	45.0–15.0	44.0 ± 16.0	42.9 ± 17.2	41.5 ± 15.1	46.0 ± 16.0	47.0 ± 16.0	35.9 ± 16.6	37.6 ± 16.7
Aortic annulus diameter (mm)	21.0 ± 2.0	21.0 ± 3.0	NR	NR	NR		23.6 ± 1.6	23.7 ± 1.6	NR	NR	24.5 ± 2.5	25.3 ± 2.6
Access site (%)	TF 74.5, TA 25.5	TF 75.7, TA 24.3	TF 100.0	TF 100.0	TF 100.0	TF 100.0	TF 99.0, TA <1.0	TF 100.0	TF 100.0	TF 100.0	TF 100.0	TF 100.0
VARC-2 outcomes definitions	yes		Yes		yes		yes		yes		yes	
Follow-up (months)	10.8 ± 9.7	12.2 ± 9.9	12		1		1		12.7 ± 2.6		1	

[1] <44% EF; RCT, randomized control trial; SC, single center; MC, multi center; RCS, retrospective cases series; PM, propensity matching; NYHA, New York Heart Association; STS-PROM, Society of Thoracic Surgeons Predicted Risk of Mortality; EuroSCORE, European System for Cardiac Operative Risk Evaluation; VARC, Valve Academic Research Consortium; EF, ejection fraction; TF, trans femoral; TA, trans apical; NR, not reported. In bold are highlighted the variables that differed significantly between study groups.

3.2. Patients Characteristic

Groups treated with ACURATE neo and SAPIEN 3 did not differ regarding patients' age ($P = 0.363$), body mass index ($P = 0.708$), NYHA III/IV status ($P = 0.115$) or left ventricle ejection fraction ($P = 0.178$). No difference was found in the baseline logistic EuroSCORE as well ($P = 0.749$). SAPIEN 3 group included significantly fewer female individuals, 59.7% vs. 64.1%, respectively ($P = 0.037$). Aortic valve baseline echo-parameters, i.e., mean trans-aortic gradient were comparable: 43.4 ± 15.8 vs. 43.6 ± 15.5 mmHg ($P = 0.861$) in ACURATE neo and SAPIEN 3, respectively (Figure 2), although the aortic annulus plane area were on average 4 mm^2 smaller in the ACURATE neo recipients 439.7 ± 62.4 vs. 446.7 ± 76.3; $P = 0.037$ as compared to SAPIEN 3. Transfemoral access was mostly widely employed during TAVR procedure; in five studies, it was used exclusively [14,16–19]. Barth et al. [15] included both transfemoral and transapical access in 75.7% vs. 24.3% and 74.5% vs. 25.5% for ACURATE neo and SAPIEN 3, respectively. For the transapical approach, ACUARATE TA device was used.

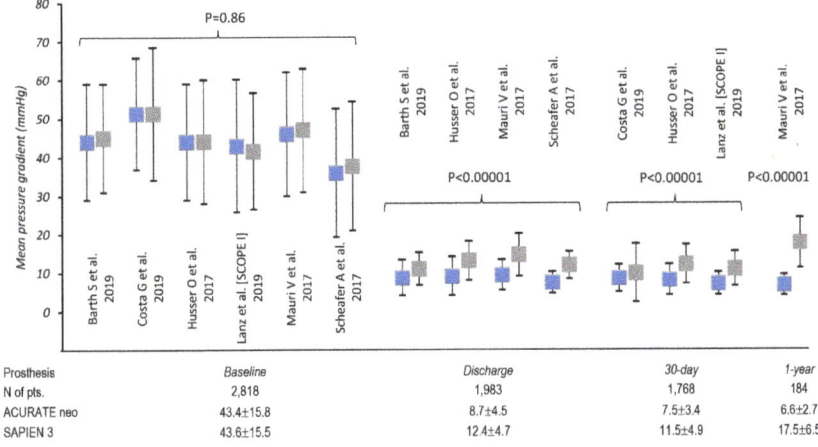

Figure 2. Analysis of mean transaortic gradients before and after transcatheter aortic valve replacement (TAVR).

3.3. Procedural Outcomes

Five studies [14,15,17–19] and 2722 patients contributed to the analysis of procedural outcomes between two devices. Both predilatation and postdilatation were more common with ACURATE neo valve; predilatation was necessary in 1124/1271 (88.4%) of cases as compared to 801/1514 (52.9%); RR 2.05, 95% CI, (1.44, 2.94) $P < 0.0001$; $I^2 = 97\%$); postdilatation: RR 3.10, 95% CI, (2.01, 4.77) $P < 0.00001$; $I^2 = 88\%$) with respective rates of 45.3% vs. 17.2% for ACURATE neo and SAPIEN 3, respectively. Figure 1 and A2. The procedures performed with ACURATE neo required significantly greater amount of contrast: 130.3 ± 56.1 mL vs. 109.7 ± 50.3 mL (MD 18.22 95% CI, (10.04, 26.40) mL; $P < 0.0001$). Figure 3). Four studies [14,15,17,19] including 1116 ACURATE neo and 1411 SAPIEN 3 cases provided data on procedure duration, which on average 3 minutes longer in the former: 60.1 ± 28.6 min. vs. $56.5.9 \pm 26.0$ min. (MD 3.06, 95% CI, (−0.66, 6.76) min) without reaching statistical significance (Figure 4). Use of >1 valve was necessary in 35 cases (26 ACURATE neo vs. nine SAPIEN 3; RR 3.24, 95% CI, (1.47, 7.13) $P = 0.004$; $I^2 = 0\%$). Incidence of cardiac tamponade was reported in three studies [14,15,18] with respective event rates of 1.0% vs. 0.7% for ACURATE neo and SAPIEN 3 valves: RR 1.17, 95% CI, (0.52, 2.63) $P = 0.70$; $I^2 = 0\%$. Early procedural complications included the following: coronary obstruction in three ACURATE neo patients and total of eight annular ruptures, 20 conversions to surgery and 20 valve malpositionings without differences between two devices.

3.4. Clinical Outcomes

Six studies [14–19] enrolling 2818 patients contributed data for the analysis of early safety as defined by VARC-2; with the corresponding rates of 13.9% (174/1256) and 12.6% (197/1562) for ACURATE neo and SAPIEN 3 valves, respectively, there were no statistical differences between two devices (RR 1.15, 95% CI, (0.94, 1.40) $P = 0.16$; $I^2 = 0$%) and pooled estimates of RCT and PS-matched studies in subgroup analysis ($P_{interaction} = 0.47$) (Figure 3a). In the pooled analysis of device success (five studies included (2634 patients.)), there were no differences between two types of valve in the pooled analysis: RR 1.01, 95% CI, (0.92, 1.10) $P = 0.89$; $I^2 = 89$%). Analyzed separately, there were strong between-subgroup differences between RCT and pooled estimate from PS-matched studies: RR 1.44, 95% CI, (1.24, 1.66); $P < 0.00001$; $I^2 = $ NA and RR 0.95, 95% CI, (0.91, 0.99); $P = 0.01$; $I^2 = 47$% with $P_{interaction} < 0.00001$ (Figure 3b).

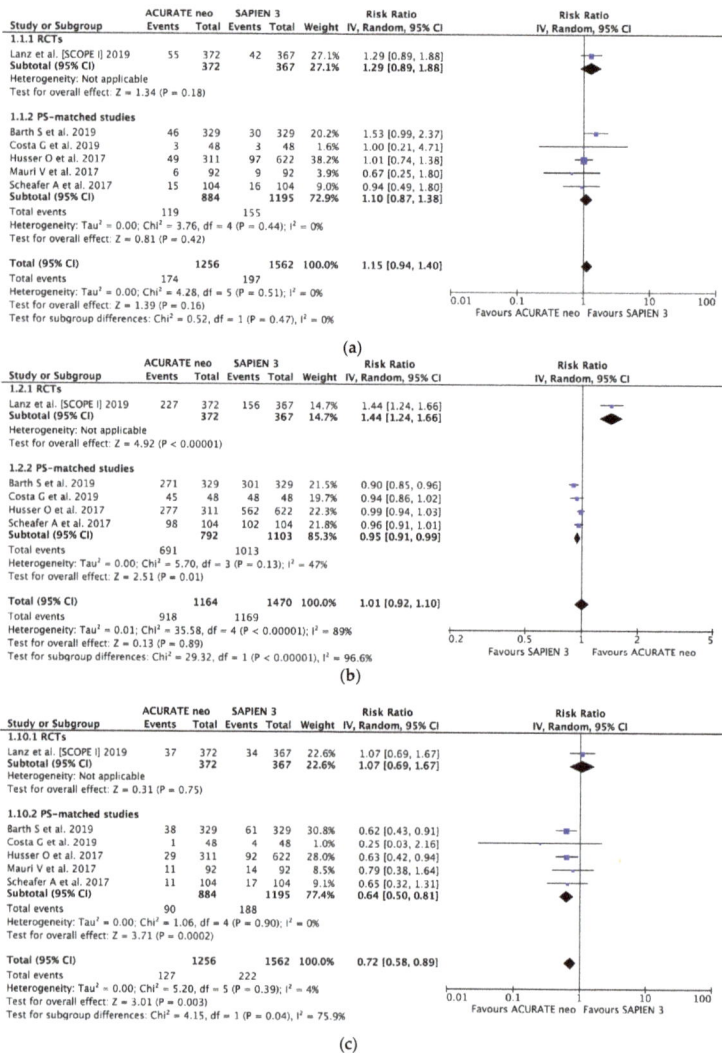

Figure 3. Individual and summary risk ratios with corresponding 95% confidence intervals for the comparison of ACURATE neo vs. SAPIEN 3 in the analysis of clinical outcomes: (**a**) early safety, (**b**) device success and (**c**) permanent pacemaker implantation.

There were no differences between ACURATE neo and SAPIEN 3 valves in terms of risk of major vascular complications (RR 1.21, 95% CI, (0.89, 1,65); $P = 0.23$; $I^2 = 6\%$; Figure 5), acute kidney injury (RR 1.28, 95% CI, (0.71, 2,31); $P = 0.42$; $I^2 = 15\%$; Figure 6), periprocedural myocardial infarction (RR 1.76, 95% CI, (0.36, 8.47); $P = 0.428$ $I^2 = 0\%$; Figures 7 and 8), stroke (RR 0.95, 95% CI, (0.57, 1.57); $P = 0.84$ $I^2 = 0\%$; Figures 9 and 10), and serious bleeding events (RR 1.23, 95% CI, (0.95, 1.61); $P = 0.12$; $I^2 = 0\%$; Figure 11).

Based on the data from six studies (2818 pts.), PPI was required nearly 30% less often after ACURATE neo implantation as compared to SAPIEN 3 (RR 0.72, 95% CI, (0.58, 0.89); $P = 0.003$; $I^2 = 75.9\%$) with corresponding frequency of 10.1% vs. 14.2%, respectively (Figure 3c). Importantly, the estimates derived from SCOPE I differed from the pooled estimates ($P_{interaction} = 0.04$) with higher rates of PPI observed in SAPIEN 3 arm in PS-matched studies (9.3% vs. 15.8%) Table 6 lists the VARC-2 derived quality criteria for PPI appraisal

3.5. Functional Outcomes

With five studies [14–16,18,19] and 1885 patients included, mild PVL occurred less frequently in SAPIEN 3 recipients, 28.0% (263 of 940), compared to ACURATE neo group, 45.5% (430 of 945); (RR 1.60, 95% CI, (1.40, 1.84) $P < 0.00001$; $I^2 = 14\%$) (Figure 4a). Moderate-to-severe PVL was uncommon in the entire series (6.5%); however, there was a significant 3.7-fold increase in moderate-to-severe PVL risk with ACURATE neo implantation: (RR 3.70, 95% CI, (2.04, 6.70) $P < 0.0001$; $I^2 = 53\%$) (Figure 4b) and corresponding incidence of 11.7% (147/1,256) and 2.3% (36/1,562) in ACURATE neo and SAPIEN 3 valves.

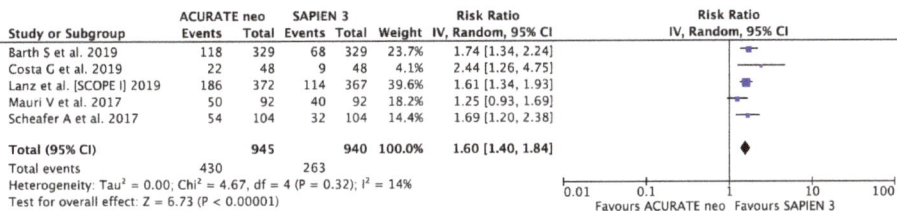

(a)

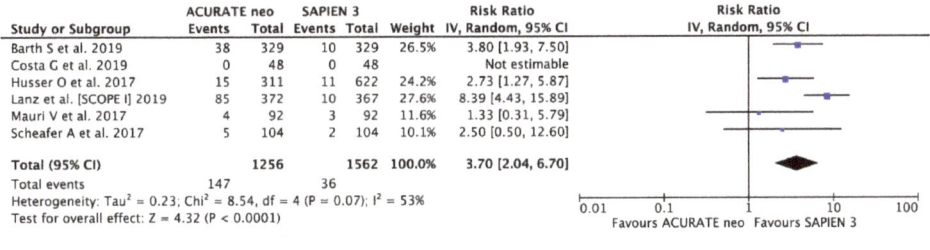

(b)

Figure 4. Individual and summary risk ratios with corresponding 95% confidence intervals for the comparison of ACURATE neo vs. SAPIEN 3 in the analysis of functional outcomes: (**a**) mild and (**b**) moderate-to-severe paravalvular leak.

Data regarding postprocedural transaortic gradient came from all six studies with 2818 patients. Mauri et al. [18] reported on 1-year transaortic gradients as well. (Figure 2). Mean postprocedural transaortic gradients were higher in SAPIEN 3 patients both at discharge and at 30 days post-op: 12.4 ± 4.7 vs. 8.7 ± 4.5 mmHg ($P < 0.00001$) and 11.5 ± 4.9 vs. 7.5 ± 3.4 mmHg ($P < 0.00001$) respectively.

3.6. All-Cause Mortality

Six studies reported on 30-day all-cause mortality. Overall, 61 (2.2%) patients died within the first 30 days, with respective rates of 2.9% and 1.6% in ACURATE neo and SAPIEN 3 groups; ACURATE neo was associated with 77% higher 30-day mortality risk (RR 1.77, 95% CI, (1.03, 3.04); $P = 0.04$; $I^2 = 0\%$) (Figure 5a and Appendix Figure 12). A random-effects meta-regression was fitted, counter-opposing all-cause mortality risk ratio against the risk difference of moderate-to-severe PVL; there was a trend for higher 30-day mortality rates with higher incidence of moderate-to-severe PVL (beta = 0.023; $P = 0.093$) (Figure 5b); similarly, a meta-regression was fitted with all-cause mortality risk ratio against the mean annulus area in the ACURATE neo arm showing a trend for lower between devices mortality ratio in smaller annuli (beta = 22.078; $P = 0.098$) (Figure 5c).

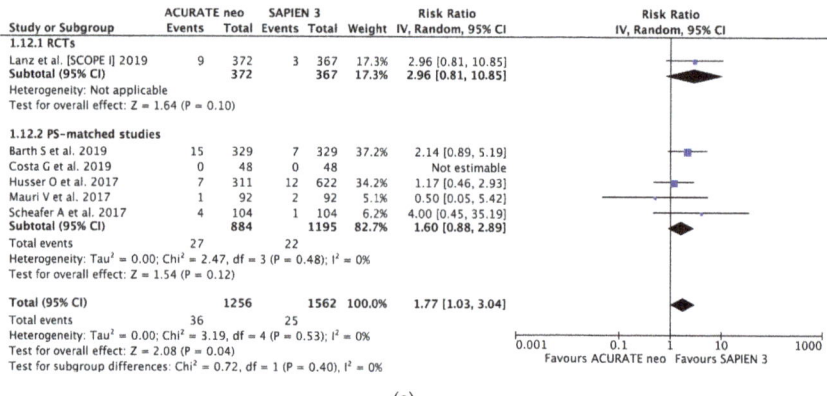

(a)

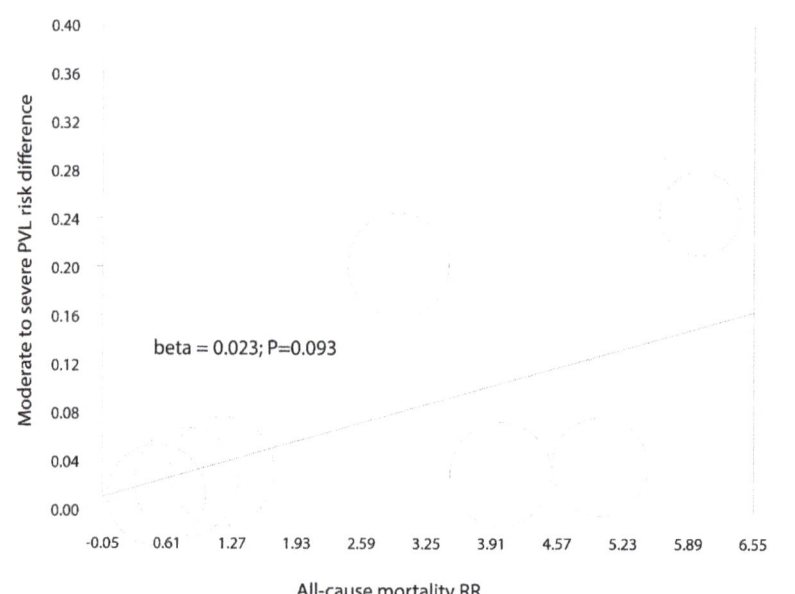

(b)

Figure 5. *Cont.*

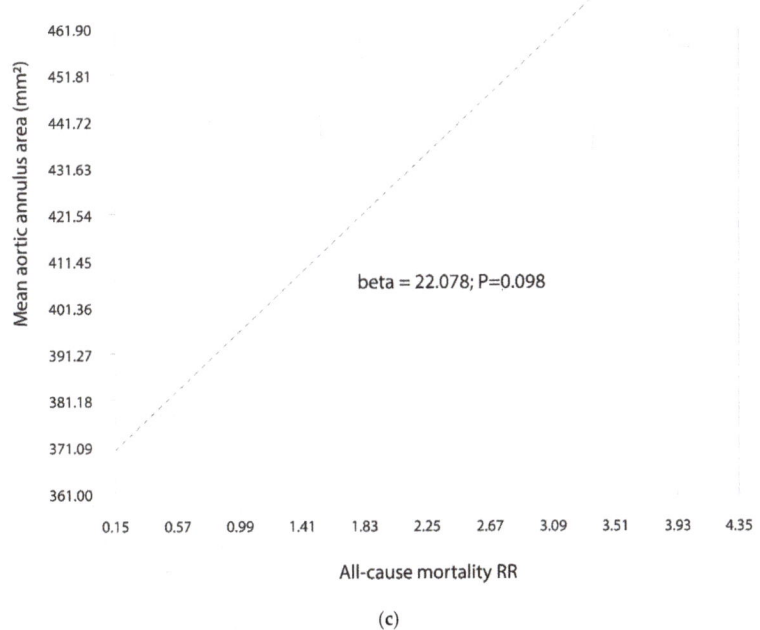

Figure 5. Individual and summary risk ratios with corresponding 95% confidence intervals for the comparison of ACURATE neo vs. SAPIEN 3 in the analysis of (**a**) 30-day all-cause mortality; (**b**,**c**) meta regression analyses.

4. Discussion

To the best of our knowledge, this is the first systematic review and meta-analysis of observational trials comparing major procedural, short-term clinical and functional outcomes between the ACURATE neo and SEPIEN 3, the next-generation transcatheter valves designed to minimize shortcomings of the earlier-generation devices. Our analysis, by pooling data from one RCT and five PS-matched studies, demonstrated excellent data regarding short-term performance of both devices. Compared populations of patients were well balanced with respect to baseline characteristics and severity of underlying valvular disease. Main findings of the current study are that the ACURATE neo implantation as compared to SAPIEN 3 was associated with lower transvalvular gradients and lower risk of permanent pacemaker implantation. Other clinical endpoints which included vascular complications, AKI, as well as life threatening and major bleeding; stroke and MIs did not differ between the two groups. The use of ACURATE neo procedures were significantly longer and required a greater amount of contrast volume. Device success and early safety combined endpoints, as defined by VARC-2 criteria, were, however, similar regardless the type of valve implanted. Importantly, the current study revealed significantly higher rates of both mild and moderate-to-severe PVL with ACURATE neo as compared to SAPIEN 3 and the latter were indirectly associated with worse survival observed in ACURATE neo group.

Previous observational studies [15–21] and, among them, the SAVI-TF (Symetis ACURATE neo Valve Implantation Using Transfemoral Access) registry [29,30] reported on excellent short-term outcomes with low complications and, in particular, PPI rates in ACURATE neo valve attributable to the design of the prosthesis. The particularly low gradients also contributed to the similar or better rates of device success for ACURATE neo and SAPIEN 3 in propensity matched comparisons. Whether the abovementioned benefits would hold true in randomized populations and further translate into improved clinical outcomes was investigated in the Safety and Efficacy of the Symetis ACURATE

Neo/TF Compared to the Edwards SAPIEN 3 Bioprosthesis trial (SCOPE I) [14]. Interestingly, the ACURATE neo valve failed to meet noninferiority for its primary endpoint of combined at 30 days against the balloon-expandable SAPIEN 3 (Edwards Lifesciences) valve. Moreover, secondary analyses demonstrated SAPIEN 3 to be superior for the composite safety and efficacy endpoint, driven by less stage 2 or 3 acute kidney injury and less paravalvular leak. Valve dysfunction requiring repeat interventions was also less common at 30 days. In particular, findings on device success need to be addressed, since the rates varied largely between RCT and the remaining PS-matched studies driven by higher patient prosthesis mismatch in the SAPIEN 3 group ($P < 0.00001$). Indeed, median mean transvalvular gradient was lower, and the median mean aortic valve area was larger, in the ACURATE neo, compared to the SAPIEN 3 group, at follow-up echocardiography in the SCOPE I trial. This may have been partially due to the fact that sizing and thus the choice of the valve process were different in the SCOPE I and the remaining studies. Some residual bias despite propensity score matching also cannot be excluded. In fact, Mauri et al. [18] reports on the sizing category was based on perimeter for ACURATE neo and annular area for SAPIEN 3, then all patients received ACURATE neo size S or SAPIEN 3 23 mm. In the study by Husser et al. [17] after PS-matching, there remained a $P = 0.003$ difference in aortic annular area; Schaefer et al. [19] reports aortic annulus size to have presented significant differences for area derived aortic annulus diameter (23.9 ± 2.8 vs. 24.8 ± 2.6 mm; $P = 0.02$) and perimeter-derived aortic annulus diameter (24.5 ± 2.5 vs. 25.3 ± 2.6 mm; $P = 0.02$), which, in consequence, led to oversizing in the ACURATE neo and undersizing SAPIEN 3 (1.5 ± 6.6 vs. −0.9 ± 6.4; $P = 0.01$ for cover index). Further, only in the SCOPE I trial, both the clinical events and functional assessment details were adjudicated by independent core lab. Independently, there were fewer PPI necessary after ACURATE neo in the PS-matched studies; since not confirmed in the SCOPE I, the supra-annular positioning of the valve must have had played, however, a much less important role than expected, and the lower PPI rates originating from skewed valve-size selection and positioning of the valve in the annulus [29]. More importantly, though, SCOPE I trial, by design, excluded over 300 patients with excessive calcification of aortic valve or left ventricular outflow tract (LVOT), which was not the case in remaining studies included in the current analysis. Presence of calcifications in both aortic annulus and LVOT could have accounted for much higher rates of PPI in the SAPIEN 3 arms across included PS-matched studies (average PPI incidence rate of 15.8%) as compared to SCOPE I trial with 9.3% rate, similarly to what has been already demonstrated for SAPIEN 3 in another meta-analysis by the same group [30].

Conversely to the abovementioned, yet still contributing to device success rates, was the higher incidence of moderate-to-severe PVL in the ACURATE neo valve, which was confirmed also in the current meta-analysis. In the next-generation devices, improved by addition an external sealing cuff or a skirt, the frequencies of mild and moderate-to-severe PVL became significantly lower as compared with the earlier-generation valves. The pooled occurrence of more than mild PVL decreased from 6.9% SAPIEN XT to 1.6% in SAPIEN 3 valve, as in a meta-analysis by Ando et al. with 2498 patients [31]. The PARTNER II SAPIEN-3 trial, which assessed early outcomes after TAVR in inoperable, high-risk and intermediate-risk patients with severe aortic stenosis, showed moderate-to-severe PVL in 3.4% and mild in 40.7% of the cases [32]. The abovementioned improvements seen in next-generation devices seem not to be the case with ACURATE neo; in the meta-analysis, we found 11.7% incidence of moderate-to-severe PVL in the ACURATE neo arm, nearly fourfold higher than in SAPIEN 3 and mild PVL in 45.5% cases, translating into 60% increased risk. Unlike the current findings, SAVI TF registry showed 4.1% of >mild PVL in 1000 patients treated with ACURATE neo which is within ranges observable for other devices [33–38]. Postdilatation was performed in 44.8% of the patients in that series, and this percentage is also comparable to 40.4%–51.9% in the current analysis, and therefore, theoretically, should not influence the outcome; on the other hand, Barth et al. [15] reports lower >mild PVL rates in one of participating centers (C) that used "zero tolerance of more than mild paravalvular leak" policy and postdilated more frequently than other centers (52.7% as compared to 12.3% and 33.3%), which translated to 3.4% rate of >mild PVL (as compared to 6.0% and 34.1% in the remaining centers). Interestingly, this center was the one to demonstrate highest one-year survival (87.4% (95% CI: 79.6–92.3) compared to 75.4% (95% CI: 60.4–85.3) and 81.3% (95% CI: 70.1–88.6)). Corroborating these estimates on larger scale and also in shorter follow-up, the current meta-analysis found an indirect link between increased rates of >mild PVL and higher mortality in the ACURATE neo arm at 30 days. While the presence of residual >mild PVL has been long shown to be associated with increased mortality in the long-term [39,40], the link between >mild PVL and 30-day mortality appears less clear, particularly for next-generation devices [12]. The abovementioned may be of importance given the fact that acute aortic insufficiency of various degree in patients with prior pure aortic stenosis and diminished LV compliance is often a cause of heart-failure exacerbation early in the sequelae [41].

An indirect link to increased mortality with ACURATE neo, as found also in meta-regression of annular area; indeed, lower between-devices mortality risk ratios between ACURATE neo and SAPIEN 3 were shown in patients with smaller annuli. An important hypothesis generated by present meta-analysis is that ACURATE neo performs differently in this setting; since we could not demonstrate excess of annual ruptures, cardiac tamponades, conversions to surgery or other periprocedural complications in either group, the explanation of this phenomenon remains to be elucidated.

Several inherent limitations to the current analysis need to be acknowledged; firstly, the majority of included studies are of an observational nature. Despite accounting for differences in the patients' baseline populations by propensity matching in all of the non-randomized reports, there remain other confounders, like learning curve, operators' experience and decision as of valve size and type that add to the risk of bias. Indeed, it cannot be refused that ACURATE neo was the preferred valve in smaller aortic annuli in PS-matched studies. Secondly, one study [15] reports on outcomes with both transfemoral ACURATE neo and transapical ACURATE TA systems. While similar in stent design and technological features, there are certain, albeit minor, differences in delivery system and biological tissue used in both devices [42]. Thirdly, only half of included studies reported follow-up longer than one month; paucity of data regarding long-term clinical and functional outcomes significantly impedes interpretation of ACURATE neo and SAPIEN 3 clinical suitability. Lastly, all but one study [14] lacked of an external core lab assessment and adjudication of echocardiographic outcomes. Finally, to better visualize the relative advantages of the contemporary-use valve systems, the results of a second similar study, SCOPE II (NCT03192813), will compare the ACURATE neo to the EVOLUT R system with respect to a composite of all-cause death and stroke at one year.

5. Conclusions

Contemporary evidence shows good short-term implantation outcomes of both ACURATE neo and SAPIEN 3 valves, with no differences in combined endpoints of device success and early safety. Implantation of ACURATE neo was associated with lower transvalvular gradients and lower risk of permanent pacemaker implantation. Moderate-to-severe PVL rates were, however, higher in ACURATE neo valve and were indirectly associated with increased 30-day all-cause mortality.

Author Contributions: Conceptualization, M.G., M.M., D.F., F.J., P.M., G.M.R., P.G.M., A.S. and M.K.; methodology, K.Z., M.P., D.P., J.K., R.L., P.S. and M.K.; software, M.K.; validation, all authors; formal analysis, M.G., G.M.R., P.G.M. and M.K.; investigation, M.G., K.Z., M.P., M.M., D.F., F.J., P.M.; resources, not available; data curation, M.G., G.M.R., P.G.M. and M.K.; writing—original draft preparation, all authors; writing—review and editing, R.L., P.S. and M.K.; visualization, M.K.; supervision, R.L., P.S. and M.K.; project administration, M.K.; funding acquisition, not available. All authors have read and agreed to the published version of the manuscript.

Conflicts of Interest: The authors declare no conflicts of interest.

Appendix A

Table A1. Checklist for meta-analyses of observational studies.

Item No.	Recommendation	Reported on Page No.
	Reporting of background should include	
1	Problem definition	2
2	Hypothesis statement	NA
3	Description of study outcome(s)	3–11
4	Type of exposure or intervention used	5
5	Type of study designs used	5
6	Study population	5
	Reporting of search strategy should include	
7	Qualifications of searchers (e.g., librarians and investigators)	Title page
8	Search strategy, including time period included in the synthesis and key words	4, Figure 1
9	Effort to include all available studies, including contact with authors	5
10	Databases and registries searched	5
11	Search software used, name and version, including special features used (e.g., explosion)	NA
12	Use of hand searching (e.g., reference lists of obtained articles)	5
13	List of citations located and those excluded, including justification	NA
14	Method of addressing articles published in languages other than English	NA
15	Method of handling abstracts and unpublished studies	NA
16	Description of any contact with authors	NA
	Reporting of methods should include	
17	Description of relevance or appropriateness of studies assembled for assessing the hypothesis to be tested	NA
18	Rationale for the selection and coding of data (e.g., sound clinical principles or convenience)	NA
19	Documentation of how data were classified and coded (e.g., multiple raters, blinding and interrater reliability)	NA
20	Assessment of confounding (e.g., comparability of cases and controls in studies where appropriate)	Table A2
21	Assessment of study quality, including blinding of quality assessors, stratification or regression on possible predictors of study results	Table A2
22	Assessment of heterogeneity	3
23	Description of statistical methods (e.g., complete description of fixed or random effects models, justification of whether the chosen models account for predictors of study results, dose-response models, or cumulative meta-analysis) in sufficient detail to be replicated	3
24	Provision of appropriate tables and graphics	yes

Table A1. Cont.

Item No.	Recommendation	Reported on Page No.
	Reporting of results should include	
25	Graphic summarizing individual study estimates and overall estimate	Figures 3–5
26	Table giving descriptive information for each study included	Table 2
27	Results of sensitivity testing (e.g., subgroup analysis)	NA
28	Indication of statistical uncertainty of findings	13–14
	Reporting of discussion should include	
29	Quantitative assessment of bias (e.g., publication bias)	NA
30	Justification for exclusion (e.g., exclusion of non-English language citations)	Figure 1
31	Assessment of quality of included studies	13, Table A2
	Reporting of conclusions should include	
32	Consideration of alternative explanations for observed results	11–13
33	Generalization of the conclusions (i.e., appropriate for the data presented and within the domain of the literature review)	14
34	Guidelines for future research	NA
35	Disclosure of funding source	Title page

From: Stroup DF, Berlin JA, Morton SC, et al. for the Meta-Analysis of Observational Studies in Epidemiology (MOOSE) Group. Meta-Analysis of Observational Studies in Epidemiology. A Proposal for Reporting. JAMA 2000; 283:2008-2012.

Table A2. Publication bias analysis.

Study (RCT)	Random sequence generation (selection bias)	Allocation concealment (selection bias)	Blinding of participants and personnel (performance bias)	Bias in measurement of interventions	Blinding of outcome assessment (detection bias)	Bias due to missing data	Incomplete outcome data (attrition bias)	Selective reporting (reporting bias)	Other bias	Overall bias
Lanz et al. [SCOPE I] 2019 [14]	Low	Unclear	High	Low	Low		Low	Low	Low	
Study (PS-matched studies)	Bias due to confounding	Bias in selection of participants into the study	Bias in measurement of interventions	Bias due to departures from intended interventions	Bias due to missing data		Bias in measurement of outcomes[1]	Bias in selection of reported result		Overall bias
Barth S et al. 2019 [15]	Serious	Serious	Low	Low	Low		Serious	Low		Moderate
Costa G et al. 2019 [16]	Serious	Low	Low	Low	Low		Serious	Low		Moderate
Husser O et al. 2017 [17]	Serious	Low	Low	Low	Low		Serious	Low		Moderate
Mauri V et al. 2017 [18]	Serious	Low	Low	Low	Low		Serious	Low		Moderate
Scheafer A et al. 2017 [19]	Serious	Low	Low	Low	Low		Serious	Low		Moderate

[1] When multiple outcomes were reported for a study, the highest level of bias at the outcome level is reported in the table.

Table A3. Inclusion and exclusion criteria. Choice of procedure and valve-type.

Study [ref]	Inclusion criteria	Exclusion criteria	Selection criteria for the procedure	Selection criteria for the valve
Barth S et al. 2019 [15]	Patients received either the ACURATE/ACURATE neo prostheses (n = 591) or the SAPIEN 3 prosthesis (n = 715).	Through nearest neighborhood matching with exact allocation for access route and center, pairs of 329 patients (250 transfemoral, 79 transapical) per group were determined.	Not reported.	Not reported.
Costa et al. 2019 [16]	All the patients treated with SAPIEN 3, Evolut R, or ACURATE neo, which could have indifferently received all the three devices according to manufacturer sizing indications.	Patients who did not performed pre-TAVI multi-detector computed tomography assessment (n = 169), patients who had a valve-in-valve implantation in a failed aortic bioprosthesis (n = 21), patients with bicuspid aortic valve (n = 28), and pure aortic regurgitation (n = 1).	Not reported.	Not reported.
Husser O et al. 2017 [17]	Patients with symptomatic, severe stenosis of the native aortic valve were treated with transfemoral TAVI using ACURATE neo (n = 311) or SAPIEN 3 (n = 810) at 3 centers in Germany.	Not reported.	The interdisciplinary heart team discussed all cases and consensus was achieved regarding the therapeutic strategy.	The interdisciplinary heart team discussed all cases and consensus was achieved regarding the therapeutic strategy.

Table A3. Cont.

Study [ref]	Inclusion criteria	Exclusion criteria	Selection criteria for the procedure	Selection criteria for the valve
Lanz J et al. 2019 [14]	Patients aged 75 years or older. With severe aortic stenosis defined by an aortic valve area (AVA) < 1 cm^2 or AVA indexed to body surface area of < 0.6 cm^2/m^2. Symptomatic (NYHA functional class > 1, angina or syncope). At increased risk for mortality if undergoing SAVR as determined by: - the heart team OR - an STS-PROM score > 10% OR - a Logistic EuroSCORE > 20%. Heart team agrees on eligibility for participation. Aortic annulus perimeter 66–85 mm AND area 338–573 mm^2 based on multi-slice computed tomography. Minimum diameter of arterial aorto-iliac-femoral axis on one side: ≥5–5 mm. Patient understand the purpose, potential risks and benefits of the trial, is able to provide written informed content and willing to participate in all parts of the follow-up.	-Non-valvular, congenital or non-calcific acquired aortic stenosis, uni- or bicuspid aortic valve. -Anatomy not appropriate for transfemoral TAVR due to degree or eccentricity of calcification or tortuosity of aorto- and iliac-femoral arteries. -Pre-existing prosthetic heart valve in aortic or mitral position. -Emergency procedures, cardiogenic shock (vasopressor dependence, mechanical hemodynamic support), or severely reduced left ventricular ejection fraction (<20%). -Concomitant planned procedure except for percutaneous coronary intervention. -Stroke or myocardial infarction (except type 2) in prior 30 days. -Planned non-cardiac surgery within 30 days after TAVR. -Severe coagulation conditions, inability to tolerate anticoagulation/antiplatelet therapy. -Evidence of intra-cardiac mass, thrombus or vegetation. -Active bacterial endocarditis or other active infection. -Hypertrophic cardiomyopathy with or without obstruction. -Contraindication to contrast media or allergy to nitinol. -Participation in another trial leading to deviations in the preparation and conduction of the intervention or the post-implantation management.	The heart team or an STS-PROM score > 10% or a Logistic EuroSCORE > 20%. Heart team agrees on eligibility for participation.	Patients were randomly assigned in a 1:1 ratio to undergo TAVI with either the ACURATE neo or the SAPIEN 3 system.

Table A3. Cont.

Study [ref]	Inclusion criteria	Exclusion criteria	Selection criteria for the procedure	Selection criteria for the valve
Mauri V et al. 2017 [18]	Inclusion criteria were small annular dimension defined as an annulus area <400 mm^2 and transfemoral TAVI with either an ACURATE neo size S or an Edwards SAPIEN 3 size 23 mm.	Not reported.	Eligibility of the individual candidate for TAVI had been decided within the local institutional heart team.	Prosthesis selection was at the discretion of the operating physicians at each center.
Schaefer A et al. 2017 [19]	A consecutive series of 104 patients received transfemoral TAVI using the ACURATE neo for treatment of severe symptomatic calcified aortic stenosis (study group) between 2012 and 2016. For comparative assessment, a matched control group of 104 patients treated by transfemoral TAVI using the Edwards SAPIEN 3 during the same time frame (2014 to 2016) was retrieved from dedicated hospital database containing a total of 1326 TAVI patients (210 SAPIEN 3 patients).	Patients unsuitable for a retrograde transfemoral approach and all valve-in-valve procedures were excluded from analysis.	Allocation of patients to TAVI followed current international recommendations after consensus of the local dedicated heart team.	Not reported.

Table A4. Patients' baseline characteristics.

Study [ref]	Intervention	HT (%)	DM (%)	PVD (%)	CKI (%)	COPD (%)	PM/ICD (%)	AF (%)	CAD (%)	MI history (%)	Stroke history (%)	Heart surgery history (%)	NYHA III/IV (%)	LVEF (%)	Mean aortic gradient (mmHg)	Aortic valve area (cm^2)	Aortic annulus diameter (mm)
Barth S et al. 2019 [15]	ACURATE neo	**93.3**	36.8	NR	2.7	15.8	NR	38.0	NR	NR	**14.0**	**14.9**	**79.0**	**53.0 ± 13.0**	**44.0 ± 15.0**	**0.68 ± 0.18**	21.0 ± 2.0
	SAPIEN 3	93.0	35.0	NR	2.7	14.9	NR	38.7	NR	NR	14.6	14.6	78.1	54.0 ± 15.0	45.0 ± 14.0	0.67 ± 0.17	21.0 ± 3.0
Costa et al. 2019 [16]	ACURATE neo	89.6	18.8	6.3	4.2	20.8	NR	12.5	NR	14.6	2.1	6.3	NR	54.5 ± 9.7	51.3 ± 14.5	NR	NR
	SAPIEN 3	89.6	27.1	4.2	2.1	14.6	NR	12.5	NR	14.6	4.2	2.1	NR	56.1 ± 9.7	51.3 ± 17.2	NR	NR
Husser O et al. 2017 [17]	ACURATE neo	NR	33.1	10.6	2.3	13.5	9.0	24.8	61.1	10.0	13.8	10.6	82.3	NR	45.0 ± 15.0	NR	NR
	SAPIEN 3	NR	32.3	11.3	1.9	17.8	10.0	26.2	62.7	10.1	12.5	8.7	78.6	NR	44.0 ± 16.0	NR	NR
Lanz J et al. 2019 [14]	ACURATE neo	92.0	29.0	12.0	4.0	9.0	12.0	36.0	59.0	10.0	13.0	9.0	77.0	56.4 ± 11.1	42.9 ± 17.2	0.7 ± 0.2	23.6 ± 1.6
	ACURATE neo	91.0	32.0	11.0	5.0	12.0	10.0	37.0	60.0	13.0	13.0	9.0	73.0	57.1 ± 10.7	41.5 ± 15.1	0.7 ± 0.2	23.7 ± 1.6
Mauri V et al. 2017 [18]	SAPIEN 3	NR	NR	NR	NR	NR	NR	NR	NR	NR	NR	NR	NR	59.0 ± 8.0	46.0 ± 16.0	NR	NR
	ACURATE neo	NR	NR	NR	NR	NR	NR	NR	NR	NR	NR	NR	NR	59.0 ± 10.0	47.0 ± 16.0	NR	NR
Schaefer A et al. 2017 [19]	SAPIEN 3	85.6	27.9	16.3	NR	17.3	NR	34.6	59.6	NR	14.4	9.6	86.5	NR	35.9 ± 16.6	0.8 ± 0.2	24.5 ± 2.5
	ACURATE neo	93.3	26.0	13.5	NR	20.2	NR	32.7	57.7	NR	11.5	5.8	88.5	NR	37.6 ± 16.7	0.8 ± 0.2	25.3 ± 2.6

HT, hypertension; DM, diabetes mellitus; PVD, peripheral vascular disease; CKI, chronic kidney injury; COPD, chronic obstructive pulmonary disease; PM/ICD, pacemaker/implantable cardioverter-defibrillator; AF, atrial fibrillation; CAD, coronary artery disease; MI, myocardial infarction; LVEF, left ventricle ejection fraction; NR, not reported. In bold are highlighted the variables that differed significantly.

Table A5. Procedural characteristics.

Study [ref]	Intervention	Anesthesia (%)	Access Site (%)	Valve sizes Implanted (%), (Mean ± SD)	Pre-Dilatation (%)	Post-Dilatation (%)	Contrast Volume (mL)	Fluoroscopy Time (min)	Procedure Duration (min)
Barth S et al. 2019 [15]	ACURATE neo	general 96.0, conscious sedation 4.0	femoral 74.5, apical 25.5	S NR M NR L NR (25.0 ± 2.0)	97.6	40.4	128 ± 54	9.2 ± 4.4	62.0 ± 24.0
	SAPIEN 3	general 96.4, conscious sedation 3.6	femoral 75.7, apical 24.3	23 mm NR 26 mm NR 29 mm NR (25.0 ± 2.0)	52.1	11.6	106 ± 43	8.5 ± 4.9	59.0 ± 26.0
Costa et al. 2019 [16]	ACURATE neo	NR	femoral 100	NR	NR	NR	NR	NR	NR
	SAPIEN 3		femoral 100	NR	NR	NR	NR	NR	NR
Husser O et al. 2017 [17]	ACURATE neo	general 52.7, conscious sedation 47.3	femoral 100	S 30.9 M 40.2 L 28.9	95.8	42.1	115.0 ± 54.0	10.0 ± 6.0	55.0 ± 30.0
	SAPIEN 3	general 54.0, conscious sedation 46.0	femoral 100	23 mm 43.9 26 mm 41.6 29 mm 14.5	74.3	23.8	104.0 ± 53.0	11.0 ± 5.9	54.0 ± 24.0
Lanz J et al. 2019 [14]	ACURATE neo	general 25.0, conscious sedation 75.0	femoral 99.0, other 1.0	S 20.0 M 43.0 L 34.0	88.0	52.0	136.0 ± 55.6	NR	53.2 ± 26.5
	SAPIEN 3	general 23.0, conscious sedation 77.0	femoral 99.0, other 1.0	23 mm 39.0 26 mm 55.0 29 mm 5.0	23.0	48.0	110 ± 45.9	NR	46.0 ± 25.9
Mauri V et al. 2017 [18]	ACURATE neo	general 100.0	femoral 100	S 100.0	94.6	31.5	NR	NR	NR
	SAPIEN 3		femoral 100	23 mm 100.0	31.5	6.5	NR	NR	NR
Schaefer A et al. 2017 [19]	ACURATE neo	conscious sedation 47.1% general 52.9%	femoral 100	S 35.6 M 38.5 L 25.9	90.3	47.6	162.6 ± 70.3	19.3 ± 9.4	94.0 ± 46.9
	SAPIEN 3	conscious sedation 34.6% general 65.4%	femoral 100	23mm 40.4 26mm 49.0 29mm 10.6	53.8	20.2	154.8±73.0	19.4±9.1	94.8±38.0

NR, not reported.

Table 6. VARC-2 derived permanent pacemaker implantation criteria quality appraisal.

Study [ref]	Presence of Pacemaker at Baseline Reported	Precision of the Indication Reported	Days Post TAVR for PPI Reported
Barth S et al. 2019 [15]	No	no	In-hospital
Costa et al. 2019 [16]	Yes	no	NA
Husser O et al. 2017 [17]	Yes	no	In-hospital and 30 days
Lanz J et al. 2019 [14]	Yes	no	30 days
Mauri V et al 2017 [18]	No	no	30 days
Schaefer A et al. 2017 [19]	No	Atrioventricular block Grade 3 or rapid progressive left bundle branch block	In-hospital

TAVR, transcatheter aortic valve replacement; PPI, permanent pacemaker implantation; NA, not available.

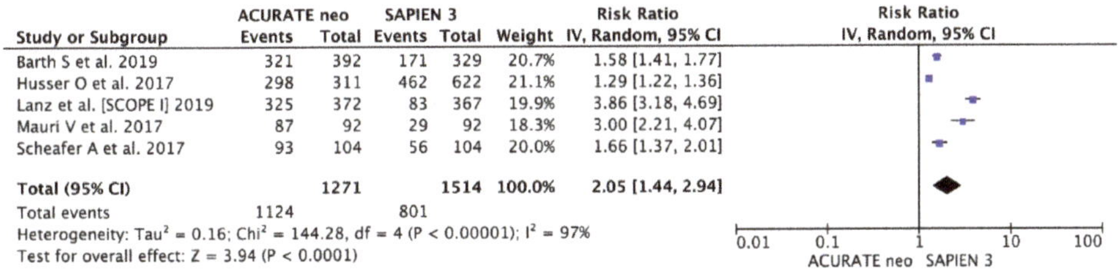

Study or Subgroup	ACURATE neo Events	Total	SAPIEN 3 Events	Total	Weight	Risk Ratio IV, Random, 95% CI
Barth S et al. 2019	321	392	171	329	20.7%	1.58 [1.41, 1.77]
Husser O et al. 2017	298	311	462	622	21.1%	1.29 [1.22, 1.36]
Lanz et al. [SCOPE I] 2019	325	372	83	367	19.9%	3.86 [3.18, 4.69]
Mauri V et al. 2017	87	92	29	92	18.3%	3.00 [2.21, 4.07]
Scheafer A et al. 2017	93	104	56	104	20.0%	1.66 [1.37, 2.01]
Total (95% CI)		**1271**		**1514**	**100.0%**	**2.05 [1.44, 2.94]**
Total events	1124		801			

Heterogeneity: Tau^2 = 0.16; Chi^2 = 144.28, df = 4 (P < 0.00001); I^2 = 97%
Test for overall effect: Z = 3.94 (P < 0.0001)

Figure 1. Procedural outcomes. Individual and summary risk ratios with corresponding 95% confidence intervals for the comparison of ACURATE neo vs. SAPIEN 3 in the analysis of predilatation.

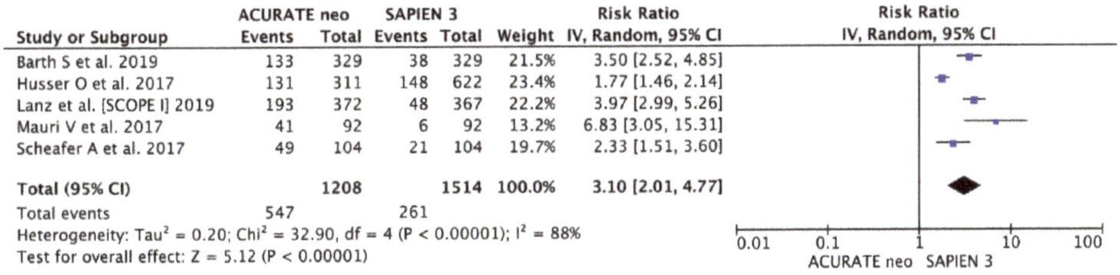

Study or Subgroup	ACURATE neo Events	Total	SAPIEN 3 Events	Total	Weight	Risk Ratio IV, Random, 95% CI
Barth S et al. 2019	133	329	38	329	21.5%	3.50 [2.52, 4.85]
Husser O et al. 2017	131	311	148	622	23.4%	1.77 [1.46, 2.14]
Lanz et al. [SCOPE I] 2019	193	372	48	367	22.2%	3.97 [2.99, 5.26]
Mauri V et al. 2017	41	92	6	92	13.2%	6.83 [3.05, 15.31]
Scheafer A et al. 2017	49	104	21	104	19.7%	2.33 [1.51, 3.60]
Total (95% CI)		**1208**		**1514**	**100.0%**	**3.10 [2.01, 4.77]**
Total events	547		261			

Heterogeneity: Tau^2 = 0.20; Chi^2 = 32.90, df = 4 (P < 0.00001); I^2 = 88%
Test for overall effect: Z = 5.12 (P < 0.00001)

Figure 2. Procedural outcomes. Individual and summary risk ratios with corresponding 95% confidence intervals for the comparison of ACURATE neo vs. SAPIEN 3 in the analysis of postdilatation.

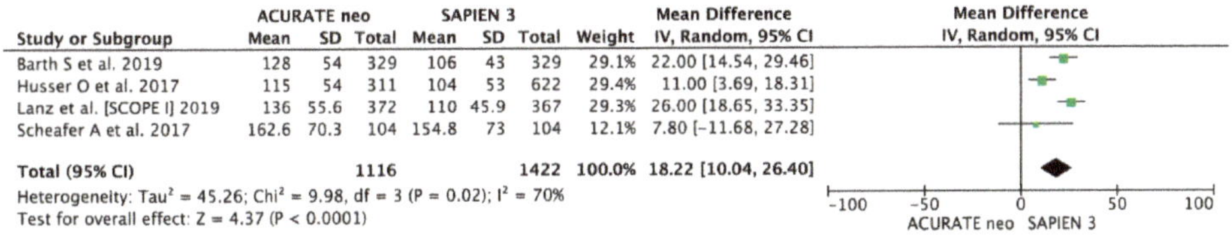

Study or Subgroup	ACURATE neo Mean	SD	Total	SAPIEN 3 Mean	SD	Total	Weight	Mean Difference IV, Random, 95% CI
Barth S et al. 2019	128	54	329	106	43	329	29.1%	22.00 [14.54, 29.46]
Husser O et al. 2017	115	54	311	104	53	622	29.4%	11.00 [3.69, 18.31]
Lanz et al. [SCOPE I] 2019	136	55.6	372	110	45.9	367	29.3%	26.00 [18.65, 33.35]
Scheafer A et al. 2017	162.6	70.3	104	154.8	73	104	12.1%	7.80 [−11.68, 27.28]
Total (95% CI)			**1116**			**1422**	**100.0%**	**18.22 [10.04, 26.40]**

Heterogeneity: Tau^2 = 45.26; Chi^2 = 9.98, df = 3 (P = 0.02); I^2 = 70%
Test for overall effect: Z = 4.37 (P < 0.0001)

Figure 3. Procedural outcomes. Detailed analysis of individual weighted mean differences (MDs) with corresponding 95% CIs on contrast volume used for the comparison of ACURATE neo vs. SAPIEN 3.

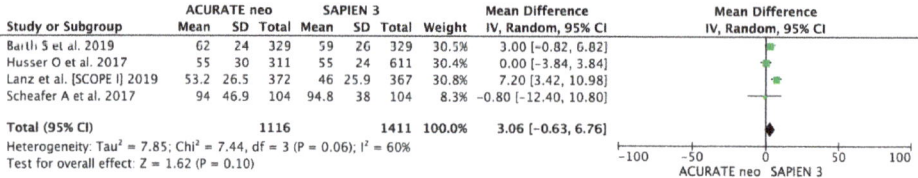

Figure 4. Procedural outcomes. Detailed analysis of individual weighted mean differences (MDs) with corresponding 95% CIs on procedure duration for the comparison of ACURATE neo vs. SAPIEN 3.

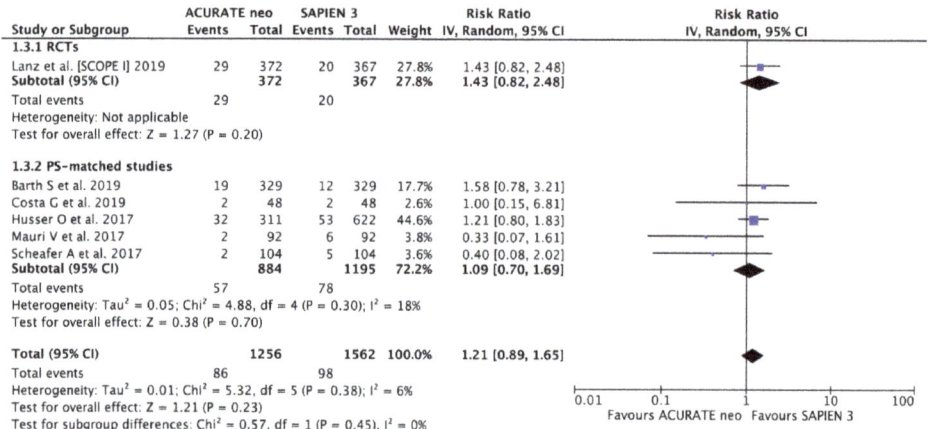

Figure 5. Clinical outcomes. Individual and summary risk ratios with corresponding 95% confidence intervals for the comparison of ACURATE neo and SAPIEN 3 in the analysis of major vascular complications.

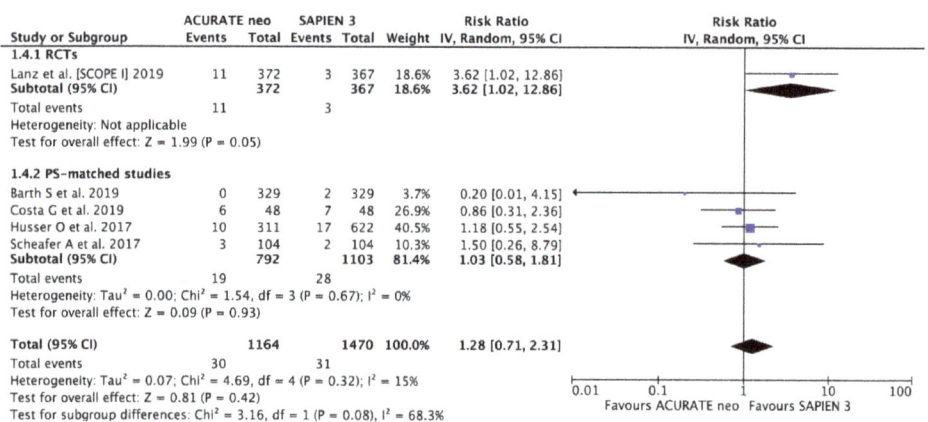

Figure 6. Clinical outcomes. Individual and summary risk ratios with corresponding 95% confidence intervals for the comparison of ACURATE neo and SAPIEN 3 in the analysis of acute kidney injury.

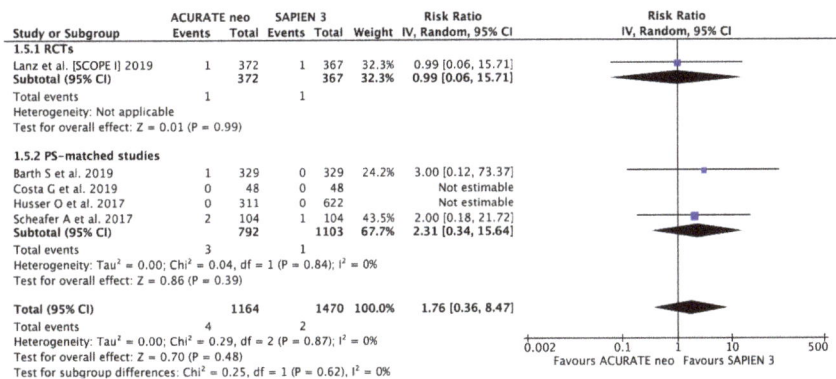

Figure 7. Clinical outcomes. Individual and summary risk ratios with corresponding 95% confidence intervals for the comparison of ACURATE neo and SAPIEN 3 in the analysis of periprocedural myocardial infarction.

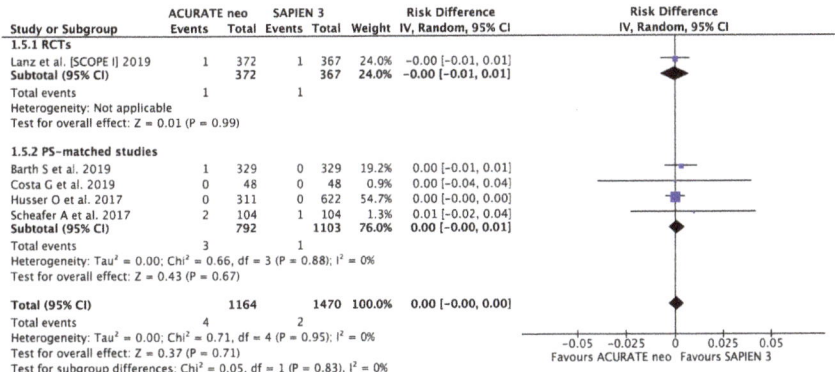

Figure 8. Clinical outcomes. Individual and summary risk ratios with corresponding 95% confidence intervals for the comparison of ACURATE neo and SAPIEN 3 in the analysis of periprocedural myocardial infarction taking into account "0 events".

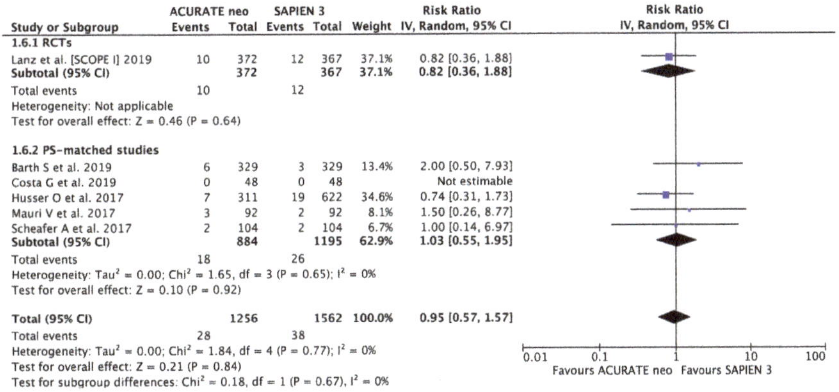

Figure 9. Clinical outcomes. Individual and summary risk ratios with corresponding 95% confidence intervals for the comparison of ACURATE neo and SAPIEN 3 in the analysis of stroke.

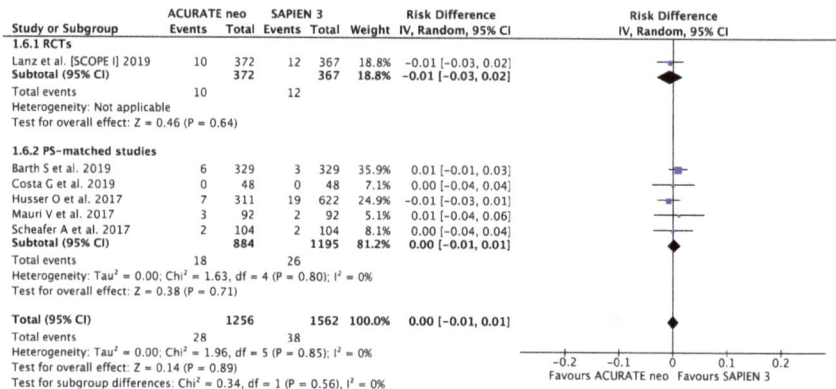

Figure 10. Clinical outcomes. Individual and summary risk ratios with corresponding 95% confidence intervals for the comparison of ACURATE neo and SAPIEN 3 in the analysis of stroke taking into account "0 events".

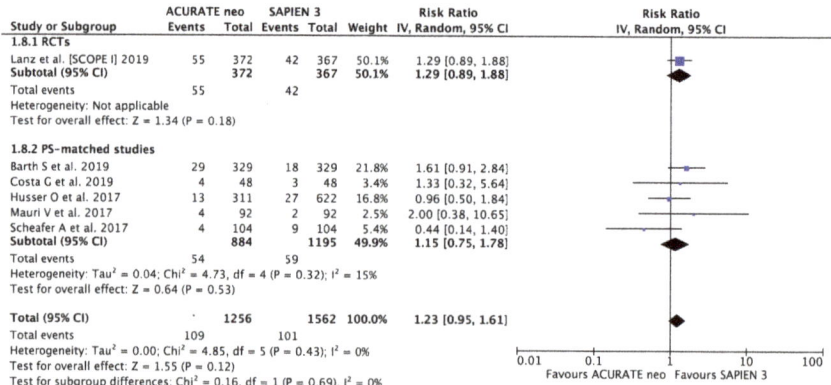

Figure 11. Clinical outcomes. Individual and summary risk ratios with corresponding 95% confidence intervals for the comparison of ACURATE neo and SAPIEN 3 in the analysis serious bleeding events.

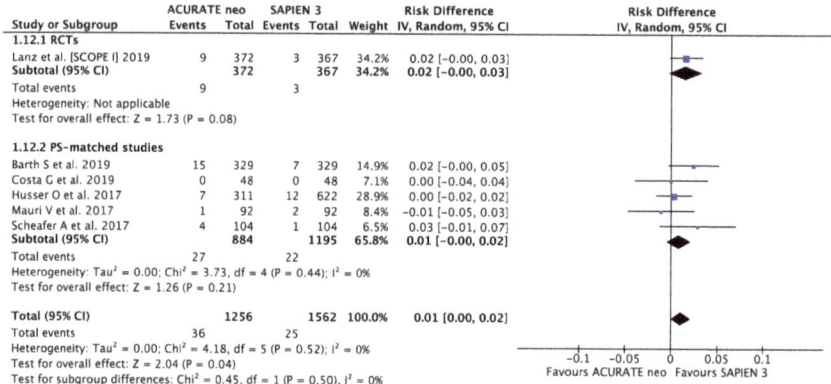

Figure 12. Clinical outcomes. Individual and summary risk ratios with corresponding 95% confidence intervals for the comparison of ACURATE neo and SAPIEN 3 in the analysis of 30-day all-cause mortality taking into account "0 events".

References

1. Cribier, A.; Eltchaninoff, H.; Bash, A.; Borenstein, N.; Tron, C.; Bauer, F.; Derumeaux, G.; Anselme, F.; Laborde, F.; Leon, M.B. Percutaneous transcatheter implantation of an aortic valve prosthesis for calcific aortic stenosis: First human case description. *Circulation* **2002**, *106*, 3006–3008. [CrossRef]
2. Smith, C.R.; Leon, M.B.; Mack, M.J.; Miller, D.C.; Moses, J.W.; Svensson, L.G.; Tuzcu, E.M.; Webb, J.G.; Fontana, G.P.; Makkar, R.R.; et al. Transcatheter versus surgical aortic-valve replacement in high-risk patients. *N. Engl. J. Med.* **2011**, *364*, 2187–2198. [CrossRef] [PubMed]
3. Adams, D.H.; Popma, J.J.; Reardon, M.J.; Yakubov, S.J.; Coselli, J.S.; Deeb, G.M.; Gleason, T.G.; Buchbinder, M.; Hermiller, J., Jr.; Kleiman, N.S.; et al. Transcatheter aortic-valve replacement with a self-expanding prosthesis. *N. Engl. J. Med.* **2014**, *370*, 1790–1798. [CrossRef] [PubMed]
4. Webb, J.G.; Pasupati, S.; Humphries, K.; Thompson, C.; Altwegg, L.; Moss, R.; Sinhal, A.; Carere, R.G.; Munt, B.; Ricci, D.; et al. Percutaneous transarterial aortic valve replacement in selected high-risk patients with aortic stenosis. *Circulation* **2007**, *116*, 755–763. [CrossRef]
5. Leon, M.B.; Smith, C.R.; Mack, M.; Miller, D.C.; Moses, J.W.; Svensson, L.G.; Tuzcu, E.M.; Webb, J.G.; Fontana, G.P.; Makkar, R.R.; et al. Transcatheter aortic-valve implantation for aortic stenosis in patients who cannot undergo surgery. *N. Engl. J. Med.* **2010**, *363*, 1597–1607. [CrossRef]
6. Thourani, V.H.; Kodali, S.; Makkar, R.R.; Herrmann, H.C.; Williams, M.; Babaliaros, V.; Smalling, R.; Lim, S.; Malaisrie, S.C.; Kapadia, S.; et al. Transcatheter aortic valve replacement versus surgical valve replacement in intermediate-risk patients: A propensity score analysis. *Lancet* **2016**, *387*, 2218–2225. [CrossRef]
7. Leon, M.B.; Smith, C.R.; Mack, M.J.; Makkar, R.R.; Svensson, L.G.; Kodali, S.K.; Thourani, V.H.; Tuzcu, E.M.; Miller, D.C.; Herrmann, H.C.; et al. Transcatheter or Surgical Aortic-Valve Replacement in Intermediate-Risk Patients. *N. Engl. J. Med.* **2016**, *374*, 1609–1620. [CrossRef]
8. Reardon, M.J.; Van Mieghem, N.M.; Popma, J.J.; Kleiman, N.S.; Sondergaard, L.; Mumtaz, M.; Adams, D.H.; Deeb, G.M.; Maini, B.; Gada, H.; et al. Surgical or Transcatheter Aortic-Valve Replacement in Intermediate-Risk Patients. *N. Engl. J. Med.* **2017**, *376*, 1321–1331. [CrossRef]
9. Mack, M.J.; Leon, M.B.; Thourani, V.H.; Makkar, R.; Kodali, S.K.; Russo, M.; Kapadia, S.R.; Malaisrie, S.C.; Cohen, D.J.; Pibarot, P.; et al. Transcatheter Aortic-Valve Replacement with a Balloon-Expandable Valve in Low-Risk Patients. *N. Engl. J. Med.* **2019**, *380*, 1695–1705. [CrossRef]
10. Nishimura, R.A.; Otto, C.M.; Bonow, R.O.; Carabello, B.A.; Erwin, J.P., 3rd; Fleisher, L.A.; Jneid, H.; Mack, M.J.; McLeod, C.J.; O'Gara, P.T.; et al. 2017 AHA/ACC Focused Update of the 2014 AHA/ACC Guideline for the Management of Patients With Valvular Heart Disease: A Report of the American College of Cardiology/American Heart Association Task Force on Clinical Practice Guidelines. *Circulation* **2017**, *135*, e1159–e1195. [CrossRef]
11. Van Belle, E.; Juthier, F.; Susen, S.; Vincentelli, A.; Dallongeville, J.; Iung, B.; Eltchaninoff, H.; Laskar, M.; Leprince, P.; Lievre, M.; et al. Response to letter regarding article, "postprocedural aortic regurgitation in balloon-expandable and self-expandable transcatheter aortic valve replacement procedures: Analysis of predictors and impact on long-term mortality: Insights from the FRANCE2 registry". *Circulation* **2015**, *131*, e16–e17. [CrossRef]
12. Kodali, S.K.; Williams, M.R.; Smith, C.R.; Svensson, L.G.; Webb, J.G.; Makkar, R.R.; Fontana, G.P.; Dewey, T.M.; Thourani, V.H.; Pichard, A.D.; et al. Two-year outcomes after transcatheter or surgical aortic-valve replacement. *N. Engl. J. Med.* **2012**, *366*, 1686–1695. [CrossRef]
13. Jones, B.M.; Tuzcu, E.M.; Krishnaswamy, A.; Popovic, Z.; Mick, S.; Roselli, E.E.; Gul, S.; Devgun, J.; Mistry, S.; Jaber, W.A.; et al. Prognostic significance of mild aortic regurgitation in predicting mortality after transcatheter aortic valve replacement. *J. Thorac. Cardiovasc. Surg.* **2016**, *152*, 783–790. [CrossRef]
14. Lanz, J.; Kim, W.K.; Walther, T.; Burgdorf, C.; Mollmann, H.; Linke, A.; Redwood, S.; Thilo, C.; Hilker, M.; Joner, M.; et al. Safety and efficacy of a self-expanding versus a balloon-expandable bioprosthesis for transcatheter aortic valve replacement in patients with symptomatic severe aortic stenosis: A randomised non-inferiority trial. *Lancet* **2019**, *394*, 1619–1628. [CrossRef]
15. Barth, S.; Reents, W.; Zacher, M.; Kerber, S.; Diegeler, A.; Schieffer, B.; Schreiber, M.; Lauer, B.; Kuntze, T.; Dahmer, M.; et al. Multicentre propensity-matched comparison of transcatheter aortic valve implantation using the ACURATE TA/neo self-expanding versus the SAPIEN 3 balloon-expandable prosthesis. *EuroIntervention* **2019**, *15*, 884–891. [CrossRef]

16. Costa, G.; Buccheri, S.; Barbanti, M.; Picci, A.; Todaro, D.; Di Simone, E.; La Spina, K.; D'Arrigo, P.; Criscione, E.; Nastasi, M.; et al. Outcomes of three different new generation transcatheter aortic valve prostheses. *Catheter. Cardiovasc. Interv.* **2019**. [CrossRef]
17. Husser, O.; Kim, W.K.; Pellegrini, C.; Holzamer, A.; Walther, T.; Mayr, P.N.; Joner, M.; Kasel, A.M.; Trenkwalder, T.; Michel, J.; et al. Multicenter Comparison of Novel Self-Expanding Versus Balloon-Expandable Transcatheter Heart Valves. *JACC Cardiovasc. Interv.* **2017**, *10*, 2078–2087. [CrossRef]
18. Mauri, V.; Kim, W.K.; Abumayyaleh, M.; Walther, T.; Moellmann, H.; Schaefer, U.; Conradi, L.; Hengstenberg, C.; Hilker, M.; Wahlers, T.; et al. Short-Term Outcome and Hemodynamic Performance of Next-Generation Self-Expanding Versus Balloon-Expandable Transcatheter Aortic Valves in Patients With Small Aortic Annulus: A Multicenter Propensity-Matched Comparison. *Circ. Cardiovasc. Interv.* **2017**, *10*. [CrossRef]
19. Schaefer, A.; Linder, M.; Seiffert, M.; Schoen, G.; Deuschl, F.; Schofer, N.; Schneeberger, Y.; Blankenberg, S.; Reichenspurner, H.; Schaefer, U.; et al. Comparison of latest generation transfemoral self-expandable and balloon-expandable transcatheter heart valves. *Interact. Cardiovasc. Thorac. Surg.* **2017**, *25*, 905–911. [CrossRef]
20. Moriyama, N.; Vento, A.; Laine, M. Safety of Next-Day Discharge After Transfemoral Transcatheter Aortic Valve Replacement With a Self-Expandable Versus Balloon-Expandable Valve Prosthesis. *Circ. Cardiovasc. Interv.* **2019**, *12*, e007756. [CrossRef]
21. Pagnesi, M.; Kim, W.K.; Conradi, L.; Barbanti, M.; Stefanini, G.G.; Zeus, T.; Pilgrim, T.; Schofer, J.; Zweiker, D.; Testa, L.; et al. Transcatheter Aortic Valve Replacement With Next-Generation Self-Expanding Devices: A Multicenter, Retrospective, Propensity-Matched Comparison of Evolut PRO Versus Acurate neo Transcatheter Heart Valves. *JACC Cardiovasc. Interv.* **2019**, *12*, 433–443. [CrossRef]
22. Stroup, D.F.; Berlin, J.A.; Morton, S.C.; Olkin, I.; Williamson, G.D.; Rennie, D.; Moher, D.; Becker, B.J.; Sipe, T.A.; Thacker, S.B. Meta-analysis of observational studies in epidemiology: A proposal for reporting. Meta-analysis Of Observational Studies in Epidemiology (MOOSE) group. *JAMA* **2000**, *283*, 2008–2012. [CrossRef]
23. Liberati, A.; Altman, D.G.; Tetzlaff, J.; Mulrow, C.; Gotzsche, P.C.; Ioannidis, J.P.; Clarke, M.; Devereaux, P.J.; Kleijnen, J.; Moher, D. The PRISMA statement for reporting systematic reviews and meta-analyses of studies that evaluate health care interventions: Explanation and elaboration. *PLoS Med.* **2009**, *6*, e1000100. [CrossRef]
24. Higgins, J.P.; Altman, D.G.; Gotzsche, P.C.; Juni, P.; Moher, D.; Oxman, A.D.; Savovic, J.; Schulz, K.F.; Weeks, L.; Sterne, J.A.; et al. The Cochrane Collaboration's tool for assessing risk of bias in randomised trials. *BMJ* **2011**, *343*, d5928. [CrossRef]
25. Sterne, J.A.; Hernan, M.A.; Reeves, B.C.; Savovic, J.; Berkman, N.D.; Viswanathan, M.; Henry, D.; Altman, D.G.; Ansari, M.T.; Boutron, I.; et al. ROBINS-I: A tool for assessing risk of bias in non-randomised studies of interventions. *BMJ* **2016**, *355*, i4919. [CrossRef]
26. Kappetein, A.P.; Head, S.J.; Genereux, P.; Piazza, N.; van Mieghem, N.M.; Blackstone, E.H.; Brott, T.G.; Cohen, D.J.; Cutlip, D.E.; van Es, G.A.; et al. Updated standardized endpoint definitions for transcatheter aortic valve implantation: The Valve Academic Research Consortium-2 consensus document. *J. Am. Coll. Cardiol.* **2012**, *60*, 1438–1454. [CrossRef]
27. Higgins, J.P.; Thompson, S.G.; Deeks, J.J.; Altman, D.G. Measuring inconsistency in meta-analyses. *BMJ* **2003**, *327*, 557–560. [CrossRef]
28. Wan, X.; Wang, W.; Liu, J.; Tong, T. Estimating the sample mean and standard deviation from the sample size, median, range and/or interquartile range. *BMC Med. Res. Methodol.* **2014**, *14*, 135. [CrossRef]
29. Sathananthan, J.; Hensey, M.; Fraser, R.; Landes, U.; Blanke, P.; Hatoum, H.; Dasi, L.P.; Sedaghat, A.; Bapat, V.N.; Leipsic, J.; et al. Implications of hydrodynamic testing to guide sizing of self-expanding transcatheter heart valves for valve-in-valve procedures. *Catheter. Cardiovasc. Interv.* **2019**. [CrossRef]
30. Gozdek, M.; Ratajczak, J.; Arndt, A.; Zieliński, K.; Pasierski, M.; Matteucci, M.; Fina, D.; Jiritano, F.; Meani, P.; Raffa, G.M.; et al. Transcatheter aortic valve replacement with Lotus and Sapien 3 prosthetic valves: A systematic review and meta-analysis. *J. Thorac. Dis.* **2020**. (ahead of print).
31. Ando, T.; Briasoulis, A.; Holmes, A.A.; Taub, C.C.; Takagi, H.; Afonso, L. Sapien 3 versus Sapien XT prosthetic valves in transcatheter aortic valve implantation: A meta-analysis. *Int. J. Cardiol.* **2016**, *220*, 472–478. [CrossRef]

32. Kodali, S.; Thourani, V.H.; White, J.; Malaisrie, S.C.; Lim, S.; Greason, K.L.; Williams, M.; Guerrero, M.; Eisenhauer, A.C.; Kapadia, S.; et al. Early clinical and echocardiographic outcomes after SAPIEN 3 transcatheter aortic valve replacement in inoperable, high-risk and intermediate-risk patients with aortic stenosis. *Eur. Heart J.* **2016**, *37*, 2252–2262. [CrossRef]
33. Noble, S.; Stortecky, S.; Heg, D.; Tueller, D.; Jeger, R.; Toggweiler, S.; Ferrari, E.; Nietlispach, F.; Taramasso, M.; Maisano, F.; et al. Comparison of procedural and clinical outcomes with Evolut R versus Medtronic CoreValve: A Swiss TAVI registry analysis. *EuroIntervention* **2017**, *12*, e2170–e2176. [CrossRef]
34. Naber, C.K.; Pyxaras, S.A.; Ince, H.; Frambach, P.; Colombo, A.; Butter, C.; Gatto, F.; Hink, U.; Nickenig, G.; Bruschi, G.; et al. A multicentre European registry to evaluate the Direct Flow Medical transcatheter aortic valve system for the treatment of patients with severe aortic stenosis. *EuroIntervention* **2016**, *12*, e1413–e1419. [CrossRef]
35. Wendler, O.; Schymik, G.; Treede, H.; Baumgartner, H.; Dumonteil, N.; Ihlberg, L.; Neumann, F.J.; Tarantini, G.; Zamarano, J.L.; Vahanian, A. SOURCE 3 Registry: Design and 30-Day Results of the European Postapproval Registry of the Latest Generation of the SAPIEN 3 Transcatheter Heart Valve. *Circulation* **2017**, *135*, 1123–1132. [CrossRef]
36. Thomas, M.; Schymik, G.; Walther, T.; Himbert, D.; Lefevre, T.; Treede, H.; Eggebrecht, H.; Rubino, P.; Michev, I.; Lange, R.; et al. Thirty-day results of the SAPIEN aortic Bioprosthesis European Outcome (SOURCE) Registry: A European registry of transcatheter aortic valve implantation using the Edwards SAPIEN valve. *Circulation* **2010**, *122*, 62–69. [CrossRef]
37. Naber, C.K.; Pyxaras, S.A.; Ince, H.; Latib, A.; Frambach, P.; den Heijer, P.; Wagner, D.; Butter, C.; Colombo, A.; Kische, S. Real-world multicentre experience with the Direct Flow Medical repositionable and retrievable transcatheter aortic valve implantation system for the treatment of high-risk patients with severe aortic stenosis. *EuroIntervention* **2016**, *11*, e1314–e1320. [CrossRef]
38. Kowalewski, M.; Gozdek, M.; Raffa, G.M.; Slomka, A.; Zielinski, K.; Kubica, J.; Anisimowicz, L.; Kowalewski, J.; Landes, U.; Kornowski, R.; et al. Transcatheter aortic valve implantation with the new repositionable self-expandable Medtronic Evolut R vs. CoreValve system: Evidence on the benefit of a meta-analytical approach. *J. Cardiovasc. Med.* **2019**, *20*, 226–236. [CrossRef]
39. Tamburino, C.; Capodanno, D.; Ramondo, A.; Petronio, A.S.; Ettori, F.; Santoro, G.; Klugmann, S.; Bedogni, F.; Maisano, F.; Marzocchi, A.; et al. Incidence and predictors of early and late mortality after transcatheter aortic valve implantation in 663 patients with severe aortic stenosis. *Circulation* **2011**, *123*, 299–308. [CrossRef]
40. Kodali, S.; Pibarot, P.; Douglas, P.S.; Williams, M.; Xu, K.; Thourani, V.; Rihal, C.S.; Zajarias, A.; Doshi, D.; Davidson, M.; et al. Paravalvular regurgitation after transcatheter aortic valve replacement with the Edwards sapien valve in the PARTNER trial: Characterizing patients and impact on outcomes. *Eur. Heart J.* **2015**, *36*, 449–456. [CrossRef]
41. Gilard, M.; Eltchaninoff, H.; Iung, B.; Donzeau-Gouge, P.; Chevreul, K.; Fajadet, J.; Leprince, P.; Leguerrier, A.; Lievre, M.; Prat, A.; et al. Registry of transcatheter aortic-valve implantation in high-risk patients. *N. Engl. J. Med.* **2012**, *366*, 1705–1715. [CrossRef]
42. Choudhury, T.; Solomonica, A.; Bagur, R. The ACURATE neo transcatheter aortic valve system. *Exp. Rev. Med. Device.* **2018**, *15*, 693–699. [CrossRef]

© 2020 by the authors. Licensee MDPI, Basel, Switzerland. This article is an open access article distributed under the terms and conditions of the Creative Commons Attribution (CC BY) license (http://creativecommons.org/licenses/by/4.0/).

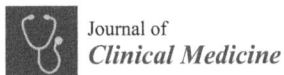

Article

Predictors for Target Vessel Failure after Recanalization of Chronic Total Occlusions in Patients Undergoing Surveillance Coronary Angiography

Martin Geyer [1,*,†], Johannes Wild [1,2,†], Marc Hirschmann [1], Zisis Dimitriadis [1], Thomas Münzel [1,3], Tommaso Gori [1,3] and Philip Wenzel [1,2,3,*]

1. Center for Cardiology, Cardiology I, University Medical Center Mainz of the Johannes Gutenberg-University Mainz, Langenbeckstr. 1, 55131 Mainz, Germany; Johannes.wild@unimedizin-mainz.de (J.W.); marc.hirschmann@icloud.com (M.H.); zisis.dimitriadis@unimedizin-mainz.de (Z.D.); tmuenzel@uni-mainz.de (T.M.); tommaso.gori@unimedizin-mainz.de (T.G.)
2. Center for Thrombosis and Hemostasis, University Medical Center Mainz of the Johannes Gutenberg-University Mainz, Langenbeckstr 1, 55131 Mainz, Germany
3. German Center for Cardiovascular Research (DZHK), Partner Site Rhine Main, Langenbeckstr. 1, 55131 Mainz, Germany
* Correspondence: martin.geyer@unimedizin-mainz.de (M.G.); wenzelp@uni-mainz.de (P.W.); Tel.: +49-6131-17-8785 (M.G.); +49-6131-17-7695 (P.W.)
† M.G. and J.W. contributed equally and should both be considered as first authors.

Received: 24 November 2019; Accepted: 7 January 2020; Published: 9 January 2020

Abstract: (1) Background: Knowledge about predictors for the long-time patency of recanalized chronic total coronary occlusions (CTOs) is limited. Evidence from invasive follow-up in the absence of acute coronary syndrome (routine surveillance coronary angiography) is scarce. (2) Methods: In a monocentric-retrospective analysis, we obtained baseline as well as periprocedural data of patients undergoing routine invasive follow-up. We defined target vessel failure (TVF) as a combined primary endpoint, consisting of re-occlusion, restenosis, and target vessel revascularization (TVR). (3) Results: We included 93 consecutive patients (15.1% female) from October 2013 to May 2018. After a follow-up period of 206 ± 129 days (median 185 (IQR 127–237)), re-occlusion had occurred in 7.5%, restenosis in 11.8%, and TVR in 5.4%; the cumulative incidence of TVF was 15.1%. Reduced TIMI-flow immediately after recanalization (OR for TVR: 11.0 (95% CI: 2.7–45.5), $p = 0.001$) as well as female gender (OR for TVR: 11.0 (95% CI: 2.1–58.5), $p = 0.005$) were found to be predictive for pathological angiographic findings at follow-up. Furthermore, higher blood values of high-sensitive troponin after successful revascularization were associated with all endpoints. Interestingly, neither the J-CTO score nor the presence of symptoms at the follow-up visit could be correlated to adverse angiographic results. (4) Conclusions: In this medium-sized cohort of patients with surveillance coronary angiography, we were able to identify reduced TIMI flow and female gender as the strongest predictors for future TVF.

Keywords: chronic total occlusion; target vessel failure; re-occlusion; surveillance coronary angiography

1. Introduction

Coronary chronic total occlusion (CTO) is defined as either absent or minimal antegrade coronary blood flow diagnosed by coronary angiography that had existed for >12 weeks [1]. According to registry data, this distinct subtype of coronary artery disease has a prevalence of up to 20% of all invasive coronary diagnostics [2]. Nevertheless, expert opinion on the optimal treatment strategy (conservative, interventional, or surgical) is still controversial. According to contemporary data on clinical practice, only about one third of all patients with a CTO are treated by revascularization (percutaneous coronary intervention (PCI) or coronary artery bypass grafting surgery (CABG)) [2]. In contrast to non-CTO PCIs with a procedural success rate of 98%, interventional CTO procedures are more complex and have a significantly lower periprocedural revascularization rate of 60% to 70% in non-specialized centers [2,3], which can exceed 90% in highly specialized units [4,5]. As a tool to assess and grade lesion difficulty as well as predicting successful guidewire crossing within 30 min in interventional recanalization, the J-CTO (Multicenter CTO Registry in Japan) score was developed and validated. The presence of five specific lesion characteristics in CTO vessels that are known to hamper revascularization success (blunt stump, occlusion length > 20 mm, calcification, vessel bending > 45 degrees, and previously failed PCI) are assigned to one point each and summarized [6]. Vessel revascularization in CTO lesions has been associated with clinical improvement of angina and a prognostic benefit regarding a lower rate of subsequent myocardial infarction and longer survival in clinical registries [7–10]. However, evidence on long-term angiographic results as well as potential predictors for vessel patency and re-occlusion post CTO-PCI is scarce. Results from other registries imply that a higher pre-interventional J-CTO score—beyond acute success—might have an impact on an increased probability for future adverse events [11,12]. Thus, the objectives of this study were (i) to investigate the incidence of long-term target vessel failure (re-occlusion, restenosis, and target vessel revascularization) as assessed by invasive follow-up in an all-comer retrospective monocentric analysis, and (ii) to identify potential predictors of future target vessel failure after successful CTO recanalization, including the J-CTO score.

2. Methods

Data of all patients consecutively treated with successful PCI for CTO-lesions in our center between October 2013 to September 2017 that had an elective control coronary angiography until May 2018 were included in this retrospective analysis. Surveillance angiography after a follow-up period of 3 to 12 months was routinely recommended after successful recanalization of a CTO vessel in accordance with the guidelines for high-risk lesions [13]. Patients primarily undergoing urgent invasive control for acute coronary syndrome at a follow-up instead of the elective control coronary angiography were excluded from the analysis. From October 2013 to September 2017, recanalization of CTO lesions by PCI was successfully performed in 201 cases in our center. For this retrospective analysis, data of 100 patients of this cohort with an invasive follow-up in our center were available (49.8%). Seven patients were excluded because of either an extremely long latency from the index procedure to follow-up ($n = 3$) and/or because of acute coronary syndrome as an indication for repeated invasive coronary angiography ($n = 5$) in order to prevent potential bias by findings not solely grounded on previously recommended routine control. All subjects were adult individuals (≥18 years) with pre-existing fluoroscopic evidence of a chronically occluded coronary vessel. The choice of the interventional approach (antegrade vs. retrograde recanalization, radial or femoral access) and material for intervention at the index visit (e.g., guiding catheters, guidewires, PCI balloons, and stents) was subject to the discretion of the operator.

Patients' characteristics, clinical features (angina pectoris: Defined as chest discomfort as classified by Canadian Cardiovascular Society (CCS) class >2; symptoms: Defined as the presence of angina pectoris CCS class >2 and/or dyspnea NYHA (New York Heart Association) class >1; echocardiographic baseline parameters; proof of vitality of the region of the CTO), comorbidities, cardiovascular risk factors, as well as features of the PCI procedure (e.g., treated vessel, dose of contrast dye and radiation, fluoroscopy and procedural duration, J-CTO score and its subfactors (lesion entry, length, bending, and previously failed PCI attempt) of the lesion, number and length of used stent material), periprocedural levels of biomarkers (e.g., high-sensitive troponin I, creatinine, C-reactive protein), and clinical and angiographic findings at the invasive follow-up visit were gathered and analyzed. For a detailed protocol to quantify the J-CTO score, see [6]. Adipositas was defined as BMI (Body mass index) ≥ 30 kg/m^2, according to the WHO definition. Renal impairment was defined as a glomerular filtration rate < 60 mL/min*1.73m^2. The grade of a potential restenosis at the follow-up coronary angiography was retrospectively reassessed and the diameter loss in comparison to the reference vessel diameter was quantified in a semi-automatic manner by the Quantitative Coronary Analysis (QCA) tool (Philips Healthcare, Andover, MA, USA) for this study. Additionally, TIMI flow—as defined by the Thrombolysis in Myocardial Infarction Trial, quantified in Grades 0–3—was recorded semi-quantitatively for the time points directly after the index procedure and at the follow-up visit.

The primary endpoints of the retrospective analysis of our patient cohort study were defined as follows:

(1) Re-occlusion: Defined as TIMI flow grade 0, as assessed by fluoroscopy of the treated vessel at the timepoint of surveillance coronary angiography.
(2) Restenosis: Defined as the recurrence of lumen loss >50% in the CTO vessel as quantified retrospectively by QCA (including re-occlusion).
(3) Target vessel failure (TVF): Defined as a combined endpoint by the presence of re-occlusion, restenosis, or target vessel revascularization (defined as a necessity for a repeated PCI within the former CTO vessel).

We compared baseline parameters and values of clinical, fluoroscopic, and laboratory findings during index hospitalization (CTO PCI procedure) and at the timepoint of invasive follow-up and assigned patients to groups dependent on the presence of each singular endpoint as well as the combined endpoint at the time of follow-up surveillance coronary angiography. Continuous variables are presented as a mean ± standard deviation or as a median and interquartile range and categorial variables are expressed as percentages. Continuous variables found not to follow a normal distribution when tested with the modified Kolmogorov–Smirnov test (Lilliefors test) and Shapiro–Wilk-test were compared using the Wilcoxon matched-pairs signed rank test or the Wilcoxon–Mann–Whitney test for comparison between each two groups. Normally distributed continuous variables were compared using the Students' t-test and categorical variables with Fisher's exact or Chi^2 test, as appropriate.

Logistic regression analyses were performed in order to identify potential predictors for the occurrence of endpoints. Odds ratios (ORs) are given with the corresponding 95% confidence intervals (CIs). Logistic regressions were calculated by a univariate and a multivariate model, which was adjusted for age, diabetes, hyperlipidemia, smoking, hypertension, and a positive family history of cardiovascular disease. Receiver operating characteristics (ROCs) curves were calculated for the sensitivity and specificity of the J-CTO score to predict each individual endpoint, and the areas under the curve (AUC) are presented with the corresponding 95% CI. p values < 0.05 (two-sided) were considered to be statistically significant. Statistical analysis was conducted using SPSS software version 24 (SPSS Inc., Chicago, IL, USA).

Since the study involved only an anonymized, retrospective analysis of diagnostic standard data, ethics approval was not required according to German law.

3. Results

At the time of the index procedure, the 93 patients included in our analysis had a mean age of 65.6 ± 11.0 years old, 15.1% of them were female, and they had been symptomatic (angina or dyspnea) before intervention in 81.7% of the cases. The predominant target vessel for CTO intervention was the right coronary artery in 54.8% of the cases and the mean J-CTO score was 1.49 ± 1.09. Most predominant cardiovascular risk factors comprised arterial hypertension (79.6%), smoking (57.0%), and hyperlipidemia (59.1%) as well as a history of previous PCI (74.2%). A detailed overview of the baseline characteristics of all included subjects is displayed in Table 1. A mean of 2.2 ± 1.1 stents were implanted over an average lesion length of 56.6 ± 30.5 mm. One patient (1.1%) received treatment with a drug-eluting balloon alone without additional stent implantation; in all other patients, second-generation drug-eluting stents or scaffolds (in 76 cases (82.8%), everolimus-eluting stents (EESs); in 4 cases (4.3%), biolimus eluting stents; in 9 cases (9.7%), everolimus-eluting bioresorbable vascular scaffolds (BVSs), and in 3 cases (3.2%), a combination of EESs and BVSs) were used to treat the lesion. No patient was treated by POBA (plain old balloon angioplasty). Three patients (3.2%) encountered periinterventional acute renal failure, and one patient (1.1%) had relevant bleeding at the site of vascular access; in all other patients, no relevant major adverse events during the index visit were recorded. In total, 95.7% ($n = 89$) of the recanalizations were performed via the antegrade approach and primary vascular access was via the radial artery in 62.4% of cases ($n = 58$). In accordance with the guidelines [8], 89.2% (83 patients) were treated with dual anti-platelet therapy alone, and 10 cases (10.8%) with a combination of antiplatelet therapy and an oral anticoagulant. The time elapsed from the index procedure to invasive follow-up was, on average, 206 ± 129 days (median 185 (IQR 127–237 days)).

Table 1. Baseline characteristics ($n = 93$).

Parameter	n (%)	Mean ± SD	Median (IQR)
Age at procedure (years)		65.6 ± 11.0	66.5 (58.2/74.6)
female gender	14 (15.1%)		
Angina before intervention	53 (57.0%)		
Symptoms before intervention	76 (81.7%)		
multivessel disease	80 (86.0%)		
previous CABG	10 (10.8%)		
previous PCI	70 (74.2%)		
Diabetes	31 (33.3%)		
Smoking	53 (57.0%)		
Hyperlipidemia	55 (59.1%)		
Family history of CAD	24 (25.8%)		
arterial hypertension	74 (79.6%)		
peripheral artery disease	9 (9.7%)		
cerebral artery disease	8 (8.6%)		
renal insufficiency	6 (6.4%)		
hyperthyroidism	13 (14.0%)		
weight (KG)		90.2 ± 20.3	87.3 (78.0/100.8)
height (meters)		1.74 ± 0.10	1.76 (1.68/1.80)
Body mass index (kg/m^2)		25.8 ± 4.8	24.9 (22.8/28.4)
Adipositas	14 (21.2%)		
mean LVEF (%)		50.5 ± 9.6	55.0 (45.0/55.0)
reduced LVEF at baseline	19 (29.7%)		
proof of vitality of CTO region prior to intervention	52 (57.8%)		
CTO vessel			
LAD	19 (20.4%)		
LCX	23 (24.7%)		
RCA	51 (54.8%)		
J-CTO Score		1.49 ± 1.09	1.0 (1.0/2.0)
Components of the J-CTO Score			
Entry	27 (29.0%)		
Calcification	47 (50.5%)		
Bending > 45°	25 (26.9%)		
Lesion Length > 20 mm	29 (31.2%)		
Retry Lesion	12 (12.9%)		

Abbreviations: CABG: coronary artery bypass grafting, PCI: percutaneous coronary intervention, CTO: chronic total occlusion, LVEF: left ventricular ejection fraction. LAD: left anterior descending artery, LCX: left circumflex artery, RCA: right coronary artery. IQR: Interquartile Range, SD: standard deviation.

We compared patients' clinical and periinterventional characteristics, including gender, coronary vascular risk factors, renal impairment, left ventricular ejection fraction, duration and cumulative fluoroscopy dose, stent length and number, periinterventional biomarkers, and symptoms, at baseline and follow-up for each individual endpoint, and the cumulative endpoint. The incidence of re-occlusion was low (7.5%, $n = 7$) and re-stenosis of the former CTO lesion (including re-occlusion) was observed in 11.8% ($n = 11$). In five patients (5.4%), TVR was performed (two patients with treatment within the former CTO lesion, in three patients with de novo stenosis adjacent to the former CTO lesion). Thus, the incidence of the combined endpoint TVF was 15.1% ($n = 14$). Detailed results are presented in Table 2 (for enhanced results, see Supplementary Materials Table S1).

Table 2. Patients' baseline, periprocedural, and follow-up characteristics stratified for endpoints.

	Re-Occlusion ($n = 7$)	No Re-Occlusion ($n = 86$)	p-Value	Restenosis ($n = 11$)	No Restenosis ($n = 82$)	p-Value	TVF ($n = 14$)	No TVF ($n = 79$)	p-Value
Baseline parameters									
female gender	28.6	14.0	0.283	36.4	12.2	0.058	35.7	11.3	0.034
Age at procedure	65.1 ± 6.9	65.6 ± 11.3	0.843	65.6 ± 7.5	65.6 ± 11.5	0.988	60.6 ± 13.4	66.5 ± 10.4	0.063
Reduced LVEF	20.0	30.5	1.000	22.2	30.9	0.713	30.0	29.6	1.000
LVEF baseline	51.8 ± 6.6	50.4 ± 9.8	0.923	51.0 ± 6.4	50.5 ± 10.0	0.667	50.4 ± 6.4	50.6 ± 10.1	0.466
Angina at baseline	57.1	57.0	1.000	54.5	57.3	1.000	50.0	58.2	0.574
Symptoms at baseline	100	80.2	0.342	100.0	79.3	0.206	92.9	79.7	0.453
Body Mass Index	23.6 ± 2.1	25.9 ± 4.9	0.356	23.1 ± 2.7	26.1 ± 4.9	0.130	23.8 ± 4.8	26.1 ± 4.8	0.158
J-CTO Score	1.86 ± 1.07	1.47 ± 1.09	0.307	1.55 ± 1.21	1.49 ± 1.08	0.843	1.60 ± 1.82	1.49 ± 1.05	0.889
J-CTO Score ≥ 3	28.6	22.1	0.654	37.5	22.0	0.707	28.6	21.5	0.511
Periprocedural characteristics									
CTO vessel			0.332			0.969			0.811
- LAD	28.6	19.8		18.2	20.7		14.3	21.5	
- LCx	42.9	23.3		27.3	24.4		28.6	24.1	
- RCA	28.6	57.0		54.5	54.9		57.1	54.40	
Reduced TIMI-flow post intervention	100.0	8.1	<0.001	90.9	4.9	<0.001	71.4	5.1	<0.001
Stent length (mm)	36.3 ± 41.1	58.3 ± 29.2	0.044	38.2 ± 36.2	59.1 ± 29.0	0.020	43.0 ± 35.9	59.0 ± 29.0	0.042
Stent number	1.6 ± 1.6	2.2 ± 1.0	0.065	1.6 ± 1.4	2.2 ± 1.0	0.040	1.9 ± 1.3	2.2 ± 1.0	0.183
Fluoroscopy dose (cgy*dm)	8062 ± 4148	7363 ± 6308	0.351	7547 ± 4697	7398 ± 6352	0.677	7134 ± 4324	7465 ± 6449	0.830
Fluoroscopy time (min)	29.6 ± 18.0	26.0 ± 15.9	0.570	30.8 ± 18.8	25.7 ± 15.6	0.388	30.2 ± 18.0	25.6 ± 15.6	0.347
Duration (total) (min)	165.1 ± 26.8	123.8 ± 44.8	0.006	154.6 ± 44.0	123.2 ± 44.0	0.013	144.4 ± 45.7	123.8 ± 44.4	0.056
Contrast volume (mL)	277.4 ± 159.4	240.7 ± 103.1	0.662	279.2 ± 141.2	238.8 ± 102.4	0.372	263.8 ± 132.2	239.9 ± 103.2	0.576
Periinterventional CK (u/L)	178.3 ± 141.2	116.0 ± 94.9	0.276	132.7 ± 120.8	118.8 ± 96.6	0.929	123.5 ± 108.9	119.9 ± 98.9	0.802
High-sensitive Troponin I periinterventional (pg/mL)	1126.3 ± 1560.6	412.0 ± 1391.4	0.013	771.4 ± 1255.7	420.7 ± 1425.5	0.013	662.4 ± 1124.7	425.5 ± 1451.3	0.044
Creatinine periinterventional (mg/dL)	0.93 ± 0.11	1.16 ± 0.97	0.412	0.96 ± 0.14	1.17 ± 0.99	0.636	0.96 ± 0.13	1.18 ± 1.01	0.580
CrP periinterventional (mg/L)	37.0 ± 59.5	7.77 ± 15.7	0.238	23.6 ± 47.7	8.1 ± 16.4	0.712	21.8 ± 45.6	8.1 ± 16.5	0.685
Symptoms at follow-up									
Angina	28.6	32.5	1.000	36.4	31.6	0.741	35.7	31.6	0.763
Symptoms	42.9	53.4	0.704	54.5	52.4	1.000	50.0	53.2	1.000

values presented as percentages or mean values ± SD. Abbreviations: LVEF: left ventricular ejection fraction, CTO: chronic total occlusion, LAD: left anterior descending artery, LCx: left circumflex artery, RCA: right coronary artery, CrP: c-reactive protein, CK: creatin kinase. TVF: Target Vessel Failure.

When comparing baseline characteristics as well as periprocedural factors of the index procedure of patients encountering endpoints to those without adverse outcomes at the time of follow-up, we identified several parameters with statistically significant differences between the patient groups. Patients with reduced TIMI flow of the target vessel directly at the end of the index procedure were statistically significantly overrepresented in the groups encountering each of the endpoints. We observed a significantly greater incidence of re-occlusion (100% vs. 8.1%, $p < 0.001$), restenosis (90.9% vs. 4.9%, $p < 0.001$), and the combined endpoint (71.4% vs. 5.1%, $p < 0.001$). Furthermore, the patients reaching the endpoints had higher periprocedural levels of high-sensitive troponin I (1126.3 ± 1560.6 vs. 412.0 ± 1391.4, $p = 0.006$ for re-occlusion, 771.4 ± 1255.7 vs. 420.7 ± 1425.5, $p = 0.013$ for restenosis, and 662.4 ± 1124.7 vs. 425.5 ± 1451.3, $p = 0.044$ for TVF), and the cumulative length of implanted stents was significantly shorter (36.3 ± 41.1 vs. 58.3 ± 29.2, $p = 0.044$ for re-occlusion, 38.2 ± 36.2 vs. 59.1 ± 29.0 mm, $p = 0.020$ for restenosis, 43.0 ± 35.9 vs. 59.0 ± 29.0 mm, $p = 0.042$ for TVF). Other factors with statistically significant differences between the groups encountering endpoints were a lower number of implanted stents for restenosis, as well as a longer cumulative duration of the CTO index procedure both for re-occlusion and restenosis. Patients with female gender were significantly overrepresented in the target vessel failure group at follow-up (35.7% vs. 11.3%, $p = 0.034$)—a similar trend could also be observed for restenosis and re-occlusion, although this did not reach statistical significance (for details, see Table 2).

We performed logistic regression analyses to assess the odds ratios of independent predictors for each individual endpoint, including TVF, and adjusted those further for general cardiovascular risk factors (age, diabetes, hyperlipidemia, smoking, hypertension, and family history of cardiovascular disease) in a multivariate model. The results are presented in Table 3 (for further detailed calculations, see online Supplementary Materials Table S1). Individual factors as potential predictors for TVF comprised—as expected—reduced TIMI flow at the end of the index procedure all endpoints for re-occlusion (OR: 20.36 (95% CI: 3.21–129.00), $p = 0.001$), restenosis (OR: 21.29 (95% CI: 4.28–105.97), $p < 0.01$), and the combined endpoint/TVF (OR: 11.00 (95% CI: 2.66–45.45), $p = 0.001$). Female gender proved to be a predictor for the occurrence of restenosis (OR: 8.88 (95% CI: 1.58–49.89), $p = 0.013$) as well as target vessel failure (OR: 11.03 (95% CI: 2.08–58.47), $p = 0.005$). Of note, a lower BMI was assessed to be predictive regarding the endpoints of restenosis (OR: 0.73 (95% CI: 0.55–0.98), $p = 0.037$) and TVF (OR: 0.80 (95% CI: 0.65–0.99), $p = 0.037$).

The J-CTO score at the index procedure as well as the presence of its singular factors could not be correlated with the later occurrence of any of the singular endpoints or TVF. Neither was there any statistically significant difference between the groups reaching the endpoints and those without adverse events, nor were any ORs statistically significant (Figure 1). In order to further determine the sensitivity and specificity to predict each individual end point by the J-CTO score, we computed ROC curves. The AUC for re-occlusion was calculated as 0.61 (95% CI 0.40–0.82), for restenosis as 0.52 (95% CI 0.32–0.71), and for TVF as 0.51 (95% CI 0.33–0.70) (see online Supplementary Materials Figure S1), further documenting that the J-CTO score could not predict later adverse outcomes in our cohort. Interestingly, the presence of typical angina pectoris and/or dyspnea at the time of follow-up did also not have any correlation with the co-incidence of re-occlusion, restenosis, or TVR (see Table 2).

Table 3. Multivariate regression analysis (odds ratios) for re-occlusion, restenosis, and TVF.

	Re-Occlusion		Restenosis		TVF	
	OR (95% CI)	p-Value	OR (95% CI)	p-Value	OR (95% CI)	p-Value
Baseline parameters						
female gender	3.77 (0.54–26.43)	0.182	8.88 (1.58–49.89)	0.013	11.03 (2.08–58.47)	0.005
Age at procedure	0.99 (0.91–1.08)	0.822	1.00 (0.93–1.07)	0.995	0.95 (0.90–1.01)	0.080
Reduced LVEF	0.43 (0.04–5.09)	0.426	0.49 (0.08–3.10)	0.449	0.70 (0.13–3.87)	0.680
LVEF baseline	1.92 (0.91–1.16)	0.713	1.01 (0.92–1.10)	0.895	1.00 (0.92–1.09)	0.956
Angina at baseline	0.96 (0.19–4.79)	0.957	0.78 (0.20–2.97)	0.712	0.70 (0.21–2.40)	0.704
Symptoms at baseline	not calculable		not calculable		8.65 (0.62–121.31)	0.109
Body Mass Index	0.79 (0.57–1.09)	0.147	0.73 (0.55–0.98)	0.037	0.80 (0.65–0.99)	0.037
J-CTO-Score	1.42 (0.64–3.16)	0.394	1.03 (0.54–1.95)	0.929	1.11 (0.62–1.98)	0.728
J-CTO Score ≥ 3	1.40 (0.21–8.99)	0.721	1.26 (0.27–5.84)	0.768	1.35 (0.33–5.45)	0.676
Periprocedural characteristics						
CTO vessel						
-LAD	0.50 (0.18–1.38)	0.180	0.98 (0.37–2.14)	0.797	0.97 (0.43–2.19)	0.936
-LCx						
-RCA						
Reduced TIMI-flow post intervention	20.36 (3.21–129.00)	0.001	21.29 (4.28–105.97)	<0.001	11.00 (2.66–45.45)	0.001
Stent length (mm)	0.97 (0.94–1.00)	0.081	0.98 (0.95–1.00)	0.051	0.98 (0.95–1.00)	0.060
Stent number	0.52 (0.21–1.29)	0.156	0.58 (0.28–1.17)	0.125	0.70 (0.38–1.29)	0.255
Fluoroscopy dose (cgy*dm)	1.00 (1.00–1.00)	0.748	1.00 (1.00–1.00)	0.871	1.00 (1.00–1.00)	0.868
Fluoroscopy time (min)	1.02 (0.97–1.07)	0.470	1.02 (0.99–1.07)	0.233	1.03 (0.99–1.06)	0.185
Duration (total) (min)	1.02 (1.00–1.04)	0.025	1.02 (1.00–1.03)	0.030	1.01 (1.00–1.03)	0.056
Contrast volume (mL)	1.00 (1.00–1.01)	0.287	1.00 (1.00–1.01)	0.200	1.00 (1.00–1.01)	0.486
Periinterventional CK (u/L)	1.01 (1.00–1.01)	0.153	1.00 (0.99–1.01)	0.757	1.00 (0.99–1.01)	0.973
High-sensitive Troponin I periinterventional (pg/mL)	1.00 (1.00–1.00)	0.286	1.00 (1.00–1.00)	0.247	1.00 (1.00–1.00)	0.459
Creatinine periinterventional (mg/dL)	0.07 (0.00–8.94)	0.284	0.12 (0.00–4.57)	0.256	0.22 (0.01–5.91)	0.366
CrP periinterventional (mg/L)	1.03 (1.00–1.06)	0.049	1.02 (1.00–1.05)	0.067	1.02 (1.00–1.04)	0.103
Symptoms at follow-up						
Angina	0.75 (0.13–4.45)	0.750	1.24 (0.30–5.07)	0.762	0.99 (0.28–3.59)	0.992
Symptoms	0.69 (0.14–3.36)	0.642	1.27 (0.34–4.71)	0.723	0.92 (0.28–3.01)	0.891

Abbreviations: LVEF: left ventricular ejection fraction, CTO: chronic total occlusion, LAD: left anterior descending artery, LCx: left circumflex artery, RCA: right coronary artery, CrP: c-reactive protein, CK: creatin kinase. TVF: Target Vessel Failure.

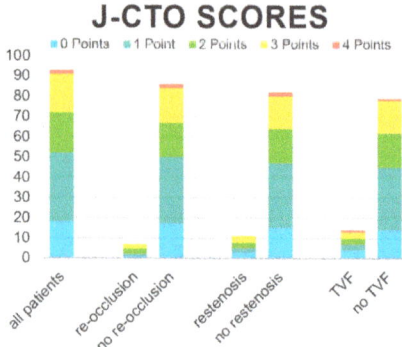

Figure 1. Distribution of the J-CTO score in all patients in the groups reaching endpoints. J-CTO scores were calculated for the whole study group and stratified for all single endpoints and the combined endpoint. In our study, the distribution of J-CTO scores did not differ significantly between groups (for details, see the text).

4. Discussion

Over the last years, percutaneous recanalization procedures of CTO lesions have been introduced into daily clinical practice in most PCI centers. Successful intervention in CTO lesions has been attributed to clinical as well as prognostic benefit [7–9]. Yet, follow-up data, including invasive control coronary angiography, as well as evidence on potential predictors for long-term success are rare.

The key findings of this retrospective study are as follows: In a monocentric retrospective analysis with routinely recommended invasive follow-up of intermediate to difficult CTO lesions (mean J-CTO score 1.49 ± 1.09), re-occlusion rates tended to be low. Yet, the incidence of adverse findings, like restenosis, target lesion revascularization, and the combined endpoint target vessel failure, was moderate but still relevant. Of all clinical parameters entered in the analysis, reduced TIMI flow of the target vessel at the end of the index procedure was the strongest predictor of the endpoints at the follow-up visit. Furthermore, patients with higher periinterventional levels of high-sensitive troponin I as well as a shorter cumulative length of implanted stents were overrepresented in the groups with a later occurrence of adverse events at the timepoint of surveillance coronary angiography. Female patients were at a higher risk for TVF. Interestingly, the pre-procedural J-CTO score was not predictive of the occurrence of later restenosis, re-occlusion, or TLV in our cohort.

Other retrospective analyses have aimed to identify potential predictors for later cardiac adverse events in cohorts of patients that underwent PCI for CTO lesions. In a retrospective analysis of 249 patients with a mean (non-invasive) follow-up of 19.8 ± 13.1 months, a higher J-CTO score was found to be associated with a higher rate of major adverse cardiovascular events (MACEs) [11]. Although the baseline characteristics in this cohort were mainly comparable (age 63 ± 11 years vs. 65.6 ± 11.0 years in our study, 70.3% vs. 84.9% male, right coronary artery as the target vessel in 49.4% vs. 54.8%, J-CTO score 1.8 ± 1.0 vs. 1.49 ± 1.09), the study design was distinctly different, which might account for the controversial findings. The follow-up was also survey based without surveillance coronary angiography and the endpoints were also determined differently by MACEs (cardiovascular or unknown cause of death, myocardial infarction, TVR by PCI or CABG). In another large European multi-center retrospective analysis of a total of 1395 patients with a mean follow-up of 23 months, female sex, high J-CTO score ≥ 3, and prior PCI as well as reduced left ventricular function were found to be correlated with a higher incidence of MACEs [12].

In our analysis, we identified female gender as a risk factor for TVF. Although some registries generated evidence that women derive the same benefit from CTO-PCI as men in regard to clinical benefit [14], female gender was found to be a predictor of PCI-related complications as well as MACEs in other retrospective studies too [12,15,16]. The reason for this observation remains unclear but may include differences in the hormonal status between men and women. Yet, this finding might strengthen the recommendation on optimal patient pre-selection. This should comprise of routine use of non-invasive testing for myocardial ischemia prior to recanalization attempts, especially in female patients who appear to be at elevated risk for future TVF.

Only a very few studies have assessed the mechanisms and predictors of target vessel failure in CTO patients. In a prospective multicenter noninferiority trial comparing the use of a sirolimus-Eluting stent (SES) to an Everolimus-eluting stent (EES) on 330 patients with total coronary occlusions, the incidence of re-occlusion (2.2% in the SES vs. 1.4% in the EES group) and re-stenosis (8.0% vs. 2.1%) was distinctly lower than in our study group [17]. The follow-up rate was high, with 85% in comparison to nearly 50% in our study. Yet, a less strict definition of total coronary occlusion (estimated duration of occlusion ≥ 4 weeks) was utilized for this trial, which might partially account for the different findings. In a monocentric retrospective Korean registry on 235 patients with PCI for CTO with an invasive follow-up rate of 61.3% after 6 months, a longer occlusion length was found to be predictive for a higher incidence of TVR [16].

In our PCI center from which we recruited the study population, surveillance invasive follow-up was routinely recommended but only opted for in nearly 50% of the individuals. According to European Guidelines [13], follow-up coronary angiography might be routinely performed in high-risk coronary setups. The strategy of routine invasive follow-up is discussed controversially because of limited evidence and—in contrast to the situation in Europe—American guidelines abstain from a recommendation [18]. One prospective randomized multicenter study in Japan ((Randomized Evaluation of Routine Follow-up Coronary Angiography after Percutaneous Coronary Intervention Trial) ReACT Trial) on 700 patients could not find evidence of a clinical benefit for a general angiographic follow-up at least in a normal risk patient cohort [19]. Of course, it remains controversial whether CTO-PCIs resemble a high-risk PCI collective (not further explained in the European guidelines) and, furthermore, an impact on further clinical benefit by this strategy of an early invasive follow-up and treatment of probably non-symptomatic re-stenosis remains hypothetic up to now. Nevertheless, our study provides evidence that surveillance coronary angiography might be justified after recanalization of CTO lesions, especially in the presence of specific factors predictive of TVF. Clinical findings, such as ongoing symptoms alone, with definite exclusion of acute coronary syndrome, might not be helpful to stratify patients at risk of potential TVF.

Some limitations of our study merit consideration: First, the design is a monocentric retrospective analysis with a mid-term follow-up. Due to the observational nature of the study, the follow-up rate was only 49.8%, which might further account for a potential selection bias, which has to be taken into account in the interpretation of our results. BVS were used for treatment in some cases, which are not available anymore. Although routine surveillance invasive follow-up was recommended in all patients, symptomatic individuals could be overrepresented at the follow-up visit, as the prevalence of angina pectoris and dyspnea at the time of follow-up was higher in comparison to other registries [12]. Indication for TVR was based on individual assessment of the interventional operator and not mandatorily grounded on further non-invasive or invasive evaluation of the stenosis (e.g., measurement of fractional flow reserve, intracoronary imaging like optical coherence tomography or intravascular ultrasound) and a potential clinical and prognostic benefit of these interventions has not been studied. Larger prospective randomized studies with defined protocol, including intracoronary imaging or flow measurements, for surveillance coronary angiography would be desirable. Furthermore, patients with female gender were relevantly underrepresented (15.1%), yet at a comparable extent to most published CTO registries [11,12,14–16].

5. Conclusions

In this retrospective monocentric cohort of patients undergoing routine follow-up coronary angiography after CTO recanalization, we found evidence that reduced TIMI flow at the end of the index procedure as well as female gender could be predictors of later angiographic adverse outcome (TVF). Furthermore, patients with a shorter cumulative length of implanted stents and higher periinterventional levels of high-sensitive troponin I were overrepresented in the group of patients encountering re-occlusion, restenosis, and TVF at the timepoint of invasive follow-up. In contrast to other registers, we could not prove any correlation between the initial J-CTO score of the treated CTO lesion and the later occurrence of any of the endpoints. Remarkably, symptoms at the time of follow-up coronary angiography could not be attributed to adverse angiographic results. Based on the still relevant rate of TVF, even in populations of intermediate lesion complexity, such as ours, routine invasive follow-up after CTO procedures appears to be justified and should rather be guided by the presence of risk predictors, and not by the occurrence of angina (with the exception of acute coronary syndrome). Thus, our present work might stress a potential beneficial value of routine surveillance coronary angiography after CTO interventions, especially for females and patients with reduced TIMI flow at the end of the index procedure.

Supplementary Materials: The following are available online at http://www.mdpi.com/2077-0383/9/1/178/s1, Figure S1: ROC (receiver operating characteristics) curves for the J-CTO score vs. endpoints, Table S1: Detailed results for baseline, periprocedural, and follow-up data as well as uni- and multivariate regressions analysis stratified for the incidence of endpoints.

Author Contributions: Conceptualization, M.G., J.W. and P.W.; methodology, M.G. and P.W.; validation, M.G. and P.W.; formal analysis, M.G., M.H., T.G. and P.W.; resources, M.G., T.M., Z.D. and P.W.; data curation, M.G., J.W. and M.H.; writing—original draft preparation, M.G.; writing—review and editing, P.W., T.G., Z.D. and T.M.; supervision and project administration, P.W. and T.M. All authors have read and agreed to the published version of the manuscript.

Funding: This work is partially supported by the German Federal Ministry of Education and Research (Bonn, Germany; grant number BMBF 01EO1503).

Acknowledgments: This work contains results that are part of the doctoral thesis of Marc Hirschmann. T.M., T.G. and P.W. are PIs of the DZHK (German Center for Cardiovascular Research), Partner Site Rhine-Main, Mainz, Germany.

Conflicts of Interest: The authors declare no conflict of interest. The funders had no role in the design of the study; in the collection, analyses, or interpretation of data; in the writing of the manuscript, or in the decision to publish the results.

References

1. Strauss, B.H.; Shuvy, M.; Wijeysundera, H.C. Revascularization of Chronic Total Occlusions. *J. Am. Coll. Cardiol.* **2014**, *64*, 1281–1289. [CrossRef] [PubMed]
2. Fefer, P.; Knudtson, M.L.; Cheema, A.N.; Galbraith, P.D.; Osherov, A.B.; Yalonetsky, S.; Gannot, S.; Samuel, M.; Weisbrod, M.; Bierstone, D.; et al. Current perspectives on coronary chronic total occlusions: The Canadian Multicenter Chronic Total Occlusions Registry. *J. Am. Coll. Cardiol.* **2012**, *59*, 991–997. [CrossRef] [PubMed]
3. Rathore, S.; Matsuo, H.; Terashima, M.; Kinoshita, Y.; Kimura, M.; Tsuchikane, E.; Nasu, K.; Ehara, M.; Asakura, Y.; Katho, O.; et al. Procedural and in-hospital outcomes after percutaneous coronary interventions for chronic total occlusion of coronary arteries 2002 to 2008: Impact of novel guidewire techniques. *J. Am. Coll. Cardiol. Intv.* **2009**, *2*, 489–497. [CrossRef] [PubMed]
4. Brilakis, E.S.; Banerjee, S.; Karmpaliotis, D.; Lombardi, W.L.; Tsai, T.T.; Shunk, K.A.; Kennedy, K.F.; Spertus, J.A.; Holmes, D.R., Jr.; Grantham, J.A. Procedural outcomes of chronic total occlusion percutaneous coronary intervention. A report from the NCDR (national cardiovascular data registry). *J. Am. Coll. Cardiol. Intv.* **2015**, *8*, 245–253. [CrossRef] [PubMed]
5. Christopoulos, G.; Karmpaliotis, D.; Alaswad, K.; Yeh, R.W.; Jaffer, F.A.; Wyman, R.M.; Lombardi, W.L.; Menon, R.V.; Grantham, J.A.; Kandzari, D.E.; et al. Application and outcomes of a hybrid approach to chronic total occlusion percutaneous coronary intervention in a contemporary multicenter US registry. *Int. J. Cardiol.* **2015**, *98*, 222–228. [CrossRef] [PubMed]
6. Morino, Y.; Abe, M.; Morimoto, T.; Kimura, T.; Hayashi, Y.; Muramatsu, T.; Ochiai, M.; Noguchi, Y.; Kato, K.; Shibata, Y.; et al. Predicting successful guidewire crossing through chronic total occlusion of native coronary lesions within 30 minutes. *J. Am. Coll. Cardiol. Intv.* **2011**, *4*, 213–221. [CrossRef] [PubMed]

7. Hoye, A.; van Domburg, R.T.; Sonnenschein, K.; Serruys, P.W. Percutaneous coronary interventions for chronic total occlusions: The Thoraxcenter experience 1992–2002. *Eur. Heart J.* **2005**, *26*, 2630–2636. [CrossRef] [PubMed]
8. Suero, J.A.; Marso, S.P.; Jones, P.G.; Laster, S.B.; Huber, K.C.; Giorgi, L.V.; Johnson, W.L.; Rutherford, B.D. Procedural outcomes and long-term survival among patients undergoing percutaneous coronary intervention of a chronic total occlusion in native coronary arteries: A 20-year experience. *J. Am. Coll. Cardiol.* **2001**, *38*, 409–414. [CrossRef]
9. George, S.; Cockburn, J.; Clayton, T.C.; Ludman, P.; Cotton, J.; Spratt, J.; Redwood, S.; de Belder, M.; de Belder, A.; Hill, J.; et al. Long-term follow-up of elective chronicl total coronary occlusion angioplasty. *J. Am. Coll. Cardiol.* **2014**, *64*, 235–243. [CrossRef] [PubMed]
10. Jones, D.A.; Rathod, K.S.; Pavlidis, A.N.; Gallagher, S.M.; Astroulakis, Z.; Lim, P.; Sirker, A.; Knight, C.J.; Dalby, M.C.; Malik, I.S.; et al. Outcomes after chronic total occlusion percutaneous coronary interventions: An observational study of 5496 patients from the Pan-London CTO Cohort. *Coron. Artery Dis.* **2018**, *29*, 557–563. [CrossRef] [PubMed]
11. Forounzandeh, F.; Suh, J.; Stahl, E.; Ko, Y.A.; Lee, S.; Joshi, U.; Sabharwal, N.; Almuwaqqat, Z.; Gandhi, R.; Lee, H.S.; et al. Performance of J-CTO and PROGRESS CTO-Scores in predicting angiographic success and long-term outcomes of percutaneous coronary interventions for chronic total occlusions. *Am. J. Cardiol.* **2018**, *121*, 14–20. [CrossRef] [PubMed]
12. Galassi, A.R.; Sianos, G.; Werner, G.S.; Escaned, J.; Tomasello, S.D.; Boukhris, M.; Castaing, M.; Büttner, J.H.; Bufe, A.; Kalnins, A.; et al. Retrograde recanalization of chronic total occlusions in Europe. *J. Am. Coll. Cardiol.* **2015**, *65*, 2388–2400. [CrossRef] [PubMed]
13. Neumann, F.J.; Sousa-Uva, M.; Ahlsson, A.; Alfonso, F.; Banning, A.P.; Benedetto, U.; Byrne, R.A.; Collet, J.P.; Falk, V.; Head, S.J.; et al. 2018 ESC/EACTS Guidelines on myocardial revascularization. *Eur. Heart J.* **2019**, *40*, 87–165. [CrossRef] [PubMed]
14. Pershad, A.; Gulati, M.; Karmpaliotis, D.; Moses, J.; Nicholson, W.J.; Nugent, K.; Tang, Y.; Sapontis, J.; Lombardi, W.; Grantham, J.A.; et al. A sex stratified outcome analysis from the OPEN-CTO registry. *Catheter. Cardiovasc. Interv.* **2019**, *93*, 1041–1047. [CrossRef]
15. Toma, A.; Stähli, B.E.; Gick, M.; Ferenc, M.; Mashayekhi, K.; Buettner, H.J.; Neumann, F.J.; Gebhard, C. Temporal changes in outcomes of women and men undergoing percutaneous coronary intervention for chronic total occlusion: 2005–2013. *Clin. Res. Cardiol.* **2018**, *107*, 449–459. [CrossRef]
16. Ahn, J.; Rha, S.W.; Choi, B.; Choi, S.Y.; Byun, J.K.; Mashaly, A.; Abdelshafi, K.; Park, Y.; Jang, W.Y.; Kim, W.; et al. Impact of chronic total occlusion length on six-month angiographic and 2-year clinical outcomes. *PLoS ONE* **2018**, *13*, 30198571. [CrossRef] [PubMed]
17. Teeuwen, K.; van der Schaaf, R.; Adraenssens, T.; Koolen, J.J.; Smits, C.; Henriques, J.P.S.; Vermeersch, P.H.; Tjon Joe Gin, R.M.; Schölzel, B.E.; Kelder, J.C.; et al. Randomized multicenter trial investigating angiographic outcomes of hybrid sirolimus-eluting stents with biodegradable polymer compared with everolimus-eluting stents with durable polymer in chronic total occlusions. *J. Am. Coll. Cardiol. Intervn.* **2017**, *10*, 133–143. [CrossRef] [PubMed]
18. Levine, G.N.; Bates, E.R.; Blankenship, J.C.; Bailey, S.R.; Bittl, J.A.; Cercek, B.; Chambers, C.E.; Ellis, S.G.; Guyton, R.A.; Hollenberg, S.M.; et al. 2011 ACCF/AHA/SCAI Guideline for percutaneous coronary intervention: Executive summary. *Circulation* **2011**, *124*, 2474–2609. [CrossRef]
19. Shiomi, H.; Morimoto, T.; Kitaguchi, S.; Nakagawa, Y.; Ishii, K.; Haruna, Y.; Takamisawa, I.; Motooka, M.; Nakao, K.; Matsuda, S.; et al. The ReACT Trial. Randomized evaluation of routine follow-up coronary angiography after percutaneous coronary intervention trial. *J. Am. Coll. Cardiol. Intv.* **2017**, *10*, 109–117. [CrossRef] [PubMed]

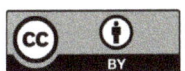

© 2020 by the authors. Licensee MDPI, Basel, Switzerland. This article is an open access article distributed under the terms and conditions of the Creative Commons Attribution (CC BY) license (http://creativecommons.org/licenses/by/4.0/).

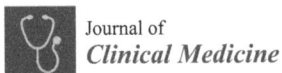

Article

Assessment of Global Longitudinal and Circumferential Strain Using Computed Tomography Feature Tracking: Intra-Individual Comparison with CMR Feature Tracking and Myocardial Tagging in Patients with Severe Aortic Stenosis

Emilija Miskinyte [1,†], Paulius Bucius [1,2,†], Jennifer Erley [1], Seyedeh Mahsa Zamani [1], Radu Tanacli [1], Christian Stehning [3], Christopher Schneeweis [4], Tomas Lapinskas [2], Burkert Pieske [1,5,6], Volkmar Falk [5,7], Rolf Gebker [1], Gianni Pedrizzetti [8], Natalia Solowjowa [7] and Sebastian Kelle [1,5,6,*]

1. Department of Internal Medicine/Cardiology, German Heart Center Berlin, 13353 Berlin, Germany
2. Department of Cardiology, Medical Academy, Lithuanian University of Health Sciences, 50161 Kaunas, Lithuania
3. Philips Healthcare, 22335 Hamburg, Germany
4. Klinik für Kardiologie und Internistische Intesivmedizin, Krankenhaus der Augustinerinnen, 50678 Köln, Germany
5. DZHK (German Centre for Cardiovascular Research), Partner Site Berlin, 10785 Berlin, Germany
6. Department of Internal Medicine/Cardiology, Charité Campus Virchow Clinic, 13353 Berlin, Germany
7. Department of Cardiothoracic Surgery, German Heart Center Berlin, 13353 Berlin, Germany
8. Department of Engineering and Architecture, University of Trieste, 34127 Trieste, Italy
* Correspondence: kelle@dhzb.de; Tel.: +49-30-4593-1182
† Both authors contributted equally.

Received: 26 July 2019; Accepted: 5 September 2019; Published: 10 September 2019

Abstract: In this study, we used a single commercially available software solution to assess global longitudinal (GLS) and global circumferential strain (GCS) using cardiac computed tomography (CT) and cardiac magnetic resonance (CMR) feature tracking (FT). We compared agreement and reproducibility between these two methods and the reference standard, CMR tagging (TAG). Twenty-seven patients with severe aortic stenosis underwent CMR and cardiac CT examinations. FT analysis was performed using Medis suite version 3.0 (Leiden, The Netherlands) software. Segment (Medviso) software was used for GCS assessment from tagged images. There was a trend towards the underestimation of GLS by CT-FT when compared to CMR-FT (19.4 ± 5.04 vs. 22.40 ± 5.69, respectively; $p = 0.065$). GCS values between TAG, CT-FT, and CMR-FT were similar ($p = 0.233$). CMR-FT and CT-FT correlated closely for GLS ($r = 0.686$, $p < 0.001$) and GCS ($r = 0.707$, $p < 0.001$), while both of these methods correlated moderately with TAG for GCS ($r = 0.479$, $p < 0.001$ for CMR-FT vs. TAG; $r = 0.548$ for CT-FT vs. TAG). Intraobserver and interobserver agreement was excellent in all techniques. Our findings show that, in elderly patients with severe aortic stenosis (AS), the FT algorithm performs equally well in CMR and cardiac CT datasets for the assessment of GLS and GCS, both in terms of reproducibility and agreement with the gold standard, TAG.

Keywords: systemic disease; cardiac computed tomography; cardiac magnetic resonance; feature tracking; tagging; myocardial deformation; strain

1. Introduction

Multiple systemic and neuromuscular diseases can affect the cardiovascular system at some point in their course. A wide variety of pathological processes fall under these definitions, some of which have pathognomonic cardiovascular manifestations [1]. However, non-specific manifestations, such as a subtle decline in regional or global myocardial function, are also common [2]. It can often go unnoticed until the ejection fraction (EF) starts to decline or clinical symptoms of heart failure begin to develop. Recently, myocardial strain has emerged as an imaging technique that adds information about myocardial function beyond the left ventricular ejection fraction (LVEF) [3]. Furthermore, recent studies have shown early reduction in myocardial strain in multiple systemic and neuromuscular disorders, such as amyloidosis [4], systemic sclerosis [5], rheumatoid arthritis [6], and Duchenne muscular dystrophy [7]. These data suggest that deformation imaging could become an important tool for the early identification of cardiac involvement in these patients.

Due to its availability, speckle tracking echocardiography (STE) is the most widely used method for strain assessment. However, the accuracy and feasibility of STE is highly dependent on image quality [8], warranting the need for alternatives in certain patients. Cardiac magnetic resonance (CMR) not only allows for myocardial strain assessment, overcoming the shortcomings of echocardiography, but also offers tissue characterization ability that is second to none. Thus, it is an important tool in the diagnostic work-up of patients with systemic connective tissue disorders [9]. A recently developed cardiac magnetic resonance feature tracking (CMR-FT) technique has been validated against the gold standard myocardial tagging (TAG) and is now considered a preferred CMR tool for strain assessment [10]. The main advantage of CMR-FT is that it can be applied to steady-state free precession (SSFP) cine loops that are used in routine clinical practice, therefore not requiring additional image acquisition. Interestingly, although developed for CMR, the FT algorithm can also be applied to cardiac computed tomography (CT) datasets to assess myocardial strain [11,12]. Naturally, strain assessment from cardiac CT datasets has started to gain popularity.

In this study, we used a single commercially available software solution to acquire global strain parameters via computed tomography feature tracking (CT-FT) and CMR-FT in a cohort of patients with severe aortic stenosis (AS). We compared agreement and reproducibility of global longitudinal (GLS) and global circumferential strain (GCS) between both these methods and the reference standard, TAG.

2. Experimental Section

2.1. Study Population

Twenty-six patients (14 females and 12 males, mean age 80.59 ± 5.87 years) with severe AS referred to our institution for transcathether aortic valve replacement (TAVR) were enrolled in this study. Further demographic and clinical data of the study population are listed in Table 1. AS was diagnosed and graded echocardiographically according to the latest European Society of Cardiology and European Association for Cardiothoracic Surgery guidelines [13]. All subjects underwent clinically indicated CMR and cardiac CT examinations. This study complies with the Declaration of Helsinki. Institutional Review Board approval was not necessary because it was a retrospective analysis of clinical data. According to local law, all individuals signed an informed consent form before entering the clinical CMR and cardiac CT. None of the observers could identify patient information when analyzing the data.

2.2. Cardiac Computed Tomography Acquisition

Contrast-enhanced, retrospectively electrocardiography (ECG)-gated cardiac scans were performed using a 2 × 128-slice multi-detector computed tomography scanner (Somatom Definition Flash, Siemens AG, Erlangen, Germany). The following study protocol was used: tube voltage 100, 120 kV, tube current 320 ref. mAs/rotation, rotation time 280 ms, slice collimation of 128 × 0.6 mm, with a temporal resolution of 75 ms, slice width of 0.75 mm, reconstruction increment of 0.4 mm, and reconstruction kernel B30f. Images were acquired in a cranio-caudal direction, from above the aortic sinuses to below the diaphragm.

Table 1. Demographic and clinical data of the study population.

Variables.	$n = 27$ Mean ± SD or n (%)
Age	22.40 ± 5.69
Male	18.91 ± 5.97
Body mass index (kg/m^2)	26.60 ± 3.60
Heart rate	67.59 ± 10.27
Clinical history	
Hypertension	25 (92.56%)
CAD	16 (59.25%)
Myocardial infarction	6 (22.22%)
History of CABG	5 (18.51%)
Stroke	4 (14.81%)
Diabetes mellitus type 2	6 (22.22%)
COPD	5 (18.51%)

Abbreviations: CAD: coronary artery disease; CABG: coronary artery bypass graft; COPD: chronic obstructive pulmonary disease.

2.3. Cardiac Magnetic Resonance Acquisition

CMR acquisitions were made using a 1.5 Tesla magnetic resonance imaging (MRI) scanner (Achieva, Philips Healthcare, Best, The Netherlands). Signals were received using a five-element phased array cardiac coil. A four-lead vector ECG was used for R-wave triggering. A balanced steady-state free precession (bSSFP) sequence with breath hold was acquired in long-axis (LAX) two-, three-, and four-chamber views, as well as a short-axis (SAX) stack. This was used for volumetric and FT analysis. Acquisition parameters used were a repetition time (TR) of 3.3 ms, echo time (TE) of 1.6 ms, flip angle of 60°, acquisition voxel size of $1.8 \times 1.7 \times 8.0$ mm^3, and 30 phases per cardiac cycle. The complementary spatial modulation of magnetization (CSPAMM) technique was used to acquire tagging images in three short-axis planes (basal, medial, and apical) with a temporal resolution of 35 ms, spatial resolution of 1.4×1.4 mm, and a slice thickness of 8 mm.

2.4. Cardiac CT Data Analysis

Original three-dimensional (3D) datasets were analyzed offline using the commercially available Medis Suite version 3.0 (Leiden, The Netherlands) software package to generate two-dimensional (2D) cine loops of three LAX slices (i.e., two-, three-, and four-chamber), three SAX slices (i.e., basal, mid, and apical), and a SAX stack with a slice thickness of 0.75 mm and a reconstruction increment of 0.4 mm. Images were generated with temporal resolution of 10 phases per cardiac cycle in 10% increments from early systole (0% cardiac cycle) to end-diastole (90% cardiac cycle). Care was taken to make sure that 2D cardiac CT reconstructions closely matched the anatomical locations of the images used for CMR analysis. End-systolic and end-diastolic cardiac phases were chosen visually. Endocardial and epicardial borders in the SAX stack were outlined manually to calculate the volumetric parameters, which were indexed to body surface area (BSA). Left ventricular mass index (LVMi), left ventricular end-diastolic volume index (LVEDVi), left ventricular end-systolic volume index (LVESVi), left ventricular stroke volume index (LVSVi), and left ventricular ejection fraction (LVEF) were calculated. Global longitudinal strain (GLS) was assessed by averaging the peak systolic strain values of 17 segments extracted from three LAX images, while global circumferential strain (GCS) was acquired from three SAX images using a 16-segment model.

2.5. CMR Data Analysis

bSSFP images were analyzed using Medis Suite version 3.0 (Leiden, The Netherlands) software in the same manner as cardiac CT images to determine LVMi, LVEDVi, LVESVi, LVSVi, LVEF, GLS, and GCS. Tagged images were analyzed using commercially available software Segment version 2.2 R6960. Endocardial and epicardial borders were manually outlined at an end-systolic timeframe in three short-axis slices (i.e., basal, mid, and apical). After applying an automatic propagation algorithm, quality of tracking was visually assessed, and changes were made as needed. GCS was derived using a 16-segment model by averaging the peak systolic values. TAG data of one of the subjects could not be analyzed due to breathing artefacts, therefore 26 patients were used for GCS comparisons.

Due to the counter-intuitive increase of strain in more diseased subjects, we chose to report absolute values for easier interpretation.

2.6. Statistics

Data analysis was performed using commercially available software (GraphPad Prism 8, GraphPad Software, San Diego, CA, USA). The Shapiro–Wilk test was used to assess the normality of distribution of continuous variables. Unpaired Student's *t*-test was used to compare differences between cardiac CT and MRI derived volumetric parameters and GLS. One-way ANOVA was used to compare differences in GCS between the three modalities. Pearson's correlation coefficient and Bland–Altman analysis were used to assess inter-method agreement. Intra- and interobserver variability were assessed using two-way mixed intra-class correlation coefficient (ICC), Bland–Altman analysis, and coefficient of variance (CoV). This was defined as the standard deviation of the differences divided by the mean, in keeping with previous studies [14]. Agreement levels were defined according to previous studies [15] as follows: excellent if ICC > 0.74, good if ICC = 0.6-0.74, fair if ICC = 0.4–0.59, poor if ICC < 0.4. *p*-values of <0.05 were considered statistically significant.

3. Results

3.1. Volumetric Assessment

Values of volumetric assessment are represented in Table 2. LVEDVi, LVESVi, LVSVi, LVEF, and LVMi values were similar between CMR and cardiac CT. There was excellent correlation between the two techniques in LVEDVi ($r = 0.913$, $p < 0.001$), LVESVi ($r = 0.879$, $p < 0.001$), LVEF ($r = 0.791$, $p < 0.001$), and LVMi ($r = 0.971$, $p < 0.001$), with good correlation for LVSVi ($r = 0.619$, $p < 0.001$). Results of the Bland–Altman analysis of volumetric measurements are shown in the figures (Figures 1a–d and 2).

Table 2. Values of volumetric assessment of the LV by CMR and CCT.

Measurement	CMR	CCT	*p*-Value
LVEF (%)	64.57 ± 14.55	59.15 ± 14.82	0.181
LVEDVi (mL/m^2)	72.60 ± 27.22	80.35 ± 26.42	0.374
LVESVi (mL/m^2)	28.62 ± 21.21	35.79 ± 23.39	0.293
LVSVi (mL/m^2)	43.98 ± 11.65	44.56 ± 8.13	0.933
LVMi (g/m^2)	62.13 ± 20.51	66.04 ± 19.42	0.471

Values are expressed as mean ± SD. Abbreviations: CCT: cardiac computed tomography; CMR: cardiac magnetic resonance; LVEF: left ventricular ejection fraction; LVEDVi: left ventricular end-diastolic volume index; LVESVi: left ventricular end-systolic volume index; LVMi: left ventricular mass index; LVSVi: left ventricular stroke volume index.

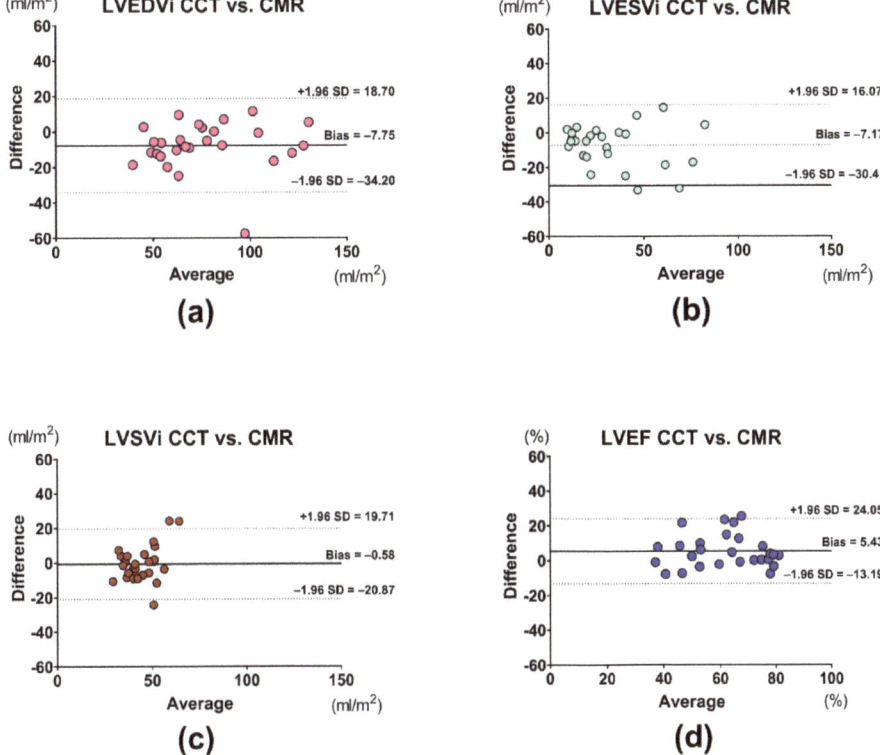

Figure 1. Bland–Altman analyses of (**a**) LVEDVi, (**b**) LVESVi, (**c**) LVSVi, and (**d**) LVEF assessment between CMR and CCT. Abbreviations: CCT: cardiac computed tomography; CMR: cardiac magnetic resonance; LVEF: left ventricular ejection fraction; LVEDVi: left ventricular end-diastolic volume index; LVESVi: left ventricular end-systolic volume index; LVSVi: left ventricular stroke volume index.

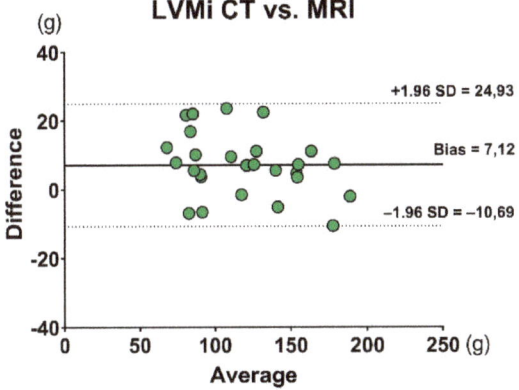

Figure 2. Bland–Altman analysis of LVMi assessment between CMR and CCT. Abbreviations: CCT: cardiac computed tomography; CMR: cardiac magnetic resonance; LVMi: left ventricular mass index.

3.2. Strain Assessment

Figures 3 and 4 show examples of GLS and GCS assessment in the same patient using different strain-assessment techniques. Strain values from each technique are represented in Table 3. GLS showed a trend towards being lower in CT-FT vs. CMR-FT (19.40 ± 5.04 vs. 22.40 ± 5.69, $p = 0.065$). GCS values were similar between all techniques ($p = 0.233$). There was good correlation between CMR-FT and CT-FT derived GLS ($r = 0.686$, $p < 0.001$) and GCS ($r = 0.707$, $p < 0.001$), while both of these methods had moderate correlation with TAG for GCS ($r = 0.479$, $p < 0.001$ for CMR-FT vs. TAG; $r = 0.548$ for CT-FT vs. TAG). Bland–Altman analysis revealed similarly wide limits of agreement (LOA) between all techniques in both GLS and GCS (Figure 5a–d and Table 4).

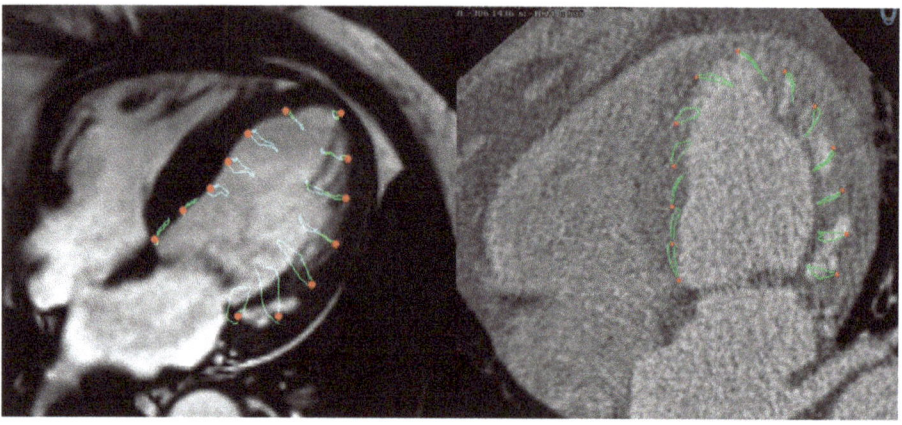

Figure 3. Assessment of GLS from the four-chamber long-axis (LAX) view in the same subject using CMR-FT (**left**) and CT-FT (**right**).

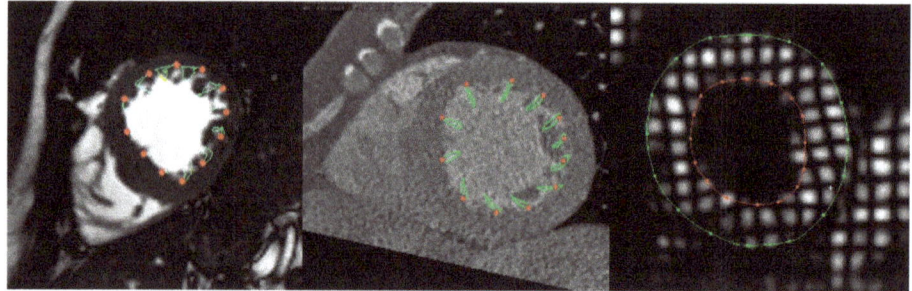

Figure 4. Assessment of GCS in the same subject from the mid-ventricular short-axis (SAX) view using CMR-FT (**left**), CT-FT (**middle**), and TAG (**right**).

Table 3. Values of strain assessment of the LV by CMR and CCT.

Measurement	CMR-FT	CT-FT	TAG
GLS (%)	22.40 ± 5.69	19.4 ± 5.04	N/A
GCS (%)	18.91 ± 5.97	18.13 ± 4.63	16.66 ± 3.38

Values are expressed as mean ± SD. Abbreviations: LV: left ventricular; CCT: cardiac computed tomography; GLS: global longitudinal strain, GCS: global circumferential strain, CMR-FT: cardiac magnetic resonance feature tracking, CT-FT: computed tomography feature tracking; TAG: myocardial tagging.

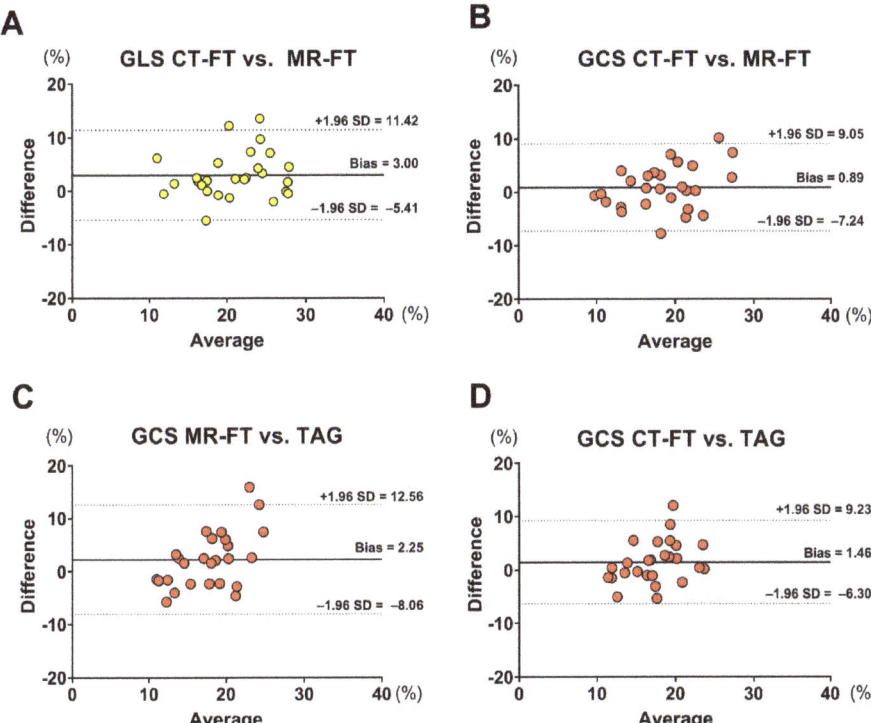

Figure 5. Bland–Altman analysis of the (**a**) GLS assessment between CT-FT and MR-FT; (**b**) GCS assessment between CT-FT and MR-FT; (**c**) GCS assessment between MR-FT and TAG; and (**d**) GCS assessment between CT-FT and TAG. Abbreviations: MR-FT: magnetic resonance feature tracking; CT-FT: computed tomography feature tracking; TAG: myocardial tagging; GLS: global longitudinal strain; GCS: global circumferential strain.

Table 4. Tabular representation of Bland–Altman and Pearson's correlation analyses for strain assessment.

Measurement	Comparison	Bias (%)	LOA (%)	Pearson's R
GLS	CMR-FT vs. CT-FT	3.003	±8.415	0.6860
GCS	CMR-FT vs. CT-FT	0.888	±8.16	0.7067
GCS	CMR-FT vs. TAG	2.250	±10.31	0.4799
GCS	CT-FT vs. TAG	1.468	±7.77	0.5484

Abbreviations: GLS: global longitudinal strain; GCS: global circumferential strain; CMR-FT: cardiac magnetic resonance feature tracking; CT-FT: computed tomography feature tracking; LOA: limits of agreement; TAG: myocardial tagging.

3.3. Intraobserver and Interobserver Reproducibility

The results of the reproducibility analyses are presented in Table 5. Intraobserver and interobserver agreement was excellent for all techniques. CMR-FT had worse intraobserver reproducibility for GLS (LOA ±2.4% vs. ±4.36%; CoV 6.8% vs. 10.1%) but performed better in interobserver comparison (LOA ±3.16% vs. ±5.5%; CoV 7.4% vs. 16.1%). TAG had superior reproducibility compared to the FT-based imaging technique for GCS, while FT-based techniques had similar results in interobserver and intraobserver comparisons.

Table 5. Reproducibility comparison of GLS and GCS between CMR-FT, CT-FT, and TAG.

		Bias (%)	Limits of Agreement (±)	CoV (%)	ICC (95% CI)
		\multicolumn{4}{c}{Intraobserver reproducibility}			
		\multicolumn{4}{c}{CMR-FT}			
GLS		0.09	4.36	10.1	0.960 (0.837–0.990)
GCS		−2.44	4.8	13.1	0.931 (0.439–0.985)
		\multicolumn{4}{c}{CT-FT}			
GLS		−0.08	2.4	6.8	0.983 (0.932–0.996)
GCS		−0.05	5.0	14.4	0.949 (0.801–0.987)
		\multicolumn{4}{c}{TAG}			
GCS		−0.08	1.26	3.9	0.992 (0.969–0.998)
		\multicolumn{4}{c}{Interobserver reproducibility}			
		\multicolumn{4}{c}{CMR-FT}			
GLS		0.03	3.16	7.4	0.982 (0.926–0.995)
GCS		−2.3	6.6	18.1	0.922 (0.629–0.981)
		\multicolumn{4}{c}{CT-FT}			
GLS		1.25	5.5	16.1	0.866 (0.501–0.966)
GCS		0.39	5.1	14.6	0.940 (0.759–0.985)
		\multicolumn{4}{c}{TAG}			
GCS		0.48	1.72	5.4	0.981 (0.918–0.995)

Abbreviations: GLS: global longitudinal strain; GCS: global circumferential strain; CMR-FT: cardiac magnetic resonance feature tracking; CT-FT: computed tomography feature tracking; TAG: myocardial tagging; CoV: coefficient of variance; ICC: intra-class correlation coefficient.

4. Discussion

4.1. Main Findings

To our knowledge, this is the first study that compared CT-FT derived strain values to CMR-FT and TAG. The main findings of our study were as follows.

i. There was good correlation between CMR-FT and CT-FT for GLS and GCS assessment, while GCS derived from both CMR-FT and CT-FT had a moderate correlation with TAG;
ii. The intra- and interobserver reproducibility of CMR-FT and CT-FT were excellent;
iii. There were no significant differences between cardiac CT and CMR for the volumetric assessment of the LV.

In the past decade, multiple methods to assess myocardial strain parameters from cardiac CT datasets have emerged. Most use tissue tracking algorithms originally developed for CMR or echocardiography to track either endocardial or epicardial borders of the left ventricular (LV) in 2D cine loops generated from 3D cardiac CT datasets. As with CMR and echocardiography, these methods allow for the quantification of well-studied global strain parameters, GLS, GCS, and global radial strain (GRS). In 2010, Helle-Valle et al. used a multimodality tissue tracking algorithm, originally developed for analysis of echocardiographic images, to assess GRS in a cohort of ischemic heart disease patients ($n = 20$). They demonstrated that the results of this method had good correlation with GRS derived from TAG ($r = 0.68$) and that the method has the ability to discern scarred LV segments [16]. Buss et al. used a similar feature tracking algorithm in a cohort of congestive heart failure patients ($n = 27$) to obtain and compare global strain parameters from cardiac CT and transthoracic echocardiography datasets. They found close correlation for GRS ($r = 0.97$), GCS ($r = 0.94$), and GLS ($r = 0.93$) between these modalities [12]. In the largest study to date ($n = 123$), Fukui et al. compared FT-derived GLS in a cohort of severe AS patients and found moderate correlation between cardiac CT and transthoracic echocardiography (TTE) ($r = 0.62$) [11].

Another method, developed specifically for cardiac CT, allows for the quantification of a cardiac CT-specific 3D principal strain. First, images of neighboring phases are interpolated using a motion coherent algorithm to reduce noise and improve motion coherence. Interpolated images are then analyzed using image and model matching algorithms to create a 3D motion-vector matrix of the LV [17]. Voxels of interest can then be chosen within this matrix to derive either a regional or global principal strain. Unlike 2D strain parameters, 3D principal strain encompasses deformation in all directions. It, thus, incorporates longitudinal, circumferential, and radial components. It is expressed as a positive value [18]. In a recent study, Ammon et al. found a close correlation ($r = -0.8$) between 3D principal strain and STE-derived GLS in a cohort ($n = 35$) of severe AS patients [19].

As previously noted, in the present study, we used a commercially available feature tracking software to measure GLS and GCS from cardiac CT datasets and compared it to CMR-FT and TAG in a cohort of patients with severe AS. We found a strong correlation between CT-FT and CMR-FT, but CT-FT tended to underestimate both GLS (22.40 ± 5.69 vs. 19.4 ± 5.04, $p = 0.065$) and GCS (18.91 ± 5.97 vs. 18.13 ± 4.63, $p = 0.233$). Previous authors have noticed a similar underestimation when comparing cardiac CT-derived strain to STE [12,19]. This underestimation could be driven by low temporal resolution of cardiac CT-derived cine loops. As shown by Rösner et al., accuracy of STE-derived strain measurements is dependent on the temporal resolution of the recordings [20]. They found systematic underestimation of strain parameters at temporal resolutions of less than 30 frames/cardiac cycle. Indeed, our 2D cine cardiac CT reconstructions had a temporal resolution of 10 frames/cardiac cycle, while CMR cine loops were acquired at 30 frames/cardiac cycle. To our knowledge, the performance of feature tracking at lower temporal resolutions has not been investigated yet, thus further studies are needed.

Interestingly, despite having a lower temporal resolution, when compared with TAG (the reference standard strain assessment technique), CT-FT and CMR-FT had similar correlation and LOA for GCS assessment. Additionally, reproducibility analysis revealed similar results for both FT-based techniques. If TAG data are taken as the ground truth, these findings suggest that FT algorithm performs equally well on both CMR and cardiac CT datasets.

Additionally, due to its angle independency and high temporal and spatial resolutions, CMR is the gold standard technique for the functional assessment of the heart [21]. However, despite having the worse temporal resolution, cardiac CT has been shown to have a close correlation and good agreement with CMR for the assessment of LV volumes in multiple studies [22–24], indicating that these methods can be used interchangeably for volumetric assessment. Our results agree with these findings.

4.2. Clinical Implications

There is an increasing number of patients who have implanted cardiac devices, and this decreases the feasibility of CMR due to potential artefacts or the inability to condition these devices. Our results imply that cardiac CT datasets are non-inferior to CMR datasets for the assessment of GLS and GCS using the FT algorithm. Furthermore, ours and multiple previous studies have shown potential interchangeability of volumetric measurements between cardiac CT and CMR. With further advancements in technology and an increase in temporal resolution, a cardiac CT might be used as a convenient follow-up tool to previous CMR assessments for both volumetric and strain measurements in patients with implanted cardiac devices.

4.3. Limitations

Naturally, there are certain limitations in our study. Firstly, this was a small-scale single-center trial. Secondly, we only had TAG acquisitions for short-axis slices, therefore we could not compare FT-derived GLS to a reference standard imaging technique. However, previous studies suggest that

CMR-FT has similar correlation and agreement to TAG for both GCS and GLS [25]. Thirdly, we did not have STE-derived strain parameters for a more comprehensive inter-modality comparison. Finally, given the retrospective nature of this trial and limited availability of high quality CT and CMR acquisitions that were made within a short timeframe in other populations, the trial was performed in a highly selected population of patients with severe AS. Thus, further studies are required to confirm these findings in more diverse cohorts.

5. Conclusions

Our findings show that the FT algorithm performs equally well in both CMR and cardiac CT datasets for the assessment of GLS and GCS, both in terms of reproducibility and agreement with the gold standard, TAG. In the clinical routine, cardiac CT might be used as a convenient follow-up tool to previous CMR assessments for both volumetric and strain measurements in patients with implanted cardiac devices.

Author Contributions: Conceptualization: S.K., B.P., and V.F.; methodology: S.K. and G.P.; validation: E.M., P.B., J.E., S.M.Z., R.T., and C.S. (Christopher Schneeweis); formal analysis: P.B.; investigation: C.S. (Christian Stehning) and N.S.; resources: S.K. and R.G.; data curation: S.M.Z.; writing—original draft preparation: P.B., N.S., and E.M.; writing—review and editing: all authors; visualization: P.B.; supervision: S.K. and T.L.; project administration: S.K.; funding acquisition: S.K. and B.P.

Funding: This research did not receive any specific grants from funding agencies in the public, commercial, or not-for-profit sectors.

Acknowledgments: We thank the technicians of the German Heart Center Berlin for the performance of high-quality CMR and cardiac CT examinations.

Conflicts of Interest: T.L. received support from the Hospital of Lithuanian University of Health Sciences. T.L., S.K., V.F., and B.P. received support from the DZHK (German Center for Cardiovascular Research), Partner Site Berlin. S.K. was supported by Philips Healthcare and Siemens. C.S. is an employee of Philips Healthcare. V.F. reports grants and other support from Abbott, Medtronic, Boston Scientific, and Edwards Lifesciences, as well as other support from Biotronik, Berlin Heart, and Novartis Pharma, outside of the submitted work. V.F. is also on the advisory board for Medtronic, Berlin Heart, Novartis Pharma, and Boston Scientific. G.P. is shareholder of a company that develops deformation imaging software for Medis BV.

References

1. Caforio, A.L.P.; Adler, Y.; Agostini, C.; Allanore, Y.; Anastasakis, A.; Arad, M.; Böhm, M.; Charron, P.; Elliott, P.M.; Eriksson, U.; et al. Diagnosis and management of myocardial involvement in systemic immune-mediated diseases: A position statement of the European Society of Cardiology Working Group on Myocardial and Pericardial Disease. *Eur. Heart J.* **2017**, *38*, 2649–2662. [CrossRef] [PubMed]
2. Prasad, M.; Hermann, J.; Gabriel, S.E.; Weyand, C.M.; Mulvagh, S.; Mankad, R.; Oh, J.K.; Matteson, E.L.; Lerman, A. Cardiorheumatology: Cardiac involvement in systemic rheumatic disease. *Nat. Rev. Cardiol.* **2015**, *12*, 168–176. [CrossRef] [PubMed]
3. Pedrizzetti, G.; Lapinskas, T.; Tonti, G.; Stoiber, L.; Zaliunas, R.; Gebker, R.; Pieske, B.; Kelle, S. The Relationship Between EF and Strain Permits a More Accurate Assessment of LV Systolic Function. *JACC Cardiovasc. Imaging* **2019**, *3033*. [CrossRef] [PubMed]
4. Pagourelias, E.D.; Mirea, O.; Duchenne, J.; Van Cleemput, J.; Delforge, M.; Bogaert, J.; Kuznetsova, T.; Voigt, J.-U. Echo Parameters for Differential Diagnosis in Cardiac Amyloidosis: a head-to-head comparison of deformation and nondeformation parameters. *Circ. Cardiovasc. Imaging* **2017**, *10*, e005588. [CrossRef] [PubMed]
5. Guerra, F.; Stronati, G.; Fischietti, C.; Ferrarini, A.; Zuliani, L.; Pomponio, G.; Capucci, A.; Danieli, M.G.; Gabrielli, A. Global longitudinal strain measured by speckle tracking identifies subclinical heart involvement in patients with systemic sclerosis. *Eur. J. Prev. Cardiol.* **2018**, *25*, 1598–1606. [CrossRef] [PubMed]
6. Fine, N.M.; Crowson, C.S.; Lin, G.; Oh, J.K.; Villarraga, H.R.; Gabriel, S.E. Evaluation of myocardial function in patients with rheumatoid arthritis using strain imaging by speckle-tracking echocardiography. *Ann. Rheum Dis.* **2014**, *73*, 1833–1839. [CrossRef] [PubMed]

7. Cho, M.-J.; Lee, J.-W.; Lee, J.; Shin, Y.B. Evaluation of Early Left Ventricular Dysfunction in Patients with Duchenne Muscular Dystrophy Using Two-Dimensional Speckle Tracking Echocardiography and Tissue Doppler Imaging. *Pediatr. Cardiol.* **2018**, *39*, 1614–1619. [CrossRef] [PubMed]
8. Obokata, M.; Nagata, Y.; Wu, V.C.-C.; Kado, Y.; Kurabayashi, M.; Otsuji, Y.; Takeuchi, M. Direct comparison of cardiac magnetic resonance feature tracking and 2D/3D echocardiography speckle tracking for evaluation of global left ventricular strain. *Eur. Heart J. Cardiovasc. Imaging* **2016**, *17*, 525–532. [CrossRef]
9. Mavrogeni, S.; Markousis-Mavrogenis, G.; Koutsogeorgopoulou, L.; Kolovou, G. Cardiovascular magnetic resonance imaging: Clinical implications in the evaluation of connective tissue diseases. *J. Inflamm. Res.* **2017**, *10*, 55–61. [CrossRef]
10. Scatteia, A.; Baritussio, A.; Bucciarelli-Ducci, C. Strain imaging using cardiac magnetic resonance. *Heart Fail. Rev.* **2017**, *22*, 465–476. [CrossRef]
11. Fukui, M.; Xu, J.; Abdelkarim, I.; Sharbaugh, M.S.; Thoma, F.W.; Althouse, A.D.; Pedrizzetti, G.; Cavalcante, J.L. Global longitudinal strain assessment by computed tomography in severe aortic stenosis patients—Feasibility using feature tracking analysis. *J. Cardiovasc. Comput. Tomogr.* **2019**, *13*, 157–162. [CrossRef] [PubMed]
12. Buss, S.J.; Schulz, F.; Mereles, D.; Hosch, W.; Galuschky, C.; Schummers, G.; Stapf, D.; Hofmann, N.; Giannitsis, E.; Hardt, S.E.; et al. Quantitative analysis of left ventricular strain using cardiac computed tomography. *Eur. J. Radiol.* **2014**, *83*, e123–e130. [CrossRef] [PubMed]
13. Baumgartner, H.; Falk, V.; Bax, J.J.; De Bonis, M.; Hamm, C.; Holm, P.J.; Lung, B.; Lancellotti, P.; Lansac, E.; Rodriguez Munoz, D.; et al. 2017 ESC/EACTS Guidelines for the management of valvular heart disease. *Eur. Heart J.* **2017**, *38*, 2739–2791. [CrossRef] [PubMed]
14. Morton, G.; Schuster, A.; Jogiya, R.; Kutty, S.; Beerbaum, P.; Nagel, E. Inter-study reproducibility of cardiovascular magnetic resonance myocardial feature tracking. *J. Cardiovasc. Magn. Reson.* **2012**, *14*, 43. [CrossRef] [PubMed]
15. Oppo, K.; Leen, E.; Angerson, W.J.; Cooke, T.G.; McArdle, C.S. Doppler perfusion index: An interobserver and intraobserver reproducibility study. *Radiology* **1998**, *208*, 453–457. [CrossRef] [PubMed]
16. Helle-Valle, T.M.; Yu, W.C.; Fernandes, V.R.S.; Rosen, B.D.; Lima, J.A.C. Usefulness of radial strain mapping by multidetector computer tomography to quantify regional myocardial function in patients with healed myocardial infarction. *Am. J. Cardiol.* **2010**, *106*, 483–491. [CrossRef] [PubMed]
17. Tanabe, Y.; Kido, T.; Kurata, A.; Sawada, S.; Suekuni, H.; Kido, T.; Yokoi, T.; Uetani, T.; Inoue, K.; Miyagawa, M.; et al. Three-dimensional maximum principal strain using cardiac computed tomography for identification of myocardial infarction. *Eur. Radiol.* **2017**, *27*, 1667–1675. [CrossRef] [PubMed]
18. Marwan, M.; Ammon, F.; Bittner, D.; Röther, J.; Mekkhala, N.; Hell, M.; Schuhbaeck, A.; Gitsioudis, G.; Feryrer, R.; Schlundt, C.; et al. CT-derived left ventricular global strain in aortic valve stenosis patients: A comparative analysis pre and post transcatheter aortic valve implantation. *J. Cardiovasc. Comput. Tomogr.* **2018**, *12*, 240–244. [CrossRef] [PubMed]
19. Ammon, F.; Bittner, D.; Hell, M.; Mansour, H.; Achenbach, S.; Arnold, M.; Marwan, M. CT-derived left ventricular global strain: A head-to-head comparison with speckle tracking echocardiography. *Int. J. Cardiovasc. Imaging* **2019**, *35*, 1701–1707. [CrossRef] [PubMed]
20. Rösner, A.; Barbosa, D.; Aarsæther, E.; Kjønås, D.; Schirmer, H.; D'hooge, J. The influence of frame rate on two-dimensional speckle-tracking strain measurements: A study on silico-simulated models and images recorded in patients. *Eur. Heart J. Cardiovasc. Imaging* **2015**, *16*, 1137–1147. [CrossRef] [PubMed]
21. Schulz-Menger, J.; Bluemke, D.A.; Bremerich, J.; Flamm, S.D.; Fogel, M.A.; Friedrich, M.G.; Kim, R.J.; von Knobelsdorff-Brenkenhoff, F.; Kramer, C.M.; Pennell, D.J.; et al. Standardized image interpretation and post processing in cardiovascular magnetic resonance: Society for Cardiovascular Magnetic Resonance (SCMR) Board of Trustees Task Force on Standardized Post Processing. *J. Cardiovasc. Magn. Reson.* **2013**, *15*, 35. [CrossRef] [PubMed]
22. Greupner, J.; Zimmermann, E.; Grohmann, A.; Dübel, H.-P.; Althoff, T.; Borges, A.C.; Rutsch, W.; Schlattmann, P.; Hamm, B.; Dewey, M. Head-to-Head Comparison of Left Ventricular Function Assessment with 64-Row Computed Tomography, Biplane Left Cineventriculography, and Both 2- and 3-Dimensional Transthoracic Echocardiography. *J. Am. Coll. Cardiol.* **2012**, *59*, 1897–1907. [CrossRef] [PubMed]
23. Wu, Y.-W.; Tadamura, E.; Yamamuro, M.; Kanao, S.; Okayama, S.; Ozasa, N.; Toma, M.; Kimura, T.; Komeda, M.; Togashi, K. Estimation of global and regional cardiac function using 64-slice computed

tomography: A comparison study with echocardiography, gated-SPECT and cardiovascular magnetic resonance. *Int. J. Cardiol.* **2008**, *128*, 69–76. [CrossRef] [PubMed]

24. Sarwar, A.; Shapiro, M.D.; Nasir, K.; Nieman, K.; Nomura, C.H.; Brady, T.J.; Cury, R.C. Evaluating global and regional left ventricular function in patients with reperfused acute myocardial infarction by 64-slice multidetector CT: A comparison to magnetic resonance imaging. *J. Cardiovasc. Comput. Tomogr.* **2009**, *3*, 170–177. [CrossRef] [PubMed]

25. Cao, J.J.; Ngai, N.; Duncanson, L.; Cheng, J.; Gliganic, K.; Chen, Q. A comparison of both DENSE and feature tracking techniques with tagging for the cardiovascular magnetic resonance assessment of myocardial strain. *J. Cardiovasc. Magn. Reson.* **2018**, *20*, 26. [CrossRef] [PubMed]

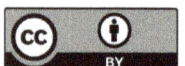

© 2019 by the authors. Licensee MDPI, Basel, Switzerland. This article is an open access article distributed under the terms and conditions of the Creative Commons Attribution (CC BY) license (http://creativecommons.org/licenses/by/4.0/).

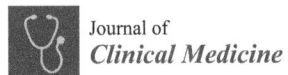

Article

Progenitor Cells Derived from Drain Waste Product of Open-Heart Surgery in Children

Tak-Wah Wong [1,2,3], Chung-Dann Kan [4], Wen-Tai Chiu [5], Kin Lam Fok [6], Ye Chun Ruan [6,†], Xiaohua Jiang [6,7], Junjiang Chen [6,†], Chiu-Ching Kao [1], I-Yu Chen [1], Hui-Chun Lin [1], Chia-Hsuan Chou [1,8], Chou-Wen Lin [9,‡], Chun-Keung Yu [8,10,11], Stephanie Tsao [1], Yi-Ping Lee [8], Hsiao Chang Chan [6,7] and Jieh-Neng Wang [12,*]

1. Department of Dermatology, National Cheng Kung University Hospital, College of Medicine, National Cheng Kung University, Tainan 704, Taiwan
2. Department of Biochemistry and Molecular Biology, College of Medicine, National Cheng Kung University, Tainan 701, Taiwan
3. Center of Applied Nanomedicine, National Cheng Kung University, Tainan 701, Taiwan
4. Department of Surgery, Institute of Cardiovascular Research Center, National Cheng Kung University Hospital, College of Medicine, National Cheng Kung University, Tainan 704, Taiwan
5. Department of Biomedical Engineering, National Cheng Kung University, Tainan 701, Taiwan
6. Epithelial Cell Biology Research Center, School of Biomedical Sciences, Faculty of Medicine, the Chinese University of Hong Kong, Shatin, Hong Kong
7. Key Laboratory for Regenerative Medicine, Ministry of Education of the People's Republic of China, Shatin, HongKong
8. Institute of Basic Medical Sciences, College of Medicine, National Cheng Kung University, Tainan 704, Taiwan
9. Biomedical Technology and Device Research Laboratories, Industrial Technology Research Institute, Liuo-Jia, Tainan 734, Taiwan
10. Department of Microbiology and Immunology, Center of Infectious Disease and Signaling Research, College of Medicine, National Cheng Kung University, Tainan 701, Taiwan
11. National Laboratory Animal Center, National Applied Research Laboratories, Taipei 11529, Taiwan
12. Department of Pediatrics, National Cheng Kung University Hospital, College of Medicine, National Cheng Kung University, Tainan 704, Taiwan
* Correspondence: jiehneng@mail.ncku.edu.tw; Tel.: +886-6-235-3535 (ext. 4189)
† Present address: Department of Biomedical Engineering, Hong Kong Polytechnic University, Kowloon, Hong Kong.
‡ Present address: Gold Medal Glycine Tomentella Hayata Biological Technology Company, Tainan 73052, Taiwan.

Received: 4 June 2019; Accepted: 10 July 2019; Published: 12 July 2019

Abstract: Human cardiac progenitor cells isolated from the same host may have advantages over other sources of stem cells. The aim of this study is to establish a new source of human progenitor cells collected from a waste product, pericardiac effusion fluid, after open-heart surgery in children with congenital heart diseases. The fluid was collected every 24 h for 2 days after surgery in 37 children. Mononuclear cells were isolated and expanded in vitro. These pericardial effusion-derived progenitor cells (PEPCs) exhibiting cardiogenic lineage markers, were highly proliferative and enhanced angiogenesis in vitro. Three weeks after stem cell transplantation into the ischemic heart in mice, cardiac ejection fraction was improved significantly without detectable progenitor cells. Gene expression profiles of the repaired hearts revealed activation of several known repair mechanisms including paracrine effects, cell migration, and angiogenesis. These progenitor cells may have the potential for heart regeneration.

Keywords: congenital heart disease; cardiac surgery; open heart; progenitor cells; regeneration; stem cells

1. Introduction

Despite the recent advances in molecular medicine and health care; cardiac diseases, including both adult and congenital heart diseases, are still the leading cause of morbidity and mortality throughout the world [1]. Congenital heart disease (CHD) is the most common congenital anomalies in newborns [2]. Globally, there are around 1.35 million neonates born with CHD every year over the last 15 years. The highest CHD birth prevalence is reported in Asian countries with 9.3 per 1000 live births which is one of the leading causes of perinatal and infant death from congenital malformations [3]. Approximately 25 percent of these neonates require surgery or catheter-based intervention in the first year of life [4]. The prognosis of CHD is good with 83% of patients are free from reoperation for 20 years and the overall survival rate was 86%, including early mortality [5]. However, multiple-stage operations are needed to correct the defects in cases with complex CHD. Lui et al. pointed out the misperception that CHD is cured by surgery [6]. CHD patients are at increased risk of developing myocardial ischemia or premature coronary artery disease (CAD) while growing up. The number of adult CHD patients continues to increase by 5% per year, there are now more than 1 million patients in the United States [6]. Owing to the lack of effective treatment strategy after severe cardiac injury in these patients, stem cell-based therapies may be a potential therapeutic strategy [7,8].

A variety of stem cell populations have been explored for their potential to promote cardiac repair and regeneration. The results are controversial since each type of stem cell has its own profile of advantages, limitations, and translational practicability. The most frequently studied stem cell populations in cardiac diseases include embryonic stem cells (ESC), bone marrow-derived stem cells (BMSC), tissue-specific stem cells (TSSC), and the most recently inducible pluripotent stem cells (iPS). ESCs are conceptually attractive for cardiac repair because of the potential to differentiate into different cell types in a damaged heart. Despite the recent success of ESCs engraftment and repairing injured myocardium in a primate model of myocardial infarction [9], translation into clinical use has been hindered by ESCs' genetic instability, potential tumorigenic and immunogenic properties, and ethical considerations related to the origin of these cells [7]. BMSCs are composed of several cell populations that have the capacity to differentiate into various cell types, including hematopoietic stem cells (HSC), mesenchymal stem cells (MSC), endothelial progenitor stem cells (EPC), and others. Each cell type has been reported to improve cardiac function on top of standard therapy in cardiac diseases. Most clinical trials to date have used total bone marrow mononuclear cells, which comprise HSCs, MSCs, and monocytes [7]. Promising results from Cochrane Heart Group enrolled more than a thousand patients with heart diseases but debates continued because of a high degree of heterogeneity in the results [10,11]. It is still too early to draw conclusions on the efficacy of BMSCs [12]. TSSC, such as adipose tissue-derived stem cells (ADS) [13] and umbilical cord blood-derived stem cells (UBS) [14], appeared to be attractive in the treatment of cardiac diseases. Early promising results in clinical trials have been shown in ADS treated cardiac damages [13]. However, the tumorigenic potential of these cells cannot be totally excluded [13]. UBS is still in the early recruitment stages of the clinical trial [14].

Resident cardiac progenitor cells expanded from heart biopsy in the early clinical trial showed promising results [15]. These cells have exhibited robust cardiovascular differentiation potential. However, an invasive heart biopsy is not easily accepted by parents of CHD patients. Human iPS cells provide new revenue for sufficient stem cells in the treatment of heart failure. Yet the safety in clinical applications remains to be determined [16]. Taken together, while multiple clinical trials of stem cell therapy worldwide on adult or congenital heart diseases suggest that stem cell therapy is safe with modest improvement in cardiac functioning and structural remodeling [7,16], the right source of stem cells remains one of the major challenges in this field. A new source of stem cells, which is free of ethical conflict, easy to isolate and propagate, and with cardiac regenerative potential, is desirable for cell-based therapy in the treatment of CHD.

Draining of blood and effusion from the mediastinum and pleural space following open-heart surgery is critical to establish adequate evacuation of fluid after surgery [17]. Surgical drainage is usually left in place for 3 to 4 days until the fluid is decreased to less than 50 ml per day with stable hemodynamic and respiratory functions. In this study, we explored the possibility of the isolation and expansion of progenitor cells from pericardial effusion drained after open-heart surgery in children with congenital heart diseases. We named these cells pericardial effusion-derived progenitor cells (PEPCs).

2. Materials and Methods

2.1. Isolation and Expansion of Progenitor Cells from Open-Heart Surgery Drain Fluids

All human studies were conducted according to the principles expressed in the Helsinki Declaration and approved by the institutional review board. Thirty-seven patients with congenital heart diseases aged 3 days to 43 months (mean 9.7 ± 9.2 months, Table S1) and scheduled for open-heart surgery were recruited after signing informed consent by their parents. Immediately after cardiac surgery, drain tubes were inserted into pericardial space to relieve fluid accumulation around the heart. Drain fluids were collected every 24 h for 2 days after the operation in an aseptic container (Figure 1) containing 300 mL of cold saline and was kept at 4 °C. Cells were centrifuged at 1500 rpm for 10 min at 4 °C and re-suspended in 30 ml cold RPMI medium (Gibco, Invitrogen, Carlsbad, CA, USA). Mononuclear cells were isolated with Ficoll-Paque (GE Healthcare, Buckinghamshire, UK) by following the manufacturer's instruction. They were cultured directly without sorting on a fibronectin-coated 48-well plate with cardiosphere medium [15] (300 µL/well) consisting of 35% IMDM and 65% DMEM/F-12 Mix (Gibco, Invitrogen, Carlsbad, CA, USA), 3.5% FBS, 1% penicillin-streptomycin, 1% L-glutamine, 0.1mM 2-mercaptoethanol, thrombin, 1× B-27, 80 ng/mL bFGF, 25 ng/mL EGF, and 4 ng/mL cardiotrophin-1. On the second and third day, 200 µL of the supernatant with RBCs and white blood cells were replaced carefully with freshly prepared medium without disturbing the loosely attached cells. The procedure was repeated every 3 days to completely remove the RBCs and unattached cells. Cells were expanded in a ratio of 1:2 in 5–7 days thereafter.

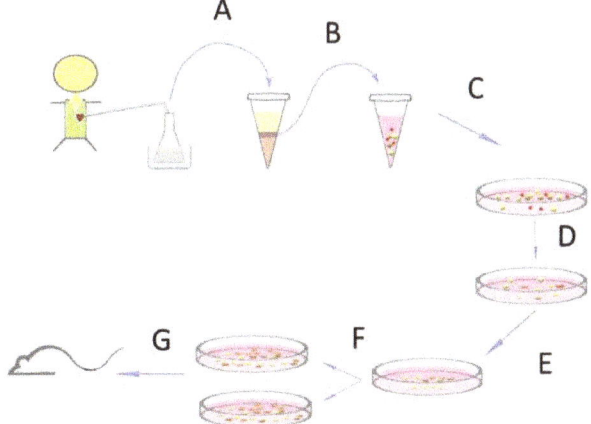

Figure 1. Schematic drawing of the isolation and expansion procedures for human pericardial effusion-derived progenitor cells (PEPCs). (**A**) Drain fluid was collected on the first and second day after open-heart surgery in a drain bottle containing 300 mL of 4 °C normal saline. The bottle was kept at 4 °C during collection. (**B**) Mononuclear cells were collected by density gradient centrifugation with Ficoll-Paque. (**C**) The mononuclear cells with red blood and white blood cells were plated on a fibronectin-coated plate and cultured in cardiosphere medium. (**D**) The red blood and white blood cells were removed by serial medium supplement every 3 days. (**E**) Spindle-like cells were noted as early as 3 days while cardiospheres appear around 7 days after seeding. (**F**) Further cell expansions to obtain sufficient cell number for transplantation. (**G**) PEPCs were injected into peri-infarction regions of a mouse heart.

2.2. Flow Cytometry

Cells isolated on day 1 and day 2 from cardiac surgery drain fluid were analyzed with flow cytometry to study the early surface marker expression. Cells with a higher passage (>5) were used to study the chronological changes of surface markers. All experiments were done with a FACSCalibur (BD Biosciences, San Jose, CA, USA) flow cytometer. Data were analyzed with free software WinMDI 2.8. Monoclonal antibodies used for cell surface markers analyses included fluorescein isothiocyanate (FITC)-conjugated anti-human CD34, phycoerythrin (PE)-conjugated anti-human CD133 (MACS, Bergisch Gladbach, Germany), allophycocyanin (APC)-conjugated anti-human CD117, PE-conjugated anti-human CD31, and CD45 (BD Pharmingen, San Diego, CA, USA), FITC-mouse IgG2aκ, APC-mouse IgG1κ, and PE-mouse IgG1κ isotype controls (BD Pharmingen, San Diego, CA, USA).

2.3. Cell Culture and Conditioned Medium for Angiogenesis Assay

Human fibroblasts from neonatal foreskin (HS68, Bioresource Collection and Research Center, Taipei, Taiwan) were cultured in DMEM with 10% fetal calf serum, 5% streptomycin and penicillin. Primary human umbilical vein endothelial cells (HUVEC) were purchased from the same center and were cultured in Medium 199 (Life Technologies, Taipei, Taiwan). Conditioned medium (CM) was collected 48 h in serum-free DMEM for fibroblasts, serum-free Medium 199 for HUVEC, and serum-free culture medium for PEPCs, respectively. CM was pooling from 100 µL of medium with 2×10^4 cells in each well of a 96-well plate and stored at −20 °C until used. Twenty thousand HUVEC cells were seeded on a 96-well plate pre-coated with basement membrane matrix (Matrigel Matrix Growth Factor Reduced^{TM}, BD Biosciences, Taipei, Taiwan). They were plated either with 100 µL complete Medium 199 as the positive control, with 100 µL FBS-free Medium 199 as the negative control, or with 100 µL CM. To evaluate the mechanism of angiogenesis elicited by PEPCs, neutralizing antibodies 0.04 µg/100 µL anti-VEGF (R&D, Minneapolis, MN, USA), or 0.8 µg/100 µL anti-HGF (Abcam, Billerica, MA, USA), or 50 µg/mL thalidomide (Sigma-Aldrich, St. Louis, MO, USA) was added to CM on a shaker for 1 hour at room temperature. Cells were imaged after 18 h with a digital camera coupled to a microscope. Five different areas were taken from one well. Images were analyzed with Image J software (Version 1.52p, National Institutes of Health, Bethesda, MD, USA) and the total vessel length was measured with AngioTool Software (version 0.6a, National Cancer Institute, Bethesda, MD, USA) [18]. Each condition was triplicated and at least three independent experiments were performed.

2.4. Cardiac Infarction in Mice

All animal studies were performed in compliance with the US Department of Health and Human Services Guide for the Care and Use of Laboratory Animals and approved by the institutional review board. Adult male SCID-beige mice, aged 10 to 20 weeks, were purchased from the animal center of National Taiwan University, Taipei, Taiwan. The left main descending branch of the coronary artery was ligated with a 7-0 prolene suture [15]. To minimize the number of mice used for the experiments and to compare results from different assays, PEPCs at passage 6 from three randomly selected patients were used in all following experiments. Either PEPCs or lentivirus-transduced PEPCs (10^5 cells in a total volume of 10 µL phosphate-buffered saline (PBS)) were injected at two sites bordering the infarcts (5 µl each) immediately after vessels ligation. 8 mice were injected with PEPCs, while the other 6 mice were injected with lentivirus-transduced PEPCs for in vivo bioluminescence imaging. Transduced or non-transduced (both $n = 8$) human fetal skin fibroblasts (WS1, Bioresource Collection and Research Center, Taipei, Taiwan) and PBS ($n = 11$) were used as both positive and negative controls, respectively. WS1 is a normal skin fibroblast cell line originated from a 12-week gestation fetus. The embryonic nature of these cells is expected to have partial effects on tissue repair. These cells were grown in Eagle's Minimum Essential Medium with 10% FBS.

All mice underwent echocardiography (Philips Sonos 5500, 15 MHz probe, Eindhoven, Netherlands) to evaluate the ventricular function on the day before operation (baseline, day 0),

2 days, 1 week, 2 weeks, and 3 weeks after surgery. Ventricular wall thickness and chamber dimensions were measured using a short-axis parasternal view at the level of the papillary muscles. Left ventricular ejection fraction (LVEF) and fractional area were calculated from 2D long-axis views taken through the infarcted area. Mice were sedated with isoflurane during all procedures. Data were collected by averaging three separate measurements during each examination. Mice were euthanized at 3 weeks.

2.5. Transplanted Cell Tracing with Optical Bioluminescence Imaging and Alu Sequence

Cardiac bioluminescence imaging was performed using the Xenogen IVIS 50 system (Hopkinton, MA, USA). After intraperitoneal injection of reporter probe D-luciferin (150 mg luciferin/kg), animals were imaged for 1–10 min under anesthesia. The same mice were scanned weekly for 3 weeks. Imaging signals were quantified in units of maximum photons per second per square centimeter per steradian (photons/sec/cm^2/sr) as described [19]. To test the possibility that a small population of PEPCs might survive but not be detected by in vivo imaging, the human Alu repeat [20], acted as a marker to detect human PEPCs from infarcted hearts, was amplified by PCR.

2.6. Virus Production and Cell Transduction

PEPCs were transduced with luciferase gene as a tracer. The plasmid pLLB13 was constructed by inserting the Mef I-and Xba I-digested luciferase DNA fragment, PCR-amplified from pGL4.10 (Promega, USA) using both the 5'-primer (5'-CGAACTCAATTGCCACCATGGAAGATGCC-3') and 3'primer (5'-CCCGACTCTAGAATTATTACACGGC-3'), into pLenti6/Ubc/V5-DEST (Invitrogen, Carlsbad, CA, USA) from which the 1752-bp fragment between EcoR I and Xba I restriction enzyme sites had been removed. Lentivirus production and transduction of PEPCs were performed as suggested by the manufacturer. Briefly, lentivirus was produced by transfecting 293FT cells (Invitrogen, Carlsbad, CA, USA) with both pLLB13 and ViroPower Packaging Mix (Invitrogen, Carlsbad, CA, USA) in the presence of Lipofectamine 2000 (Invitrogen, Carlsbad, CA, USA). The lentivirus was harvested three days later with a titer of 2×10^6 transducing units. They were then used to transduce PEPCs in the presence of 6 µg/mL polybrene and 0.5 µg/mL blasticidin.

2.7. Immunocytochemistry and Histological Analysis

Spindle shape PEPCs and cardiosphere-like cell clusters were collected for immunostaining. Cells were fixed with 3.7% buffered paraformaldehyde, permeabilized with 0.5% Triton X-100 for 15 min and then blocked with goat serum (Zymed, San Diego, CA, USA) for 30 min at 37 °C. Cells were incubated with antibodies including mouse anti-CD105 (R&D Systems, Inc., Minneapolis, MN), anti-CX43 (Chemicon, Temecula, CA, USA), anti-sarcomeric actin (Abcam, Cambridge, UK), rabbit anti-CD117, anti-Ki67 (Abcam, Cambridge, UK) for 12 h at 4 °C, followed by an hour room temperature incubation with Alexa 488 or Alexa 489 conjugated secondary anti-mouse/anti-rabbit IgG antibodies (Molecular Probes, Eugene, OR, USA). Cell nucleus was stained with 4', 6-diamidino-2-phenylindole (DAPI) (Sigma). The fluorophore was excited by a laser at 405 nm; 488 nm or 543 nm and detected by a scanning confocal microscope (Olympus FV-1000, Tokyo, Japan). The specificity of all antibodies used in this study was examined with isotype-specific immunoglobulins at the same protein concentration as a negative control. Mouse hearts were excised, fixed in 10% formaldehyde or fresh frozen, and sectioned in 5-µm slices. Tissue sections were stained with a hematoxylin-eosin reagent or Masson's trichrome. Tissue infarct zone was calculated from Masson's trichrome-stained sections by tracing the infarct borders manually [15] and then by using ImageJ software to calculate the percent of infarct myocardium by a researcher who blinded to the study.

2.8. Gene Expression in Mouse Heart after Cell Transplantation

To realize the crosstalk between implanted PEPCs and mouse cardiomyocytes, mouse hearts treated with PBS, human fibroblasts, and PEPCs were collected 3 weeks after surgery for DNA microarray analysis. Each group contained at least 3 mice. Mouse hearts were excised and frozen stored at −80 °C. The whole ventricular portion of each ischemic heart was used for RNA extraction. RNA was extracted after stabilizing in RNA later-ICE (Ambion, Foster City, CA, USA) by following the manufacturer's instruction. Affymetrix cDNA microarray (Mouse Gene 1.0 ST Array GeneChip, Santa Clara, CA, USA) with 28,853 genes was used for whole-genome analysis. Gene expression level differences were analyzed with methods developed by Tusher VG et al. [21]. SYBR green master mix and 7500 Fast Real-Time PCR systems were used to confirm the gene expression (Applied Biosystems, Foster City, CA, USA). 18s RNA or GAPDH was used as an internal control.

2.9. Statistics Analysis

The Pearson product–moment correlation coefficient method was used to identify the patient parameter that might be independently associated with cell growth and cell isolation. One-way analysis of variance (ANOVA) was performed to determine whether there were significant differences between the different treatments. Bonferroni *t*-test was applied for multiple pairwise comparisons among individual groups. The Student's *t*-test was used to compare differences in two groups when the variables were normally distributed and Mann–Whitney rank sum test when data were not normally distributed. Data were analyzed using SigmaStat (Systat Software Inc. San Jose, CA, USA) version 3.11. A *p*-value less than 0.05 was considered significant. Data were calculated with at least three separated independent experiments.

3. Results

3.1. Isolation of PEPCs from Drain Fluid after Open-Heart Surgery

Figure 1 depicts the methods of collection and propagation of PEPCs from the drain fluids. The average cells yield for the first 24-hour drain fluid was $6.3 \pm 3.0 \times 10^6$, and $2.2 \pm 1.4 \times 10^6$ for the second 24-hour. On 6–7 days-in-vitro (DIV), the morphology of the loosely attached cells changed. Spindle-like cells spread out on the culture dish while loosely attached cells began to form cell clumps resembling the morphology of a cardiosphere (Figure 2A). Subsequently, the culture showed robust growth. Spindle-like cells became confluent with cardiospheres growing on top on 14 DIV (Figure 2B). Of note, initial cell density affected cell growth [22]. With a higher culture density ($2 \times 10^4/\mu L$), spindle-like cells appeared on day 3 while cardiospheres appeared around day 7 after seeding. However, with a lower density ($2 \times 10^2/\mu L$), spindle-like cells appeared around day 7 while cardiopspheres emerged around 2–3 weeks. Importantly, PEPCs culture could be established from all 37 patients (3-day-old to 43-month-old, median 9-month-old) included in the study (Table S1), suggesting that this protocol was reproducible regardless of the patient's sex, age, and disease conditions (r = 0, Pearson product–moment correlation coefficient). The doubling time of these cells was 4.56 ± 1.8 days.

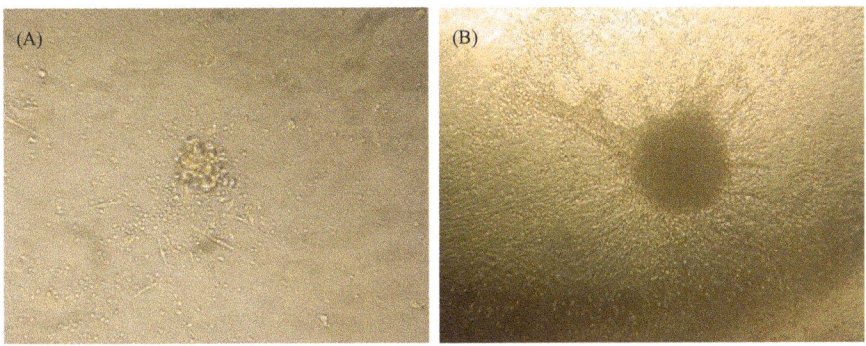
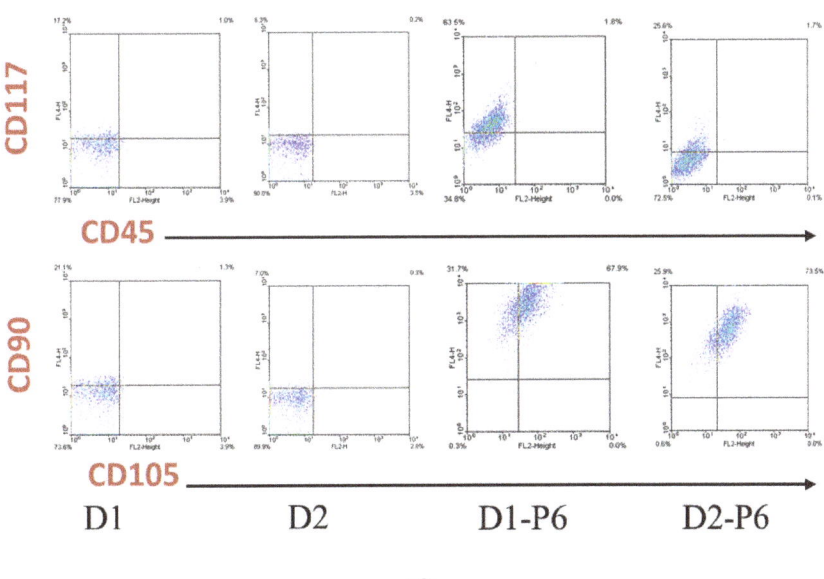

Figure 2. Cont.

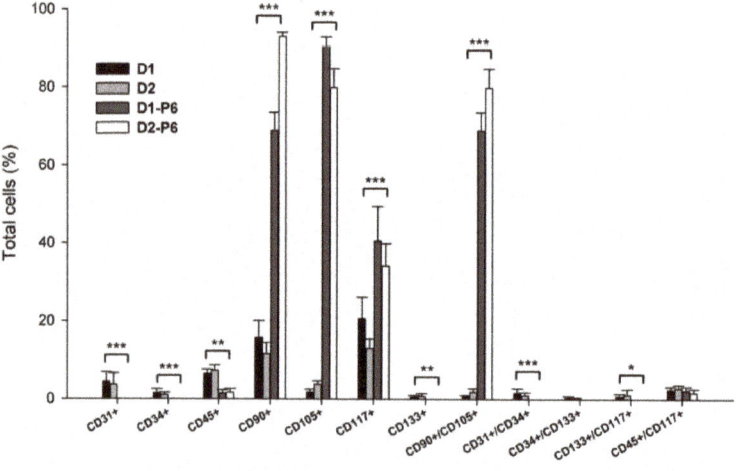

(D)

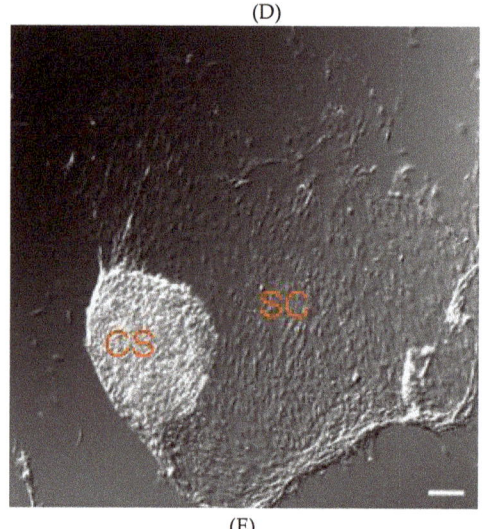

(E)

Figure 2. *Cont.*

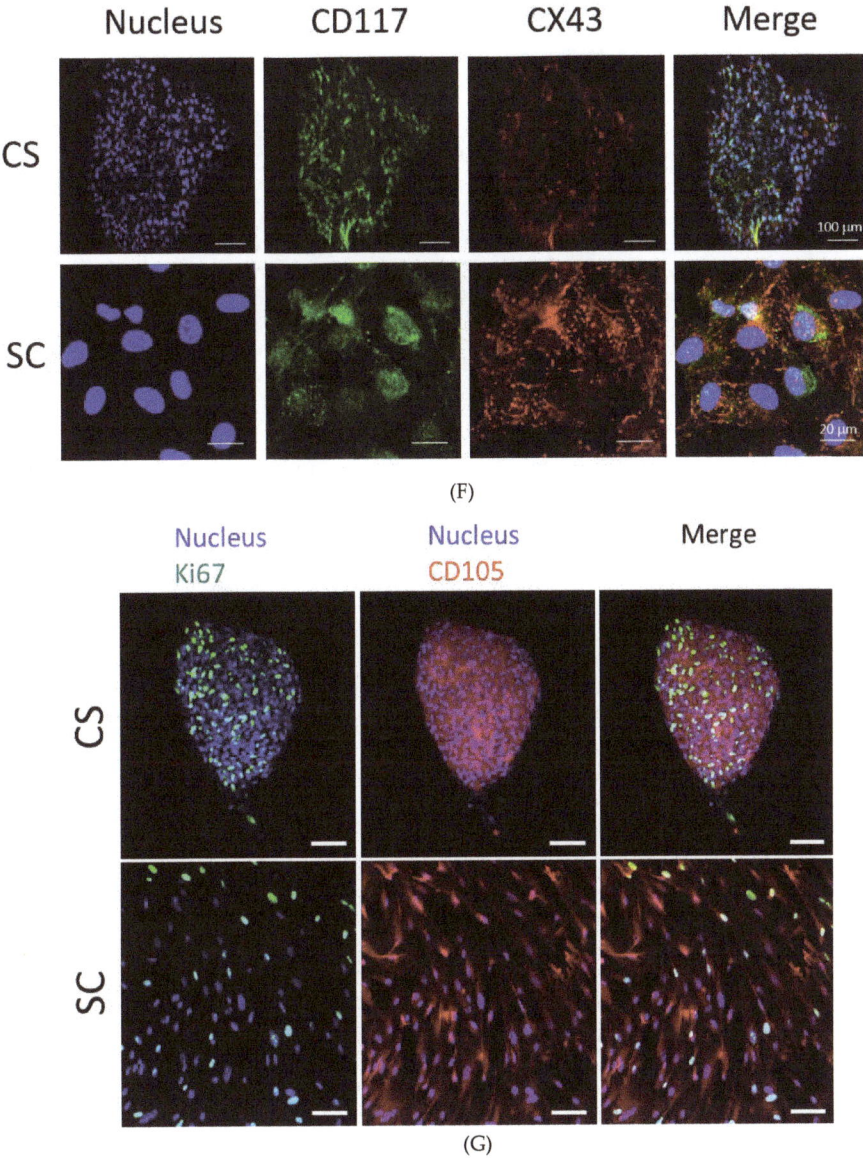

Figure 2. Cont.

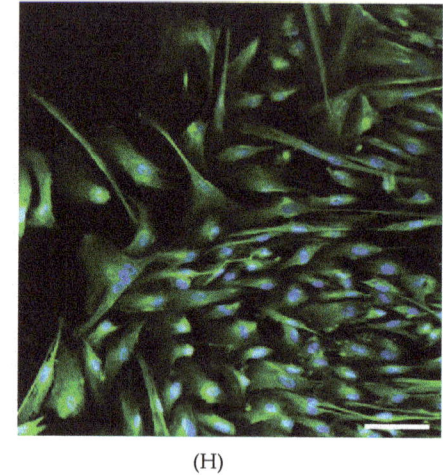

(H)

Figure 2. PEPCs are highly proliferating cells and express cardiac lineage potential after in vitro culture. (**A**) Spindle-like cells and cardiosphere-like cell clusters appeared 7 days after cell seeding. (**B**) Day 14 culture showed robust growth of spindle cells and cardiospheres. (**C**) FACS analysis, either from day 1 (D1) or day 2 (D2) drain fluid collections, showed increased expression of stem cell factor receptor (CD117), CD90, and CD105 after 6 cell passages (D1–P6, D2–P6) compared with their corresponding primary cells (D1 and D2). (**D**) The expression of CD31, CD34, CD45, and CD133 decreased with increased cell passages (* $p < 0.05$, ** $p < 0.01$, *** $p < 0.001$). (**E**) Differential interference contrast (DIC) image of cultured human PEPCs showed two distinct cell morphologies: cardiosphere-like (CS) and spindle-like cell (SC) on the fibronectin-coated plate. (**F**) and (**G**) Confocal immunofluorescence images of CS and SC cells stained with CD117, connexin (CX) 43, Ki67, CD105, (**H**) α-sarcomeric actin. Nuclei were counterstained with 4′, 6-diamidino-2-phenylindole (DAPI). Scale bar = 200 μm in E and G, and scale bar = 50μm in H.

3.2. PEPCs Differentiate toward Cardiovascular Lineage

PEPCs collected directly from patients' day 1 or day 2 ($n = 11$ in each group) after surgery expressed similar, if not all, cell surface markers including CD31, CD34, CD45, CD90, CD105, CD117 (c-kit), and CD133 (Figure 2C,D) at variable levels (no significant difference, $p > 0.05$). Day 1 PEPCs contained surface markers including CD31 (4.4 ± 2.4%), CD34 (1.4 ± 1.2%), CD45 (6.4 ± 3.7%), CD90 (15.8 ± 12.3%), CD105 (1.8 ± 1.8%), CD117 (20.7 ± 18.1%), and CD133 (0.5 ± 0.4%), CD31/CD34 (1.6 ± 1.1%), CD34/CD133 (0.3 ± 0.4), CD45/CD117 (2.4 ± 2.5%), CD90/CD105 (0.7 ± 0.6%), CD117/CD133 (0.7 ± 0.7%). After six in vitro passages, the expressions of CD45 decreased to 1.4% while no expression of CD31, CD34, and CD133. CD90 (68.9%), CD105 (90.6%), and CD117 (40.6%) increased dramatically. Co-expression of surface markers CD45/CD117 was about the same (2.2 ± 1.0%) while CD90/CD105 increased significantly to 68.9 ± 4.7%. The present in vitro culture and passage condition might favor the expansion of a distinct population progenitor cells.

PEPCs including cardiospheres (CS) and spindle-like cells (SC) (Figure 2E) proliferated rapidly by a doubling time of 5–7 days during in vitro expansion. Consistent with this observation, immunofluorescence staining of Ki67 showed strong signals in both CS and SC (Figure 2G). PEPCs also expressed various cardiac stem cell and lineage-specific cell surface markers. In general, SC exhibited antigenic markers similar to those of the CS. As shown in Figure 2F, cells from both CS and SC populations express CD117, indicating the presence of progenitor cells [23]. The majority of PEPCs expressed markers indicative of cardiovascular lineages including CD105 [24], connexin (CX) 43 [25], and α-sarcomeric actin [15] (Figure 2F–H).

3.3. In Vitro Angiogenesis of PEPCs

Conditioned medium from PEPCs enhanced angiogenesis of HUVEC in vitro. Figure 3 shows PEPCs condition medium significant enhanced HUVEC to form tubes (Figure 3C) in comparison to serum-free medium control (Figure 3A) or serum-free conditioned medium from fibroblasts (Figure 3B). The efficacy of PEPCs conditioned medium promoting tube formation was the same as medium supplemented with 10% serum (Figure 3D). The enhancement was inhibited by anti-HGF, anti-VEGF, and thalidomide (Figure 3E,F, * $p < 0.05$, *** $p < 0.001$).

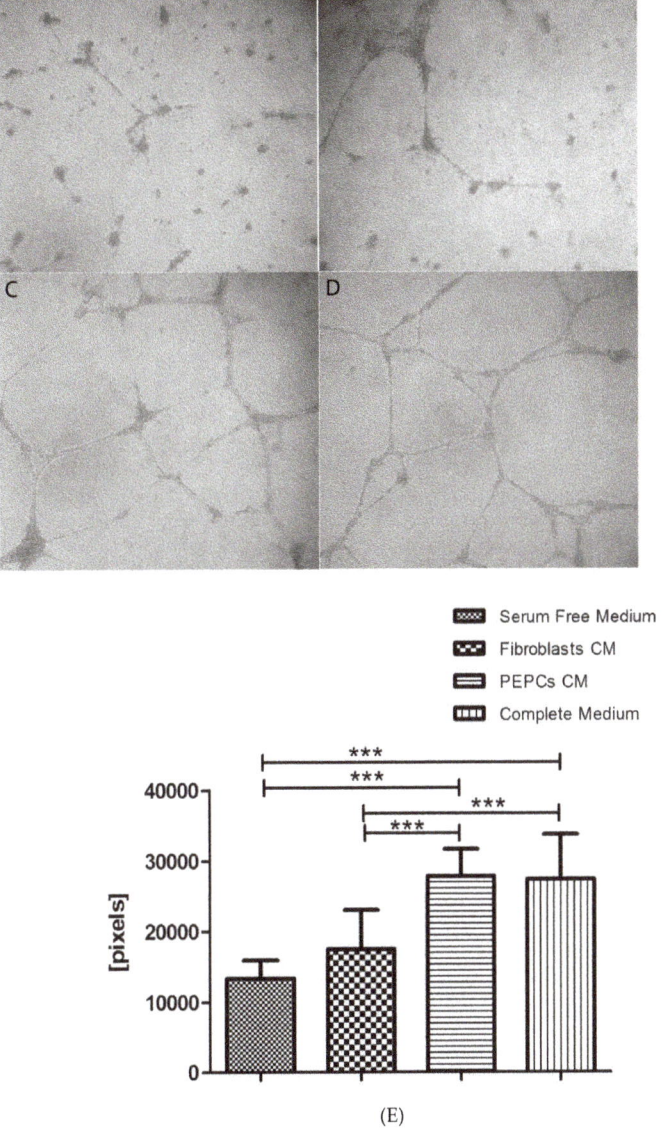

(E)

Figure 3. *Cont.*

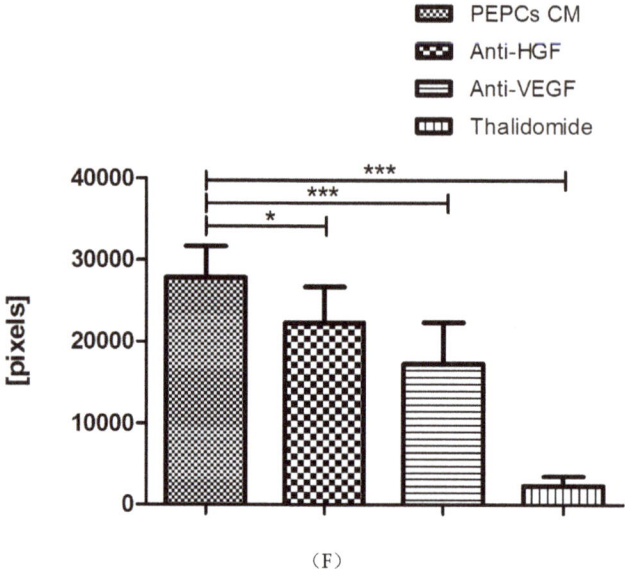

(F)

Figure 3. PEPCs conditioned medium enhanced angiogenesis in vitro. (**A**) Twenty thousand HUVEC cells were seeded on a 96-well plate pre-coated with basement membrane matrix. Cells were imaged after 18 h with a digital camera coupled to a microscope. HUVEC cells cultured in serum-free medium showed no tube formation. (**B**) Few vascular networks formed in serum-free conditioned medium from fibroblasts. (**C**) Well-formed vascular networks developed in cells cultured in PEPCs conditioned medium. (**D**) Cells cultured in completed medium (positive control) showed vascular networks as in PEPCs conditioned medium. (**E**) The total vessel length in pixels under different conditions. Data were pooled from three independent experiments expressed as average ± SD. (**F**) The enhancement was inhibited by anti-HGF, anti-VEGF and thalidomide (* $p < 0.05$; *** $p < 0.001$).

3.4. Therapeutic Potential of PEPCs and Cell Fate in Ischemic Heart Repair

Three weeks after injection of PEPCs into the margins of ischemic myocardium in mice, echocardiography revealed a significant improvement of cardiac ejection fraction compared to the PBS and fibroblast treated mice (Figure 4A,B; * $p < 0.05$). The regeneration ability was further quantified in sections stained with Masson trichrome to discriminate viable from fibrous tissue (Figure 4C–F). Ischemic hearts with PBS (negative control, Figure 4C) or fibroblasts (positive cell control, Figure 4D) transplantation showed significant heart dilatation. PEPC transplanted hearts had a smaller blue-stained (fibrous) infarct zone (25 ± 9%) compared to the hearts transplanted with fibroblasts (35 ± 7%; $p < 0.01$) or PBS-treated hearts (49 ± 17%; *** $p < 0.001$, Figure 4F).

In vivo luciferase signals from injected PEPCs declined from day 3 to day 15, and completely undetectable at day 22 after transplantation, advocating human PEPCs might not survive in injured mice hearts (Figure 4G,H). It may of interest to analyze whether any difference in cardiac repair ability between luciferase-transduced cells and non-transduced cells. However, the small sample size limited further subpopulation analysis. The absence of human cells was further confirmed by undetectable human Alu repeats in PEPC-treated infarct mouse heart (Figure 4I).

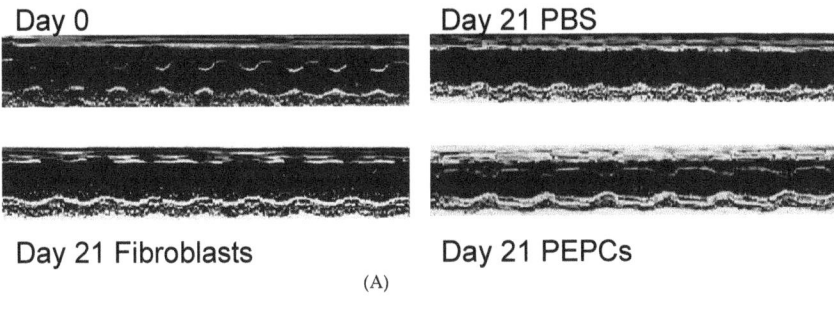

(A)

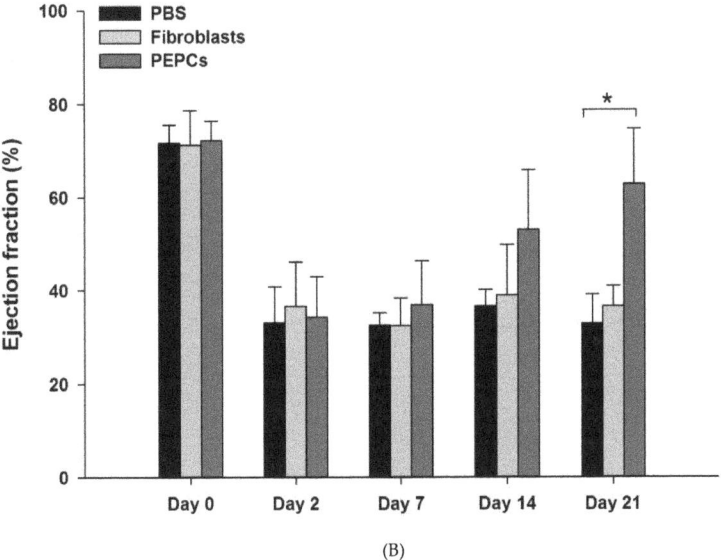

(B)

Figure 4. *Cont.*

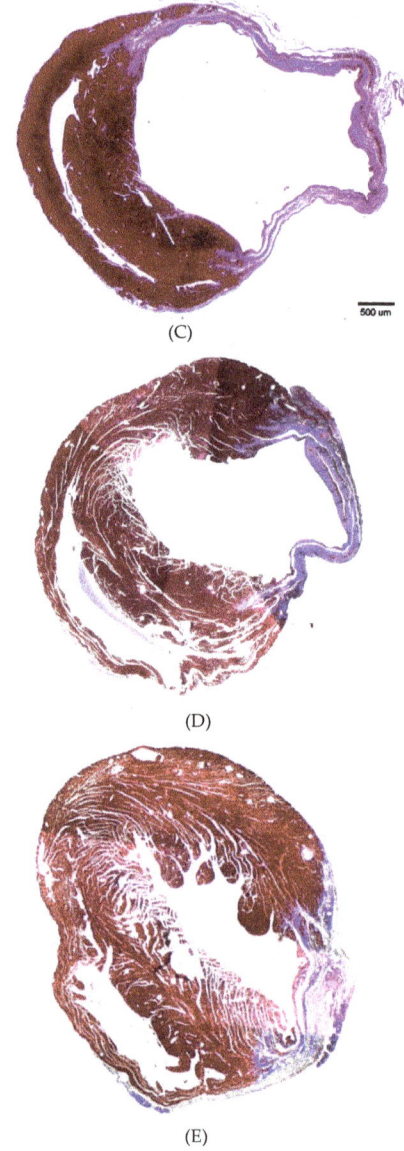

(C)

(D)

(E)

Figure 4. *Cont.*

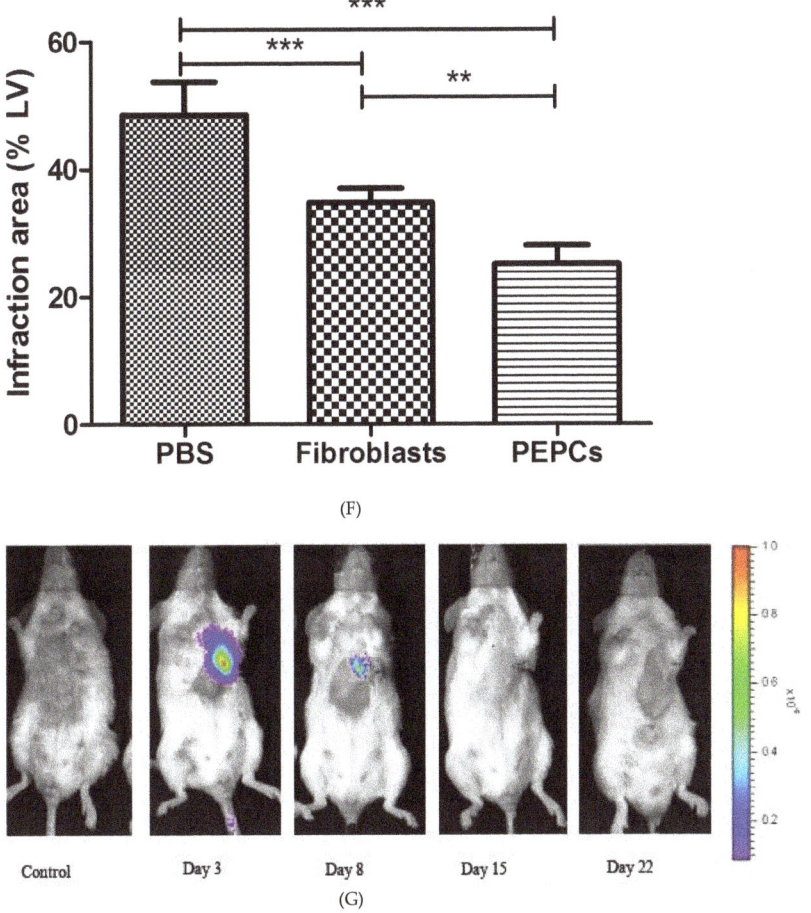

Figure 4. Cont.

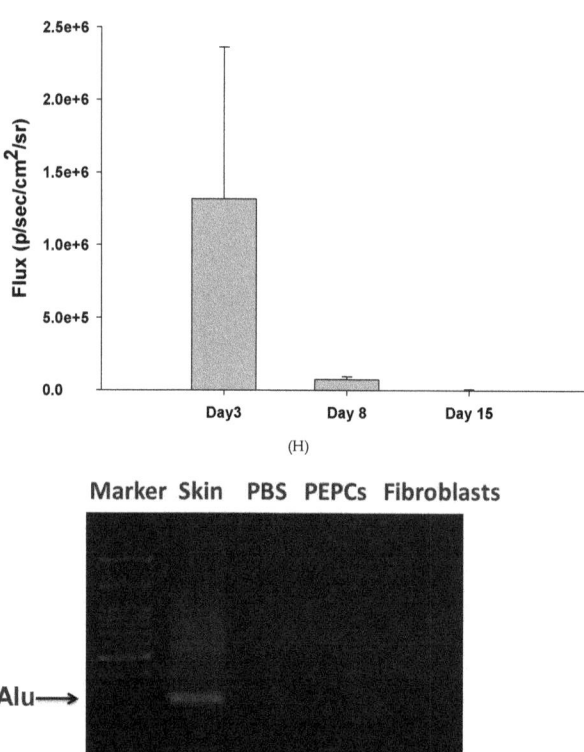

Figure 4. PEPCs restore cardiac functions and initiate tissue regeneration after transplantation into an ischemic heart. (**A**) Long-axis views from an echocardiogram performed 21 days post-infarction showed improvement of cardiac contractility after PEPCs transplantation ($n = 14$) compared to fibroblasts ($n = 16$) and PBS ($n = 11$). (**B**) Left ventricle ejection fractions were improved in mice injected with PEPCs (* $p < 0.05$). (**C**) Masson trichrome stain of ischemic heart in which viable tissue stains red whereas fibrous tissue stained blue, representative heart 3 weeks after PBS injection ($n = 11$); (**D**) fibroblasts transplanted ($n = 10$); and (**E**) PEPCs transplanted ($n = 10$). (**F**) Percent of infarction area in ischemic heart (** $p < 0.01$, *** $p < 0.001$) 3 weeks after cell transplantation. (**G**) In vivo imaging of PEPCs fate after transplantation. A representative mouse injected with 1×10^5 PEPCs showed significant bioluminescence activity on day 3, which decreased progressively over the following 3 weeks. (**H**) Quantitative analysis of signals from all animals transplanted with PEPCs (signal activity is expressed as photons/sec/cm2/sr), $n = 8$ in PEPCs transplanted mice. (**I**) No human Alu sequence was detected in mouse heart 3 weeks after PEPCs transplantation.

3.5. Paracrine Effects of PEPCs on Ischemic Heart Repair

To define the key components involved in the sustain effect of PEPCs on cardiac repair in the ischemic heart mouse model, we performed a whole genome microarray pooled from three ventricles of the mouse hearts in each group treated with PBS, human fibroblasts or PEPCs 22 days after transplantation. The heat map (baseline cutoff of ± 1.5fold change) indicated there are 95 genes regulated in the PEPCs-treated ischemic heart compared to human fibroblast-injected and PBS-injected controls (Figure 5A). Of these, 54 genes were upregulated and 41 genes were downregulated (Table S2).

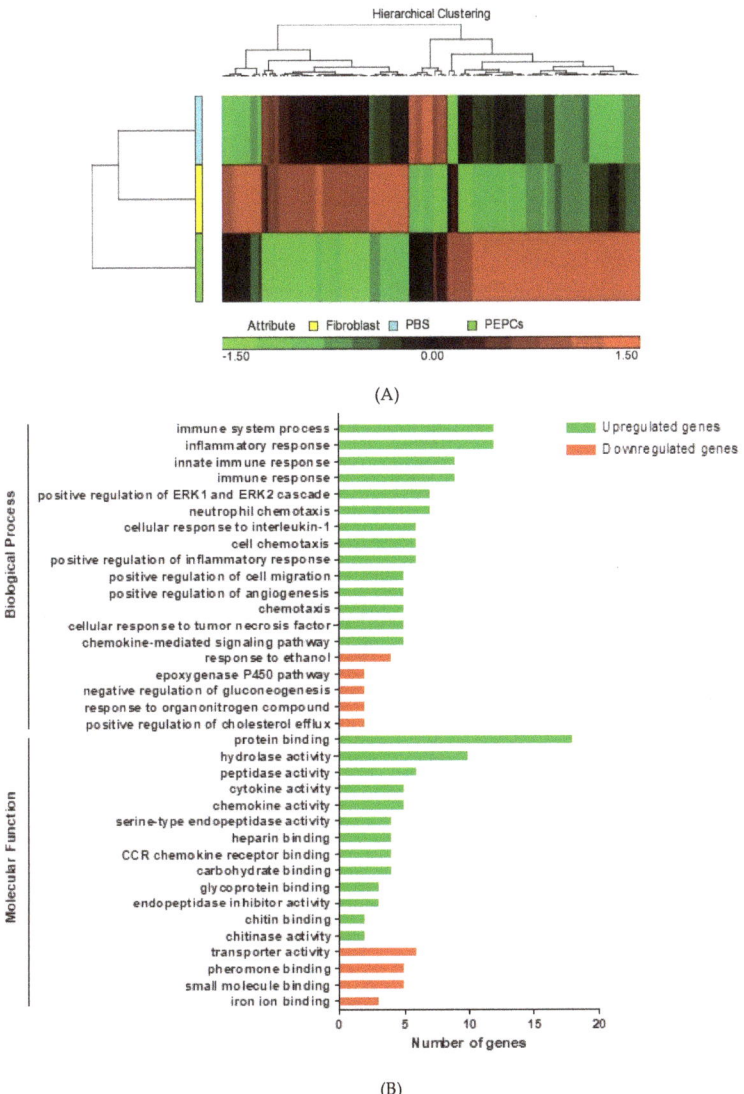

Figure 5. The difference of microarray gene expression profile after PEPCs-injected ischemic heart. (**A**) Hierarchical clustering heatmap displaying genes that were upregulated (red) or downregulated (green) in response to PEPCs, fibroblasts or PBS exposure (>1.5-fold change). (**B**) Gene ontology enrichment analysis of 95 differentially expressed genes revealed the enriched biological process and molecular function. Representative gene ontology terms listed on the bar plot have enrichment *p* values < 0.05 and the horizontal axis was the gene count.

Gene ontology analysis revealed several pathways to be significantly overrepresented in the PEPCs-treated group, including pathways involved in the immune and inflammatory response, cytokine and chemokine activity as well as paracrine signaling (Figure 5B). Particularly, genes involved in neutrophil chemotaxis such as chemokine ligands and cell adhesion such as integrins and cluster of differentiation molecules, were upregulated in PEPCs-treated ischemic hearts. Various cytokines including integrin subunit beta 2 (ITGB2) and matrix metalloproteinase-3 (MMP-3), which have been implicated in promoting angiogenesis and cell migration in the ischemic hearts [26] were increased in the PEPCs-treated group. The increased immune complements and chemokine receptors induced by PEPCs at a later time point when PEPCs were physically absent in the ischemic site suggested an enhanced homing or recruitment of host stem cells and other cell types that might contribute to ischemic heart repair [27].

4. Discussion

In this study, we found cells isolated from congenital heart disease patients' own pericardial effusion for pressure relief after cardiac surgery may have potential to treat their heart disease in the future. We named these cells as PEPCs because the drainage tube was inserted in this space to relieve pressure after the operation. The PEPCs may be originated from heart, bone marrow or fibroblasts. Further studies are needed to clarify their origin. Agarwal U et al. found an age-dependent effect of human pediatric cardiac progenitor cells isolated from juvenile heart failure patients in repairing right ventricular heart failure in a rat [28]. They divided children undergoing reconstructive surgeries into three groups based on age: neonate (1 day to 1 month), infant (1 month to 1 year), and child (1 to 5 years). Injection of neonatal cardiac progenitor cells exerting the maximum beneficial effect compared with cells from infant and child. All patients in our study are younger than 4 years old (median 9 months). PEPCs could be established from all 37 patients regardless of age, sex, and disease types in our study. However, more patients are needed to confirm age effects in the future.

During the process of PEPCs culture, two critical points could determine the efficiency of PEPCs expansion: (1) initial cell density affects the cell growth and the formation of cardiospheres, and (2) a mixed cell population at the beginning of culture benefits cell growth. Initially, we tried to culture PEPCs after purifying the $CD117^+$ cells through FACS cell sorting. Although $CD117^+$ cells have been demonstrated to represent cardiac stem cells, this subpopulation of cells grew very slowly and failed to form cardiospheres. The unfavorable cell growth of this subpopulation might attribute to a low cell density and lack of cytokines/growth factors release from other cells. We decided to culture PEPCs without cell sorting. The suspended RBC and white blood cells were removed gradually by serial changing of the medium. A highly heterogeneous population of cells, possibly including inflammatory cells, mesenchymal stem/progenitor cells, and endothelial stem/progenitor cells at the initiation of PEPCs culture might provide a better milieu for subsequent PESCs expansion by mimicking host environment. This is in line with the observation by Smith RR et.al. in the establishment of cardiosphere-derived cells from cardiac biopsy without antigenic selection. The authors speculate that a mixed cell population might be advantageous for progenitor cell proliferation and function more potent than CD117 or CD90 purified stem cell subsets after injection into infarct areas [29]. It is also true in adipose tissue-derived stem cells in vitro [22]. Sukho P. et al. showed a higher cell seeding density in the presence of inflammatory cytokines enhances endothelial cell proliferation and fibroblast migration [22].

This study is focusing on how to isolate potential progenitor cells from surgery byproduct. The limitation of the present study is the lack of a sophisticated analysis of cell function and lineage assays by differentiation PEPCs with different culture media and a head-to-head comparison with another more established cardiac stem/progenitor cell. Nevertheless, PEPCs are heterogeneous in nature, exhibiting a phenotypic signature distinct from that reported for cardiac resident stem cell [15] and mesenchymal stem cells [16]. In the present study, day 1 and day 2 primary cells expressed CD117, the receptor for stem cell factor; and CD105, the regulatory component of the transforming growth factor-beta receptor complex which is important for angiogenesis [24]. A small portion (<5%) of cells expressed CD31. CD31 is also known as platelet/endothelial cell adhesion molecule-1 (PECAM-1) and can be found on the surface of platelets, monocytes, neutrophils, and some types of T-cells [30]. Less than 2% of cells expressed CD34 (hematopoietic progenitor cell antigen) which is associated with the selection and enrichment of hematopoietic stem cells for bone marrow transplants clinically but may express in different progenitor cells [31]. Around 7% PEPCs expressed CD45, a leukocyte common antigen and an essential regulator of T and B-cell antigen receptor signaling. The surface markers data implies a mixed cell population in the fresh isolates. Around 3% PEPCs expressed CD105 and 7% expressed CD45 while cardiac resident stem cells express almost 100% CD105 and do not express CD45 [15]. However, more than 70% PEPCs expressed CD90 and CD105 without expression of CD34 after in vitro expansion to passage 6. Our results are in agreement with recent studies that CD105$^+$ MSC isolated from human heart improved ventricular ejection function in ischemic mouse heart and improved functional recovery by an ischemic limb after cells implantation [24]. MSC usually reveals a negative expression of CD34 and CD45 surface markers [32]. Colony-forming units-fibroblasts (CFU-Fs) also can repair myocardial damages [33]. The fibroblasts we used for in vivo study were originated from fetal skin. It was reasonable to expect some therapeutic effects in the ischemic heart as we showed in Figure 4D. However, these cells are CD117 negative cells. Taken together, we conclude that PEPCs may represent a distinct progenitor cell type. However, more studies are needed to clarify PEPCs as a new progenitor cell.

The safety and efficacy of clinical trials of stem cell therapy in myocardial infarction patients are encouraging yet remain in dispute [7,16]. Despite the potential uses of ideally matched autologous cardiogenic cells from PEPCs transplantation, certain risks such as tumor formation and sudden death need to be concerned before clinical application. No tumors formed or sudden death happened in the PEPCs-treated mice. The use of cells with early passage (passage 6) for expansion may minimize the risk of tumor transformation of PEPCs [34,35]. However, a long-term follow up in vivo and more experiments are needed to confirm the results.

The delay of cell harvesting to cell transplantation is one of the practical limitations in cell therapy. PEPCs expanded after six passages were used for cell therapy in eight ischemic hearts to achieve a homogenous cell background in mice. After expansion in vitro, 90% PEPCs expressed CD105 which may play a major role in therapeutic efficacy and cardiomyogenic differentiation [36]. The first 24 h drain fluid contained 6 million cells which may enough for cell therapy. It is of interest to study if the primary cells without expansion or cells with a lower passage expansion will have better or similar regenerative efficacy. We did not examine electrophysiology in PEPCs. The expression of connexin 43, a gap junction protein which plays a crucial role in the synchronized contraction, and α-sarcomeric actin, a major constituent of the contractile apparatus of cardiomyocytes [37,38] have been used as indicators for the electrical coupling potential [15]. PEPCs express both proteins, suggesting the potential to differentiate toward cardiomyocytes with electrically coupling potential. Nevertheless, long-term engraftment of implant cells may be unnecessary for cell therapy in cardiac repair and regeneration [29]. Indirect stimulation of the reparative response through paracrine effects has been one of the major hypotheses of cardiac regeneration in the first and second-generation cell therapy for myocardial infarction [16,39]. Bone marrow stem cell secretome analysis has revealed more than 100 soluble intrinsic paracrine factors, the restorative potential of which includes myocardial protection, angiogenesis, modulation of remodeling, increase in cardiomyocyte proliferation, and activation of resident progenitor cells [40]. The beneficial effects in reducing scars, reducing inflammation [41] and enhancing heart regeneration were mainly derived from indirect mechanisms such as paracrine effects [42], and exosomes secreted by cardiosphere-derived cells [43]. The recognition of dominant indirect mechanism opens a new research paradigm that secretory factors from stem cells may have potential in the regeneration of the ischemic heart [43]. However, the studying of the secretome of PECPs in vitro may not reflect the long-term effects in vivo, though it may explain the enhanced angiogenesis in Figure 3. The paracrine activity may require multiple cell type in the microenvironment. Therefore, we have used microarray to probe for differential gene expression in the infarction site. The microarray experiment at 3 weeks after transplantation revealed the upregulation of genes involved in chemotaxis, angiogenesis, and cell migration in PEPCs-transplanted heart, indicating that the long-term effect of PEPCs transplantation could trigger endogenous paracrine signaling that facilitates homing or recruitment of host stem cells and other cell types for ischemic heart repair.

5. Conclusions

In the present study, we have established a simple method for the isolation and propagation of progenitor cells from pericardial effusion which supposed to be discarded after heart surgery. Results from cardiac repair in mice suggested the potential of PEPCs in cell-based therapy in CHD. The PEPCs isolated and expanded by this method appear to have some pragmatic advantages. First, PEPCs are easy to harvest from drain fluids, the byproduct of open-heart surgery. Isolating and propagating cells without the need for cell sorting makes this technique simple and reduces the risk of contamination. Second, the yield of PEPCs is at least comparable, if not higher, to that previously reported for cardiosphere-derived cells obtained from endomyocardial biopsy (average 3 million in 4 weeks). Third, PEPCs are isolated from the same patient that will not raise an ethical issue and immune rejection for his/her future cell therapy. PEPCs may represent a new potential source for cell therapy in treating CHD with its easy harvesting protocol and potential in cardiac repairs. However, the functional characterization and differentiation of PEPCs into other cell types and the long-term safety needs to be investigated before the future application of PEPCs in the clinic.

Supplementary Materials: The following are available online at http://www.mdpi.com/2077-0383/8/7/1028/s1, Table S1. Patients' demographic data, Table S2. Differentially expressed genes in PEPCs-treated ischemic heart mice model.

Author Contributions: Study conception and design: J.N.W., C.D.K., W.T.C. and T.W.W.; Acquisition of data: J.N.W., C.D.K., W.T.C., K.L.F., Y.R., X.J., J.C., C.C.K., I.Y.C., S.T. and Y.P.L.; Analysis and interpretation of data: K.L.F., I.Y.C., H.C.L., C.H.C., C.W.L., C.K.Y., H.C.C. and T.W.W.; Drafting of the manuscript: J.N.W., W.T.C., H.C.C. and T.W.W.; Critical revision: J.N.W., W.T.C, H.C.C. and T.W.W.

Funding: This work was supported by the Ministry of Science and Technology (MOST) grants 1002627E033001; 1072321B006008; National Cheng Kung University (NCKU) B106-K028, B107-K048; National Cheng Kung University Hospital (NCKUH) 10703019, and the Center of Applied Nanomedicine, National Cheng Kung University from the Featured Areas Research Center Program within the framework of the Higher Education Sprout Project by the Ministry of Education (MOE) in Taiwan to T.W.W.; MOST grants 972314B006018MY2, 106-2218-E-006-020, NCKUH 10705004 to C.D.K.; MOST grant 105-2628-B-006-003-MY3 to W.T.C.; Focused Investment Scheme and Li Ka Shing Institute of Health Science of the Chinese University of Hong Kong to H.C.C. and GRF2010/2011 (CUHK466710) to X.J.; MOST grants 101-2314-B-006-031, 102-2314-B-006-018, 103-2314-B-006-077, NCKUH 10506007 to J.N.W.

Acknowledgments: We sincerely thank Ke-Ji Chang for technical help and Michael Hughes for critical comments on this manuscript.

Conflicts of Interest: The authors declare no conflict of interest. The study has been reported partly as a poster in the Frontiers in CardioVascular Biology 2014, 4–6 July 2014, Barcelona, Spain.

References

1. Benjamin, E.J.; Blaha, M.J.; Chiuve, S.E.; Cushman, M.; Das, S.R.; Deo, R.; de Ferranti, S.D.; Floyd, J.; Fornage, M.; Gillespie, C.; et al. Heart Disease and Stroke Statistics-2017 Update: A Report from the American Heart Association. *Circulation* **2017**, *135*, e146–e603. [CrossRef] [PubMed]
2. Zheleva, B.; Atwood, J.B. The invisible child: Childhood heart disease in global health. *Lancet* **2017**, *389*, 16–18. [CrossRef]
3. Wren, C.; Irving, C.A.; Griffiths, J.A.; O'Sullivan, J.J.; Chaudhari, M.P.; Haynes, S.R.; Smith, J.H.; Hamilton, J.R.; Hasan, A. Mortality in infants with cardiovascular malformations. *Eur. J. Pediatr.* **2012**, *171*, 281–287. [CrossRef] [PubMed]
4. Oster, M.E.; Lee, K.A.; Honein, M.A.; Riehle-Colarusso, T.; Shin, M.; Correa, A. Temporal trends in survival among infants with critical congenital heart defects. *Pediatrics* **2013**, *131*, e1502–e1508. [CrossRef] [PubMed]
5. Erikssen, G.; Liestol, K.; Seem, E.; Birkeland, S.; Saatvedt, K.J.; Hoel, T.N.; Dohlen, G.; Skulstad, H.; Svennevig, J.L.; Thaulow, E.; et al. Achievements in congenital heart defect surgery: A prospective, 40-year study of 7038 patients. *Circulation* **2015**, *131*, 337–346; discussion 346. [CrossRef] [PubMed]
6. Lui, G.K.; Fernandes, S.; McElhinney, D.B. Management of cardiovascular risk factors in adults with congenital heart disease. *J. Am. Heart Assoc.* **2014**, *3*, e001076. [CrossRef] [PubMed]

7. Behfar, A.; Crespo-Diaz, R.; Terzic, A.; Gersh, B.J. Cell therapy for cardiac repair—Lessons from clinical trials. *Nat. Rev. Cardiol.* **2014**, *11*, 232–246. [CrossRef] [PubMed]
8. Mathur, A.; Fernandez-Aviles, F.; Dimmeler, S.; Hauskeller, C.; Janssens, S.; Menasche, P.; Wojakowski, W.; Martin, J.F.; Zeiher, A.; Investigators, B. The consensus of the Task Force of the European Society of Cardiology concerning the clinical investigation of the use of autologous adult stem cells for the treatment of acute myocardial infarction and heart failure: Update 2016. *Eur. Heart J.* **2017**. [CrossRef] [PubMed]
9. Chong, J.J.; Yang, X.; Don, C.W.; Minami, E.; Liu, Y.W.; Weyers, J.J.; Mahoney, W.M.; Van Biber, B.; Cook, S.M.; Palpant, N.J.; et al. Human embryonic-stem-cell-derived cardiomyocytes regenerate non-human primate hearts. *Nature* **2014**, *510*, 273–277. [CrossRef] [PubMed]
10. Fisher, S.A.; Brunskill, S.J.; Doree, C.; Mathur, A.; Taggart, D.P.; Martin-Rendon, E. Stem cell therapy for chronic ischaemic heart disease and congestive heart failure. *Cochrane Database Syst. Rev.* **2014**, CD007888. [CrossRef]
11. Nowbar, A.N.; Mielewczik, M.; Karavassilis, M.; Dehbi, H.M.; Shun-Shin, M.J.; Jones, S.; Howard, J.P.; Cole, G.D.; Francis, D.P.; Group, D.W. Discrepancies in autologous bone marrow stem cell trials and enhancement of ejection fraction (DAMASCENE): Weighted regression and meta-analysis. *BMJ* **2014**, *348*, g2688. [CrossRef] [PubMed]
12. Abbott, A. Doubts over heart stem-cell therapy. *Nature* **2014**, *509*, 15–16. [CrossRef] [PubMed]
13. Dykstra, J.A.; Facile, T.; Patrick, R.J.; Francis, K.R.; Milanovich, S.; Weimer, J.M.; Kota, D.J. Concise Review: Fat and Furious: Harnessing the Full Potential of Adipose-Derived Stromal Vascular Fraction. *Stem Cells Transl. Med.* **2017**, *6*, 1096–1108. [CrossRef] [PubMed]
14. Roura, S.; Pujal, J.M.; Galvez-Monton, C.; Bayes-Genis, A. The role and potential of umbilical cord blood in an era of new therapies: A review. *Stem Cell Res. Ther.* **2015**, *6*, 123. [CrossRef] [PubMed]
15. Smith, R.R.; Barile, L.; Cho, H.C.; Leppo, M.K.; Hare, J.M.; Messina, E.; Giacomello, A.; Abraham, M.R.; Marban, E. Regenerative potential of cardiosphere-derived cells expanded from percutaneous endomyocardial biopsy specimens. *Circulation* **2007**, *115*, 896–908. [CrossRef] [PubMed]
16. Cambria, E.; Pasqualini, F.S.; Wolint, P.; Gunter, J.; Steiger, J.; Bopp, A.; Hoerstrup, S.P.; Emmert, M.Y. Translational cardiac stem cell therapy: Advancing from first-generation to next-generation cell types. *NPJ Regen. Med.* **2017**, *2*, 17. [CrossRef] [PubMed]
17. Cheung, E.W.; Ho, S.A.; Tang, K.K.; Chau, A.K.; Chiu, C.S.; Cheung, Y.F. Pericardial effusion after open-heart surgery for congenital heart disease. *Heart* **2003**, *89*, 780–783. [CrossRef]
18. Zudaire, E.; Gambardella, L.; Kurcz, C.; Vermeren, S. A computational tool for quantitative analysis of vascular networks. *PLoS ONE* **2011**, *6*, e27385. [CrossRef]
19. Li, Z.; Wu, J.C.; Sheikh, A.Y.; Kraft, D.; Cao, F.; Xie, X.; Patel, M.; Gambhir, S.S.; Robbins, R.C.; Cooke, J.P. Differentiation, survival, and function of embryonic stem cell derived endothelial cells for ischemic heart disease. *Circulation* **2007**, *116*, I46–I54. [CrossRef]
20. Nelson, D.L.; Ledbetter, S.A.; Corbo, L.; Victoria, M.F.; Ramirez-Solis, R.; Webster, T.D.; Ledbetter, D.H.; Caskey, C.T. Alu polymerase chain reaction: A method for rapid isolation of human-specific sequences from complex DNA sources. *Proc. Natl. Acad. Sci. USA* **1989**, *86*, 6686–6690. [CrossRef]
21. Tusher, V.G.; Tibshirani, R.; Chu, G. Significance analysis of microarrays applied to the ionizing radiation response. *Proc. Natl. Acad. Sci. USA* **2001**, *98*, 5116–5121. [CrossRef] [PubMed]
22. Sukho, P.; Kirpensteijn, J.; Hesselink, J.W.; van Osch, G.J.; Verseijden, F.; Bastiaansen-Jenniskens, Y.M. Effect of Cell Seeding Density and Inflammatory Cytokines on Adipose Tissue-Derived Stem Cells: An in Vitro Study. *Stem Cell Rev.* **2017**, *13*, 267–277. [CrossRef] [PubMed]
23. Gude, N.A.; Sussman, M.A. Chasing c-Kit through the heart: Taking a broader view. *Pharmacol. Res.* **2017**. [CrossRef] [PubMed]
24. Czapla, J.; Matuszczak, S.; Wisniewska, E.; Jarosz-Biej, M.; Smolarczyk, R.; Cichon, T.; Glowala-Kosinska, M.; Sliwka, J.; Garbacz, M.; Szczypior, M.; et al. Human Cardiac Mesenchymal Stromal Cells with CD105+CD34- Phenotype Enhance the Function of Post-Infarction Heart in Mice. *PLoS ONE* **2016**, *11*, e0158745. [CrossRef] [PubMed]
25. Britz-Cunningham, S.H.; Shah, M.M.; Zuppan, C.W.; Fletcher, W.H. Mutations of the Connexin43 gap-junction gene in patients with heart malformations and defects of laterality. *N. Engl. J. Med.* **1995**, *332*, 1323–1329. [CrossRef]

26. Keck, M.; van Dijk, R.M.; Deeg, C.A.; Kistler, K.; Walker, A.; von Ruden, E.L.; Russmann, V.; Hauck, S.M.; Potschka, H. Proteomic profiling of epileptogenesis in a rat model: Focus on cell stress, extracellular matrix and angiogenesis. *Neurobiol. Dis.* **2018**, *112*, 119–135. [CrossRef]
27. Yagi, H.; Soto-Gutierrez, A.; Parekkadan, B.; Kitagawa, Y.; Tompkins, R.G.; Kobayashi, N.; Yarmush, M.L. Mesenchymal stem cells: Mechanisms of immunomodulation and homing. *Cell Transplant.* **2010**, *19*, 667–679. [CrossRef]
28. Agarwal, U.; Smith, A.W.; French, K.M.; Boopathy, A.V.; George, A.; Trac, D.; Brown, M.E.; Shen, M.; Jiang, R.; Fernandez, J.D.; et al. Age-Dependent Effect of Pediatric Cardiac Progenitor Cells After Juvenile Heart Failure. *Stem Cells Transl. Med.* **2016**, *5*, 883–892. [CrossRef]
29. Marban, E. Breakthroughs in cell therapy for heart disease: Focus on cardiosphere-derived cells. *Mayo Clin. Proc.* **2014**, *89*, 850–858. [CrossRef]
30. Privratsky, J.R.; Newman, D.K.; Newman, P.J. PECAM-1: Conflicts of interest in inflammation. *Life Sci.* **2010**, *87*, 69–82. [CrossRef]
31. Sidney, L.E.; Branch, M.J.; Dunphy, S.E.; Dua, H.S.; Hopkinson, A. Concise review: Evidence for CD34 as a common marker for diverse progenitors. *Stem Cells* **2014**, *32*, 1380–1389. [CrossRef] [PubMed]
32. Singh, A.; Singh, A.; Sen, D. Mesenchymal stem cells in cardiac regeneration: A detailed progress report of the last 6 years (2010–2015). *Stem Cell Res. Ther.* **2016**, *7*, 82. [CrossRef] [PubMed]
33. Chong, J.J.; Chandrakanthan, V.; Xaymardan, M.; Asli, N.S.; Li, J.; Ahmed, I.; Heffernan, C.; Menon, M.K.; Scarlett, C.J.; Rashidianfar, A.; et al. Adult cardiac-resident MSC-like stem cells with a proepicardial origin. *Cell Stem Cell* **2011**, *9*, 527–540. [CrossRef] [PubMed]
34. Peterson, S.E.; Garitaonandia, I.; Loring, J.F. The tumorigenic potential of pluripotent stem cells: What can we do to minimize it? *Bioessays* **2016**, *38* (Suppl. 1), S86–S95. [CrossRef] [PubMed]
35. Lee, A.S.; Tang, C.; Rao, M.S.; Weissman, I.L.; Wu, J.C. Tumorigenicity as a clinical hurdle for pluripotent stem cell therapies. *Nat. Med.* **2013**, *19*, 998–1004. [CrossRef] [PubMed]
36. Cheng, K.; Ibrahim, A.; Hensley, M.T.; Shen, D.; Sun, B.; Middleton, R.; Liu, W.; Smith, R.R.; Marban, E. Relative roles of CD90 and c-kit to the regenerative efficacy of cardiosphere-derived cells in humans and in a mouse model of myocardial infarction. *J. Am. Heart Assoc.* **2014**, *3*, e001260. [CrossRef] [PubMed]
37. Smits, A.M.; van Vliet, P.; Metz, C.H.; Korfage, T.; Sluijter, J.P.; Doevendans, P.A.; Goumans, M.J. Human cardiomyocyte progenitor cells differentiate into functional mature cardiomyocytes: An in vitro model for studying human cardiac physiology and pathophysiology. *Nat. Protoc.* **2009**, *4*, 232–243. [CrossRef]
38. Rupp, S.; Badorff, C.; Koyanagi, M.; Urbich, C.; Fichtlscherer, S.; Aicher, A.; Zeiher, A.M.; Dimmeler, S. Statin therapy in patients with coronary artery disease improves the impaired endothelial progenitor cell differentiation into cardiomyogenic cells. *Basic Res. Cardiol.* **2004**, *99*, 61–68. [CrossRef]
39. Gnecchi, M.; Zhang, Z.; Ni, A.; Dzau, V.J. Paracrine mechanisms in adult stem cell signaling and therapy. *Circ. Res.* **2008**, *103*, 1204–1219. [CrossRef]
40. Korf-Klingebiel, M.; Kempf, T.; Sauer, T.; Brinkmann, E.; Fischer, P.; Meyer, G.P.; Ganser, A.; Drexler, H.; Wollert, K.C. Bone marrow cells are a rich source of growth factors and cytokines: Implications for cell therapy trials after myocardial infarction. *Eur. Heart J.* **2008**, *29*, 2851–2858. [CrossRef]
41. Gallet, R.; de Couto, G.; Simsolo, E.; Valle, J.; Sun, B.; Liu, W.; Tseliou, E.; Zile, M.R.; Marban, E. Cardiosphere-derived cells reverse heart failure with preserved ejection fraction (HFpEF) in rats by decreasing fibrosis and inflammation. *JACC Basic Transl. Sci.* **2016**, *1*, 14–28. [CrossRef] [PubMed]
42. Marban, E.; Cheng, K. Heart to heart: The elusive mechanism of cell therapy. *Circulation* **2010**, *121*, 1981–1984. [CrossRef] [PubMed]
43. Gallet, R.; Dawkins, J.; Valle, J.; Simsolo, E.; de Couto, G.; Middleton, R.; Tseliou, E.; Luthringer, D.; Kreke, M.; Smith, R.R.; et al. Exosomes secreted by cardiosphere-derived cells reduce scarring, attenuate adverse remodelling, and improve function in acute and chronic porcine myocardial infarction. *Eur. Heart J.* **2017**, *38*, 201–211. [CrossRef] [PubMed]

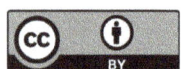

© 2019 by the authors. Licensee MDPI, Basel, Switzerland. This article is an open access article distributed under the terms and conditions of the Creative Commons Attribution (CC BY) license (http://creativecommons.org/licenses/by/4.0/).

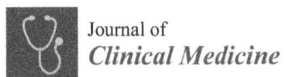

Article

Hybrid Coronary Percutaneous Treatment with Metallic Stents and Everolimus-Eluting Bioresorbable Vascular Scaffolds: 2-Years Results from the GABI-R Registry

Tommaso Gori [1,2,*], Stephan Achenbach [3], Thomas Riemer [4], Julinda Mehilli [5,6], Holger M. Nef [7], Christoph Naber [8], Gert Richardt [9], Jochen Wöhrle [10], Ralf Zahn [11], Till Neumann [12], Johannes Kastner [13], Axel Schmermund [14], Christian Hamm [7,15] and Thomas Münzel [1,2] for the GABI-R Study Group

[1] Zentrum für Kardiologie, University Medical Center, Johannes Gutenberg University Mainz, 55131 Mainz, Germany; tmuenzel@uni-mainz.de
[2] German Centre for Cardiovascular Research, partner site Rhine Main, 55131 Mainz, Germany
[3] Department of Cardiology, Friedrich-Alexander University Erlangen-Nürnberg, 91054 Erlangen, Germany; achenbach@uni-erlangen.de
[4] IHF GmbH-Institut für Herzinfarktforschung, 67063 Ludwigshafen, Germany; riemer@ihf.de
[5] Department of Cardiology, Munich University Clinic, LMU, 80539 Munich, Germany; mehilli@lmu.de
[6] German Centre for Cardiovascular Research, partner site Munich Heart Alliance, 80539 Munich, Germany
[7] Department of Cardiology, University of Giessen, Medizinische Klinik I, 35392 Giessen, Germany; h.nef@me.com (H.M.N.); hamm@neuheim.de (C.H.)
[8] Klinik für Kardiologie und Angiologie, Elisabeth-Krankenhaus, 45138 Essen, Germany; naber@contilia.de
[9] Herzzentrum, Segeberger Kliniken GmbH, 23795 Bad Segeberg, Germany; richrdt@segeberg.de
[10] Department of Internal Medicine II, University of Ulm, 89081 Ulm, Germany; woehrle@ulm.de
[11] Abteilung für Kardiologie, Herzzentrum Ludwigshafen, 67063 Ludwigshafen, Germany; zahn@klinikum.de
[12] Department of Cardiology, University of Essen, 45138 Essen, Germany; neumann@uniwien.at
[13] Department of Cardiology, University of Vienna Medical School, 1090 Wien, Austria; kastner@viennw.at
[14] Bethanien Hospital, 60389 Frankfurt, Germany; schmermund@ccb.de
[15] Department of Cardiology, Kerckhoff Heart and Thorax Center, 61231 Bad Nauheim, Germany
* Correspondence: tomgori@hotmail.com

Received: 2 May 2019; Accepted: 29 May 2019; Published: 30 May 2019

Abstract: The limitations of the first-generation everolimus-eluting coronary bioresorbable vascular scaffolds (BVS) have been demonstrated in several randomized controlled trials. Little data are available regarding the outcomes of patients receiving hybrid stenting with both BVS and drug-eluting stents (DES). Of 3144 patients prospectively enrolled in the GABI-Registry, 435 (age 62 ± 10, 19% females, 970 lesions) received at least one BVS and one metal stent (hybrid group). These patients were compared with the remaining 2709 (3308 lesions) who received BVS-only. Patients who had received hybrid stenting had more frequently a history of cardiovascular disease and revascularization ($p < 0.05$), had less frequently single-vessel disease ($p < 0.0001$), and the lesions treated in these patients were longer ($p < 0.0001$) and more frequently complex. Accordingly, the incidence of periprocedural myocardial infarction ($p < 0.05$) and that of cardiovascular death, target vessel and lesion failure and any PCI at 24 months was lower in the BVS-only group (all $p < 0.05$). The 24-months rate of definite and probable scaffold thrombosis was 2.7% in the hybrid group and 2.8% in the BVS-only group, that of stent thrombosis in the hybrid group was 1.86%. In multivariable analysis, only implantation in bifurcation lesions emerged as a predictor of device thrombosis, while the device type was not associated with this outcome ($p = 0.21$). The higher incidence of events in patients receiving hybrid stenting reflects the higher complexity of the lesions in these patients; in patients treated with a hybrid strategy, the type of device implanted did not influence patients´ outcomes.

Keywords: coronary artery disease; drug eluting stents; stent bioresorbable

1. Introduction

A number of randomized controlled trials comparing the outcomes of drug eluting stents compared to first-generation everolimus-eluting coronary bioresorbable vascular scaffolds (BVS) have shown the limitations of this novel type of devices [1–4]. When compared with drug eluting stents (DES), the mechanical limitations of BVS, including thicker and wider struts, lower radial strength, and limited expansion capabilities [5,6] represent important limitations for the treatment of complex lesions, including ostial or calcific ones, bifurcations, and lesions in small vessels. Supporting this concept, a number of post-hoc analyses have shown that this type of lesions represents predictors for BVS failure [7–9] unless a dedicated implantation technique is used [10,11]. Additionally, lesions in the left main, in by-pass grafts, and restenotic lesions have been excluded from the CE certification from the very beginning.

Based on these considerations, some authors have advocated for the use of a hybrid approach, which consists of limiting the use of BVS to settings in which the use of BVS is allowed (or considered to be safe) [12]. While this strategy is in conflict with the concept of "vascular regeneration" which represents the foundation of the use of BVS, it might still have the theoretical advantage that vessels (e.g., the proximal segments) in which long-term complications are clinically more relevant, would be "stent-free" after device resorption. Independently of the clinical rationale supporting the use of hybrid stenting, this setting however allows a direct head-to-head comparison of the outcomes of the device types independently of patients' characteristics and clinical presentation.

The multicenter German-Austrian ABSORB Registry (GABI-R) was designed to monitor the usage of BVS in everyday practice. Details on this international registry have been published elsewhere [13]. In the current analysis, we set out to assess the incidence of clinical events in patients receiving hybrid percutaneous coronary interventions.

2. Methods

Between November 2013 and January 2016, consecutive patients undergoing implantation of at least one BVS (Absorb; Abbott Vascular, Santa Clara, CA, USA) were enrolled in a prospective single-arm registry in 92 GABI-R centers. Details on the methods for patients' inclusion and follow-up in this observational registry have been previously published [13–15]. The study was conducted in accordance with the provisions of the Declaration of Helsinki and with the International Conference on Harmonization Good Clinical Practices, the protocol was approved by each local ethics committee (first Vote: Ethic committee of the Justus Liebig Universität Giessen 190/13) and all patients provided written, informed consent. Clinicaltrial.gov NCT02066623

2.1. Objective of the Study

The objective of this study was to investigate the outcome of patients receiving hybrid stenting with at least one drug eluting stent and one bioresorbable scaffold.

2.2. Procedures

Lesion preparation, BVS implantation, postdilation and use of intracoronary imaging, as well as medical therapy, were left to the operator's discretion. The protocol recommended use of pre- and postdilation. High-pressure dilation was defined as dilation with ≥14ATM. Antiplatelet therapy consisted of aspirin (loading dose 250–500 mg and maintenance dose 100 mg/day) and clopidogrel (loading dose at least 300 mg and maintenance dose 75 mg/day), prasugrel (loading dose 60 mg and maintenance dose 10 mg), or ticagrelor (loading dose 180 mg and maintenance dose 90 mg bid). Dual antiplatelet therapy was recommended for at least 12 months.

2.3. Definitions

For the purpose of the present analysis, hybrid stenting was defined as implantation of at least one Absorb BVS and one metallic stent (BMS or DES) in the same patient. The primary endpoint of the present study was the incidence of definite/probable device thrombosis in lesions/patients treated with BVS compared to metallic stents.

Procedural success was defined as visually estimated residual stenosis <30% with thrombolysis in myocardial infarction flow grade III. Other definitions were based on the Academic Research Consortium (ARC) criteria [16]. Scaffold thrombosis was defined as definite or probable. Cardiac death was defined as death from immediate cardiac causes or complications related to the procedure as well as any death in which a cardiac cause could not be excluded. Myocardial infarction (MI) was defined according to the World Health Organization extended definition. Target lesion failure (TLF) was defined as a composite of cardiac death, target vessel MI, and clinically-driven target lesion revascularization (TLR). Target vessel failure (TVF) was defined as a composite of cardiac death, target-vessel MI, and clinically driven target vessel revascularization (TVR).

2.4. Data Management and Outcomes of Interest

Data in the GABI-R were collected electronically via an internet-based application and centralized by the IHF GmbH-Institut für Herzinfarktforschung (Ludwigshafen, Germany). Patients were contacted by telephone at 30 days, six months and two years using standardized questionnaires. Follow-up, source verification, quality controls were performed centrally. All events were adjudicated and classified by an independent event adjudication committee.

2.5. Statistical Analysis

Data are presented as mean ± standard deviation, absolute frequencies and percentages, or median (lower, upper quartile) as appropriate. Data are presented per patient and per lesion. Odds-ratios (95% confidence limits) are presented to characterize the differences in event frequencies among groups. The incidence of events in the periprocedural interval and at each of the follow-up times was tested with Pearson's Chi-squared test. Concerning device thrombosis, testing for differences on patient level had to face a highly unbalanced design: There was no reference group for DES/BMS-only treatment. Thus, we implemented a loglinear model for an incomplete contingency table and three factors: BVS thrombosis, stent thrombosis, and hybrid treatment, accounting for interactions between the treatment and device type. To compare times to event (= device thrombosis) and assess the impact of the device type and hybrid stenting on outcomes, a proportional-hazard model ("Cox regression") on stent level was implemented. Intra-subject correlations were considered by using a robust sandwich estimate aggregating stent residuals to subject level. This multiple regression model included the device type as a main factor and additional pre-defined predictor variables that have been previously shown to be associated with scaffold/stent thrombosis in the GABI-R: Total stent length, lesion type, bifurcation lesion, and time of implantation (before or after January 2015). Missing values were imputed either by random drawing from the standardized empirical distribution (in case of missing times-to-event), by modal values (binary) or by median values (metrical variables). A two-tailed p value <0.05 was considered to indicate statistical significance. Statistical analyses were performed using the SAS® software, version 9.4 for Windows. Copyright © 2002–2012 SAS Institute Inc. SAS and all other SAS Institute Inc. product or service names are registered trademarks or trademarks of SAS Institute Inc., Cary, NC, USA.

3. Results

3.1. Patient Characteristics

CONSORT flow diagrams are presented in Figure 1 (left and right panel). Of 3144 (4278 lesions) patients included in the GABI-R registry who received at least one BVS and whose two-years vital status was known, 2709 (3308 lesions) were treated with scaffolds only (BVS-only group) while 435 (970 lesions) were treated with at least one additional metallic stent (hybrid group).

Patient characteristics are presented in Table 1. Patients in the hybrid group consistently showed characteristics compatible with a higher complexity: Glomerular filtration rate was lower ($p < 0.05$), the prevalence of prior PCI ($p < 0.01$), myocardial infarction ($p < 0.01$), multivessel disease ($p < 0.0001$), male sex ($p < 0.05$) were all higher in the hybrid group and there was a trend towards older age and higher diabetes prevalence in this group (both = 0.06). In line with this, procedure duration, contrast use, radiation time, and the number of lesions treated per patient were larger in the hybrid group (all $p < 0.0001$). DAPT with prasugrel was used more commonly in the hybrid group ($p < 0.05$). The prevalence of smoking was higher in the BVS-only group ($p < 0.05$).

Table 1. Baseline characteristics of the cohort.

	Total (Hybrid + BVS-Only) $n = 3144$	Hybrid Group $n = 435$	BVS Only $n = 2709$	p Value
Female gender	22.9% (721/3144)	19.1% (83/435)	23.6% (638/2709)	<0.05
Age (years, rounded)	60.87 ± 11.02	61.91 ± 10.36,	60.7 ± 11.11	0.06
Diabetes mellitus	20.9% (651/3117)	24.2% (105/433)	20.3% (546/2684)	0.06
Current smoker	34.9% (1039/2978)	30.4% (128/421)	35.6 % (911/2557)	<0.05
Arterial hypertension	73.4% (2274/3100)	75.3% (324/430)	73% (1950/2670)	0.31
Hypercholesterolemia	56.5% (1702/3010)	59.6% (243/408)	56.1% (1459/2602)	0.19
Glomerular filtration rate	79.39 ± 23.68, $n = 1590$	75.33 ± 22.55, $n = 165$	79.86 ± 23.77, $n = 1425$	<0.05
History of myocardial infarction	22.2% (687/3094)	27.4% (117/427)	21.4% (570/2667)	<0.01
History of PCI	33.9% (1044/3079)	39.6% (169/427)	33% (875/2652)	<0.01
History of aorto-coronary bypass surgery	2.5% (79/3131)	3% (13/433)	2.4% (66/2698)	0.49
History of CAD	41.1% (1137/2768)	44% (178/405)	40.6% (959/2363)	0.20
History of stroke	2.7% (85/3143)	3% (13/435)	2.7% (72/2708)	0.69
Acute coronary syndrome at presentation	51.4% (1617/3143)	47.8% (208/435)	52% (1409/2708)	0.10
Stable angina pectoris	33.5% (1053/3143)	33.1% (144/435)	33.6% (909/2708)	0.85
Left ventricular ejection fraction	56.09 ± 10.5, $n = 1930$	54.84 ± 10.15, $n = 282$	56.31 ± 10.55, $n = 1648$	<0.05
1-vessel CAD	41.9% (1317/3144)	20% (87/435)	45.4% (1230/2709)	<0.0001
2-vessels CAD	31% (974/3144)	35.6% (155/435)	30.2% (819/2709)	<0.05
3-vessel CAD	27.1% (852/3144)	44.4% (193/435)	24.3% (659/2709)	<0.0001

Values are mean ± SD or % (absolute number/number of available records); CAD = coronary artery disease; PCI = percutaneous coronary intervention, CBR = clinical BVS restenosis.

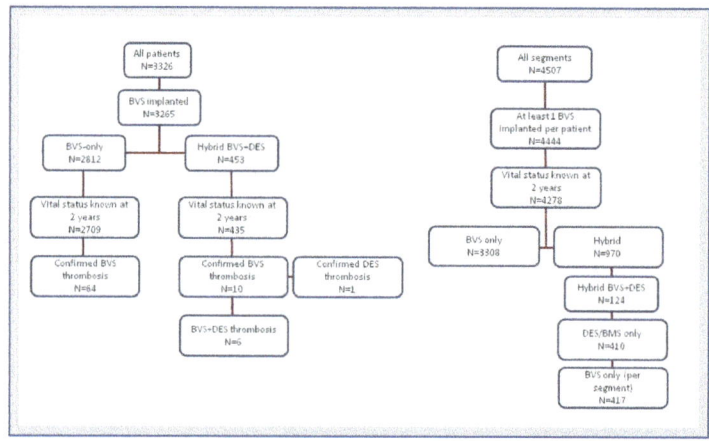

Figure 1. Study flow per patient (**left** panel) and per lesion (**right**).

Lesion characteristics are presented in Table 2. A total of 4962 BVS/Stents (4349 BVS, 631 in the hybrid group and 3718 in the BVS-only group, and 613 stents, all in the hybrid group) were implanted.

The large majority of metallic stents were DES (total of DES used: 610), and only three BMS were used. Interventions in the hybrid group were more frequent in the LAD, those in the BVS-only group were more frequent in the RCA ($p < 0.0001$ and $p < 0.05$). Compatible with the above differences between groups, all parameters expressing lesion complexity were more frequent in the hybrid group: The prevalence of B2 ($p < 0.05$), C1 ($p < 0.0001$), C2 ($p < 0.05$) lesions, bifurcation lesions ($p < 0.0001$), chronic total occlusions ($p < 0.0001$), lesions with severe tortuosity ($p < 0.05$), presence of calcium ($p < 0.05$), and lesion length ($p < 0.0001$) were higher in the hybrid group than in the BVS only group. Predilatation was performed in 93.5% of BVS-only treated patients and 85.7% of patients treated with hybrid-PCI ($p < 0.0001$). The use of high-pressure inflations, scoring balloons, rotablator, was more frequent in the hybrid group ($p < 0.001$). In contrast, postdilation was performed more frequently (73.6% compared to 68.4% in BVS-only patients.

Table 2. Angiographic and procedural characteristics.

	Total (Hybrid + BVS-Only)	Hybrid Group	BVS Only	p Value
Procedure duration, minutes	58.90 ± 28.91, n = 3141	77.83 ± 35.96, n = 435	55.85 ± 26.38, n = 2706	<0.0001
Radiation time, minutes	11.84 ± 8.22, n = 3143	18.05 ± 10.64, n = 435	10.84 ± 7.28, n = 2708	<0.0001
Amount of contrast medium, mL	174.76 ± 74.65, n = 3140	223.40 ± 91.21, n = 435	166.94 ± 68.50, n = 2705	<0.0001
IVUS	3% (94/3142)	2.8% (12/435)	3% (82/2707)	0.76
OCT	4.5% (141/3142)	4.6% (20/435)	4.5% (121/2707)	0.90
Per lesion				
Treated segments	4278	970	3308	
Lesions treated with BRS only	87.3% (3670/4204)	43.8% (417/951)	100% (3253/3253)	
Lesions treated with stents only	9.8% (410/4204)	43.1% (410/951)	0% (0/3253)	
Intervention in LAD	74.7% (1582/2118)	84.7% (287/339)	72.8% (1295/1779)	<0.0001
Intervention in LCX	59.6% (813/1363)	63.8% (153/240)	58.8% (660/1123)	0.15
Intervention in RCA	68.4% (1051/1537)	62.8% (155/247)	69.5% (896/1290)	<0.05
Graft	23.8% (5/21)	0% (0/1)	25% (5/20)	0.57
Lesion type				
A	26.5% (1133/4270)	19.4% (187/964)	28.6% (946/3306)	<0.0001
B1	37% (1579/4270)	36.1% (348/964)	37.2% (1231/3306)	0.52
B2	19.6% (836/4270)	21.9% (211/964)	18.9% (625/3306)	<0.05
C1	12.6% (539/4270)	17% (164/964)	11.3% (375/3306)	<0.0001
C2	4.3% (183/4270)	5.6% (54/964)	3.9% (129/3306)	<0.05
De novo lesion	94.2% (4025/4272)	92.9% (897/966)	94.6% (3128/3306)	<0.05
Ostial lesion	0.8% (36/4272)	0.5% (5/966)	0.9% (31/3306)	0.21
Bifurcation lesion	2.9% (123/4272)	5.5% (53/966)	2.1% (70/3306)	<0.0001
100% stenosis	5.6% (241/4272)	5.7% (55/966)	5.6% (186/3306)	0.94
Chronic total occlusion	37.3% (90/241)	63.6% (35/55)	29.6% (55/186)	<0.0001
Severe tortuosity	1.2% (52/4263)	1.9% (18/961)	1% (34/3302)	<0.05
No calcification	35.9% (1533/4270)	33.2% (320/964)	36.7% (1213/3306)	<0.05
% Stenosis	86.30 ± 11.73, n = 4275	84.92 ± 11.93, n = 968	86.71 ± 11.65, n = 3307	<0.0001
Imaging	3.2% (136/4275)	1.8% (17/968)	3.6% (119/3307)	<0.01
FFR	5.2% (223/4262)	6.7% (64/961)	4.8% (159/3301)	<0.05
RVD	2.95 ± 0.63, n = 93	3.15 ± 0.43, n = 11	2.92 ± 0.64, n = 82	0.26
Lesion length	17.12 ± 9.30, n = 4258	18.84 ± 10.51, n = 956	16.62 ± 8.85, n = 3302	<0.0001
Lesion length >34 mm	5.6% (238/4258)	8.4% (80/956)	4.8% (158/3302)	<0.0001
Any lesion preparation	91.7% (3921/4274)	85.7% (830/968)	93.5% (3091/3306)	<0.0001
Pre-dilatation	100% (3920/3921)	100% (830/830)	100% (3090/3091)	0.60
High pressure balloon	43% (1680/3908)	49.3% (408/828)	41.3% (1272/3080)	<0.0001
Non-compliant balloon	73% (1215/1665)	85.3% (348/408)	69% (867/1257)	<0.0001
Use of scoring balloon	3% (116/3921)	5.4% (45/830)	2.3% (71/3091)	<0.0001
Rotablation	0.2% (6/3921)	0.6% (5/830)	0% (1/3091)	<0.0001
Stent/BVS size, mm	3.07 ± 0.59, n = 4960	3.03 ± 0.45, n = 1243	3.08 ± 0.63, n = 3717	<0.001
Postdilatation performed	72.4% (3093/4271)	68.4% (660/965)	73.6% (2433/3306)	<0.01
High-pressure Postdilation	89.5% (2766/3090)	86.9% (573/659)	90.2% (2193/2431)	<0.05
PSP-technique	6.4% (244/3794)	12.6% (68/541)	5.4% (176/3253)	<0.0001
Procedural success	99% (4229/4273)	98.7% (954/967)	99.1% (3275/3306)	0.27
Glycoprotein IIb/IIIa inhibitors	8% (252/3143)	6.7% (29/435)	8.2% (223/2708)	0.26
Medical therapy at discharge				
Aspirin	97.3% (3056/3141)	95.9% (417/435)	97.5% (2639/2706)	<0.05
P2Y12-receptor inhibitorsClopidogrel	44% (1351/3068)	41.2% (175/425)	44.5% (1176/2643)	0.2
Prasugrel	34.1% (1045/3068)	38.6% (164/425)	33.3% (881/2643)	<0.05
Ticagrelor	21.9% (672/3068)	20.2% (86/425)	22.2% (586/2643)	0.37

Values are mean ± SD, median (quartiles) or % (absolute number/number of available records); BVS = bioresorbable vascular scaffold; CBR = clinical BVS restenosis; DES = drug eluting stent; PCI = percutaneous coronary intervention.

Lesion and procedural characteristics in the hybrid group are presented in Table 3. Of the 970 lesions in patients in the hybrid group, 417 (43.8%) had been treated with BVS only, 410 (43.1%) with DES/BMS only and there was a total of 124 lesions treated with overlapping hybrid strategy (2.9% of the total, 12.8% of the lesions treated in patients who received hybrid revascularization). An additional 19 were not classified in the database. When lesions treated with BVS-only were compared to lesions treated with DES/BMS only, BVS-only lesions were longer, more frequently type C2 (both $p < 0.05$), and there was a trend towards more frequent chronic total occlusions ($p = 0.06$). Only the prevalence of bifurcation lesions was higher in the DES/BMS-treated lesions ($p < 0.0001$). There was a total of 25 Medina 1,1,1 lesions, and 2 Medina 0,1,1 lesions in the hybrid group. There were only three cases of hybrid bifurcation stenting (metallic stent + BVS in the same bifurcation lesion). In terms of procedural parameters, larger predilation balloons, imaging and postdilation were used more frequently in BVS-treated lesions ($p < 0.01$, $p < 0.05$ and $p < 0.0001$). Procedural success was 99% in both groups.

Table 3. Lesion-level analysis, bioresorbable vascular scaffold (BVS)-treated lesions compared to lesions treated with metallic stents in the hybrid group.

	Total	BVS Only	DES/BMS Stent Only	p Value	OR (95%-CI)
Number of lesions	827	417	410		
Stenosis (%) before PCI	84.42 ± 11.94, $n = 827$	84.47 ± 11.36, $n = 417$	84.37 ± 12.51, $n = 410$	0.69	
RVD (mm)	2.96 ± 0.29, $n = 6$	2.96 ± 0.24, $n = 3$	2.95 ± 0.39, $n = 3$	1	
Lesion length (mm)	18.01 ± 9.9, $n = 815$	18.6 ± 9.66, $n = 411$	17.41 ± 10.1, $n = 404$	<0.05	
Lesion length >34 mm	6.5 % (53/815)	6.8% (28/411)	6.2% (25/404)	0.72	1.11 (0.63–1.94)
Morphology					
A	20.4% (168/823)	21.4% (89/416)	19.4% (79/407)	0.48	1.13 (0.80–1.59)
B1	36.2% (298/823)	36.8% (153/416)	35.6% (145/407)	0.73	1.05 (0.79–1.40)
B2	22.6% (186/823)	20% (83/416)	25.3% (103/407)	0.07	0.74 (0.53–1.02)
C1	15.6% (128/823)	15.1% (63/416)	16% (65/407)	0.74	0.94 (0.64–1.37)
C2	5.2% (43/823)	6.7% (28/416)	3.7% (15/407)	<0.05	1.89 (0.99–3.59)
De novo vessel	93% (767/825)	93.8% (391/417)	92.2% (376/408)	0.37	1.28 (0.75–2.19)
In-stent re-stenosis	1% (8/825)	0.5 % (2/417)	1.5% (6/408)	0.15	0.32 (0.06–1.61)
Bifurcation	5.9% (49/825)	2.4% (10/417)	9.6% (39/408)	<0.0001	0.23 (0.11–0.47)
Complete occlusion	5.3% (44/825)	6.2% (26/417)	4.4% (18/408)	0.24	1.44 (0.78–2.67)
CTO	61.4% (27/44)	73.1% (19/26)	44.4% (8/18)	0.06	3.39 (0.95–12.09)
Ostial lesion	0.6% (5/825)	0.2% (1/417)	1% (4/408)	0.17	0.24 (0.03–2.18)
Severe tortuosity	2% (16/820)	1.2% (5/416)	2.7% (11/404)	0.12	0.43 (0.15–1.26)
No calcification	33.7% (277/823)	36.3% (151/416)	31% (126/407)	0.11	1.27 (0.95–1.7)
Mild	43.7% (360/823)	44.2% (184/416)	43.2% (176/407)	0.78	1.04 (0.79–1.37)
Moderate	18.2% (150/823)	15.9% (66/416)	20.6% (84/407)	0.08	0.73 (0.51–1.04)
Severe	4.4% (36/823)	3.6% (15/416)	5.2% (21/407)	0.28	0.69 (0.35–1.35)

Table 3. Cont.

	Total	BVS Only	DES/BMS Stent Only	p Value	OR (95%-CI)
		Procedural Characteristics			
Pre-dilatation	100% (693/693)	100% (396/396)	100% (297/297)	n.d.	
High pressure balloon	51.1% (353/691)	52.3% (207/396)	49.5% (146/295)	0.47	1.12 (0.83–1.51)
Maximum balloon diameter (mm)	2.75 ± 0.46, $n = 689$	2.79 ± 0.41, $n = 395$	2.69 ± 0.5, $n = 294$	<0.01	
Scoring balloon	5.8% (40/693)	6.8% (27/396)	4.4% (13/297)	0.17	1.6 (0.81–3.15)
Rotablation	0.6% (4/693)	0.5% (2/396)	0.7% (2/297)	0.77	0.75 (0.10–5.35)
Post-dilatation	66.8% (551/825)	85.5% (355/415)	47.8% (196/410)	<0.0001	
High pressure balloon	86.5% (476/550)	89.9% (319/355)	80.5% (157/195)	<0.01	
Intravasc. imaging (IVUS/OCT/QCA) after PCI	1.6% (13/827)	2.6% (11/417)	0.5% (2/410)	<0.05	
Procedural success	99% (819/827)	99% (413/417)	99% (406/410)	0.98	

Values are mean ± SD or % (absolute number/number of available records).

3.2. Clinical Outcomes

The incidence of periprocedural myocardial infarction ($p < 0.05$, OR 4.2(1.2–14.9)) and vessel perforation ($p < 0.001$, OR 4.9(1.8–13.2)) was higher in the hybrid group. Otherwise, there was no difference in the incidence of periprocedural events.

At 30 days (Table 4), the incidence of cardiovascular death, target vessel and target lesion failure were higher in the hybrid group. Similarly, at 24-month follow-up (follow up available in 98.4% of the patients), the incidence of cardiovascular death ($p < 0.05$, OR 2.3(1.0–5.2)), target vessel failure ($p < 0.01$, OR 1.7(1.2–2.3)) and target lesion failure ($p < 0.05$, OR 1.6(1.1–2.3)), and that of any PCI ($p < 0.05$, OR 1.4(1.1–1.8)), were higher in the hybrid group.

There was no significant difference ($p = 0.13$) in the incidence of target lesion revascularization (estimates and confidence limits presented in Figure 2).

A total of 17 definite/probable stent thromboses occurred in the hybrid group during the 24-months follow-up: In six cases, they affected both (at least) a DES and a BVS in the same patient; in four cases, they only affected a BVS, and in one case only one DES.

Figure 3A,B show the two-years incidence, as well as estimates and confidence limits for the incidence of stent and BVS thrombosis in both the hybrid and BVS-only group. Before testing for differences, effects of the device type and hybrid treatment had to be separated and adjusted for possible interactions. Thereafter, with regard to treatment strategy, only a trend towards a higher incidence of BVS thrombosis remained in the BVS-only group ($p = 0.07$). With regards to the device type, BVS and stent thrombosis rates did not differ significantly, neither within the hybrid group ($p = 0.22$), between hybrid and BVS-only group ($p = 0.31$), nor pooled over all treatments ($p = 0.07$).

In the multivariable analysis, only the implantation in bifurcation lesions emerged as an independent predictor of device thrombosis (Table 5). In separate analyses neither acute coronary syndrome at index nor the implantatation technique used modified this association ($p = 0.241$ and $p = 0.637$, respectively).

Table 4. Clinical Outcomes.

	Total (n = 3144)	Hybrid Stenting (n = 435)	BVS Only (n = 2709)	p Value	OR (95%-CI)
		Periprocedural complications			
Death	0% (0/3143)	0% (0/435)	0% (0/2708)	n.d.	-
MI	0.3% (10/3143)	0.9% (4/435)	0.2% (6/2708)	<0.05	4.18 (1.17–14.87)
CABG - emergency operation	0% (0/3143)	0% (0/435)	0% (0/2708)	n.d.	-
Coronary thrombosis	0.4% (12/3143)	0.9% (4/435)	0.3% (8/2708)	0.05	3.13 (0.94–10.45)
Coronary perforation	0.5% (16/3140)	1.6% (7/435)	0.3% (9/2705)	<0.001	4.9 (1.82–13.22)
		30-days follow-up			
All-cause mortality	0.51% (16/3144)	1.15% (5/435)	0.41% (11/2709)	<0.05	2.85 (0.99–8.25)
Cardiovascular mortality	0.32% (10/3144)	0.92% (4/435)	0.22% (6/2709)	< 0.05	4.18 (1.18–14.88)
Scaffold thrombosis Definite	0.86% (27/3144)	1.15% (5/435)	0.81% (22/2709)	0.48	1.42 (0.53–3.77)
- Probable	0.35% (11/3144)	0.69% (3/435)	0.3% (8/2709)	0.20	2.34 (0.62–8.87)
Stent thrombosis Definite	0.23% (1/435)	0.23% (1/435)		-	-
- Probable	0.69% (3/435)	0.69% (3/435)		-	-
Any myocardial infarction	1.43% (45/3144)	1.84% (8/435)	1.37% (37/2709)	0.44	1.35 (0.63–2.93)
Target vessel related MI	1.18% (37/3144)	1.61% (7/435)	1.11% (30/2709)	0.37	1.46 (0.64–3.35)
Target lesion revascularization	1.08% (34/3144)	1.38% (6/435)	1.03% (28/2709)	0.52	1.34 (0.55–3.25)
Target lesion failure	1.49% (47/3144)	2.76% (12/435)	1.29% (35/2709)	<0.05	2.17 (1.12–4.21)
Target vessel failure	1.72% (54/3144)	2.99% (13/435)	1.51% (41/2709)	<0.05	2 (1.07–3.77)
		24-months follow-up			
Follow-up available	98.4% (3094/3144)	97.2% (423/435)	98.6% (2671/2709)		
All-cause mortality	3.06% (96/3135)	4.37% (19/435)	2.85% (77/2700)	0.09	1.56 (0.93–2.6)
Cardiovascular mortality	0.96% (30/3135)	1.84% (8/435)	0.81% (22/2700)	<0.05	2.28 (1.01–5.16)
Scaffold thrombosis Definite	2% (54/2694)	1.33% (5/375)	2.11% (49/2319)	0.32	0.63 (0.25–1.58)
- Probable	0.78% (21/2688)	1.33% (5/377)	0.69% (16/2311)	0.19	1.93 (0.7–5.29)
Stent thrombosis Definite	0.53% (2/374)	0.53% (2/374)		-	-
- Probable	1.33% (5/377)	1.33% (5/377)		-	-
Any myocardial infarction	5.07% (137/2703)	5.31% (20/377)	5.03% (117/2326)	0.82	1.06 (0.65–1.72)
Target vessel related MI	3.37% (91/2700)	3.19% (12/376)	3.4% (79/2324)	0.84	0.94 (0.51–1.74)
Target lesion revascularization	6% (162/2698)	7.71% (29/376)	5.73% (133/2322)	0.13	1.38 (0.91–2.09)
Target lesion failure	7.19% (195/2711)	10.24% (39/381)	6.7% (156/2330)	<0.05	1.59 (1.1–2.3)
Target vessel failure	10.21% (277/2714)	14.7% (56/381)	9.47% (221/2333)	<0.01	1.65 (1.2–2.26)
Any PCI	18.52% (505/2727)	23.02% (87/378)	17.79% (418/2349)	<0.05	1.38 (1.06–1.79)

Values are mean ± SD or % (absolute number/number of available records); BRS = bioresorbable vascular scaffold; CI = confidence interval; PCI = percutaneous coronary intervention; OR = Odds ratio.

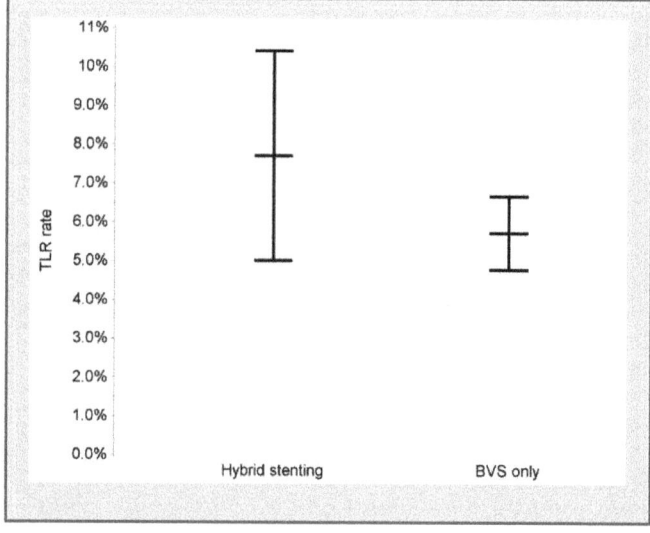

Figure 2. Two-years rates of target lesion revascularization. Comparison of Patients treated with hybrid vs. BVS-only strategy.

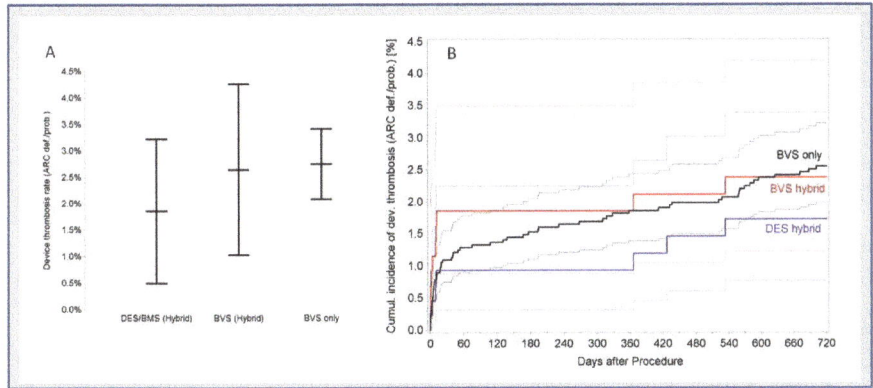

Figure 3. (**A**) Two-years incidence of device thrombosis. There was no difference among lesions treated with BVS only, metal stents only, or hybrid strategies; (**B**) cumulative incidence curves showing an overlap of the confidence intervals.

Table 5. Multivariate analysis of the predictors of definite/probable device thrombosis.

	Analysis of Maximum Likelihood Estimates				
Parameter	Parameter Estimate	Standard Error	Chi-Square	Pr > ChiSq	Hazard Ratio
Device type	0.44883	0.36030	1.5518	0.2129	1.566
Total stent length	0.21102	0.16178	1.7015	0.1921	1.235
Lesion type B2/C	−0.32342	0.26101	1.5354	0.2153	0.724
Implantation after Jan. 2015	−0.33539	0.23905	1.9683	0.1606	0.715
Bifurcation	1.04114	0.48421	4.6233	0.0315	2.832

4. Discussion

The GABI-R is a large international registry on the use of BVS. In the present analysis, we investigate the characteristics and outcomes of patients who received hybrid stenting (i.e., at least one BVS and at least one metallic stent). The major findings of the current analysis include: (i) Patients treated with hybrid stent/scaffold therapy had a more complex presentation and worse outcomes than those treated with BVS alone; (ii) During a two-years follow-up, the incidence of adverse events at the level of the lesions treated with BVS was not worse than that of the lesions treated with metallic stents.

The concept of a vascular scaffold that provides temporary mechanical support and is resorbed during follow-up to avoid a permanent unnecessary foreign body remains an attractive concept for percutaneous coronary intervention. Although initial randomized trials reported non-inferiority as compared to metallic drug-eluting stents [17,18], with signals that these devices might also be used in more complex lesion [19–22], more recent trials have consistently demonstrated a higher incidence of adverse events both early and late after implantation [3,4,23]. Mechanistic evidence shows that these increased rates might depend on the technique used at the time of implantation, inadequate selection of lesions, and, importantly, on the mechanical limitations of the devices, including increased strut thickness, reduced expansion limits, reduced radial resistance [6,8]. Further, particular settings, such as chronic total occlusions, acute coronary syndromes, treatment of ostial lesions and a lack of care at the time of implantation have all been associated with increased events, including thrombosis and restenosis [3,24–28]. Based on these notions, the general recommendation is that patients who have been treated with BVS should prolong their dual antiplatelet therapy until complete resorption of the device. This recommendation is likely to be particularly important in patients treated for complex lesions, such as those presented here. Knowledge of these limitations lead to the hypothesis that, by avoiding implantation in the presence of adverse lesion characteristics (e.g., long lesions with proximal or distal reference vessel diameters unsuitable for BVSs, very calcific or bifurcation lesions) may represent an adequate compromise between the benefit of the BVS and the risk of adverse events.

Interestingly, this setting also allows within-patients comparison of the outcomes, i.e., removes the confounding influence of differences in patient-related risk factors among groups.

Beyond any consideration on the safety of the devices implanted, it might be hypothesized that the use of BVS might be more advantageous in long and proximal segments, which might thereafter regain the possibility to adjust their diameter in response to biochemical and physical stimuli. Calcific lesions, in contrast, might have theoretically less potential for regeneration. Thrombotic lesions might also represent a setting for BVS, allowing "plaque stabilization" as previously reported [29]. The use of BVS in CTO lesions has also been reported, but no data are available regarding the capacity of these lesions to regenerate [30]. In the present database, lesions treated with BVS-only were indeed longer and more frequently of type C (thrombotic). There was a trend towards less calcific lesions being treated with BVS-only, but this difference remains speculative. Finally, in theory there is also a rationale for the use of BVS in ostial or bifurcation lesions to limit (in time) the risks associated with malapposed struts, but the evidence on their (lack of) safety in these settings clearly discouraged their use [31]. Based on the instructions for use, in the present database, bifurcation lesions were almost exclusively treated with metallic stents.

Reports on the short-term outcomes of this so-called hybrid stenting strategy (the use of both metallic stents and BVS in the same patient or lesion) have been previously published [32–35]. Collectively, these studies reported that the use of a hybrid approach might be an acceptable compromise to overcome the limitations of BVS. In the present study, we report data from a larger database with longer follow-up. In our study, the incidence of events was similar between BVS and metallic stents, while treatment of complex patients and lesions (particularly bifurcation lesions) remained an independent predictor of events. These findings confirm the hypothesis that a hybrid approach, in which more complex settings are treated with DES, might be a feasible option, although its rationale needs to be validated. While polymeric devices of the first generation (Absorb, Abbott vascular) have been removed from the market following the evidence of increased adverse events, the present results might also apply to other similar devices for which data from large databases are not available. Further, they provide a perspective for novel devices of this type.

5. Limitations

The GABI-R was a prospective registry designed to provide information on the real-life use of BVS and is therefore affected by the limitations of this type of study design. Centralized data monitoring, quality assessment, and follow-up were however performed to limit these issues. With regards to the present analysis, hybrid treatment of lesions complicates the adjudications of the events to one or the other device type. For this reason, the comparison of the incidence of device thrombosis was limited to lesions treated with only one type of device. Despite the size of the database, conclusions on very rare subsets (e.g., bifurcation lesions treated with hybrid strategy) were not possible. As well, data on the antiplatelet regimen at the time of the event are missing. The present data should not be directly extrapolated to second-generation BVS. However, they provide an insight that a prudent strategy of hybrid stenting might allow combining the benefit of bioresorbable devices with the safety of standard metallic stents also in more complex settings. The impact of a correct implantation technique has been demonstrated in a number of papers, including those from our group [8,18,24,25,27,28]. Unfortunately, the absence of a central quantitative coronary analysis in the present database does not allow clear conclusions to this regard. Finally, the comparison of the outcomes within hybrid patients removes patient-related confounders but not lesion-related confounders, which would be better addressed in trials with a randomization at lesion level.

6. Conclusions

We report on the outcome of patients undergoing BVS and DES implantation, a particularly complex subset among patients treated with BVS. In this database, which is one of the largest ones worldwide on the use of BVS, the type of device implanted did not influence patients' outcomes.

Hybrid stenting is a negotiation between the concept of "full vascular regeneration" and the mechanical limitations of these novel devices. Whether the use of metallic stents, although limited as compared to a full-metal strategy, compromises the benefits of BVS remains however to be discussed. Whether the use of a hybrid strategy with newer (and safer) scaffolds will present any advantage as compared to a full-DES strategy, will need to be studied in the future.

Author Contributions: Conceptualization, H.N. and T.G.; Methodology, T.G. and H.N.; Formal Analysis, T.G.; Writing—Original Draft Preparation, T.G.; Supervision, H.N.; Revision for intellectual content: S.A., T.R., J.M., C.N., G.R., J.W., R.Z., T.N., J.K., A.S., C.H., T.M.

Funding: The GABI Registry is supported by Abbott Vascular, and is conducted by IHF GmbH—Institut für Herzinfarktforschung, Ludwigshafen, Germany.

Conflicts of Interest: Holger Nef: Research grants (institutional) and speaker honoraria—Abbott Vascular, Gert Richart: Advisory board—Abbott Vascular, Stephan Achenbach: Research grants (institutional)—Abbott Vascular and Siemens Healthcare, Julinda Mehilli: Speaker´s honoraria and advisory board—Abbot Vascular, research grant (institutional)—Abbott Vascular; Axel Schmermund: Speaker honorarium—Abbott Vascular, Christian Hamm: Speaker honorarium—Abbott Vascular. Tommaso Gori: Research grants (institutional), advisory board and speaker honoraria—Abbott Vascular. Other authors did not report conflicts of interest.

References

1. Kereiakes, D.J.; Ellis, S.G.; Metzger, C.; Caputo, R.P.; Rizik, D.G.; Teirstein, P.S.; Litt, M.R.; Kini, A.; Kabour, A.; Marx, S.O.; et al. 3-Year Clinical Outcomes With Everolimus-Eluting Bioresorbable Coronary Scaffolds: The ABSORB III Trial. *J. Am. Coll. Cardiol.* **2017**, *70*, 2852–2862. [CrossRef]
2. Mahmoud, A.N.; Barakat, A.F.; Elgendy, A.Y.; Schneibel, E.; Mentias, A.; Abuzaid, A.; Elgendy, I.Y. Long-Term Efficacy and Safety of Everolimus-Eluting Bioresorbable Vascular Scaffolds Versus Everolimus-Eluting Metallic Stents: A Meta-Analysis of Randomized Trials. *Circ. Cardiovasc. Interv.* **2017**, *10*, e005286. [CrossRef] [PubMed]
3. Polimeni, A.; Anadol, R.; Munzel, T.; Indolfi, C.; De Rosa, S.; Gori, T. Long-term outcome of bioresorbable vascular scaffolds for the treatment of coronary artery disease: a meta-analysis of RCTs. *BMC Cardiovasc. Disord.* **2017**, *17*, 147. [CrossRef] [PubMed]
4. Wykrzykowska, J.J.; Kraak, R.P.; Hofma, S.H.; van der Schaaf, R.J.; Arkenbout, E.K.; Ijsselmuiden, A.J.; Elias, J.; van Dongen, I.M.; Tijssen, R.Y.G.; Koch, K.T.; et al. Bioresorbable Scaffolds versus Metallic Stents in Routine PCI. *N. Engl. J. Med.* **2017**, *376*, 2319–2328. [CrossRef]
5. Foin, N.; Lee, R.; Mattesini, A.; Caiazzo, G.; Fabris, E.; Kilic, I.D.; Chan, J.N.; Huang, Y.; Venkatraman, S.S.; Di Mario, C.; et al. Bioabsorbable vascular scaffold overexpansion: insights from in vitro post-expansion experiments. *EuroIntervention* **2016**, *11*, 1389–1399. [CrossRef] [PubMed]
6. Ormiston, J.A.; Webber, B.; Ubod, B.; Darremont, O.; Webster, M.W. An independent bench comparison of two bioresorbable drug-eluting coronary scaffolds (Absorb and DESolve) with a durable metallic drug-eluting stent (ML8/Xpedition). *EuroIntervention* **2015**, *11*, 60–67. [CrossRef]
7. Anadol, R.; Lorenz, L.; Weissner, M.; Ullrich, H.; Polimeni, A.; Münzel, T.; Gori, T. Characteristics and outcome of patients with complex coronary lesions treated with bioresorbable scaffolds Three years follow-up in a cohort of consecutive patients. *EuroIntervention* **2018**, *14*, e1011–e1019. [CrossRef]
8. Ellis, S.G.; Gori, T.; Serruys, P.W.; Nef, H.; Steffenino, G.; Brugaletta, S.; Munzel, T.; Feliz, C.; Schmidt, G.; Sabaté, M. Clinical, Angiographic, and Procedural Correlates of Very Late Absorb Scaffold Thrombosis: Multistudy Registry Results. *JACC. Cardiovasc. Interv.* **2018**, *11*, 638–644. [CrossRef] [PubMed]
9. Wohrle, J.; Nef, H.M.; Naber, C.; Achenbach, S.; Riemer, T.; Mehilli, J.; Münzel, T.; Schneider, S.; Markovic, S.; Seeger, J.; et al. Predictors of early scaffold thrombosis: results from the multicenter prospective German-Austrian ABSORB RegIstRy. *Coron. Artery Dis.* **2018**, *29*, 389–396. [CrossRef]
10. Regazzoli, D.; Latib, A.; Ezhumalai, B.; Tanaka, A.; Leone, P.P.; Khan, S.; Kumar, V.; Rastogi, V.; Ancona, M.B.; Mangieri, A.; et al. Long-term follow-up of BVS from a prospective multicenter registry: Impact of a dedicated implantation technique on clinical outcomes. *Int. J. Cardiol.* **2018**, *270*, 113–117. [CrossRef] [PubMed]
11. Anadol, R.; Gori, T. The mechanisms of late scaffold thrombosis. *Clin. Hemorheol. Microcirc.* **2017**, *67*, 343–346. [CrossRef] [PubMed]

12. Tanaka, A.; Jabbour, R.J.; Mitomo, S.; Latib, A.; Colombo, A. Hybrid Percutaneous Coronary Intervention With Bioresorbable Vascular Scaffolds in Combination With Drug-Eluting Stents or Drug-Coated Balloons for Complex Coronary Lesions. *JACC. Cardiovasc. Interv.* **2017**, *10*, 539–547. [CrossRef]
13. Nef, H.; Wiebe, J.; Achenbach, S.; Münzel, T.; Naber, C.; Richardt, G.; Mehilli, J.; Wöhrle, J.; Neumann, T.; Biermann, J.; et al. Evaluation of the short- and long-term safety and therapy outcomes of the everolimus-eluting bioresorbable vascular scaffold system in patients with coronary artery stenosis: Rationale and design of the German-Austrian ABSORB RegIstRy (GABI-R). *Cardiovasc. Revasc. Med.* **2016**, *17*, 34–37. [CrossRef] [PubMed]
14. Nef, H.M.; Wiebe, J.; Kastner, J.; Mehilli, J.; Muenzel, T.; Naber, C.; Neumann, T.; Richardt, G.; Schmermund, A.; Woehrle, J.; et al. Everolimus-eluting bioresorbable scaffolds in patients with coronary artery disease: Results from the German-Austrian ABSORB RegIstRy (GABI-R). *EuroIntervention* **2017**, *13*, 1311–1318. [CrossRef]
15. Mehilli, J.; Achenbach, S.; Woehrle, J.; Baquet, M.; Riemer, T.; Muenzel, T.; Nef, H.; Naber, C.; Richardt, G.; Zahn, R.; et al. Clinical restenosis and its predictors after implantation of everolimus-eluting bioresorbable vascular scaffolds: results from GABI-R. *EuroIntervention* **2017**, *13*, 1319–1326. [CrossRef]
16. Cutlip, D.E.; Windecker, S.; Mehran, R.; Boam, A.; Cohen, D.J.; van Es, G.A.; Steg, P.G.; Morel, M.A.; Mauri, L.; Vranckx, P.; et al. Clinical end points in coronary stent trials: a case for standardized definitions. *Circulation* **2007**, *115*, 2344–2351. [CrossRef]
17. Kimura, T.; Kozuma, K.; Tanabe, K.; Nakamura, S.; Yamane, M.; Muramatsu, T.; Saito, S.; Yajima, J.; Hagiwara, N.; Mitsudo, K.; et al. A randomized trial evaluating everolimus-eluting Absorb bioresorbable scaffolds vs. everolimus-eluting metallic stents in patients with coronary artery disease: ABSORB Japan. *Eur. Heart J.* **2015**, *36*, 3332–3342. [CrossRef]
18. Stone, G.W.; Gao, R.; Kimura, T.; Kereiakes, D.J.; Ellis, S.G.; Onuma, Y.; Cheong, W.F.; Jones-McMeans, J.; Su, X.; Zhang, Z.; et al. 1-year outcomes with the Absorb bioresorbable scaffold in patients with coronary artery disease: a patient-level, pooled meta-analysis. *Lancet* **2016**, *387*, 387–1277. [CrossRef]
19. De Ribamar Costa, J.; Abizaid, A.; Bartorelli, A.L.; Whitbourn, R.; Jepson, N.; Perin, M.; Steinwender, C.; Stuteville, M.; Ediebah, D.; Sudhir, K.; et al. One-year clinical outcomes of patients treated with everolimus-eluting bioresorbable vascular scaffolds versus everolimus-eluting metallic stents: a propensity score comparison of patients enrolled in the ABSORB EXTEND and SPIRIT trials. *EuroIntervention* **2016**, *12*, 1255–1262. [CrossRef] [PubMed]
20. La Manna, A.; Chisari, A.; Giacchi, G.; Capodanno, D.; Longo, G.; Di Silvestro, M.; Capranzano, P.; Tamburino, C. Everolimus-eluting bioresorbable vascular scaffolds versus second generation drug-eluting stents for percutaneous treatment of chronic total coronary occlusions: Technical and procedural outcomes from the GHOST-CTO registry. *Catheter Cardiovasc. Interv.* **2016**, *88*, E155–E163. [CrossRef]
21. Tamburino, C.; Capranzano, P.; Gori, T.; Latib, A.; Lesiak, M.; Nef, H.; Caramanno, G.; Naber, C.; Mehilli, J.; Di Mario, C.; et al. 1-Year Outcomes of Everolimus-Eluting Bioresorbable Scaffolds Versus Everolimus-Eluting Stents: A Propensity-Matched Comparison of the GHOST-EU and XIENCE V USA Registries. *JACC. Cardiovasc. Interv.* **2016**, *9*, 9–440. [CrossRef]
22. Lesiak, M.; Zawada-Iwanczyk, S.; Lanocha, M.; Klotzka, A.; Lesiak, M. Bioresorbable scaffolds for complex coronary interventions. *Minerva Cardioangiol.* **2018**, *66*, 477–488. [PubMed]
23. Sorrentino, S.; Giustino, G.; Mehran, R.; Kini, A.S.; Sharma, S.K.; Faggioni, M.; Farhan, S.; Vogel, B.; Indolfi, C.; Dangas, G.D. Everolimus-Eluting Bioresorbable Scaffolds Versus Everolimus-Eluting Metallic Stents. *J. Am. Coll. Cardiol.* **2017**, *69*, 3055–3066. [CrossRef]
24. Dimitriadis, Z.; Polimeni, A.; Anadol, R.; Geyer, M.; Weissner, M.; Ullrich, H.; Münzel, T.; Gori, T. Procedural Predictors for Bioresorbable Vascular Scaffold Thrombosis: Analysis of the Individual Components of the "PSP" Technique. *J. Clin. Med.* **2019**, *8*, 93. [CrossRef] [PubMed]
25. Gori, T.; Polimeni, A.; Indolfi, C.; Räber, L.; Adriaenssens, T.; Münzel, T. Predictors of stent thrombosis and their implications for clinical practice. *Nat. Rev. Cardiol.* **2019**, *16*, 243–256. [CrossRef]
26. Polimeni, A.; Anadol, R.; Münzel, T.; De Rosa, S.; Indolfi, C.; Gori, T. Predictors of bioresorbable scaffold failure in STEMI patients at 3years follow-up. *I. J. Cardiol.* **2018**, *268*, 68–74.
27. Polimeni, A.; Weissner, M.; Schochlow, K.; Ullrich, H.; Indolfi, C.; Dijkstra, J.; Anadol, R.; Münzel, T.; Gori, T. Incidence, Clinical Presentation, and Predictors of Clinical Restenosis in Coronary Bioresorbable Scaffolds. *JACC. Cardiovasc. Interv.* **2017**, *10*, 1819–1827. [CrossRef]

28. Sorrentino, S.; De Rosa, S.; Ambrosio, G.; Mongiardo, A.; Spaccarotella, C.; Polimeni, A.; Sabatino, J.; Torella, D.; Caiazzo, G.; Indolfi, C. The duration of balloon inflation affects the luminal diameter of coronary segments after bioresorbable vascular scaffolds deployment. *BMC Cardiovasc. Disord.* **2015**, *15*, 169. [CrossRef] [PubMed]
29. Brugaletta, S.; Gomez-Lara, J.; Garcia-Garcia, H.M.; Heo, J.H.; Farooq, V.; van Geuns, R.J.; Chevalier, B.; Windecker, S.; McClean, D.; Thuesen, L. Analysis of 1 year virtual histology changes in coronary plaque located behind the struts of the everolimus eluting bioresorbable vascular scaffold. *Int. J. Cardiovasc. Imaging* **2012**, *28*, 1307–1314. [CrossRef] [PubMed]
30. Polimeni, A.; Anadol, R.; Münzel, T.; Geyer, M.; De Rosa, S.; Indolfi, C.; Gori, T. Bioresorbable vascular scaffolds for percutaneous treatment of chronic total coronary occlusions: a meta-analysis. *BMC Cardiovasc. Disord.* **2019**, *19*, 59. [CrossRef]
31. Gori, T.; Wiebe, J.; Capodanno, D.; Latib, A.; Lesiak, M.; Pyxaras, S.A.; Mehilli, J.; Caramanno, G.; Di Mario, C.; Brugaletta, S.; et al. Early and midterm outcomes of bioresorbable vascular scaffolds for ostial coronary lesions: insights from the GHOST-EU registry. *EuroIntervention* **2016**, *12*, e550–556. [CrossRef] [PubMed]
32. Gil, R.J.; Bil, J.; Pawłowski, T.; Yuldashev, N.; Kołakowski, L.; Jańczak, J.; Jabłoński, W.; Paliński, P. The use of bioresorbable vascular scaffold Absorb BVS(R) in patients with stable coronary artery disease: one-year results with special focus on the hybrid bioresorbable vascular scaffolds and drug eluting stents treatment. *Kardiol. Pol.* **2016**, *74*, 627–633. [CrossRef] [PubMed]
33. Rigatelli, G.; Avvocata, F.D.; Ronco, F.; Giordan, M.; Roncon, L.; Caprioglio, F.; Grassi, G.; Faggian, G.; Cardaioli, P. Edge-to-Edge Technique to Minimize Ovelapping of Multiple Bioresorbable Scaffolds Plus Drug Eluting Stents in Revascularization of Long Diffuse Left Anterior Descending Coronary Artery Disease. *J. Interv. Cardiol.* **2016**, *29*, 275–284. [CrossRef] [PubMed]
34. Karbassi, A.; Kassaian, S.E.; Poorhosseini, H.; Salarifar, M.; Jalali, A.; Nematipour, E.; Kazazi, E.H.; Alidoosti, M.; Hajizeinali, A.M.; Tokaldani, M.L. Selective versus exclusive use of drug-eluting stents in treating multivessel coronary artery disease: a real-world cohort study. *Tex. Heart Inst. J.* **2014**, *41*, 477–483. [CrossRef]
35. Naganuma, T.; Latib, A.; Ielasi, A.; Panoulas, V.F.; Sato, K.; Miyazaki, T.; Colombo, A. No more metallic cages: an attractive hybrid strategy with bioresorbable vascular scaffold and drug-eluting balloon for diffuse or tandem lesions in the same vessel. *Int. J.Cardiol.* **2014**, *172*, 618–619. [CrossRef] [PubMed]

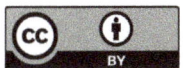

© 2019 by the authors. Licensee MDPI, Basel, Switzerland. This article is an open access article distributed under the terms and conditions of the Creative Commons Attribution (CC BY) license (http://creativecommons.org/licenses/by/4.0/).

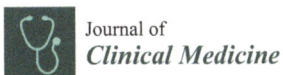

Article

Incidental Finding of Strut Malapposition Is a Predictor of Late and Very Late Thrombosis in Coronary Bioresorbable Scaffolds

Niklas F. Boeder [1,2], Melissa Weissner [2], Florian Blachutzik [1], Helen Ullrich [2], Remzi Anadol [2], Monique Tröbs [3], Thomas Münzel [2], Christian W. Hamm [1], Jouke Dijkstra [4], Stephan Achenbach [3], Holger M. Nef [1,†] and Tommaso Gori [2,*,†]

1. Medical Clinic I, University Hospital of Giessen, Klinikstrasse 33, 35392 Giessen, Germany; niklas.boeder@innere.med.uni-giessen.de (N.F.B.); Florian.Blachutzik@innere.med.uni-giessen.de (F.B.); christian.hamm@innere.med.uni-giessen.de (C.W.H.); holger.nef@innere.med.uni-giessen.de (H.M.N.)
2. Zentrum für Kardiologie, University Hospital Mainz, Langenbeckstrasse 1, 55131 Mainz, Germany and German Center for Cardiac and Vascular Research (DZHK), Standort Rhein-Main; melissaweissner@web.de (M.W.); hullrich@students.uni-mainz.de (H.U.); remzi.anadol@unimedizin-mainz.de (R.A.); tmuenzel@uni-mainz.de (T.M.)
3. Department of Cardiology, University Hospital of Erlangen, Ulmenweg 18, 91054 Erlangen, Germany; monique.troebs@uk-erlangen.de (M.T.); stephan.achenbach@uk-erlangen.de (S.A.)
4. Department of Radiology, Leiden University Medical Center, P.O. Box 9600 (mailstop C2-S), 2300 Leiden, The Netherlands; j.dijkstra@lumc.nl

* Correspondence: tommaso.gori@unimedizin-mainz.de; Tel.: +49-6131-17-2829; Fax: +49-6131-17-6428
† These authors contributed equally.

Received: 19 March 2019; Accepted: 25 April 2019; Published: 27 April 2019

Abstract: Malapposition is a common finding in stent and scaffold thrombosis (ScT). Evidence from studies with prospective follow-up, however, is scarce. We hypothesized that incidental observations of strut malapposition might be predictive of late ScT during subsequent follow-up. One hundred ninety-seven patients were enrolled in a multicentre registry with prospective follow-up. Optical coherence tomography (OCT), performed in an elective setting, was available in all at 353 (0–376) days after bioresorbable scaffold (BRS) implantation. Forty-four patients showed evidence of malapposition that was deemed not worthy of intervention. Malapposition was not associated with any clinical or procedural parameter except for a higher implantation pressure ($p = 0.0008$). OCT revealed that malapposition was associated with larger vessel size, less eccentricity (all $p < 0.01$), and a tendency for more uncovered struts ($p = 0.06$). Late or very late ScT was recorded in seven of these patients 293 (38–579) days after OCT. OCT-diagnosed malapposition was a predictor of late and very late scaffold thrombosis ($p < 0.001$) that was independent of the timing of diagnosis. We provide evidence that an incidental finding of malapposition—regardless of the timing of diagnosis of the malapposition—during an elective exam is a predictor of late and very late ScT. Our data provide a rationale to consider prolonged dual antiplatelet therapy if strut malapposition is observed.

Keywords: stent thrombosis; bioresorbable scaffold; optical coherence tomography

1. Introduction

Bioresorbable scaffolds (BRS) were introduced to offer transient vessel support after coronary angioplasty while avoiding long-term risks associated with permanent metallic stents [1]. However, the BRS with by far the most clinical experience, the everolimus-eluting Absorb BRS (Abbott Vascular, Santa Clara, CA, USA), showed an unexpectedly high incidence of scaffold thrombosis (ScT) both early and late after implantation in a number of single- and multicentre observational studies [2–6] and was ultimately removed from the market. Incomplete expansion of the BRS is believed to convey the highest risk of early ScT and implantation techniques aimed to achieve full expansion of the device were shown to reduce the incidence of early ScT [7]. In contrast, studies based on quantitative coronary angiography provided evidence that undersizing (i.e., choice of a BRS smaller than the reference vessel) is strongly associated with late adverse events [8,9]. The mechanism(s) of this association remain speculative, however, it can be hypothesized that malapposition and the resulting disturbances in blood flow dynamics might play a role.

While the mechanistic rationale for the association of malapposition and late stent/scaffold thrombosis is solid [10,11], evidence to date is limited to observational studies in which malapposition was frequently found in cases of ScT [12–16]. Therefore, the aim of this study was to investigate whether incidental observation of scaffold malapposition would predict subsequent late and very late ScT.

2. Methods

2.1. Objective of the Study

The hypothesis of the study was that incidental optical coherence tomography (OCT) evidence of scaffold malapposition (observed in an elective setting and not deemed worthy of intervention at the time of OCT) might predict the occurrence of ScT during subsequent follow-up.

2.2. Patients

Consecutive patients treated at three high-volume centres in Germany (University of Mainz; University of Giessen; University of Erlangen) with Absorb BRS between April 2012 and March 2016 who satisfied the following criteria were included in this multicentre registry:

- Patients had undergone elective OCT at the end of the implantation procedure, during non-target vessel-staged procedures, or in the setting of elective invasive exams.
- In none of these patients was there evidence of ischemia in the region perfused by the vessel treated with BRS and OCTs had been performed as elective controls after implantation of these novel devices.
- An experienced interventionalist (based on current experts' recommendations [17]) reviewed the OCT and saw no clinical indication for the re-treatment of these lesions.

Patient and procedural data were entered retrospectively after inclusion in the study. Follow-up data were acquired prospectively by trained medical staff during clinical visits and telephone interviews. Referring cardiologists, general practitioners, and patients were contacted whenever necessary for further information. All data were internally audited at each centre by trained local staff and were entered retrospectively into the multicentre database in an anonymized way according to national privacy policies and laws and following the requirements of the local ethics committees. Data were audited centrally for consistency and plausibility and queries were generated when necessary.

2.3. Definitions

Frequency domain-OCT was performed using the Ilumien Optis system (St. Jude Medical, Inc., Minneapolis, MN, USA). OCT imaging catheters were inserted distally to the treated segments and the pullback was recorded until either the guiding catheter was reached or the maximum pullback length was completed. If necessary, two sequential pullbacks were acquired to image the scaffolded segment.

OCT measurements were made offline using the QCU-CMS software (Medis, Leiden, Netherlands) by trained staff using standardized operating procedures. Longitudinal cross-sections were analysed at 1 mm intervals within the stented lesion and 5 mm proximally and distally to the scaffold. Among others, the following quantitative parameters were determined: The percentage of incomplete strut apposition (ISA) at 1 mm intervals calculated as a percentage of the total number of malapposed struts divided by the total number of struts; malapposition distance, length, and area; the eccentricity index computed as the ratio between the minimum and maximum diameters; the symmetry index defined as the difference between maximum scaffold diameter and minimum scaffold diameter divided by the maximum scaffold diameter; presence of evaginations, peri-strut low intensity areas (PSLIA), and microvessels. Evaginations were defined as any outwards protrusion in the luminal vessel contour beyond the struts' abluminal surface between well-apposed struts. Strut discontinuity/disruptions were diagnosed if there was evidence of isolated (malapposed) struts or groups of struts that did not fit the normal circular geometry of the scaffold in one or more than one cross section by more than 33% of the distance between the centre of gravity and the lumen. Further, cases where there was evidence of a clear gap (frames without any strut) were also diagnosed as strut discontinuity [18].

Definitions are described in detail in [19]. Briefly, malapposition was defined as a lack of contact of at least 1 strut with the underlying vessel wall (at least 150 μm, in the absence of a side branch) with evidence of blood flow behind the strut. It was classified as "major" malapposition if there was evidence of at least 30% of the struts in one frame. Neovessels were defined as sharply delimitated, signal-poor lacunae that extended over multiple contiguous frames. Peri-strut low intensity areas (PSLIAs) were defined as homogeneous, non-signal-attenuating zones around struts that were of lower intensity than the surrounding tissue. Peri-strut intensity was measured at the mid-strut at a depth of 150 μm from the lumen and at equal distance between two contiguous struts based on intensity of the "key" component of the CMYK (cyan, magenta, yellow, and key) colour model based on raw cross-sectional images. Quantitative assessment was obtained at 5 mm proximal and distal to the BRS to measure the proximal and distal reference vessel area (RVA). RVA was calculated as the mean of the 2 largest luminal areas 5 mm proximal and distal to the BRS edge [20]. If no meaningful value for proximal or distal RVA was obtained, the largest luminal cross-sectional area at either end was used. Incomplete expansion was defined as a minimum scaffold area of at least 90% in both the proximal and distal halves of the scaffold relative to the closest reference segment.

ScT was centrally adjudicated and classified as definite, probable, and possible according to the Academic Research Consortium criteria based on the analysis of original documents [21]. Definite ScT required angiographic or autopsy confirmation with thrombus originating in the BRS or in the segment 5mm proximal or distal to the BRS. Probable ScT was considered to have occurred after intracoronary stenting in the following cases: any unexplained death within the first 30 days or any myocardial infarction—irrespective of the time after the index procedure—that is related to documented acute ischemia in the region of the implanted BRS without angiographic confirmation, in the absence of any other obvious cause. Possible ScT was considered to have occurred with any unexplained death from 30 days after intracoronary stenting until the end of trial follow-up.

2.4. Statistical Analysis

Statistical analysis was performed using IBM SPSS Statistics (SPSS Statistics 23, IBM Deutschland GmbH, Ehningen, Germany). Categorical data are presented as absolute numbers and percentages. Continuous variables are given as mean (SD) or median (IQR). The frequencies of categorical variables were compared by the Pearson chi-square test and the distribution of continuous variables was compared by the Mann–Whitney–Wilcoxon test. No imputation was performed. A Kaplan–Meier curve was used to plot time-to-event curves and the hypothesis that malapposition could be associated with incident ScT was tested using a log-rank test. Exploratory univariate and multivariable Cox regression analysis was performed to evaluate the impact of each of the above parameters on the occurrence of ScT. Potential covariates were prioritized for data analysis (a list of the covariates is presented in Supplementary Tables S4–S6). To address the impact of the timing of the OCT diagnosis on the association between malapposition and ScT, the period until diagnosis of malapposition was grouped into early (diagnosis within 48 h after implantation of BRS), mid (diagnosis from day 3 but not later than 30 days after implantation of BRS), and late (later than 30 days after the implantation of

BRS). This variable was also entered into the Cox model. The threshold for statistical significance was $p < 0.05$.

3. Results

3.1. Patient Characteristics

A total of 197 patients (219 lesions) who underwent elective OCT within 353 (0–376) days after BRS implantation were enrolled in the study (Table 1). One hundred and thirty-two patients were treated in Mainz, 36 in Giessen, and 29 in Erlangen. Follow-up was complete (100%) at a median of 1059 (1009–1110) days, during which 7 patients presented with late or very late ScT 579 [341–623] days after implantation and 293 (38–579) days after OCT. Diagnosis of ScT was supported by OCT-imaging in 5 cases and was based on angiography alone in two patients.

Table 1. Baseline characteristics of the cohort.

Baseline Characteristic	Late or Very Late Scaffold Thrombosis ScT (n = 7)	No ScT (n = 190)	p
Age (years)	58.3 ± 9.1	61.8 ± 11.9	0.37
Male Sex (%)	85.7	81.6	0.78
Hypertension (%)	100	77.9	0.16
Diabetes mellitus (%)	14.3	20.5	0.69
Current smoker (%)	43.9	36.8	0.74
Family history (%)	14.3	30.0	0.37
Hyperlipoproteinaemia (%)	43.9	47.4	0.81
Prior revascularization (%)	71.4	34.7	0.04 *
Prior bypass surgery (%)	0	3.7	0.06
Prior percutaneous intervention (%)	71.4	33.2	0.04 *
Prior stroke/TIA (%)	0	3.2	0.63
eGFR (mean ± SD, ml/min)	91.4 ± 30.8	85.4 ± 20.2	0.74
Left ventricular ejection fraction (mean ± SD, %)	54.3 ± 7.9	54 ± 8.2	0.96
Acute coronary syndrome (%)	71.4	51.4	0.30
Clinical indication			
- Stable angina (%)	28.6	37.4	0.57
- ST-elevation myocardial infarction (%)	42.9	22.1	0.29
- Non-ST-elevation myocardial infarction (%)	28.6	24.9	0.82
- Unstable angina (%)	0	13.8	0.20
Number of vessels treated	1.6 ± 0.8	1.1 ± 0.4	0.01 *
Number of scaffolds per lesion	1.0 ± 0	1.2 ± 0.5	0.25
Number of scaffolds per patient	1.7 ± 1.1	1.3 ± 0.7	0.23
Chronic total occlusion (%)	0	6.8	0.47
Lesion type AHA/ACC classification B/C2 (%)	85.7	63.5	0.22
Dual antiplatelet therapy (DAPT)			0.58
- Clopidogrel (%)	14.3	31.2	
- Prasugrel (%)	14.3	52.4	
- Ticagrelor (%)	71.4	16.4	

* = statistically significant; eGFR = estimated Glomerular filtration rate; AHA/ACC = American Heart Association/American College of Cardiology.

Patients with late or very late ScT showed similar characteristics with respect to age, sex, and cardiovascular risk profile. A history of prior revascularization was more frequent in ScT patients (71.4% vs. 34.7%; $p = 0.04$). The majority of BRS were implanted in the setting of an acute coronary syndrome (71.4% vs. 51.4%; $p = 0.30$) with no difference between the groups. While control patients tended to have a higher number of scaffolds per lesion (1.0 ± 0 vs. 1.2 ± 0.5; $p = 0.25$), the number of treated vessels (1.6 ± 0.8 vs. 1.1 ± 0.4; p = 0.01) was higher in the ScT group. Parameters of lesion complexity were comparable between the groups.

Procedural characteristics divided by the incidence of ScT are shown in Table S1. The strategy used for implantation was not different between ScT patients and reference patients; pre-dilatation was performed in almost all cases (100% vs. 99.5%; p = 0.85) with comparable inflation pressures (13.4 ± 1.9 vs. 13.2 ± 2.3 atm; p = 0.75). All ScTs (except for one, occurring during clopidogrel therapy at 38 days after index) were observed after scheduled cessation of dual antiplatelet therapy (DAPT).

3.2. Optical Coherence Tomography (OCT) Characteristics

The timing of OCT from the index procedure is presented in Figure 1. OCT characteristics are shown in Table 2. Total scaffold length did not differ significantly between ScT patients and reference patients (35.4 ± 29.2 vs. 27.4 ± 16.5 mm; p = 0.96). At the patient level, there was no difference in scaffold nominal diameter, however, at lesion level, scaffolds that displayed an ScT during follow-up had a greater minimum (3.2 ± 0.22 vs. 3.0 ± 0.35 mm; p = 0.01) and maximum scaffold diameter (3.4 ± 0.24 vs. 3.1 ± 0.34 mm; p = 0.04). In line with this, the maximum (12.3 ± 2.5 vs. 9.1 ± 3.1 mm^2; p = 0.005) and minimum (6.3 ± 1.0 vs. 4.8 ± 1.9 mm^2; p = 0.82) lumen areas were significantly larger in ScT patients. The incidence of PSLIA and neovessels as well as BRS asymmetry and eccentricity were similar between ScT and reference patients (Table 2). Strut discontinuities were more frequently observed in the ScT patients (42.9% vs. 5.9%; p < 0.001). Furthermore, uncovered (42.9% vs. 5.9%; p < 0.001) and malapposed struts (85.7% vs. 20.1%; p < 0.001) were observed significantly more frequently in BRS that later developed ScT. Malapposition area, distance, and length were not different in patients with compared with those without ScT.

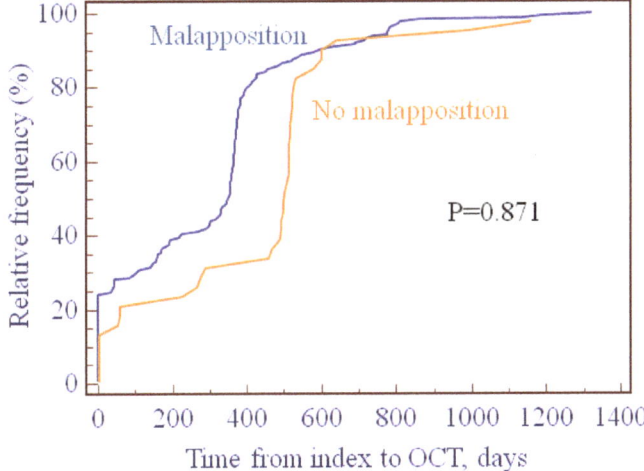

Figure 1. Timing of OCT from index procedure. There was no difference between patients with or without malapposition (p = 0.871).

Baseline characteristics and procedure-related parameters of patients with and without malapposition can be found in Tables S2 and S3 (supplementary materials). The presence of malapposition was not associated with any of the other OCT characteristics. Patients with malapposition, however, showed a larger lumen area (8.4 ± 2.5 vs. 11.6 ± 3.8 mm; p < 0.001) and more eccentricity (0.68 ± 0.09 vs. 0.61 ± 0.12; p < 0.001) and tended to have uncovered struts more frequently (p = 0.06, Table S8, supplementary materials).

Table 2. Optical coherence tomography (OCT) findings.

Optical Coherence Finding	Late or Very Late ScT (n = 7)	No ScT (n = 190)	p
Number of struts	1080 ± 485	1059 ± 837	0.38
Number of frames	116.1 ± 84	120.4 ± 49	0.24
Pullback length (mm)	19.1 ± 8.1	21.1 ± 5.4	0.35
Maximum lumen area (mm^2)	12.3 ± 2.5	9.1 ± 3.1	0.005 *
Minimum lumen area (mm^2)	6.3 ± 1.0	4.8 ± 1.9	0.02 *
Average lumen area (mm^2)	8.96 ± 1.03	6.6 ± 2.20	0.003 *
Maximum lumen asymmetry	0.28 ± 0.10	0.27 ± 0.11	0.82
Maximum scaffold asymmetry	0.24 ± 0.012	0.24 ± 0.09	0.91
Maximum lumen eccentricity	0.62 ± 0.11	0.66 ± 0.10	0.29
Maximum scaffold eccentricity	0.66 ± 0.10	0.72 ± 0.08	0.07
Peri-strut low intensity area (PSLIA) (%)	20.0	5.4	0.18
Microvessels (%)	42.9	31.0	0.51
Fractures (%)	57.1	33.5	0.20
Uncovered scaffold struts (%)	42.9	5.8	<0.001 *
Malapposition (>30% in one frame, without side) (%)	71.4	15.3	<0.001 *
Any malapposition per patient (%)	85.7	20.1	<0.001 *
Malapposition length (mm)	2.33 ± 1.5	2.76 ± 1.8	0.67
Malapposition maximum area (mm^2)	1.56 ± 0.69	2.3 ± 1.9	0.64
Number of malapposed segments	1.83 ± 1.17	1.7 ± 0.99	0.88
Malapposition distance (mm)	0.52 ± 0.25	0.89 ± 0.77	0.22
Evagination (%)	57.1	27.5	0.08

* = statistically significant.

3.3. Analysis of the OCT Predictors of Scaffold Thrombosis

Figure 2 illustrates the relationship between OCT evidence of malapposition and subsequent ScT. The log rank test p was <0.001.

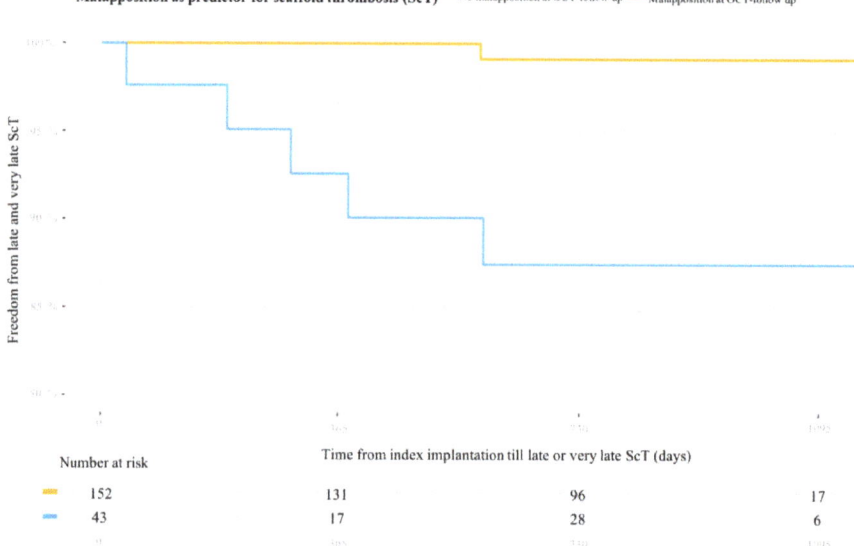

Figure 2. Kaplan–Meier curve illustrating the association between incidental finding of malapposition during elective follow-up OCT and incidence of late and very late ScT.

Multivariable Cox regression identified both malapposition diagnosed early (within 48 hours) after the index procedure (HR = 24.1, 95% CI = 1.5–387.6, p = 0.03) and later than day 30 (HR = 20.9, 95% CI = 2.5–179.7, p < 0.001) as independent predictors of ScT. Further exploratory univariate and multivariable Cox regression analysis (Tables S4–S7, supplementary materials) showed that the presence of malapposition (p = 0.049, hazard ratio (HR) 10.56 (1.0–110.68)) was the only independent predictor of ScT. The presence of uncovered struts and the number of vessels treated showed a threshold association (p = 0.05).

3.4. OCT Evidence at the Time of ScT

OCT observations at the time of ScT were collected in a separate retrospective registry. These data are presented in Appendix A.

4. Discussion

The principal findings of this study are: (1) Malapposition was identified as predictor of late and very late ScT in patients treated with BRS; this association was demonstrated for both "major" malapposition (defined as evidence of at least 30% of the struts in one frame) and for any degree of malapposition. This association was valid when malapposition was diagnosed either at implantation or >30 days thereafter. (2) The presence of uncovered struts showed a threshold association with the incidence of ScT during follow-up in multivariate analysis. (3) In an analysis of thrombi detected by OCT (see supplementary materials), evidence of malapposition was more frequent in late/very late ScT than in early ScT. This evidence was associated with larger vessel and scaffold sizes.

BRS were introduced to overcome long-term limitations of metallic stents; however, evidence from a number of registries and randomized controlled studies showed BRS to be associated with increased risk of both early and late ScT [2,4,22]. Importantly, early ScT was often shown to be associated with procedural issues (including suboptimal vessel sizing and incomplete scaffold/vessel expansion) [23]. In line with this, improvement in implantation techniques proved to be associated with reduced rates of such events [24,25]. Later, evidence was reported of late and very late ScT, i.e., at a time when the benefits of the resorbable device over metallic stents were supposed to be realized [2,4,22]. Importantly, malapposition, often associated with strut discontinuity and uncovered struts, emerged as the strongest association of very late ScT in OCT case series [13,15,16]. Although the mechanisms of this form of disruption in the geometry of the scaffold remain unknown and are probably different from case to case, the persistence of early malapposed (often uncovered) struts, or the development of late malapposition/evaginations, both resulting in struts not being embedded in the vascular wall, appear to be a prerequisite for evolution of adverse scaffold geometry. Similar data are also available for metallic stents; malapposition was the leading finding in the Bern and PESTO registries of stent thrombosis and among the three leading mechanisms in the PRESTIGE registry [26,27].

Stent malapposition results in disturbances in blood flow dynamics, adluminal areas of high shear stress, and abluminal areas of low shear stress and recirculation [10,11]. These disturbances are in turn associated with impaired strut coverage by endothelial cells ("strut healing"), strongly influence the local levels of blood viscosity, and stimulate platelet activation and neointima formation [28,29] that might amplify the supposedly higher thrombogenicity of scaffolds [30].

Despite this rationale and retrospective evidence, prospective follow-up data on the role of malapposition in determining an increased risk of late thrombosis in BRS remain limited to first-generation drug-eluting stents, in which the occurrence of late acquired malapposition at any time between imaging assessment and stent thrombosis complicates any assessment. In a meta-analysis by Hassan et al, the odds ratio for the risk of stent thrombosis in patients with diagnosed late acquired malapposition was 6.51 (1.34–34.91); however, the data were heterogeneous, with three trials supporting this conclusion and the other two leaning in the other direction. These considerations have a further level of complexity with respect to BRS use, where it would be expected that the resorption of the malapposed struts would limit their thrombogenic potential. Gomez-Lara et al. [31] performed an

OCT sub-study of the ABSORB trial Cohort B, in which BRS having a 3 mm diameter were deployed. The incidence of malapposed struts in vessels with a final distal maximal lumen diameter >3.3 mm was higher than in cases in which the final lumen diameter was smaller. In addition, we previously reported that undersizing at the time of implantation and BRS implantation in vessels larger than 3.5 mm are predictors of late/very late ScT. In contrast, oversizing and small reference vessel diameters (RVDs) were predictors of early ScT [18]. The current data provide a possible mechanism related to this observation, suggesting that malapposition, even when it is diagnosed incidentally and regardless of the length of time from implantation, is a predictor of late and very late ScT and should therefore trigger mechanical/pharmacological intervention.

In our database, total scaffold length, uncovered struts, minimum lumen area, and the number of vessels treated did not affect the chances of ScT in our cohort, although the regression model should be analyzed with caution as the covariate/case ratio may have led to overmodeling [32].

5. Limitations

There are several limitations associated with this study. First, its registry nature, with retrospective collection of patients' data and prospective follow-up, has clear inherent limitations, and the evidence provided here (particularly given the small sample size and event rate) should be seen as hypothesis generating, particularly with regard to the exploratory multivariate analysis. A strictly prospective study design to investigate malapposition as a causal factor of scaffold thrombosis would be complex from an ethical perspective. OCT follow-up was not performed at fixed time points and was not repeated, so any conclusion on the nature (early versus late acquired) of malapposition was impossible. Further, the Bern registry emphasized the importance of the longitudinal extent of malapposition (>1 mm) and suggested a cut-off >300 μm for the strut-vessel wall distance [33]. These cases are usually treated in the clinical routine and were not included in the present database. The present study expands this evidence to suggest that findings of scaffold malapposition, even those that appear as "minor" and not worthy of intervention, are indeed associated with ScT. Importantly, fluid dynamic models demonstrate that, particularly for thick struts with quadratic profile, a smaller malapposition distance might actually have the largest hemodynamic effect [28,29]. ScT is a complex phenomenon in which vessel, scaffold architecture, structure, and a number of patient characteristics play a role and it is likely that larger cohorts would have allowed identification of other clinical or procedural parameters and possible causes and mechanisms. For our analysis, late and very late ScT were pooled. However, all late ScT occurred at a time at which resorption would have already started and the two groups of patients did not differ in any of the key features. The definition of strut fracture has not yet been validated and an analysis of different types of fractures goes beyond the scope of this study. We therefore limited the definition of fracture to cases where discontinuity, altered geometry (see example in the supplement data), and/or a gap within the scaffold was evident. Our data apply to "thick strut" scaffolds; no conclusion on the importance of malapposition in (thin-strut) metallic stents can be inferred. Finally, the cross-sectional nature of our observation does not allow mechanistic insight. The (non-significantly) higher incidence of ST-segment elevation myocardial infarctions (STEMIs) at index in the patients presenting with malapposition points out the importance (and complexity) of vessel sizing in this setting.

6. Conclusions

We provide the first evidence that an incidental finding of malapposition—regardless of the timing of diagnosis of the malapposition—during an elective exam is a predictor of late and very late ScT. Whether mechanical correction of this finding also reduces events is unknown and will require further studies. However, this evidence suggests that prolonging dual antiplatelet therapy in these cases would be a prudent strategy.

J. Clin. Med. **2019**, *8*, 580

Supplementary Materials: The following are available online at http://www.mdpi.com/2077-0383/8/5/580/s1, Table S1: Procedural characteristics of the prospective follow-up observational cohort, Table S2: Baseline characteristics of patients depending on presence of malapposition, Table S3: Procedural characteristics depending on presence of malapposition, Table S4: Univariate analysis of baseline characteristics for primary endpoint (late or very late ScT), Table S5: Univariate analysis of procedural characteristics for primary endpoint (late or very late ScT), Table S6: Univariate analyse of OCT findings for primary endpoint (late or very late ScT), Table S7: Multivariable Cox regression analysis for primary endpoint (late or very late ScT), Table S8: OCT findings depending on presence of malapposition, Table S9: Baseline characteristics of patients with ScT, Table S10: Procedural characteristics in the retrospective cohort of patients with ScT, Table S11: OCT findings in the retrospective cohort (OCT at the time of ScT), Table S12: Dual antiplatelet regime in the cases in which OCT was diagnosed at the time of ScT.

Author Contributions: Conceptualization, N.B., H.N., and T.G.; methodology, T.G. and N.B.; software, M.W., F.B., H.U., R.A., and M.T.; validation, R.A., J.D., and M.W.; formal analysis, N.B., T.G.; investigation, C.H., T.M., H.N., and S.A.; data curation, N.B., M.W., and H.U.; writing—original draft preparation, T.G., H.N., and N.B.; visualization, T.G. and N.B.; supervision, T.G. and T.M.; project administration, T.M.

Acknowledgments: The authors thank Elizabeth Martinson, Ph.D., for editorial assistance.

Conflicts of Interest: T.M., T.G., and H.N. have received speaker fees and research grants from Abbott Vascular. T.G. works in DZHK. C.H. received advisory fees from Abbott Vascular and is member of Medtronic advisory board. The other authors have no conflict to declare. Abbott Vascular had no role in any phase of this research.

Appendix A

A.1. Retrospective Cohort: Malapposition at the Time of Scaffold Thrombosis (ScT)

Optical coherence tomography (OCT) recordings of consecutive patients with ScT were collected in an additional retrospective registry study (Figure A1). Observations in cases of late/very late ScT were compared with those in patients with early ScT.

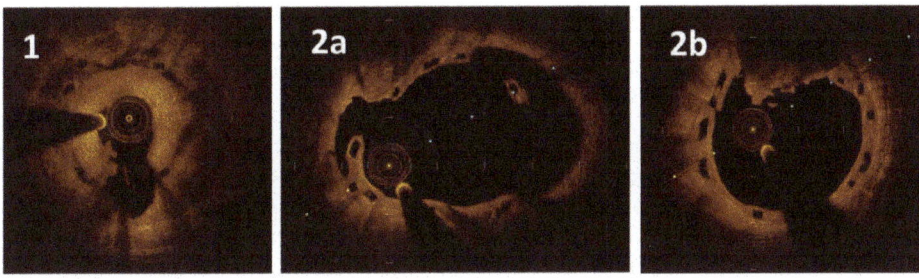

Figure A1. Representative images of cases of late/very late scaffold thrombosis (ScT) (*n* = 9). The panels are numbered according to the patient number. Case **1**: ScT 563 days after index. The patient presented with ST-segment elevation myocardial infarction (STEMI). Optical coherence tomography (OCT) shows a homogeneous layer within the bioresorbable scaffold (BRS), suggestive of neointima, evidence of white thrombus (7 o'clock), and a large signal-poor, peri-strut, low intensity area (from 1 to 5 o'clock) with increased attenuation compatible with oedema/immature neointima. The architecture of the struts appears to be disrupted, but no gap was evident. Case **2**: ScT 349 days after index. The patient presented with non-ST-segment elevation myocardial infarction (NSTEMI). OCT revealed malapposition (**2a**) immediately contiguous to white-red thrombus (**2b**). In this case, the strut architecture was also altered (**2b**; 1 o'clock) and there was evidence of incompletely covered struts (**2a**).

A.2. Results: OCT Evidence at the Time of ScT

All patients presenting with ScT in whom an OCT was performed at the three institutions were included in a separate retrospective registry. A total of 16 patients with OCT acquisition at the time of the ScT were identified. Five of these patients were also included in the prospective follow-up observational group (31.3%). Seven patients of the retrospective cohort were classified as acute or subacute and nine as late or very late ScT (563 (49) days after implantation). Representative images of the thrombi are presented in Figure A1. All ScTs were classified as definite. Patients with late or very late ScT were more frequently female and more frequently had a history of prior revascularization. Further baseline and procedural characteristics were similar (Tables S9 and S10, supplementary materials).

OCT findings are listed in Table S11 (supplementary materials). The majority of frames showed evidence of thrombus (78 ± 37 vs. 55% ± 66%; $p = 0.18$). Incomplete expansion was seen predominantly in cases of early ScT (83.3% vs. 12.4%; $p = 0.008$). Scaffold discontinuities (0% vs. 50%; $p = 0.04$) and malapposition (16.7% vs. 87.5%; $p = 0.008$) were features of late or very late ScT. OCT parameters expressing vessel and scaffold geometry did not differ between early and late ScT (Table S11, supplementary materials). The initial dual antiplatelet therapy (DAPT) regimen in use when implanting bioresorbable scaffold (BRS) was also not different ($p = 0.66$); however, 83% of patients developed late or very late ScT while not on DAPT ($p = 0.006$ compared to early ScT cases, Table S12, supplementary materials).

References

1. Wiebe, J.; Nef, H.M.; Hamm, C.W. Current status of bioresorbable scaffolds in the treatment of coronary artery disease. *J. Am. Coll. Cardiol.* **2014**, *64*, 2541–2551. [CrossRef]
2. Ali, Z.A.; Gao, R.; Kimura, T.; Onuma, Y.; Kereiakes, D.J.; Ellis, S.G.; Chevalier, B.; Vu, M.T.; Zhang, Z.; Simonton, C.A.; et al. Three-year outcomes with the absorb bioresorbable scaffold: individual-patient-data meta-analysis from the ABSORB randomized trials. *Circulation* **2018**, *137*, 464–479. [CrossRef]
3. Arroyo, D.; Gendre, G.; Schukraft, S.; Kallinikou, Z.; Muller, O.; Baeriswyl, G.; Stauffer, J.C.; Goy, J.J.; Togni, M.; Cook, S.; et al. Comparison of everolimus- and biolimus-eluting coronary stents with everolimus-eluting bioresorbable vascular scaffolds: Two-year clinical outcomes of the EVERBIO II trial. *Int. J. Cardiol.* **2017**, *243*, 121–125. [CrossRef] [PubMed]
4. Collet, C.; Asano, T.; Miyazaki, Y.; Tenekecioglu, E.; Katagiri, Y.; Sotomi, Y.; Cavalcante, R.; de Winter, R.J.; Kimura, T.; Gao, R.; et al. Late thrombotic events after bioresorbable scaffold implantation: a systematic review and meta-analysis of randomized clinical trials. *Eur. Heart J.* **2017**, *38*, 2559–2566. [CrossRef] [PubMed]
5. Polimeni, A.; Anadol, R.; Munzel, T.; Indolfi, C.; De Rosa, S.; Gori, T. Long-term outcome of bioresorbable vascular scaffolds for the treatment of coronary artery disease: A meta-analysis of RCTs. *BMC Cardiovasc. Disord.* **2017**, *17*, 147. [CrossRef] [PubMed]
6. Wykrzykowska, J.J.; Kraak, R.P.; Hofma, S.H.; van der Schaaf, R.J.; Arkenbout, E.K.; AJ, I.J.; Elias, J.; van Dongen, I.M.; Tijssen, R.Y.G.; Koch, K.T.; et al. Bioresorbable scaffolds versus metallic stents in routine PCI. *N. Engl. J. Med.* **2017**, *376*, 2319–2328. [CrossRef]
7. Puricel, S.; Cuculi, F.; Weissner, M.; Schmermund, A.; Jamshidi, P.; Nyffenegger, T.; Binder, H.; Eggebrecht, H.; Munzel, T.; Cook, S.; et al. Bioresorbable coronary scaffold thrombosis: Multicenter comprehensive analysis of clinical presentation, mechanisms, and predictors. *J. Am. Coll. Cardiol.* **2016**, *67*, 921–931. [CrossRef] [PubMed]
8. Ellis, S.G.; Gori, T.; Serruys, P.W.; Nef, H.; Steffenino, G.; Brugaletta, S.; Munzel, T.; Feliz, C.; Schmidt, G.; Sabate, M.; et al. Clinical, angiographic, and procedural correlates of very late absorb scaffold thrombosis: Multistudy registry results. *JACC Cardiovasc. Interv.* **2018**, *11*, 638–644. [CrossRef] [PubMed]
9. Gori, T.; Weissner, M.; Gonner, S.; Wendling, F.; Ullrich, H.; Ellis, S.; Anadol, R.; Polimeni, A.; Munzel, T. Characteristics, predictors, and mechanisms of thrombosis in coronary bioresorbable scaffolds: Differences between early and late events. *JACC Cardiovasc. Interv.* **2017**, *10*, 2363–2371. [CrossRef] [PubMed]
10. Foin, N.; Gutierrez-Chico, J.L.; Nakatani, S.; Torii, R.; Bourantas, C.V.; Sen, S.; Nijjer, S.; Petraco, R.; Kousera, C.; Ghione, M.; et al. Incomplete stent apposition causes high shear flow disturbances and delay in neointimal coverage as a function of strut to wall detachment distance: Implications for the management of incomplete stent apposition. *Circ. Cardiovasc. Interv.* **2014**, *7*, 180–189. [CrossRef]
11. Foin, N.; Lu, S.; Ng, J.; Bulluck, H.; Hausenloy, D.J.; Wong, P.E.; Virmani, R.; Joner, M. Stent malapposition and the risk of stent thrombosis: Mechanistic insights from an in vitro model. *EuroIntervention* **2017**, *13*, e1096–e1098. [CrossRef]
12. Anadol, R.; Gori, T. The mechanisms of late scaffold thrombosis. *Clin. Hemorheol. Microcirc.* **2017**, *67*, 343–346. [CrossRef] [PubMed]

13. Cuculi, F.; Puricel, S.; Jamshidi, P.; Valentin, J.; Kallinikou, Z.; Toggweiler, S.; Weissner, M.; Munzel, T.; Cook, S.; Gori, T. Optical coherence tomography findings in bioresorbable vascular scaffolds thrombosis. *Circ. Cardiovasc. Interv.* **2015**, *8*, e002518. [CrossRef]
14. Kraak, R.P.; Kajita, A.H.; Garcia-Garcia, H.M.; Henriques, J.P.S.; Piek, J.J.; Arkenbout, E.K.; van der Schaaf, R.J.; Tijssen, J.G.P.; de Winter, R.J.; Wykrzykowska, J.J. Scaffold thrombosis following implantation of the ABSORB Bvs. in routine clinical practice: Insight into possible mechanisms from optical coherence tomography. *Catheter. Cardiovasc. Interv.* **2018**, *92*, E106–E114. [CrossRef]
15. Raber, L.; Brugaletta, S.; Yamaji, K.; O'Sullivan, C.J.; Otsuki, S.; Koppara, T.; Taniwaki, M.; Onuma, Y.; Freixa, X.; Eberli, F.R.; et al. Very late scaffold thrombosis: Intracoronary imaging and histopathological and spectroscopic findings. *J. Am. Coll. Cardiol.* **2015**, *66*, 1901–1914. [CrossRef] [PubMed]
16. Yamaji, K.; Ueki, Y.; Souteyrand, G.; Daemen, J.; Wiebe, J.; Nef, H.; Adriaenssens, T.; Loh, J.P.; Lattuca, B.; Wykrzykowska, J.J.; et al. Mechanisms of very late bioresorbable scaffold thrombosis: The INVEST registry. *J. Am. Coll. Cardiol.* **2017**, *70*, 2330–2344. [CrossRef] [PubMed]
17. Tamburino, C.; Latib, A.; van Geuns, R.J.; Sabate, M.; Mehilli, J.; Gori, T.; Achenbach, S.; Alvarez, M.P.; Nef, H.; Lesiak, M.; et al. Contemporary practice and technical aspects in coronary intervention with bioresorbable scaffolds: A European perspective. *EuroIntervention* **2015**, *11*, 45–52. [CrossRef] [PubMed]
18. Gori, T.; Jansen, T.; Weissner, M.; Foin, N.; Wenzel, P.; Schulz, E.; Cook, S.; Munzel, T. Coronary evaginations and peri-scaffold aneurysms following implantation of bioresorbable scaffolds: Incidence, outcome, and optical coherence tomography analysis of possible mechanisms. *Eur. Heart J.* **2016**, *37*, 2040–2049. [CrossRef] [PubMed]
19. Gori, T.; Schulz, E.; Hink, U.; Kress, M.; Weiers, N.; Weissner, M.; Jabs, A.; Wenzel, P.; Capodanno, D.; Munzel, T. Clinical, angiographic, functional, and imaging outcomes 12 months after implantation of drug-eluting bioresorbable vascular scaffolds in acute coronary syndromes. *JACC Cardiovasc. Interv.* **2015**, *8*, 770–777. [CrossRef] [PubMed]
20. Tearney, G.J.; Regar, E.; Akasaka, T.; Adriaenssens, T.; Barlis, P.; Bezerra, H.G.; Bouma, B.; Bruining, N.; Cho, J.M.; Chowdhary, S.; et al. Consensus standards for acquisition, measurement, and reporting of intravascular optical coherence tomography studies: A report from the International Working Group for Intravascular Optical Coherence Tomography Standardization and Validation. *J. Am. Coll. Cardiol.* **2012**, *59*, 1058–1072. [CrossRef] [PubMed]
21. Cutlip, D.E.; Windecker, S.; Mehran, R.; Boam, A.; Cohen, D.J.; van Es, G.A.; Steg, P.G.; Morel, M.A.; Mauri, L.; Vranckx, P.; et al. Clinical end points in coronary stent trials: A case for standardized definitions. *Circulation* **2007**, *115*, 2344–2351. [CrossRef]
22. Kereiakes, D.J.; Ellis, S.G.; Metzger, C.; Caputo, R.P.; Rizik, D.G.; Teirstein, P.S.; Litt, M.R.; Kini, A.; Kabour, A.; Marx, S.O.; et al. 3-Year clinical outcomes with everolimus-eluting bioresorbable coronary scaffolds: The ABSORB III trial. *J. Am. Coll. Cardiol.* **2017**, *70*, 2852–2862. [CrossRef]
23. Ellis, S.G.; Steffenino, G.; Kereiakes, D.J.; Stone, G.W.; van Geuns, R.J.; Abizaid, A.; Nef, H.; Cortese, B.; Testa, L.; Menichelli, M.; et al. Clinical, angiographic, and procedural correlates of acute, subacute, and late absorb scaffold thrombosis. *JACC Cardiovasc. Interv.* **2017**, *10*, 1809–1815. [CrossRef]
24. Ortega-Paz, L.; Brugaletta, S.; Sabate, M. Impact of PSP technique on clinical outcomes following bioresorbable scaffolds implantation. *J. Clin. Med.* **2018**, *7*, 27. [CrossRef] [PubMed]
25. Ortega-Paz, L.; Capodanno, D.; Gori, T.; Nef, H.; Latib, A.; Caramanno, G.; Di Mario, C.; Naber, C.; Lesiak, M.; Capranzano, P.; et al. Predilation, sizing and post-dilation scoring in patients undergoing everolimus-eluting bioresorbable scaffold implantation for prediction of cardiac adverse events: Development and internal validation of the PSP score. *EuroIntervention* **2017**, *12*, 2110–2117. [CrossRef] [PubMed]
26. Adriaenssens, T.; Joner, M.; Godschalk, T.C.; Malik, N.; Alfonso, F.; Xhepa, E.; De Cock, D.; Komukai, K.; Tada, T.; Cuesta, J.; et al. Optical coherence tomography findings in patients with coronary stent thrombosis: A report of the PRESTIGE consortium (Prevention of late stent thrombosis by an interdisciplinary global European effort). *Circulation* **2017**, *136*, 1007–1021. [CrossRef] [PubMed]
27. Souteyrand, G.; Amabile, N.; Mangin, L.; Chabin, X.; Meneveau, N.; Cayla, G.; Vanzetto, G.; Barnay, P.; Trouillet, C.; Rioufol, G.; et al. Mechanisms of stent thrombosis analysed by optical coherence tomography: Insights from the national PESTO French registry. *Eur. Heart J.* **2016**, *37*, 1208–1216. [CrossRef]
28. Chesnutt, J.K.; Han, H.C. Computational simulation of platelet interactions in the initiation of stent thrombosis due to stent malapposition. *Phys. Biol.* **2016**, *13*, 016001. [CrossRef] [PubMed]

29. Poon, E.K.W.; Thondapu, V.; Hayat, U.; Barlis, P.; Yap, C.Y.; Kuo, P.H.; Wang, Q.; Ma, J.; Zhu, S.J.; Moore, S.; et al. Elevated blood viscosity and microrecirculation resulting from coronary stent malapposition. *J. Biomech. Eng.* **2018**, *140*. [CrossRef] [PubMed]
30. Vorpahl, M.; Nakano, M.; Perkins, L.E.; Otsuka, F.; Jones, R.; Acampado, E.; Lane, J.P.; Rapoza, R.; Kolodgie, F.D.; Virmani, R. Vascular healing and integration of a fully bioresorbable everolimus-eluting scaffold in a rabbit iliac arterial model. *EuroIntervention* **2014**, *10*, 833–841. [CrossRef]
31. Gomez-Lara, J.; Diletti, R.; Brugaletta, S.; Onuma, Y.; Farooq, V.; Thuesen, L.; McClean, D.; Koolen, J.; Ormiston, J.A.; Windecker, S.; et al. Angiographic maximal luminal diameter and appropriate deployment of the everolimus-eluting bioresorbable vascular scaffold as assessed by optical coherence tomography: An ABSORB cohort B trial sub-study. *EuroIntervention* **2012**, *8*, 214–224. [CrossRef] [PubMed]
32. Harrell, F.E., Jr.; Lee, K.L.; Pollock, B.G. Regression models in clinical studies: Determining relationships between predictors and response. *J. Natl. Cancer Inst.* **1988**, *80*, 1198–1202. [CrossRef] [PubMed]
33. Taniwaki, M.; Radu, M.D.; Zaugg, S.; Amabile, N.; Garcia-Garcia, H.M.; Yamaji, K.; Jorgensen, E.; Kelbaek, H.; Pilgrim, T.; Caussin, C.; et al. Mechanisms of very late drug-eluting stent thrombosis assessed by optical coherence tomography. *Circulation* **2016**, *133*, 650–660. [CrossRef] [PubMed]

 © 2019 by the authors. Licensee MDPI, Basel, Switzerland. This article is an open access article distributed under the terms and conditions of the Creative Commons Attribution (CC BY) license (http://creativecommons.org/licenses/by/4.0/).

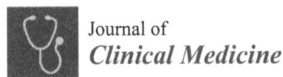

Article

Outcome of Robot-Assisted Bilateral Internal Mammary Artery Grafting via Left Pleura in Coronary Bypass Surgery

Chieh-Jen Wu [1,2], Hsin-Hung Chen [3,4], Pei-Wen Cheng [3,4], Wen-Hsien Lu [5,6], Ching-Jiunn Tseng [3,5] and Chi-Cheng Lai [7,8,*]

1. Cardiovascular Center, Kaohsiung Veterans General Hospital, Kaohsiung 813, Taiwan; cjwu@vghks.gov.tw
2. Graduate Institute of Clinical Medicine, College of Medicine, Kaohsiung Medical University, Kaohsiung 807, Taiwan
3. Department of Medical Education and Research, Kaohsiung Veterans General Hospital, Kaohsiung 813, Taiwan; shchen0910@gmail.com (H.-H.C.); peiwen420@gmail.com (P.-W.C.); cjtseng@vghks.gov.tw (C.-J.T.)
4. Yuh-Ing Junior College of Health Care & Management, Kaohsiung 821, Taiwan
5. School of Medicine, National Yang-Ming University, Taipei 112, Taiwan; whlu@vghks.gov.tw
6. Department of Pediatrics, Kaohsiung Veterans General Hospital, Kaohsiung 813, Taiwan
7. Department of Cardiology, Kaohsiung Municipal United Hospital, Kaohsiung 804, Taiwan
8. Department of Biological Sciences, National Sun Yat-Sen University, Kaohsiung 804, Taiwan
* Correspondence: llccheng@vghks.gov.tw; Tel.: +886-7-5552565 (ext. 2811); Fax: +886-7-5503272

Received: 25 February 2019; Accepted: 10 April 2019; Published: 12 April 2019

Abstract: Studies are extremely limited for the investigation of the clinical outcome of da Vinci robot-assisted bilateral internal mammary artery (BIMA) grafting in coronary artery bypass grafting (CABG) surgery. This study aimed to explore the short-term outcome of da Vinci robot-assisted BIMA grafting through the left pleural space. Relevant data were collected from patients with multi-vessel coronary artery disease receiving two kinds of CABG: a group of patients receiving da Vinci robot-assisted CABG with BIMA grafting, and another group of patients receiving sternotomy CABG with BIMA grafting. Primary endpoints, which included cardiovascular and renal endpoints, were analyzed between the groups using the chi-square test, analysis of variance test, and Kaplan–Meier analysis. Compared with the conventional group ($n = 22$), the robotic group ($n = 22$) had a significantly longer operation time (12.7 ± 1.7 vs. 8.5 ± 1.5 hours; $p < 0.01$) and a marginally lower mean of serum creatinine at baseline (1.2 ± 0.3 vs. 2.0 ± 1.7 mg/dL; $p = 0.04$). Primary endpoints (5, 22.7% vs. 12, 54.5%; $p = 0.03$) and renal endpoints (1, 4.5% vs. 7, 31.8%; $p = 0.02$) at six months were significantly reduced in the robotic group compared with the conventional group. There were no differences in cardiovascular endpoints at six months between the groups (1, 4.5% vs. 0; $p = 1.00$). The data showed that da Vinci robot-assisted BIMA grafting was safe, with equal cardiovascular events and lowered renal events at six months, as compared to conventional sternotomy BIMA grafting, despite the longer procedure time. The short-term study suggests that da Vinci robot-assisted BIMA grafting may be considered a favorable surgical option for patients with severe coronary artery disease.

Keywords: bilateral internal mammary artery; coronary artery disease; coronary artery bypass grafting; da Vinci; sternotomy; outcome

1. Introduction

International guidelines recommend coronary artery bypass grafting (CABG) surgery as a treatment option in patients with left main disease and/or multi-vessel coronary artery disease (CAD) [1–3]. Conventional CABG surgery requires sternotomy, which generates a long mid-sternal wound scar and potentiates sternal wound infection, particularly in patients receiving bilateral internal mammary artery (BIMA) grafting [4–6]. On the other hand, numerous studies have documented the clinical benefit of BIMA grafting, including prolonged graft patency [7,8], lowered adverse cardiovascular events [8,9], and improved survival [9–13]. A conflicting result obtained from a registry study showed that BIMA grafting was not associated with better outcomes compared with single internal mammary artery grafting [14]. In order to minimize surgical trauma and avoid sternotomy, a robot-assisted technique using a da Vinci operator system (Intuitive Surgical, Mountain View, CA, USA) was introduced into the field of CABG surgery. A few studies showed that robotic CABG surgeries had favorable cardiovascular outcomes [15–18]. In addition, a meta-analysis of 16 pooled studies exhibited that there were significantly fewer renal failure events in robot-assisted endoscopic CABG, as compared to conventional CABG [19]. However, no studies have reported on the composite endpoints of cardiovascular and renal events between da Vinci robot-assisted BIMA grafting and conventional BIMA grafting. Therefore, this retrospective study was designed to investigate the primary endpoints of cardiovascular and renal events between the two patient groups with severe CAD receiving robot-assisted BIMA graft via the left pleura or conventional sternotomy BIMA grafting. The present results were expected to elucidate the short-term primary outcome and help guide surgical decision in patients with severe CAD.

2. Materials and Methods

2.1. Study Design and Patient Selection

The study was a single-center, retrospective, non-randomized, and non-controlled observational study based upon the analysis of the database of a single medical center, and was designed to detect the differences in adverse events between two patient groups: Group 1 of patients receiving da Vinci robot-assisted CABG with BIMA grafting via left pleura and Group 2 of patients receiving conventional sternotomy CABG with BIMA grafting. Consecutively collected patients were those who had been angiographically diagnosed with left main disease and/or multi-vessel CAD, and thereafter received two kinds of CABG surgeries. They were matched by age. For both groups, femoral artery and vein cannulations were performed for the preparation of cardiopulmonary bypass with systemic heparinization. Beating heart CABG with BIMA skeletonization and mobilization was routinely conducted in all patients, with an on- or off-pump according to the patient's hemodynamic status and the operator's discretion. A radial artery (RA) or great saphenous vein (GSV) was harvested as a conduit with the right internal mammary artery (RIMA) for anastomosis of the left circumflex artery (LCX) and of the right coronary artery (RCA). The procedures of the two kinds of CABG surgeries are detailed below. Patients were excluded if they received an urgent CABG, received a hybrid of percutaneous coronary intervention (PCI) and CABG, received left internal mammary artery (LIMA) grafting or RIMA grafting alone, presented with ST-segment elevation myocardial infarction, or had previously been enrolled in another clinical study. All patients received a daily dose of 100 mg aspirin indefinitely, in combination with a daily dose 75 mg clopidogrel as dual antiplatelet therapy with an expected duration of at least one year after the index surgeries. Clinical follow-up was scheduled in hospital, three months, and six months after discharge for data collection. Primary endpoints consisted of a composite of cardiovascular and renal endpoints. Relevant data were recorded for patient characteristics, clinical presentations, and adverse events during the follow-up period. All patients in the two groups were thoroughly informed about the procedure preoperatively and provided written consent. The study protocol had been examined and approved by the committee of the hospital. The present study was performed in accordance with the Declaration of Helsinki and local regulatory guidelines.

2.2. Da Vinci Robot-Assisted CABG with BIMA Grafting via Left Pleura

Each beating-heart da Vinci robot-assisted CABG with unilateral BIMA grafting was performed with an on- or off-cardiopulmonary pump according to a patient's hemodynamic status by an experienced team led by a well-trained CABG surgeon with more than 15 years of CABG surgery experience. After general anesthesia and aseptic procedures, a double-lumen was intubated for single right-lung or bilateral low-volume ventilation in order to mobilize the BIMA grafts. A BIMA graft was mobilized through the left pleura using the da Vinci robot-assisted operation system, with the left chest elevated at approximately 30 degrees and with the patient in supine position. The chest cavity was insufflated with carbon dioxide to expand the surgical space. An RIMA was first mobilized through the left pleural and pre-mediastinal space with two-lung low-volume ventilation. Then, an LIMA was mobilized with single right-lung ventilation. The vessels were anastomosed by direct-vision through a left thoracotomy in the second intercostal space with a surgical wound of about 6–12 cm in length. The mobilized LIMA was anastomosed with the left anterior descending artery (LAD); the RA or GSV served as an additional conduit for connection with the RIMA and for anastomoses of the LCX-obtuse marginal branch (LCX-OM) and/or the RCA-posterior descending artery (RCA-PDA).

2.3. Conventional Sternotomy CABG with BIMA Grafting

Patients received a full mid-sternotomy for conventional CABG surgeries with BIMA grafting. The mobilized BIMA and harvested RA or GSV in each patient were anastomosed with native coronary arteries by direct-vision through a mid-sternal exposed surgical wound of about 20–30 cm in length. Similar to the da Vinci robot surgery, the RA or GSV served as an additional conduit for connection with RIMA and for anastomoses with LCX-OM and/or RCA-PDA. All patients in the two groups were treated and monitored postoperatively at the intensive care unit.

2.4. Definitions

Adverse events in hospitals were defined as wound infection, severe blood loss requiring blood transfusion, pleural effusion, pulmonary edema, and pneumonia. The definition of CAD was coronary stenosis exceeding 50% in diameter of an adjacently normal segment. Estimated glomerular filtration rate (eGFR) was calculated using the modification of diet in renal disease equation. The definition of CKD stages was according to stratified values of eGFR recommended by the guidelines [20]. Consumed units of packed red blood cells or fresh frozen plasma were defined as the sum of the blood units used in hospital. Each operator determined the use of an intra-aortic balloon pump (IABP) according the hemodynamics in the peri-operative period. Myocardial infarction (MI) was defined according to the clinical symptoms, the level of serum troponin I >5 µg/L, new eletrocardiographic changes, or echocardiographic evidence of new regional wall motion abnormality. Operation room time was defined as the time interval between the patient's arrival at the operation room and the patient's departure from the recovery room.

2.5. Primary Endpoints at Six Months

Primary endpoints in the study included cardiovascular and renal endpoints. Cardiovascular endpoints including all-cause mortality, non-fatal MI, repeated revascularization, and non-fatal hemorrhagic and ischemic stroke; renal endpoints included a rise of serum creatinine >0.5 mg/dL above the baseline value, creatinine doubling (at least a 100% raise from the basal level of serum creatinine), and occurrence of CKD stage 4 or 5. An endpoint event was confirmed by two independent physicians according to the clinical symptoms and signs, laboratory data, electrocardiographic findings, and/or diagnostic images. The follow-up period was six months.

2.6. Statistical Analysis

All variables were statistically analyzed using SPSS software version 22 (SPSS Inc., Chicago, IL, USA). All categorical data and rates are displayed as numbers (percentages), and the continuous data are shown as means ± standard deviation. Baseline and outcome data between the groups were compared using chi-square test (χ^2) or Fisher exact test for categorical variables, and the analysis of variance test for continuous variables. Kaplan–Meier analysis with log-rank test was used to detect differences in cumulative event-free survival at six months between the two groups. A p value < 0.05 with two-sided 95% confidence interval was considered statistically significant for all tests. Analysis was conducted as time to the first event involving primary endpoints, without double counting of events.

3. Results

3.1. Patient Demographic and Characteristic Data

Data for a total of 44 patients were collected from November 2010 to January 2016 (Figure 1). In this cohort, 22 patients with left main disease and/or multi-vessel CAD received da Vinci robot-assisted CABG with BIMA grafting through the left pleura. The 22 age-matched patients received conventional sternotomy CABG with BIMA grafting. Figure 2A,B show endoscopically mobilized BIMA and the minimal surgical scars after robot-assisted surgery. Figure 2C,D show a large sternotomy wound and BIMA anastomosed with coronary arteries, and a larger surgical scar after conventional sternotomy surgery. The operation time was significantly longer in robotic CABG as compared with sternotomy CABG (12.7 ± 1.7 vs. 8.5 ± 1.5 h; p < 0.01). The mean serum creatinine at baseline was marginally lower in robotic CABG compared with sternotomy CABG (1.2 ± 0.3 vs. 2.0 ± 1.7 mg/dL; p = 0.04), whereas the mean eGFR was identical between groups (57.9 ± 31.5 vs. 65.4 ± 13.6 mL/min/1.73 m^2; p = 0.32). The baseline characteristics of the two groups are shown in Table 1.

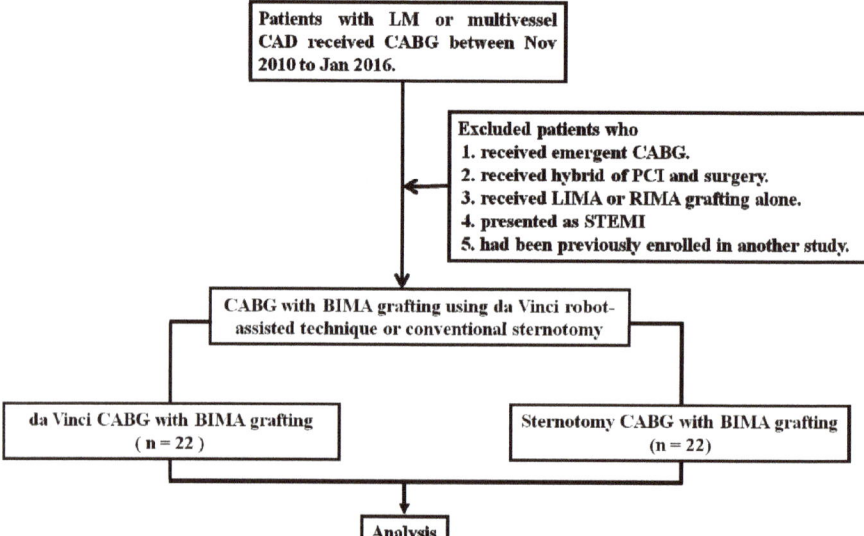

Figure 1. The patient flow chart. LM = left main; CABG = coronary artery bypass grafting; CAD = coronary artery disease; PCI = percutaneous coronary intervention; LIMA = left internal mammary artery; RIMA = right internal mammary artery; STEMI = ST-segment elevation myocardial infarction; BIMA = bilateral internal mammary artery.

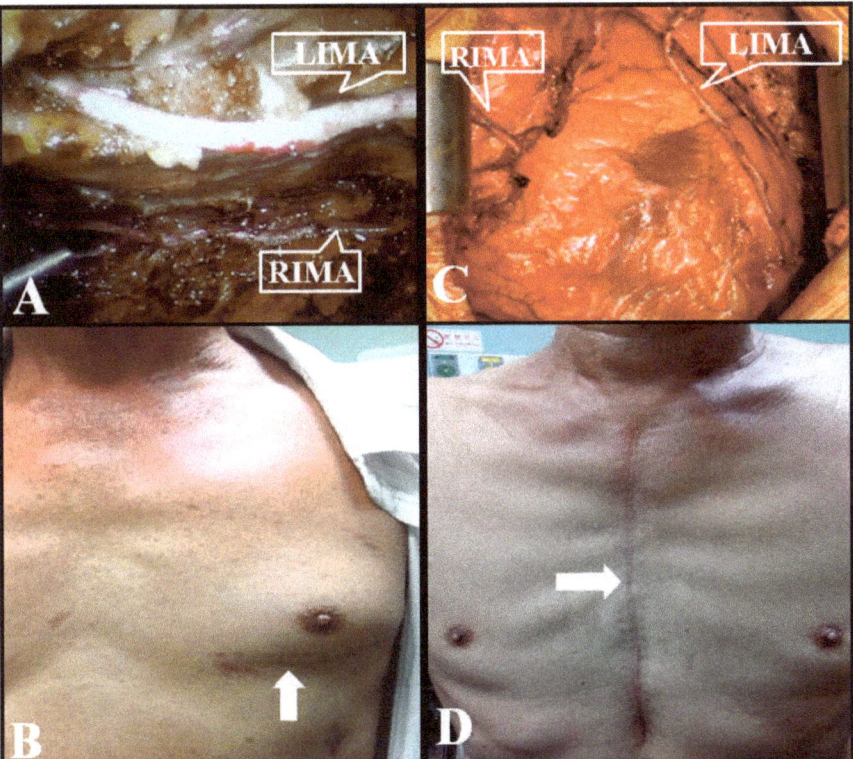

Figure 2. Wound healing in robotic and conventional sternotomy-assisted bilateral internal mammary artery grafting via the left pleura in coronary artery bypass grafting surgery. (**A**) Endoscopy shows that the left internal mammary artery (LIMA) (upper) and the right internal mammary artery (RIMA) (lower) were mobilized using the da Vinci operator system. (**B**) Surgical wounds (white arrows) of da Vinci robot-assisted CABG are small. (**C**) Finished anastomoses of LIMA (right) and RIMA (left) with coronary arteries are displayed in an explored sternal area of a sternotomy CABG. (**D**) A long mid-sternal wound scar (white arrow) is shown in a patient who had received a sternotomy CABG.

Table 1. Baseline characteristics between two surgical modalities.

	Da Vinci Robotic Surgery (n = 22)	Sternotomy Surgery (n = 22)	p Value
Male	20 (90.9)	21 (95.5)	1.00
Age (years)	61.2 ± 12.0	62.9 ± 10.5	0.63
Body mass index (kg/m^2)	26.9 ± 4.0	27.3 ± 3.2	0.70
Risk factors for CAD			
Diabetes mellitus	11 (50.0)	10 (45.5)	1.00
Hypertension	17 (77.3)	18 (81.8)	1.00
Dyslipidemia	13 (59.1)	12 (54.5)	1.00
Hyperuricemia	1 (4.5)	0 (0)	1.00
Drug allergy	5 (22.7)	1 (4.5)	0.19
Alcohol drinking	6 (23.7)	1 (4.5)	0.95
Cigarette smoking	10 (45.5)	11 (50.0)	1.00
Family history of CVD	8 (36.4)	2 (9.1)	0.03
CAD condition			
LM	10 (45.5)	13 (59.1)	0.55
TVD	17 (77.3)	20 (90.9)	0.41
DVD	5 (22.7)	2 (9.1)	0.41
Grafting conduit			
BIMA	22 (100.0)	22 (100.0)	1.00
Radial artery	19 (86.4)	19 (86.4)	1.00
GSV	3 (13.6)	3 (13.6)	1.00
Anastomosis number	3.0 ± 0.6	3.4 ± 0.7	0.34
On pump	10 (45.5)	16 (72.7)	0.12
On pump time (min)	123.9 ± 96.2	131.4 ± 59.8	0.81
Operation room time (h)	12.7 ± 1.7	8.5 ± 1.5	<0.01
Biomarkers at admission			
Hemoglobin (g/dL)	13.7 ± 1.6	12.7 ± 2.4	0.11
Creatinine (mg/dL)	1.2 ± 0.3	2.0 ± 1.7	0.04
eGFR (mL/min/1.73 m^2)	65.4 ± 13.6	57.9 ± 31.5	0.32
CKD stage			0.11
I/II	15 (68.2)	10 (45.5)	
III	7 (31.8)	7 (31.8)	
IV	0 (0)	3 (13.6)	
V	0 (0)	2 (9.1)	

Continuous data are presented as mean ± standard deviation; category data are presented as number (percentage); CABG = coronary artery bypass grafting; BMI = body mass index; CAD = coronary artery disease; CVD = cardiovascular disease; LM = left main; TVD = triple vessel disease; DVD = double vessel disease; LIMA = left internal mammary artery; RIMA = right internal mammary artery; eGFR = estimated glomerular filtration rate; CKD = chronic kidney disease.

3.2. In-Hospital Adverse Events

In-hospital adverse events did not differ between the groups ($p > 0.05$), except for a significantly lower incidence of CKD stages 4 and 5 in patients who received da Vinci robot-assisted CABG with BIMA grafting (1, 4.5% vs. 10, 45.4%, respectively; $p < 0.01$). In-hospital cardiovascular events were equal between the two groups, including death, non-fatal MI, repeated revascularization, and non-fatal stroke ($p > 0.05$). The adverse events in hospital are outlined in Table 2.

Table 2. Adverse events in hospital between two surgical modalities.

	Da Vinci Robotic Surgery (n = 22)	Sternotomy Surgery (n = 22)	p Value
Hospital stay (days)	21.0 ± 8.8	24.4 ± 14.0	0.34
ICU stay (days)	4.8 ± 3.5	5.0 ± 3.3	0.90
Ventilator weaning (days)	2.2 ± 1.8	2.3 ± 2.3	0.94
Renal events			
CKD stages IV/V	1 (4.5)	10 (22.7)	<0.01
Creatinine change >0.5 mg/dL	5 (22.7)	7 (31.8)	0.50
Doubling creatinine (mg/dL)	1 (4.8)	3 (13.6)	0.61
eGFR (mL/min/1.73 m^2) *	58.5 ± 22.1	45.5 ± 31.6	0.12
Hemodialysis	0 (0)	1 (4.5)	1.00
The lowest hemoglobin (g/dL)	11.9 ± 1.5	12.1 ± 1.5	0.57
Blood transfusion (U)			
FFP	5.3 ± 3.8	3.8 ± 4.3	0.28
PRBC	2.1 ± 2.0	1.4 ± 2.2	0.30
Adverse events	4 (18.2)	5 (27.8)	0.70
Death	0 (0)	0 (0)	1.00
Myocardial infarction	0 (0)	0 (0)	1.00
Stroke	0 (0)	0 (0)	1.00
Wound infection	1 (4.5)	1 (5.6)	1.00
Pneumonia	1 (4.5)	0 (0)	1.00
Pleural effusion	1 (4.5)	2 (11.1)	1.00
Post-operation IABP	2 (9.1)	3 (13.6)	1.00

Continuous data are presented as mean ± standard deviation; category data are presented as number (percentage); CABG = coronary artery bypass grafting; CKD = chronic kidney disease; eGFR = estimated glomerular filtration rate; FFP = fresh frozen plasma; PRBC = packed red blood cells; ICU = intensive care unit; eGFR * = indicate the lowest value of eGFR in hospital; IABP = intra-aortic balloon pump.

3.3. Primary Endpoints at Six Months

Primary endpoints at six months were significantly reduced in robotic CABG compared with sternotomy CABG (5, 22.7% vs. 12, 54.5%; $p = 0.03$) (Table 3). The finding was reinforced by the Kaplan–Meier analysis ($p = 0.03$ by log-rank test) (Figure 3). The significant reduction was mainly contributed by the fewer renal events in robotic surgery (1 vs. 7; $p = 0.02$). The cumulative rates of cardiovascular endpoints at six months were identical, including all-cause mortality (0 vs. 0; $p = 1.0$), non-fatal MI (0 vs. 1; $p = 1.0$), and non-fatal stroke (0 vs. 0; $p = 1.0$).

Table 3. Clinical outcomes at six months between two surgical modalities.

	Da Vinci Robotic Surgery (n = 22)	Sternotomy Surgery (n = 22)	p Value
Finished six months follow-up	19 (86.5)	21 (95.5)	
Primary endpoints	5 (22.7)	12 (54.5)	0.03
Cardiovascular events	1 (4.5)	0 (0)	1.00
Mortality	0 (0)	0 (0)	1.00
Myocardial infarction	1 (4.5)	0 (0)	1.00
Stoke	0 (0)	0 (0)	1.00
Renal events	1 (4.5)	7 (31.8)	0.02
CKD stages IV/V	0 (0)	7 (31.8)	0.02
Creatinine doubling	0 (0)	1 (4.5)	1.00
Creatinine change >0.5 mg/dL	1 (4.5)	5 (22.7)	0.18
Hemodialysis	0 (0)	1 (4.5)	1.00
eGFR (mL/min/1.73 m^2)	72.1 ± 19.0	56.9 ± 34.0	0.08
Re-hospitalization *	4 (18.2)	6 (27.3)	0.47

Continuous data are presented as mean ± standard deviation; category data are presented as number (percentage); CABG = coronary artery bypass grafting; * = re-hospitalizations due to any cause; primary endpoint = all-cause mortality, myocardial infarction, stock, CKD stages IV/V, and creatinine change >0.5 mg/dL.

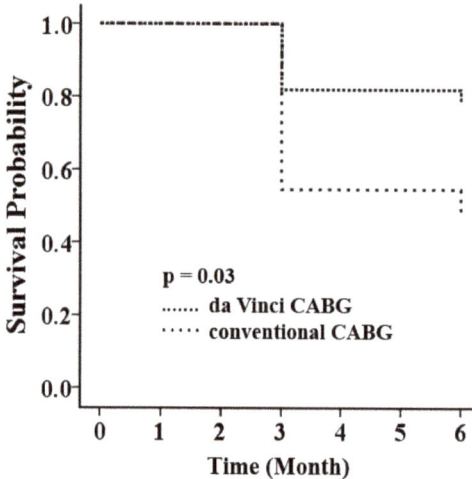

Figure 3. Kaplan–Meier survival analysis shows a significant reduction in the cumulative incidence of the composite of cardiovascular and renal endpoints at six months ($p = 0.03$ by log-rank test), including all-cause mortality, non-fatal myocardial infarction, repeated revascularization, non-fatal stroke, the presence of chronic kidney disease stage 4 or 5, creatinine doubling, and a raise of the baseline creatinine >0.5 mg/dL in patients receiving da Vinci CABG as compared with those receiving conventional CABG. CABG = coronary artery bypass grafting.

4. Discussion

The study generated three major findings: (1) primary endpoints were significantly reduced in patients receiving da Vinci robot-assisted BIMA grafting via the left pleura at six months, as compared with patients receiving sternotomy CABG with BIMA grafting; (2) the significant reduction in primary endpoints was contributed by the fewer renal events in robotic CABG. Cardiovascular endpoints were equal between the groups; (3) robotic CABG compared with conventional CABG had smaller surgical wounds but longer operation times, and identical hospital and ICU stay. The da Vinci robot-assisted CABG with BIMA grafting via the left pleura is considered a new surgical treatment option for patients with severe CAD.

Robotic CABG had a significant reduction in the rate of primary cardiovascular and renal endpoints as compared to sternotomy CABG. The relatively better renal function at baseline in da Vinci robot-assisted CABG with BIMA grafting may partially account for the significant reduction in adverse renal events in hospital and at six months. Renal dysfunction was reported to independently predict post-CABG adverse events, such as mortality and/or morbidity [21–23], and advanced renal diseases [24,25]. Compared with robotic CABG with BIMA grafting, the poorer renal function in conventional CABG possibly resulted in renal deterioration after CABG surgeries. In addition, the finding was consistent with the result obtained from a meta-analysis of 16 pooled studies which showed that robot-assisted CABG versus conventional CABG was associated with fewer renal failure events [19]. Furthermore, renal function may be preserved in off-pump CABG surgeries [26], despite the equality of cardiopulmonary pump use observed between the groups. A shorter elapsed time from coronary angiography until off-pump CABG was also reported to deteriorate renal function [27]. Nevertheless, the reason why there were fewer renal events in robotic CABG versus conventional CABG remains unclear. The finding needs to be further confirmed.

On the other hand, the two groups had identical rates of adverse cardiovascular events in hospital and at six months. The finding implicated that the da Vinci robot-assisted unilateral BIMA grafting was not inferior to the conventional BIMA grafting in terms of short-term cardiovascular outcome.

Furthermore, the data displayed satisfactory results with freedom from subsequent wound infection and post-operative ischemic stroke. A few trials indicated that BIMA harvesting may lead to a decline in blood supply to the sternum and increase the risk of sternal wound infection [4–6]. A BIMA graft-sparing aortic clamp and aortic anastomosis may reduce the risk of peri-operative ischemic stroke [8,17].

The present results disclosed that robotic CABG compared with conventional CABG had longer operation times but without longer ICU and hospital stays, and ventilation times. Similar to conventional BIMA mobilization, robot-assisted BIMA mobilization requires a longer procedure time [28,29], especially in RIMA mobilization through the left pleural and pre-mediastinal space. Unilateral BIMA grafting minimizes the surgical wounds but prolongs the operation times. The robot-assisted operation time may be shortened through collaborative team-work in a learning-curve manner [28]. This will increase operator comfort, reduce fatigue, and allow patients receiving da Vinci robot-assisted CABG with BIMA grafting to have safer interventional procedures, therefore greatly improving patient outcomes [30].

Several limitations have to be emphasized: (1) as the study had few case numbers, low event rates, short follow-up, and primary selection bias, its results should be interpreted with caution; (2) the heterogeneity at baseline and unmeasured confounders between the two different surgeries may have affected the outcomes; (3) other factors, such as hemodynamics, angiographically-proven coronary lesions, and systolic function at baseline, that differed between the two groups could have potentially influenced the outcomes, as these were not investigated in the study; (4) in the study, it was not mandatory to routinely check coronary angiograms to survey the graft patency.

In conclusion, the data showed that da Vinci robot-assisted CABG with left-pleural BIMA grafting compared with conventional sternotomy CABG with BIMA grafting did not increase in-hospital and short-term cardiovascular events but possibly lowered adverse renal events. The study suggests that the robot-assisted CABG with left-pleural BIMA grafting can be considered a new surgical option for patients with severe CAD. Further larger studies are needed to investigate long-term outcomes.

Author Contributions: The study was conceived and designed by C.-J.W., H.-H.C., P.-W.C., and C.-C.L. conducted most of the experiments with assistance from W.-H.L., and C.-J.T. The paper was written by C.-C.L., with contributions from H.-H.C. and C.-J.W.

Funding: This work was supported by funding from the Kaohsiung Veterans General Hospital (VGHKS 106-017, VGHKS107-018, VGHKS107-G01-2; to C.-J.W. and C.-C.L.) and Kaohsiung Municipal United Hospital (KMUH 10809; to C.-C.L.).

Acknowledgments: This study was supported by the Kaohsiung Veterans General Hospital. We would like to thank participating assistants for their contribution in conducting the statistical analysis, including Tina Wu and Chung Jung Chang of the cardiovascular center of Kaohsiung Veterans General Hospital.

Conflicts of Interest: The authors declare there is no conflict of interest.

References

1. Task Force, M.; Montalescot, G.; Sechtem, U.; Achenbach, S.; Andreotti, F.; Arden, C.; Budaj, A.; Bugiardini, R.; Crea, F.; Cuisset, T.; et al. 2013 ESC guidelines on the management of stable coronary artery disease: The task force on the management of stable coronary artery disease of the European society of cardiology. *Eur. Heart J.* **2013**, *34*, 2949–3003.
2. Yates, M.T.; Soppa, G.K.; Valencia, O.; Jones, S.; Firoozi, S.; Jahangiri, M. Impact of European Society of Cardiology and European Association for Cardiothoracic Surgery Guidelines on Myocardial Revascularization on the activity of percutaneous coronary intervention and coronary artery bypass graft surgery for stable coronary artery disease. *J. Thorac. Cardiovasc. Surg.* **2014**, *147*, 606–610.

3. Fihn, S.D.; Blankenship, J.C.; Alexander, K.P.; Bittl, J.A.; Byrne, J.G.; Fletcher, B.J.; Fonarow, G.C.; Lange, R.A.; Levine, G.N.; Maddox, T.M.; et al. 2014 ACC/AHA/AATS/PCNA/SCAI/STS focused update of the guideline for the diagnosis and management of patients with stable ischemic heart disease: A report of the american college of cardiology/american heart association task force on practice guidelines, and the american association for thoracic surgery, preventive cardiovascular nurses association, society for cardiovascular angiography and interventions, and society of thoracic surgeons. *J. Thorac. Cardiovasc. Surg.* **2015**, *149*, e5–e23. [PubMed]
4. He, G.W.; Ryan, W.H.; Acuff, T.E.; Bowman, R.T.; Douthit, M.B.; Yang, C.Q.; Mack, M.J. Risk factors for operative mortality and sternal wound infection in bilateral internal mammary artery grafting. *J. Thorac. Cardiovasc. Surg.* **1994**, *107*, 196–202. [PubMed]
5. Deo, S.V.; Shah, I.K.; Dunlay, S.M.; Erwin, P.J.; Locker, C.; Altarabsheh, S.E.; Boilson, B.A.; Park, S.J.; Joyce, L.D. Bilateral Internal Thoracic Artery Harvest and Deep Sternal Wound Infection in Diabetic Patients. *Ann. Thorac. Surg.* **2013**, *95*, 862–869. [CrossRef] [PubMed]
6. Dai, C.; Lu, Z.; Zhu, H.; Xue, S.; Lian, F. Bilateral Internal Mammary Artery Grafting and Risk of Sternal Wound Infection: Evidence from Observational Studies. *Ann. Thorac. Surg.* **2013**, *95*, 1938–1945. [CrossRef] [PubMed]
7. Weiss, A.J.; Zhao, S.; Tian, D.H.; Taggart, D.P.; Yan, T.D. A meta-analysis comparing bilateral internal mammary artery with left internal mammary artery for coronary artery bypass grafting. *Ann. Cardiothorac. Surg.* **2013**, *2*, 390–400. [PubMed]
8. Glineur, D.; Papadatos, S.; Grau, J.B.; Shaw, R.E.; Kuschner, C.E.; Aphram, G.; Mairy, Y.; Vanbelighen, C.; Etienne, P.Y. Complete myocardial revascularization using only bilateral internal thoracic arteries provides a low-risk and durable 10-year clinical outcome. *Eur. J. Cardio-Thorac. Surg.* **2016**, *50*, 735–741. [CrossRef]
9. Kinoshita, T.; Asai, T.; Suzuki, T.; Kambara, A.; Matsubayashi, K. Off-Pump Bilateral Versus Single Skeletonized Internal Thoracic Artery Grafting in High-Risk Patients. *Circulation* **2011**, *124*, S130–S134. [CrossRef] [PubMed]
10. Kinoshita, T.; Asai, T.; Suzuki, T. Off-pump bilateral skeletonized internal thoracic artery grafting in patients with chronic kidney disease. *J. Thorac. Cardiovasc. Surg.* **2015**, *150*, 315–321. [CrossRef] [PubMed]
11. Pettinari, M.; Sergeant, P.; Meuris, B. Bilateral internal thoracic artery grafting increases long-term survival in elderly patients. *Eur. J. Cardiothorac. Surg.* **2015**, *47*, 703–709. [CrossRef]
12. Galbut, D.L.; Kurlansky, P.A.; Traad, E.A.; Dorman, M.J.; Zucker, M.; Ebra, G. Bilateral internal thoracic artery grafting improves long-term survival in patients with reduced ejection fraction: A propensity-matched study with 30-year follow-up. *J. Thorac. Cardiovasc. Surg.* **2012**, *143*, 844–853. [CrossRef]
13. Puskas, J.D.; Sadiq, A.; Vassiliades, T.A.; Kilgo, P.D.; Lattouf, O.M. Bilateral Internal Thoracic Artery Grafting Is Associated with Significantly Improved Long-Term Survival, Even Among Diabetic Patients. *Ann. Thorac. Surg.* **2012**, *94*, 710–715. [CrossRef]
14. Dalén, M.; Ivert, T.; Holzmann, M.J.; Sartipy, U. Bilateral versus Single Internal Mammary Coronary Artery Bypass Grafting in Sweden from 1997–2008. *PLoS ONE* **2014**, *9*, e86929. [CrossRef]
15. Yang, M.; Wu, Y.; Wang, G.; Xiao, C.; Zhang, H.; Gao, C. Robotic Total Arterial Off-Pump Coronary Artery Bypass Grafting: Seven-Year Single-Center Experience and Long-Term Follow-Up of Graft Patency. *Ann. Thorac. Surg.* **2015**, *100*, 1367–1373. [CrossRef]
16. Gong, W.; Cai, J.; Wang, Z.; Chen, A.; Ye, X.; Li, H.; Zhao, Q. Robot-assisted coronary artery bypass grafting improves short-term outcomes compared with minimally invasive direct coronary artery bypass grafting. *J. Thorac. Dis.* **2016**, *8*, 459–468. [CrossRef]
17. Ishikawa, N.; Watanabe, G.; Tomita, S.; Yamaguchi, S.; Nishida, Y.; Iino, K. Robot-Assisted Minimally Invasive Direct Coronary Artery Bypass Grafting. ThoraCAB *Circ. J.* **2014**, *78*, 399–402. [CrossRef]
18. Canale, L.S.; Bonatti, J. Mammary artery harvesting using the Da Vinci Si robotic system. *Rev. Bras. Cir. Cardiovasc.* **2014**, *29*, 107–109. [CrossRef]
19. Wang, S.; Zhou, J.; Cai, J.-F. Traditional coronary artery bypass graft versus totally endoscopic coronary artery bypass graft or robot-assisted coronary artery bypass graft-meta-analysis of 16 studies. *Eur. Rev. Med. Pharmacol. Sci.* **2014**, *18*, 790–797.
20. Inker, L.A.; Astor, B.C.; Fox, C.H.; Isakova, T.; Lash, J.P.; Peralta, C.A.; Tamura, M.K.; Feldman, H.I. KDOQI US Commentary on the 2012 KDIGO Clinical Practice Guideline for the Evaluation and Management of CKD. *Am. J. Kidney Dis.* **2014**, *63*, 713–735. [CrossRef]

21. Marui, A.; Okabayashi, H.; Komiya, T.; Tanaka, S.; Furukawa, Y.; Kita, T.; Kimura, T.; Sakata, R.; CREDO-Kyoto Investigators. Impact of occult renal impairment on early and late outcomes following coronary artery bypass grafting. *Interact. Cardiovasc. Thorac. Surg.* **2013**, *17*, 638–643. [CrossRef]
22. Cooper, W.A.; O'Brien, S.M.; Thourani, V.H.; Guyton, R.A.; Bridges, C.R.; Szczech, L.A.; Petersen, R.; Peterson, E.D. Impact of renal dysfunction on outcomes of coronary artery bypass surgery: Results from the society of thoracic surgeons national adult cardiac database. *Circulation* **2006**, *113*, 1063–1070. [CrossRef] [PubMed]
23. Hillis, G.S.; Croal, B.L.; Buchan, K.G.; El-Shafei, H.; Gibson, G.; Jeffrey, R.R.; Millar, C.G.; Prescott, G.J.; Cuthbertson, B.H. Renal function and outcome from coronary artery bypass grafting: Impact on mortality after a 2.3-year follow-up. *Circulation* **2006**, *113*, 1056–1062. [CrossRef] [PubMed]
24. Rydén, L.; Sartipy, U.; Evans, M.; Holzmann, M.J. Acute Kidney Injury After Coronary Artery Bypass Grafting and Long-Term Risk of End-Stage Renal Disease. *Circulation* **2014**, *130*, 2005–2011. [CrossRef] [PubMed]
25. Brown, J.R.; Cochran, R.P.; Leavitt, B.J.; Dacey, L.J.; Ross, C.S.; MacKenzie, T.A.; Kunzelman, K.S.; Kramer, R.S.; Hernandez, F., Jr.; Helm, R.E.; et al. Multivariable Prediction of Renal Insufficiency Developing After Cardiac Surgery. *Circulation* **2007**, *116*, 139–143. [CrossRef]
26. Hayashida, N.; Teshima, H.; Chihara, S.; Tomoeda, H.; Takaseya, T.; Hiratsuka, R.; Shoujima, T.; Takagi, K.; Kawara, T.; Aoyagi, S. Does Off-Pump Coronary Artery Bypass Grafting Really Preserve Renal Function? *Circ. J.* **2002**, *66*, 921–925. [CrossRef]
27. Ji, Q.; Mei, Y.; Wang, X.; Feng, J.; Wusha, D.; Cai, J.; Zhou, Y. Effect of Elapsed Time from Coronary Angiography Until Off-Pump Coronary Artery Bypass Surgery on Postoperative Renal Function. *Circ. J.* **2012**, *76*, 2356–2362. [CrossRef]
28. Wiedemann, D.; Bonaros, N.; Schachner, T.; Weidinger, F.; Lehr, E.J.; Vesely, M.; Bonatti, J. Surgical problems and complex procedures: Issues for operative time in robotic totally endoscopic coronary artery bypass grafting. *J. Thorac. Cardiovasc. Surg.* **2012**, *143*, 639–647. [CrossRef] [PubMed]
29. Bolotin, G.; Scott, W.W., Jr.; Austin, T.C.; Charland, P.J.; Kypson, A.P.; Nifong, L.W.; Salleng, K.; Chitwood, W.R., Jr. Robotic skeletonizing of the internal thoracic artery: Is it safe? *Ann. Thorac. Surg.* **2004**, *77*, 1262–1265. [CrossRef] [PubMed]
30. Ragosta, M.; Singh, K.P. Robotic-Assisted Percutaneous Coronary Intervention: Rationale, Implementation, Case Selection and Limitations of Current Technology. *J. Clin. Med.* **2018**, *7*, 23. [CrossRef] [PubMed]

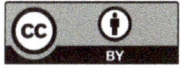

© 2019 by the authors. Licensee MDPI, Basel, Switzerland. This article is an open access article distributed under the terms and conditions of the Creative Commons Attribution (CC BY) license (http://creativecommons.org/licenses/by/4.0/).

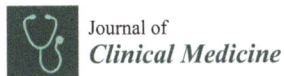

Article

Real-Life Benefit of OCT Imaging for Optimizing PCI Indications, Strategy, and Results

Dan Mircea Olinic [1,2,†], Mihail Spinu [1,*,†], Calin Homorodean [1,2,*], Mihai Claudiu Ober [2] and Maria Olinic [1,2]

1. Medical Clinic No. 1, "Iuliu Hatieganu" University of Medicine and Pharmacy, Cluj-Napoca 400006, Romania; dolinic@yahoo.com (D.M.O.); maria_olinic@yahoo.com (M.O.)
2. Interventional Cardiology Department, Emergency Clinical Hospital, Cluj-Napoca 400006, Romania; mihai_ober@yahoo.com
* Correspondence: spinu_mihai@yahoo.com (M.S.); chomorodean@yahoo.com (C.H.); Tel.: +40-746259047 (M.S.); +40-741025342 (C.H.)
† These authors contributed equally to this work.

Received: 29 January 2019; Accepted: 27 March 2019; Published: 30 March 2019

Abstract: Background: The aim of this study was to evaluate the benefit of standard practice Optical Coherence Tomography (OCT) imaging, as a complement to coronary angiography (CA), for optimizing the indications, strategy, and results of percutaneous coronary interventions (PCI). Methods: We retrospectively analyzed 182 patients with OCT imaging in a single tertiary center. Results: OCT use had a low prevalence (3.1% of 4256 CAs and 1.7% of 3027 PCIs). OCT was used post-CA in 71.5% and post-PCI in 28.5% of cases, mainly in acute coronary syndromes—95.6%. OCT was performed for borderline lesions in 43.4% of cases; lesion severity was reassessed as severe and led to PCI in 64.5% of them. OCT was performed for nonsignificant lesions in 17% of cases; lesion severity was reassessed as severe and led to PCI in 38.7% of them. OCT provided optimal selection for PCI strategy in 11% of cases. OCT identified suboptimal PCI results in 54% left main PCIs and in 48% bifurcation PCIs with optimal CA; PCI optimization was performed. In the only seven patients with suboptimal PCI, OCT revealed an optimal result in four cases, thus avoiding unneccessary optimization. In 27.3% of patients with post-CA OCT and PCI result "systematic" OCT control, a PCI optimization was indicated. Conclusion: OCT supplied a major benefit in 86.2% of cases, especially by identifying significant coroanry stenosis in CA borderline and nonsignificant lesions; OCT led to PCI indication in two-thirds and, respectively, one-third of these cases. In the post-PCI context, OCT led to an indication of PCI optimization in half of the complex left main and bifurcation lesions, as well as in a quarter of "systematic" post-PCI OCT controls.

Keywords: optical coherence tomography; percutaneous coronary interventions; borderline lesions; nonsignificant lesions; left main; bifurcations

1. Introduction

Cardiovascular diseases represent a major health burden, with coronary artery disease (CAD) as the most important cause of morbidity and mortality [1,2]. Every effort is made for improving CAD diagnosis, identifying patients with an indication for revascularization and optimal revascularization treatment through either interventional cardiology or cardiac surgery, resulting in a progressive decrease in CAD mortality [3,4].

Coronary angiography (CA) is the gold standard invasive procedure currently used for CAD diagnosis, decision-taking and assessing efficacy of percutaneous coronary interventions (PCIs) [5]. CA limitations are related to suboptimal ability to identify complicated atherosclerotic plaques and sometimes even to incorrect grading of the severity of coronary stenosis [5].

Optical coherence tomography (OCT) further improves invasive intracoronary imaging, offering new insights on the coronary wall and lumen, due to its high resolution (10 micrometers) [3,6]. OCT provides accurate characterization of atherosclerotic plaques, in terms of severity and extension, and identifies high-risk and complicated plaques, as well as coronary thrombi [5,6].

Over the last ten years, fast acquisition OCT devices and software allowed this method to be used safely, in everyday practice, as a complement to CA. OCT is therefore not only a very well recognized in vivo CAD research tool [6–8], but also an increasingly used real-life tool. Various indications have been proposed for OCT use in current clinical practice [9–11], as experience with OCT use has grown [12–14]. Recent guidelines already recommend OCT use for optimizing stent-related PCI procedures [15].

The aim of this study is to evaluate the benefit of standard practice OCT imaging, as a complement to CA for optimizing the indications, strategy and results of percutaneous coronary interventions. The study covers five years of practice of a single tertiary center from Romania.

2. Methods

2.1. Study Population

This study retrospectively analyzes the indications and benefit of OCT use in 182 patients, evaluated in a single tertiary center from Romania (Cluj County Emergency Hospital, Department of Interventional Cardiology), over a period of 5 years (January 2012–September 2017). During this interval, 4256 patients underwent CA for suspected CAD, of whom, 3027 patients also had PCI.

No exclusion criteria were considered. Informed consent was obtained before the invasive procedure. Clinical data and angiographic examinations were stored in the hospital database and in a dedicated catheterization laboratory database.

Data regarding cardiovascular risk factors [2] were obtained from patients history, physical examination, and medical records. Arterial hypertension was defined as known or newly diagnosed blood pressure values above 140/90 mmHg. Diabetes mellitus was defined as known or newly diagnosed blood fasting glucose above 126 mg/dL or glycated haemoglobin >6.5%. Dyslipidemia was defined as low-density lipoprotein cholesterol >130 mg/dL and/or triglycerides >150 mg/dL. Renal insufficiency was defined as a glomerular filtration rate <60 mL/min. Smoking habit was defined by current or recent smoking. Overweight was defined as body mass index >25 kg/m^2.

CA was performed via right radial artery in 143 (78.6%) patients, via femoral artery in 35 (19.2%) patients and transbrachial in the remaining four (2.2%) patients, on Siemens Coroskop T.O.P and Siemens Artis Zee angiographs (Siemens Healthineers, Erlangen, Germany). Severity of coronary stenosis was assessed visually and by quantitative coronary analysis (QCA). The highest degree of stenosis severity, usually the area stenosis severity provided by QCA, was considered. After CA, coronary arteries were classified as normal (without plaques), with nonsignificant lesions (<50%), with borderline lesions (50–70%) or with significant stenosis (>70%).

2.2. OCT Acquisition Technique, Analysis, and Indications

OCT images were acquired with a commercially available system (ILUMIEN OPTIS OCT Intravascular Imaging System, St. Jude Medical, St. Paul, MN, USA), using an over the wire OCT catheter (C7 Dragonfly™ and Dragonfly™ OPTIS™, St. Jude Medical, St. Paul, MN, USA). The entire length of the region of interest was scanned using the integrated automated pullback device at 20 mm/s. During image acquisition, coronary blood flow was replaced by continuous flushing of contrast medium directly from the guiding catheter. All images were recorded digitally, stored, and analyzed using proprietary software (St. Jude Medical, St. Paul, MN, USA) in concordance with standard consensus of OCT use [5].

OCT was performed by all three senior interventional cardiologists, using the predefined indications in Table 1, during working hours and, two days each week, 24/24 h, for emergency situations like acute coronary syndromes (ACS).

Table 1. Indications for OCT use, adapted from Tearney G.J. et al. [5], Räber L. et al. [10] and Karanasos A. et al. [16]. OCT: optical coherence tomography; PCI: percutaneous coronary intervention; ACS- acute coronary syndrome.

OCT Indication	Specific Area of Interest
Post-Coronary Angiography and before a first PCI procedure	
Lesion evaluation	Culprit lesion evaluation in ACS patients without coronary angiography significant stenosis
	Evaluation of lesions with angiographic haziness (suspected dissection/thrombus/calcification)
Pre-PCI assessment	Measurements of lumen diameter and lesion length for PCI devices selection (balloon/stent dimensions)
	Lesion assessment for PCI technique/strategy selection (for left main and large bifurcations)
	Evaluation of "landing zones"
	Evaluation of guide wire position (in cases of coronary dissection/chronic occlusion)
Post-PCI	
Immediate assessment of PCI result	Evaluation of stent expansion (identification of under-expansion/residual stenosis)
	Evaluation of potential vascular injury (identification of edge dissection/intra-stent thrombus/tissue protrusion)
Late evaluation of suspected stent failure	Identification and characterization of restenosis
	Identification of in stent thrombosis
	Identification of neoatherosclerosis

Indications for OCT use were the ones generally accepted at the time of the investigation (Table 1) [5,10,16]. OCT was performed either after CA, for lesion evaluation or pre-PCI strategy assessment, or after PCI, for result assessment. OCT quantification of coronary lesion severity was made using the proprietary software, as area stenosis compared to largest pre-lesion reference area. An OCT area stenosis of at least 70% was considered as significant stenosis, with an indication for PCI.

The study complies with the Declaration of Helsinki on human research.

2.3. Statistical Analysis

Categorical variables were expressed as frequencies and compared with χ^2 test. A two-sided *p*-value of 0.05 was considered significant.

3. Results

3.1. Demographic, Clinical and Angiographic Data

The investigated population includes 174 (95.6%) patients with ACS, of which 50 had ST-elevated myocardial infarction (STEMI), 39 had non-ST elevated myocardial infarction (NSTEMI), 85 had unstable angina (UA), and eight had stable CAD (SCAD). Demographic, clinical and angiographic data of OCT investigated patients are presented in Table 2 and data regarding their cardiovascular risk factors are presented in Table 3.

Table 2. Demographic, clinical and angiographic data of patients investigated by OCT (LAD—left anterior descending artery, LCX—left circumflex artery, LM—left main, RCA—right coronary artery).

		STEMI (No. of Patients) 50	NSTEMI (No. of Patients) 39	UA (No. of Patients) 85	SCAD (No. of Patients) 8	Total (No. of Patients/%) 182
Gender	Male	34	29	55	6	124 (68.1%)
	Female	16	10	30	2	58 (31.9%)
Age	<40	2	0	3	0	5 (2.7%)
	≤40–49	22	3	10	2	37 (20.3%)
	≤50–59	9	13	20	2	44 (24.2%)
	≤60–69	8	10	36	3	57 (31.3%)
	≤70–79	8	12	16	1	37 (20.3%)
	≥80	1	1	0	0	2 (1.1%)
Coronary Angiography Results	Normal	2	1	3	1	7 (3.8%)
	LM	5	6	11	0	22 (12.1%)
	1 Vessel Disease	29	8	30	2	69 (37.9%)
	2 Vessels Disease	6	7	17	3	33 (18.1%)
	3 Vessels Disease	8	17	24	2	51 (28%)
OCT Examined Vessel	LM	9	18	30	2	59 (32.4%)
	LAD	31	18	49	6	104 (57.1%)
	LCX	3	2	2	0	7 (3.8%)
	RCA	7	0	4	0	11 (6.1%)
	Venous Graft	0	1	0	0	1 (0.5%)

Table 3. Study population cardiovascular risk factors.

Hypertension	143 (78.6%)
Diabetes mellitus	46 (25.3%)
Dyslipidemia	105 (57.7%)
Renal Insufficiency	11 (6%)
Smoking habit	52 (28.6%)
Overweight	35 (19.2%)

3.2. Post Coronarography OCT

OCT was performed in two main instances: first, as a complementary imaging method after CA—130 patients (71.5% of the OCT investigations) and second, as an imaging method just used first after PCI—52 patients (28.5% of the OCT investigations) (Figure 1). Post-CA OCT was made in 3.1% of the total 4256 CAs performed in CAD patients, while post-PCI OCT was done in 1.7% of the total 3027 PCIs. OCT had two main indications, in the 130 patients post-CA group: OCT to provide accurate diagnosis and therapeutic decisions for revascularization ("decision-making OCT group")—110 patients (60.4% of the OCT investigations)—and, respectively, OCT to provide optimal selection of PCI strategy—20 patients (11% of the OCT investigations) (Figure 1).

3.2.1. "Decision-making OCT Group"

In the "decision-making OCT group" (110 patients), there were 79 patients (43.4% of the OCT investigations) with borderline (50–70%) CA lesions and 31 patients (17% of the OCT investigations) with nonsignificant lesions (<50%) or with a normal aspect on CA (Figure 1).

Borderline CA Lesions

In the 79 patients with a high clinical and electrocardiogram suspicion of CAD and with borderline CA lesions, in 77 of them with ACS (43 UAs, 17 STEMIs, and 17 NSTEMIs) and only two with SCADs an accurate decision for revascularisation could not be made based on CA alone, so OCT was performed. After performing OCT, the severity of coronary artery lesions was reassessed and graded as severe (>70%) (Figure 2A/a), with an indication for revascularization in 51 patients (64.5% of the 79 cases) (Table 4).

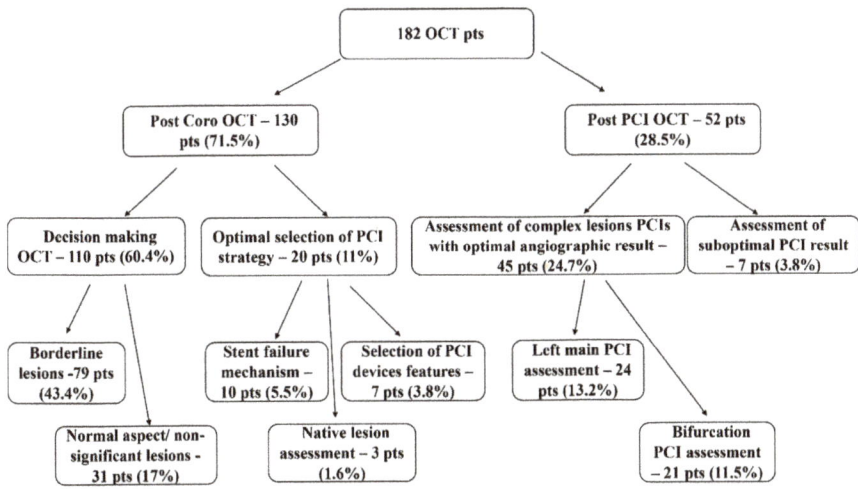

Figure 1. OCT indications. Pts: patients.

Nonsignificant Lesions or Normal Coronary Aspect

In the 31 patients with nonsignificant lesions (<50%) (Figure 2B/b and 2C/c) or with a normal coronary arteries aspect on CA (Figure 2D/d), there were 29 patients with ACS (15 STEMIs, 10 UAs, and four NSTEMIs). These ACS pts represented 15.3% of the total 189 ACS patients with nonsignificant lesions or normal coronary arteries investigated in our center, during the investigated time interval. There also were two SCAD patients. OCT identified 12 patients with significant (>70%) lesions (38.7% of the 31 cases), leading to PCI revascularization (Table 4).

When performed after CA, OCT led to revascularization in significantly more patients with borderline lesions than in ones with nonsignificant lesions or normal coronary arteries (64.5 vs. 38.7%, $p = 0.013$).

3.2.2. OCT for Optimal Selections of PCI Strategy

The second main indication for OCT, after CA, was represented by patients in whom a decision for PCI revascularization was taken after CA, but OCT was still needed on top of CA, in order to provide optimal selection of PCI strategy (Figure 1). In these 20 patients (11% of the OCT investigations), there were three indications for OCT:

- identification of stent failure mechanism (10 patients, 5.5% of the OCT investigations); OCT proved restenosis in eight and neoatherosclerosis in two patients (Figure 2E/e);
- selection of PCI devices features (seven patients, 3.8% of the OCT investigations); there were three cases of long lesions PCI (Figure 2F/f), two of left main (LM) PCI and another two of bifurcation PCI;
- comprehensive assessment of native lesions suspected of complications (three patients, 1.6% of the OCT investigations); OCT confirmed complicated atherosclerotic plaques in all three of them, with identification of thrombus in one patient.

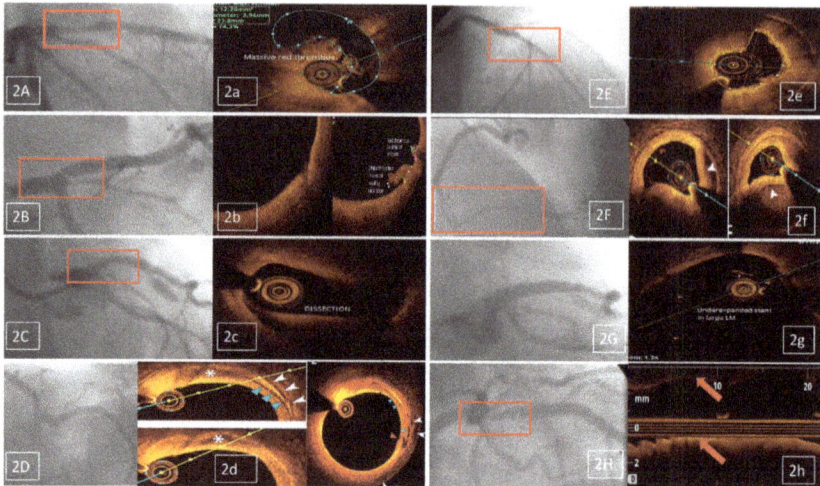

Figure 2. (**A**)—Anterior STEMI previously treated with fibrinolytic therapy—angiographically borderline lesion on proximal LAD, **a**—OCT shows massive red thrombus, with significant lumen stenosis; (**B**)—UA patient—angiographically nonsignificant lesion on ostial LAD, **b**—OCT shows signs of culprit lesion (white and red thrombus), with permeable lumen; (**C**)—Anterior STEMI patient—ostial LAD haziness of nonsignificant lesion, **c**—OCT shows coronary dissection, with significant lumen stenosis; (**D**)—Anterior STEMI patient—angiographically normal coronary aspect, **d**—OCT shows a dissection and hematoma originating from a vasa vasorum hemorrhage, being probably the underlying physiopathology of the ACS; (**E**)—NSTEMI patient at 10 years after a LCX bare metal stent implantation—angiographically intra-stent haziness, **e**—OCT shows neoatherosclerosis as the mechanism for stent failure; (**F**)—Inferior STEMI female patient—angiographically long, double lumen pattern, RCA stenosis, **f**—OCT confirms spontaneous dissection as the underlying physiopathology and guides PCI (guide wire presence in the true lumen and choice of stent's "landing zones"); (**G**)—LM PCI with excellent angiographic result, **g**—OCT shows significant malapposition; (**H**)—Suboptimal angiographic result of proximal LAD stent placement, **h**—OCT shows excellent result.

3.3. Post-PCI OCT Group

The "post-PCI" OCT group included 52 patients, with two main indications for imaging (Figure 1): assessment of complex lesions PCIs, with an optimal angiographic result—45 cases (24.7% of the OCT investigations) and assessment of suboptimal PCI results—seven cases (3.8%).

3.3.1. Assessment of Complex Lesions PCIs with Optimal Angiographic Result Included:

Left Main Lesions PCI Assessment

This group included 24 patients with LM PCI, representing 13.2% of OCT indications and 19.8% of the 121 LM PCIs performed in our center, during the investigated time interval; there were mainly ACS (nine UA, eight STEMI, and six NSTEMI) patients, while two had SCAD; OCT was performed for LM PCI control in cases of technically challenging procedures (15 cases), two stents technique (seven cases), and for important LM, LAD, or LCX decalibration (two cases); optimal OCT results were found in 11 patients, without need for LM PCI optimization; OCT imaging found malappositions (10 patients) (Figure 2G/g) and edge dissections (three patients), leading to a decision for PCI optimization (with new balloon dilatation or, respectively, new stent implantation) in these 13 out of the 24 patients (54% of the LM PCIs with optimal angiographic results) (Table 4).

Bifurcation Lesions PCI Assessment

This group included 21 patients with bifurcation PCI, representing 11.5% of OCT indications and 2.2% of the 955 bifurcation PCIs performed in our center, during the investigated time interval; there were only ACS (11 UA, seven NSTEMI, and three STEMI) patients; OCT was performed for bifurcation PCI control in cases of technically challenging procedures (11 cases) and two stents techniques (10 cases); optimal OCT results were found in 11 patients, without need for PCI optimization; OCT imaging found malappositions (six patients) and edge dissections (four patients), leading to a decision for PCI optimization in these 10 out of the 21 patients (48% of the bifurcation PCIs with optimal angiographic results) (Table 4).

3.3.2. Assessment of Suboptimal PCI Results

This group included seven patients (three STEMI, two NSTEMI, and two UA), representing only 0.23% of the 3027 PCIs performed in our center in the investigated time interval. The indication for OCT imaging was represented by

- angiographic suspicion of edge dissection (three cases); only one was confirmed by OCT, leading to PCI optimization;
- angiographic suspicion of extensive coronary dissection (one case)—unconfirmed by OCT;
- angiographic suspicion of coronary thrombus (two cases), confirmed by OCT in both cases and followed by PCI optimization;
- angiographic suspicion of significant residual stenosis in the native coronary, proximal to the stented lesion (one case), unconfirmed by OCT (Figure 2H/h).

In this group, OCT imaging revealed the presence of an optimal PCI result in four of the seven patients (57.1%), thus avoiding unneccessary PCI optimization. There were only three out of seven patients (42.8%) in whom PCI optimization was really needed.

3.4. Decision Change after OCT

For the entire group of 182 patients investigated by OCT, intracoronary imaging had a decisive benefit for optimizing interventional cardiology indications and strategy, in 157 patients (86.2%), as follows

- in all the 130 patients having OCT imaging as a complement to CA, for assessing the indication of revascularization and
- in 27 of the 52 patients investigated post-PCI (51.9% of this subgroup).

3.5. OCT Investigations not Included in This Study

There also were 44 OCT investigations performed after PCI, out of 77 cases, in patients from the "post-CA" group. In these patients, OCT catheter was already used before PCI, OCT investigations were therefore performed for PCI result control. In this group of patients, all post-PCI angiographic results were optimal, but OCT found suboptimal result and led to optimization in 12 cases (27.3%): 10 with balloon post-dilatation for stent underexpansion and two with new stent implantation for edge dissections.

Table 4. Treatment options after OCT.

Indications	Conservative Treatment No. of Patients/%	Revascularization No. of Patients/%	Total No. of Patients
Borderline lesions	28(35.5%)	51(64.5%)	79
Nonsignificant lesions or normal coronaries	19(61.3%)	12(38.7%)	31
Stent failure mechanism		10	10
Native lesion assessment		3	3
Selection of PCI devices		7	7
LM PCI control, after optimal angiography	11 (45.8%)	13 (54.2%)	24
Bifurcation PCI control, after optimal angiography	11 (52.3%)	10 (47.7%)	21
Suboptimal PCI result on angiography	4 (57.1%)	3 (42.9%)	7

4. Discussion

Multiple centers use OCT in a variety of clinical scenarios for diagnosis and therapeutic optimization in coronary interventions [9–14]. A recently issued European Association of Percutaneous Cardiovascular Interventions (EAPCI) expert consensus document on clinical use of intracoronary contained a broad array of OCT indications [10]. The ESC guidelines on myocardial revascularization [15] recommend OCT use for PCI optimization (Class IIa, Level of evidence B) and for identifying stent failure mechanism (Class IIa, Level of evidence C). A recent clinical practice survey [11] offered the perception of interventional cardiologists on the indications for OCT use and their relative prevalence. Our study provides actual evidence on real-life OCT use in a tertiary interventional cardiology center, allowing analysis of its indications and highlighting its benefits. The main benefit proved to be the identification of significant coronary stenosis, with an indication for PCI, in patients with borderline and nonsignificant coronary lesions on CA. Our study also proved OCT interest for optimizing imaging results after PCI, in complex LM and bifurcation lesions, as well as in a "systematic" post-PCI OCT control approach. This imagistic PCI optimization would translate into a better clinical outcome [5,10].

In our study, OCT proves particularly useful in the clinical setting of ACS (95.6% of the investigated patients), with 71.5% of OCTs performed as a complementary imaging method to CA, representing 3.1% of CAs in our center.

We mainly used OCT to provide accurate diagnosis and therapeutic decisions concerning revascularization (60.4% of the OCT investigations). A moderate proportion (43.4%) of the OCT investigations were performed for borderline lesions, and 17% for assessment of coronary arteries with nonsignificant lesions or with a normal aspect. Our approach is in consensus with the recent european recommendation [15] of OCT use in the up to 25% of NSTE-ACS patients with angiographically normal epicardial arteries, for identifying culprit lesions or rule out mechanisms such as dissection and haematomas (MI with nonobstructive coronary arteries, MINOCA). In ACS patients, physiological evaluation with fractional flow reserve has a limited value, with contradictory reports on safety [15,17,18] and unknown prognostic value [15].

A very important finding in our study is that OCT, performed complementary to CA, in ACS, reassessed the severity of coronary lesions and led to the indication of revascularization in 64.5% of borderline lesions, and in 38.7% of nonsignificant lesions or normal coronary arteries. This result would support inclusion of OCT imaging in the practice guidelines, in this setting.

In our study, OCT also proved useful for the control of LM PCI patients with optimal angiographic results, which accounted for 13.2% of OCT indications. In these patients, suboptimal OCT findings as malappositions and edge dissections led to PCI optimization in not less than 54% of the cases. This finding underlines the limits of angiography for LM PCI assessment and may support the need for a systematic OCT imaging in this setting. In our study, OCT was used in only 19.8% of LM PCI patients, with technically challenging procedures, a two-stent technique, or important LM, LAD, or LCX decalibration. This was in contrast to the survey on intravascular imaging use, where participants reported a 77% use for LM PCI guidance [11].

OCT was useful for optimization of bifurcation PCI, in difficult, technically challenging procedures and two-stent techniques. Despite a very good angiographic result in these patients, OCT found suboptimal results in 48% of the cases, with need for optimization. These findings support the limited existing data [19–21] regarding the need for more than angiography in bifurcation PCI. Other clinical practitioners reported a 53.5% use of IVI for guiding bifurcation PCI [11]. However, we used OCT for only 2.19% of our bifurcation PCIs (11.5% of total OCTs).

While other authors report that 79.6% of IVI evaluations are done for PCI strategy planing, in selected cases [11], this indication accounted for only 11% of OCTs, in our center. We used pre-PCI OCT for identifying stent failure mechanisms, selecting PCI devices features, and assesing native lesions.

OCT provided support in cases with suboptimal angiographic PCI results, in whom imaging proved in fact to correspond to a good PCI result, in four of the seven investigated patients. This is a rare OCT indication but its results further support that OCT imaging may overcome CA limitations.

While being available during the whole 5-year period of our study, OCT was used in only 1.7% of patients undergoing PCI. Our findings are comparable to the results of a recent large observational study, which showed a 1.3% prevalence of OCT use for PCI guiding [22].

Our relatively low prevalence of OCT use (3.1% of CA and 1.7% of PCIs) is similar to the approach of 16.6% of interventionalists in the recent clinical practice survey, that used intravascular imaging in less than 5% of their patients [11]. It is however to be noted that, in this same survey [11], 51.3% of the participants use IVI in more that 15% of patients, another 18% of participants use IVI in 5–15% of patients, and 10.3% of participants use IVI only in highly selected cases, while 3.9% of interventional cardiologists do not use any IVI [11].

Our study reports that OCT, while used in a limited number of pts submitted to CA and PCI, offer a substantial benefit for 86.2% of the investigated patients, leading to optimization of interventional cardiology indications and strategy. This is true in all patients in the post-CA group and in 51.9% of the post-PCI group.

Our results concerning OCT-related decision changes in the post-PCI LM and bifurcations complex lesions group (51.9%) are similar to the ones reported by the DOCTORS [23] trial, namely, a 50% change in procedural strategy in the OCT group. The ILUMIEN I study [24] reported 27% decision change in the post-PCI group. This low prevalence of OCT-related decision change post-PCI in the ILLUMIEN I study, can be explained by the systematic use of OCT, both pre- and post-PCI [24]. In our study, the systematic post-PCI use of OCT, in patients already having had OCT pre-PCI, led to identification of suboptimal PCI results, mainly underexpansion and edge dissection, with an indication for PCI optimization, in 27.3% of the cases, similar to the one in ILLUMIEN I study [24].

5. Study Limitations

Our study is an observational, retrospective, single-center one, with a limited sample size, without a statistical power calculation; thereby, our results should be interpreted with caution and considered hypothesis generating. Clinical follow-up of our patients is beyond the purpose of our study. Long term clinical benefit of a dual imagistic approach, using both CA and OCT, and not only CA, for the selection of PCI indications, strategy and result assessment and optimization, would require either a randomized study, or a comparison between centers using these two approaches.

6. Conclusions

The main OCT benefit is in borderline and nonsignificant lesions on CA, in whom OCT identifies significant coronary stenosis and leads to PCI indication in two-thirds and, respectively, one-third of the patients. In the post-PCI context, OCT leads to an indication of PCI optimization in half of the complex left main and bifurcation lesions, as well as in a quarter of "systematic" post-PCI OCT controls.

Author Contributions: Conceptualization, D.O. and M.S.; Methodology, C.H.; Software, M.C.O.; Validation, D.O., M.S., and M.O.; Formal Analysis, M.O.; Investigation, D.O., C.H., and M.C.O.; Resources, D.O.; Data Curation, M.S.; Writing—Original Draft Preparation, D.O. and M.S.; Writing—Review and Editing, D.O. and M.S.; Visualization, M.O.; Supervision, M.O.; Project Administration, D.O., M.S., and M.O.

Conflicts of Interest: The authors declare no conflicts of interest.

References

1. Non-Communicable Diseases Country Profiles 2018. World Health Organization: Geneva, Switzerland, 2018. Available online: apps.who.int/iris/bitstream/handle/10665/274512/9789241514620-eng.pdf (accessed on 8 October 2018).
2. Olinic, D.M.; Spinu, M.; Olinic, M.; Homorodean, C.; Tataru, D.A.; Liew, A.; Schernthaner, G.H.; Stanek, A.; Fowkes, G.; Catalano, M. Epidemiology of peripheral artery disease in Europe: VAS Educational Paper. *Int. Angiol.* **2018**, *37*, 327–334. [CrossRef] [PubMed]
3. Kim, Y.; Johnson, T.W.; Akasaka, T.; Jeong, M.H. The role of optical coherence tomography in the setting of acute myocardial infarction. *J. Cardiol.* **2018**, *72*, 186–192. [CrossRef]
4. Ha, F.J.; Giblett, J.P.; Nerlekar, N.; Cameron, J.D.; Meredith, I.T.; West, N.E.J.; Brown, A.J. Optical Coherence Tomography Guided Percutaneous Coronary Intervention. *Heart Lung Circ.* **2017**, *26*, 1267–1276. [CrossRef] [PubMed]
5. Tearney, G.J.; Regar, E.; Akasaka, T.; Adriaenssens, T.; Barlis, P.; Bezerra, H.G.; Bouma, B.; Bruining, N.; Cho, J.M.; Chowdhary, S.; et al. International Working Group for Intravascular Optical CoherenceTomography (IWG-IVOCT). Consensus standards for acquisition, measurement, and reporting of intravascular optical coherence tomography studies: A report from the International Working Group for Intravascular Optical Coherence Tomography Standardization and Validation. *J. Am. Coll. Cardiol.* **2012**, *59*, 1058–1072. [CrossRef]
6. Spînu, M.; Olinic, D.M.; Olinic, M.; Homorodean, C. In vivo imaging of complicated atherosclerotic plaque-role of optical coherence tomography (OCT). *Rom. J. Morphol. Embryol.* **2018**, *59*, 469–478. [PubMed]
7. Otsuka, F.; Joner, M.; Prati, F.; Virmani, R.; Narula, J. Clinical classification of plaque morphology in coronary disease. *Nat. Rev. Cardiol.* **2014**, *11*, 379–389. [CrossRef] [PubMed]
8. Kini, A.S.; Vengrenyuk, Y.; Yoshimura, T.; Matsumura, M.; Pena, J.; Baber, U.; Moreno, P.; Mehran, R.; Maehara, A.; Sharma, S.; et al. Fibrous cap thickness by optical coherence tomography in vivo. *J. Am. Coll. Cardiol.* **2017**, *69*, 644–657. [CrossRef]
9. Di Mario, C.; Mattesini, A. Will Optical Coherence Tomography Become the Standard Imaging Tool for Percutaneous Coronary Intervention Guidance? *JACC Cardiovasc. Interv.* **2018**, *11*, 1322–1324. [CrossRef]
10. Räber, L.; Mintz, G.S.; Koskinas, K.C.; Johnson, T.W.; Holm, N.R.; Onuma, Y.; Radu, M.D.; Joner, M.; Yu, B.; Jia, H.; et al. Clinical use of intracoronary imaging. Part 1: Guidance and optimization of coronary interventions. An expert consensus document of the European Association of Percutaneous Cardiovascular Interventions. *EuroIntervention* **2018**, *14*, 656–677. [CrossRef]
11. Koskinas, K.C.; Nakamura, M.; Räber, L.; Colleran, R.; Kadota, K.; Capodanno, D.; Wijns, W.; Akasaka, T.; Valgimigli, M.; Guagliumi, G.; et al. Current use of intracoronary imaging in interventional practice—Results of a European Association of Percutaneous Cardiovascular Interventions (EAPCI) and Japanese Association of Cardiovascular Interventions and Therapeutics (CVIT) Clinical Practice Survey. *EuroIntervention* **2018**, *14*, e475–e484. [CrossRef]
12. Homorodean, C.; Ober, M.C.; Iancu, A.C.; Olinic, M.; Tataru, D.; Spinu, M.; Olinic, D.M.; Burzotta, F.; Trani, C.; Erglis, A. How should I treat this mini-crush stenting complication? *EuroIntervention* **2017**, *13*, 1248–1252. [CrossRef]
13. Olinic, D.M.; Spinu, M.; Homorodean, C.; Olinic, M. Vasa vasorum induced LAD dissection and haematoma in an anterior STEMI patient with nearly normal angiography: The role of OCT. *Kardiol. Pol.* **2017**, *75*, 504. [CrossRef] [PubMed]
14. Homorodean, C.; Spinu, M.; Ober, M.C.; Olinic, M.; Olinic, D.M. Spontaneous coronary dissection: Optical coherence tomography insights before and after stenting. *Cardiol. J.* **2017**, *24*, 217–218. [CrossRef] [PubMed]

15. Neumann, F.J.; Sousa-Uva, M.; Ahlsson, A.; Alfonso, F.; Banning, A.P.; Benedetto, U.; Byrne, R.A.; Collet, J.P.; Falk, V.; Head, S.J.; et al. 2018 ESC/EACTS Guidelines on myocardial revascularization. *Eur. Heart J.* **2019**, *40*, 87–165. [CrossRef] [PubMed]
16. Karanasos, A.; Ligthart, J.; Witberg, K.; van Soest, G.; Bruining, N.; Regar, E. Optical Coherence Tomography: Potential Clinical Applications. *Curr. Cardiovasc. Imaging Rep.* **2012**, *5*, 206–220. [CrossRef] [PubMed]
17. Leone, A.M.; Cialdella, P.; Lassandro Pepe, F.; Basile, E.; Zimbardo, G.; Arioti, M.; Ciriello, G.; D'Amario, D.; Buffon, A.; Burzotta, F.; et al. Fractional flow reserve in acute coronary syndromes and in stable ischemic heart disease: Clinical implications. *Int. J. Cardiol.* **2019**, *277*, 42–46. [CrossRef]
18. Hakeem, A.; Almomani, A.; Uretsky, B.F. Role of fractional flow reserve in the evaluation and management of patients with acute coronary syndrome. *Curr. Opin. Cardiol.* **2017**, *32*, 767–775. [CrossRef]
19. Wolfrum, M.; De Maria, G.L.; Banning, A.P. Optical coherence tomography to guide percutaneous treatment of coronary bifurcation disease. *Expert Rev. Cardiovasc. Ther.* **2017**, *15*, 705–713. [CrossRef]
20. Onuma, Y.; Okamura, T.; Muramatsu, T.; Uemura, S.; Serruys, P.W. New implication of three-dimensional optical coherence tomography in optimising bifurcation PCI. *EuroIntervention* **2015**, *11* (Suppl. V), V71–V74. [CrossRef] [PubMed]
21. Onuma, Y.; Katagiri, Y.; Burzotta, F.; Holm, N.R.; Amabile, N.; Okamura, T.; Mintz, G.S.; Darremont, O.; Lassen, J.F.; Lefèvre, T.; et al. Joint consensus on the use of OCT in coronary bifurcation lesions by European and Japanese bifurcation clubs. *EuroIntervention* **2019**, *14*, e1568–e1577. [CrossRef] [PubMed]
22. Jones, D.A.; Rathod, K.S.; Koganti, S.; Hamshere, S.; Astroulakis, Z.; Lim, P.; Sirker, A.; O'Mahony, C.; Jain, A.K.; Knight, C.J.; et al. Angiography Alone Versus Angiography Plus Optical Coherence Tomography to Guide Percutaneous Coronary Intervention: Outcomes From the Pan-London PCI Cohort. *JACC Cardiovasc. Interv.* **2018**, *11*, 1313–1321. [CrossRef] [PubMed]
23. Meneveau, N.; Souteyrand, G.; Motreff, P.; Caussin, C.; Amabile, N.; Ohlmann, P.; Morel, O.; Lefrançois, Y.; Descotes-Genon, V.; Silvain, J.; et al. Optical coherence tomography to optimize results of percutaneous coronary intervention in patients with non-ST-elevation acute coronary syndrome: Results of the multicenter, randomized DOCTORS study (Does Optical Coherence Tomography Optimize Results of Stenting). *Circulation* **2016**, *134*, 906–917. [CrossRef] [PubMed]
24. Wijns, W.; Shite, J.; Jones, M.R.; Lee, S.W.; Price, M.J.; Fabbiocchi, F.; Barbato, E.; Akasaka, T.; Bezerra, H.; Holmes, D. Optical coherence tomography imaging during percutaneous coronary intervention impacts physician decision-making: ILUMIEN I study. *Eur. Heart J.* **2015**, *36*, 3346–3355. [CrossRef] [PubMed]

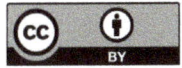

© 2019 by the authors. Licensee MDPI, Basel, Switzerland. This article is an open access article distributed under the terms and conditions of the Creative Commons Attribution (CC BY) license (http://creativecommons.org/licenses/by/4.0/).

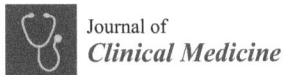

Article

Incremental Predictive Value of Longitudinal Axis Strain and Late Gadolinium Enhancement Using Standard CMR Imaging in Patients with Aortic Stenosis

Lucia Agoston-Coldea [1,2,*], Kunal Bheecarry [1], Carmen Cionca [2], Cristian Petra [1], Lelia Strimbu [3], Camelia Ober [3], Silvia Lupu [4], Daniela Fodor [1] and Teodora Mocan [5]

1. 2nd Department of Internal Medicine, Iuliu Hatieganu University of Medicine and Pharmacy, 400006 Cluj-Napoca, Romania; kunalvarmab@gmail.com (K.B.); cristian.petra@gmail.com (C.P.); dfodor@umfcluj.com (D.F.)
2. Affidea Hiperdia Diagnostic Imaging Center, 400015 Cluj-Napoca, Romania; carmen.cionca@hiperdia.ro
3. Niculae Stancioiu Heart Institute, 400001 Cluj-Napoca, Romania; lstrimbu@yahoo.com (L.S.); cami.ober@yahoo.com (C.O.)
4. 5th Department of Internal Medicine, University of Medicine and Pharmacy of Tirgu Mures, 540139 Tirgu Mures, Romania; sil_lupu@yahoo.com
5. Department of Physiology, Iuliu Hatieganu University of Medicine and Pharmacy, 400006 Cluj-Napoca, Romania; teodora_mocan@yahoo.com
* Correspondence: luciacoldea@yahoo.com; Tel.: +40-264591942; Fax: +40-264599817

Received: 26 December 2018; Accepted: 30 January 2019; Published: 1 February 2019

Abstract: To analyse the predictive ability and incremental value of left ventricular longitudinal axis strain (LAS) and late gadolinium enhancement (LGE) using standard cardiovascular magnetic resonance (CMR) imaging for the diagnosis and prognosis of severe aortic stenosis (AS) in patients with an indication for aortic valve replacement. We conducted a prospective study on 52 patients with severe AS and 52 volunteers. The evaluation protocol included standard biochemistry tests, novel biomarkers of myocardial fibrosis, 12-lead electrocardiograms and 24-hour Holter, the 6-minute walk test and extensive echocardiographic and CMR imaging studies. Outcomes were defined as the composite of major cardiovascular events (MACEs). Among AS patients, most ($n = 17$, 77.2%) of those who exhibited LGE at CMR imaging had MACEs during follow-up. Kaplan–Meier curves for event-free survival showed a significantly higher rate of MACEs in patients with LGE ($p < 0.01$) and decreased LAS ($p < 0.001$). In Cox regression analysis, only reduced LAS (hazard ratio 1.33, 95% CI (1.01 to 1.74), $p < 0.01$) and the presence of LGE (hazard ratio 11.3, 95% CI (1.82 to 70.0), $p < 0.01$) were independent predictors for MACEs. The predictive value increased if both LGE and reduced LAS were added to left ventricular ejection fraction (LVEF). None of the biomarkers of increased collagen turnover exhibited any predictive value for MACEs. LAS by CMR is an independent predictor of outcomes in patients with AS and provides incremental value beyond the assessment of LVEF and the presence of LGE.

Keywords: severe aortic stenosis; longitudinal axis strain; late gadolinium enhancement; cardiac magnetic resonance imaging

1. Introduction

Aortic stenosis (AS) is currently the most often encountered valvular heart disease in adults. The overall prevalence of this condition has recently increased as a consequence of progressive ageing of the population, reaching a maximum in patient's ≥75 years of age (2.8% of the general population) [1].

Severe AS is associated with changes in left ventricular (LV) geometry and function induced by increased afterload [2,3]. In the early stages, the constant exposure to elevated afterload leads to progressively increasing LV wall thickness, a compensatory change that temporarily relieves wall stress. At this point, LV systolic function is preserved. In later stages, compensatory mechanisms are overwhelmed by the constant exposure to increased afterload, leading to maladaptive remodelling and impaired LV systolic function [4,5]. Chronic inflammation, osteoblast activation, active valve mineralization, valvular and myocardial fibrosis occur due to the continuous exposure to increased pressure overload and are important factors in the evolution of AS [6]. Myocardial cell apoptosis [7] and the secretion of excess extracellular matrix proteins [8] favour the development of myocardial fibrosis and lead to systolic and diastolic LV dysfunction and increased ventricular stiffness [9]. Such changes are associated with a higher risk of major adverse cardiovascular events (MACEs) [10,11] and poorer outcomes in terms of clinical status and long-term survival after aortic valve replacement [12]. Changes in LV mechanics usually occur before the overt impairment of the LV systolic function, as assessed by the left ventricular ejection fraction (LVEF). Moreover, LVEF has a high inter- and intra-observer variability (14%) [13] and only becomes impaired in the late stages of the disease [14]. By contrast, global longitudinal strain has increased reproducibility, and is altered from the early stages of severe AS [15,16]. Although echocardiography is valuable, it has some limitations, and additional imaging techniques may provide incremental value for diagnostic and prognostic purposes in severe AS patients. Cardiac magnetic resonance (CMR) imaging is widely accepted as the non-invasive modality of choice for visualizing and quantifying myocardial fibrosis by late gadolinium enhancement (LGE) techniques [17]. A mid-wall pattern of fibrosis has been observed in the myocardium of up to 38% of patients with moderate or severe AS and has been associated with a more advanced hypertrophic response [10], and an eight-fold increase in mortality [10].

Recently, left ventricular longitudinal axis strain (LAS) by CMR imaging has been validated as a fast and reliable method for quantifying global LV longitudinal function [18], which does not require additional pulse sequences and off-line processing using dedicated software tools. The aim of the current pilot study was to assess the incremental value of LAS and LGE using standard CMR images for the diagnosis and prognosis of patients with severe AS undergoing aortic valve replacement.

2. Material and Methods

2.1. Study Patients

We conducted a prospective study on 128 patients with severe AS undergoing aortic valve replacement and who were examined in the 5th Department of Internal Medicine of the Iuliu Hatieganu University of Medicine and Pharmacy, Cluj-Napoca, Romania, between March 2016 and August 2018. Severe AS was defined as (1) peak aortic jet velocity ≥ 4 m/s, and/or (2) mean transvalvular gradient ≥ 40 mmHg, and/or (3) aortic valve area (AVA) ≤ 1.0 cm^2 [19,20].

Patients who had contraindications for CMR (including incompatible metallic devices, significant chronic renal disease with estimated glomerular filtration rate < 30 mL/min/1.73 m^2, or claustrophobia), other significant valvular disease, rheumatic valve disease with significant (at least moderate) mitral stenosis, post-irradiation AS, history of previous myocardial infarction with or without coronary revascularization by percutaneous coronary intervention and/or bypass, previous surgery for valvular disease, active inflammatory, infectious diseases, or neoplasia, cirrhosis, pulmonary fibrosis, poor echocardiographic window or those who did not agree to participate were excluded. The total number of excluded patients was 76 (Figure 1). Finally, 52 patients with severe AS (test group) were compared to 52 volunteers (control group), matched for age and sex, who responded to a questionnaire excluding any history of chronic heart disease, other than systemic arterial hypertension, without ongoing symptoms, normal clinical examination and normal electrocardiogram, chest radiographs, echocardiography, Holter ECG monitoring for 24 h and CMR imaging. Volunteers in the control group were recruited during the same enrolment interval as test group patients.

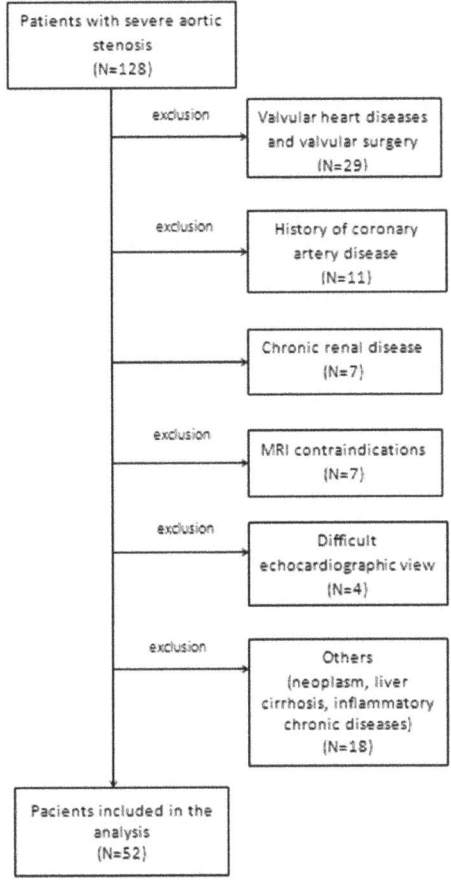

Figure 1. Patient selection and study design.

The current study was approved by the Ethics Committee of the Iuliu Hatieganu University of Medicine and Pharmacy, Cluj-Napoca—decision number 196/10.03.2016. The research was conducted in compliance with the Declaration of Helsinki. All patients were informed about the investigation protocol and signed a written consent form before being assigned to either the test or control group. Each patient underwent the same investigation protocol, including medical history, clinical examination, the recording of a 12-lead electrocardiogram, 24-h Holter monitoring, 6-min walk test (6MWT), biochemical analysis, echocardiography and CMR imaging, which were all performed during the same hospital visit.

2.2. Medical History and Clinical Examination

We recorded the medical history and cardiovascular risk factors of all enrolled subjects, including active smoking, systemic arterial hypertension, dyslipidemia, diabetes, and obesity. Coronary artery disease was considered present if myocardial infarction, angina pectoris, or revascularization (by either angioplasty or coronary artery by-pass) were performed. The New York Heart Association (NYHA) functional classification was used to assess the severity of dyspnoea. Patients with severe AS were considered symptomatic if they experienced dyspnoea, angina and/or syncope. A 12-lead electrocardiogram was recorded at enrolment and 24-h Holter monitoring was performed. The 6MWT was performed in the presence of adequately trained medical personnel following the American Thoracic Society guidelines, and the 6-min walk distance (6MWD) was reported. The risk of mortality after cardiac surgery was assessed by the EuroScore II [21] software available on www.euroscore.org.

2.3. Biochemical Analysis

Two peripheral venous blood samples were collected at enrolment from each participant and serum was separated by centrifugation. One sample was used for standard biochemistry tests, including high sensitive C reactive protein (hs-CRP) measurements, with a Beckman Coulter AU480 Chemistry Analyzer. The other serum sample was preserved at $-80\ °C$ until the end of the study and used for measuring procollagen type I C-terminal propeptide (PICP), procollagen type III N-terminal propeptide (PIIINP) and N-terminal pro-Brain Natriuretic Peptide (NT-proBNP) levels. All biomarker levels were determined by the Sandwich ELISA technique according to the manufacturer's instructions (Elabscience Biotechnology Co., Ltd., WuHan, China) For determining PICP, we used Human PICP ELISA Kits, Elabscience Biotechnology Co. PIIINP was determined using Human PIIINP ELISA Kits, and for NT-proBNP levels, Elabscience Biotechnology Co., Ltd., kits were used. Measurements were performed by a single investigator who was blinded to all clinical and imaging data. Renal function was estimated by the glomerular filtration rate (eGFR), using the Chronic Kidney Disease Epidemiology Collaboration equation, considering age, race, gender, and plasma creatinine concentration. Renal function was considered impaired at eGFR < 60 mL/min/1.73 m^2.

2.4. Echocardiography

Transthoracic echocardiography was performed in all participants to the study using a General Electric Vivid E9 (GE Health Medical, Horten, Norway) echocardiograph with a M5S 1.5/4.6 MHz active matrix-phased array transducer. Examinations were performed by two physicians (L.S. and C.O.), each with more than 10 years of experience in the field, and blinded to all clinical and laboratory data. Echocardiography data was collected and reported according to guidelines from the European Association of Echocardiography and the American Society of Echocardiography [19,20,22,23]. The severity of AS was quantified by continuous wave Doppler measurements of peak aortic flow velocity and mean transaortic gradients; AVA was calculated using the continuity equation and indexed to body surface area (BSA). LV systolic function was quantified by the LVEF (bi-plane Simpson's modified rule). LV diastolic function and right chambers dimensions and functions were assessed following global recommendations.

2.5. Cardiac Magnetic Resonance Imaging

All CMR imaging examinations were performed by two experienced examiners, one cardiologist and one radiologist (L.A.C. and C.C.), blinded to all clinical data, using specialized software (Syngo.Via, VB20A_HF04, Argus, Siemens Healthineers Global, Erlangen, Germany), as recommended [24], on a 1.5 T MR scanner (Magnetom Symphony, Siemens Medical Solutions, Erlangen, Germany) with a dedicated surface coil for radio frequency signal detection. Standard localized views and contiguous short-axis and 4-chamber cine views covering both ventricles from base to apex were first acquired by ECG-gated steady-state free precession (SSFP) sequences, in apnea (Figure 2). Pre-contrast imaging parameters were selected at the beginning of the study and a standard protocol was applied for each examination: repetition time 3.6 ms; echo time 1.8 ms; flip angle 60°; slice thickness 6 mm; field of view 360 mm; image matrix of 192 × 192 pixels; voxel size 1.9 × 1.9 × 6 mm; 25–40 ms temporal resolution reconstructed to 25 cardiac phases. The imaging plane of the aortic valve was defined by the acquisition of a systolic three-chamber view and an oblique coronal view of the aortic valve and proximal aorta. Post-contrast, standard LGE images were acquired 10 minutes after intravenous injection of 0.2 mmol/kg gadolinium contrast agent (Gadoterate meglumine or Dotarem, Guerbet, Roissy CdG, France) in long- and short axis-views, using a segmented inversion-recovery gradient-echo sequence. Inversion time was adjusted to optimize nulling of apparently normal myocardium. Brachial blood pressure was monitored during CMR SSFP acquisitions. LV end-diastolic volume (LVEDV) and end-systolic volume (LVESV), LVEF and end-diastolic LV mass (LVM) were measured on short-axis cine-SSFP images. Epicardial and endocardial borders were traced semi-automatically at end-diastole and end-systole using specialized software (Syngo.Via VB20A_HF04, Argus, Siemens Medical Solutions). AVA was measured on cross-sectional planimetric images during systole by drawing the region of interest. LV longitudinal function was assessed by LAS, defined as the difference in mitral annular displacement at end-systole vs. end-diastole, and expressed in percentages. The presence and distribution of LGE in the LV were assessed from short-axis images, using the 17-segments model, recommended by the American Heart Association [24].The pattern of LGE distribution was characterized as mid-wall, subepicardial, focal or diffuse.

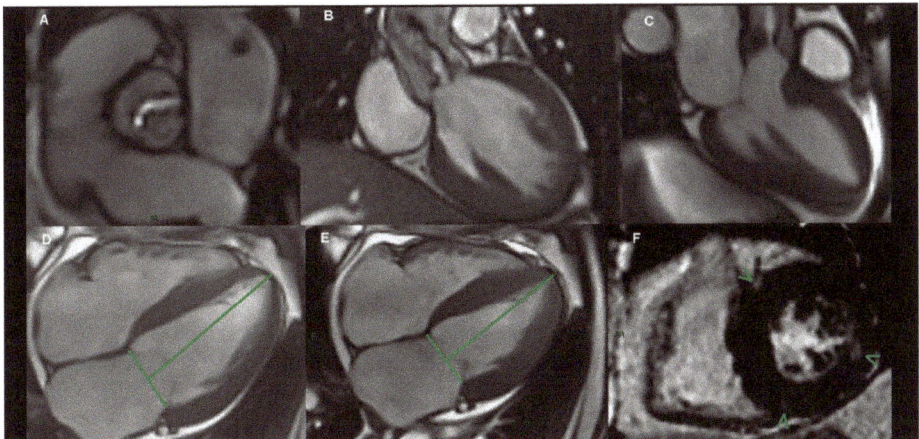

Figure 2. Cardiovascular magnetic resonance (CMR) imaging in aortic stenosis (AS) patients. (**A**) cine-SSFP (steady-state free precession) imaging of a stenotic bicuspid aortic valve; (**B**) coronal left ventricular outflow tract view acquired through-plane showing the aortic valve leaflet tips and restricted leaflet motility and resultant high velocity jet; (**C**) three-chamber view acquired through-plane showing the aortic valve leaflet tips, restricted leaflet mobility, and high velocity jet; (**D**,**E**) four-chamber view at end-diastole and end-systole acquired for longitudinal axis strain (LAS); (**F**) late gadolinium enhancement (LGE) in short-axis views of left ventricle showing focal hyper-enhancement (arrow).

2.6. Clinical Outcomes

Patients were followed-up over a median time interval of 386 days (interquartile range: 60 to 730 days) by completing a questionnaire either on hospital visits, telephone house-calls, or both. Survival analysis was performed for the combined end-point. The study end-point was a combination of major adverse cardiac events (MACE), including sudden cardiac death, non-fatal myocardial infarction, sustained ventricular arrhythmias, third-degree atrioventricular block and hospitalization for heart failure. If more than one event occurred, the most severe was selected. Hospitalizations due to non-cardiac causes were not considered in the analysis. The duration of follow-up was determined from the CMR study date until the occurrence of a MACE. The last evaluation of patient survival status was performed in August 2018 (the follow-up closing date). Complete follow-up was available for all patients.

2.7. Statistical Analysis

The normal distribution of data was tested by the Kolmogorov-Smirnoff test. Data were reported as mean and standard deviation, or median and interquartile range (IQR). Relative frequencies for categorical variables were reported as percentages. The Chi-square or Fisher's exact tests were used to compare variables between the two groups. Multiple comparisons were made using one-way ANOVA variance analysis or the Kruskall–Wallis test. Univariable and stepwise multivariable logistic regression analyses were performed to determine the association between LAS and LGE, and other variables derived from imaging modalities. The hazard ratio (HR) for the prediction of events was calculated for each of the outcomes using a Cox regression model. For each outcome of interest, we considered all of the significant variables in the univariate analysis and sought the best overall multivariate models for the composite end point, by stepwise-forward selection, with a probability to enter set at $p < 0.05$ and to remove the effect from of regression at $p < 0.05$. Event-free survival (time to first event) was generated by the Kaplan–Meier method and statistical significance was determined by the log-rank test. Receiver operating characteristic curve analysis was performed to study the predictive ability of LAS and LVEF for adverse cardio-vascular events. Results were considered statistically significant for $p < 0.05$. Cohen's Kappa inter- and intra-observer coefficient calculation was performed. Retrospective test power calculation and prospective sample size were estimated, with type I and type II variation according to sample size. The statistical analysis was performed using the MedCalc Software, version 16.1.2 (Mariakerke, Belgium).

3. Results

3.1. Baseline Characteristics

The present study was designed as a pilot study to serve as data for sample size calculation. Based on LAS numeric values and considering the threshold of alpha = 0.05, our estimation of type II beta risk stands below 0.05. However, in order to ensure the best power for inter-group tests, we have calculated a minimum necessary sample of 50 subjects /group (for type I alpha = 0.05). The study will be continued up to this limit for enabling us to decrease the type II error up to 0.05 (95% power).

All baseline characteristics of patients with AS and healthy volunteers are reported in Table 1. There were no statistically significant differences in age, gender, body surface area, systemic artery pressures, active smoking or presence of diabetes between the two groups. Patients in the test group had a poorer exercise capacity as assessed by the 6MWT.

Table 1. Baseline characteristics of patients in the test and control group.

	Test Group	Control Group	*p*-Value
Clinical characteristics	n = 52	n = 52	
Age, years	66 (7.5)	66 (7.8)	NS
Male gender, n (%)	29 (55.7)	29 (55.7)	NS
Body surface area, m^2	1.90 (0.24)	1.97 (0.13)	NS
Body-mass index, kg/m^2	28.5 (4.1)	30.2 (4.9)	NS
Heart rate, bpm	73 (11.6)	72 (8.6)	NS
Systolic blood pressure, mmHg	132 (18.1)	133 (20.3)	NS
Hypertension, n (%)	37 (71.1)	28 (53.8)	NS
Diabetes mellitus, n (%)	22 (42.3)	14 (26.9)	<0.01
Dyslipidemia, n (%)	35 (67.3)	24 (46.1)	NS
Smoking, n (%)	19 (36.5)	13 (25)	NS
6MWD, m	406 (138.1)	592 (103.9)	<0.001
Coronary artery disease, n (%)	18 (32.6)		
Chronic obstructive lung disease, n (%)	7 (11.5)		
Peripheral vascular disease, n (%)	27 (51.9)		
NYHA functional class ≥ III, n (%)	15 (28.8)		
Logistic EuroScore, %	3.8 (1.3–5.9)		

Table 1. Cont.

	Test Group	Control Group	p-Value
Medications			
β-blockers, n (%)	40 (76.9)	14 (26.9)	<0.001
ACEIs or ARBs, n (%)	45 (86.5)	10 (19.2)	<0.001
Calcium channel blockers, n (%)	6 (11.5)	13 (25)	<0.01
Statins, n (%)	38 (73)	15 (28.8)	<0.001
ASA or other antiplatelet therapy, n (%)	32 (61.5)	13 (34.6)	<0.01
Diuretics, n (%)	37 (71.1)	5 (9.6)	<0.001
Echocardiography			
Peak aortic velocity, m/s	4.45 (0.47)	1.31 (0.36)	<0.001
Peak transaortic gradient, mmHg	82.1 (17.9)	7.2 (2.7)	<0.001
Mean transaortic gradient, mmHg	52.9 (14.7)	3.6 (0.75)	<0.001
AVA index, cm^2/m^2	0.52 (0.08)	2.9 (0.08)	<0.001
E/E' ratio	9.8 (3.2)	6.5 (0.8)	<0.001
DT, ms	223 (52.2)	185 (8.8)	<0.001
sPAP, mmHg	33.4 (7.3)	26.2 (7.2)	NS
Cardiovascular magnetic resonance			
LVEDV index, mL/m^2	82.4 (21.6)	61.8 (15.0)	<0.001
LVESV index, mL/m^2	35.7 (16.6)	20.9 (5.8)	<0.001
LVM index, g/m^2	96.2 (24.3)	62.1 (16.5)	<0.001
LVEF, %	58.4 (9.7)	66.1 (4.7)	<0.001
LVM/LVEDV, g/mL	1.22 (0.35)	1.04 (0.29)	<0.01
LAV index, mL/m^2	49.1 (11.6)	25.5 (3.7)	<0.001
LAS (%)	−17.7 (3.9)	−20.5 (1.5)	<0.001
TAPSE, mm	14.9 (2.5)	19.8 (3.6)	<0.001
LGE, n (%)	30 (57.7)		
Biomarker levels			
PICP, ng/mL, IQR	1.2 (0.37–7.3)	0.42 (0.38–4.6)	<0.001
PIIINP, ng/mL, IQR	13.6 (2.5–68.3)	9.7 (2.4–29.7)	<0.01
hs-CRP, pg/mL, IQR	1.1 (0.49–1.9)	0.74 (0.16–1.1)	<0.001
NT-proBNP, pg/mL, IQR	1960 (170–9893)	210 (60–390)	<0.001
eGFR, $ml/min/1.73\ m^2$	88.1 (24.1)	89.2 (19.6)	NS

Abbreviations: n, number of patients; IQR, interquartile range; NYHA, New York Heart Association; NT-proBNP, N-terminal pro-Brain Natriuretic Peptide; hs-CRP, high sensitive C reactive protein; PICP, procollagen type I C-terminal propeptide; PIIINP, procollagen type III N-terminal propeptide; eGFR, estimated glomerular filtration rate; ACEI, angiotensin converting enzyme inhibitor; ARB, angiotensin receptor blocker; ASA, acetylsalicylic acid; LAS, left ventricular longitudinal-axis strain; LGE, left ventricular late gadolinium enhancement; LVEDV, left ventricular end-diastolic volume; LVESV, left ventricular end-systolic volume; LVM, left ventricular mass; LVEF, left ventricular ejection fraction; LAV, left atrial volume; E, peak mitral flow velocity; E', early diastolic peak myocardial velocity; DT, early diastolic filling deceleration time; sPAP, systolic pulmonary artery pressure; 6MWD, six minute walk distance; TAPSE, tricuspid annular plane systolic excursion; AVA, aortic valve area. Data are reported as mean (standard deviation) or median (IQR) or n (%).

Patients in the AS group had significantly higher levels of PICP ($p < 0.001$), PIIINP ($p < 0.01$), hs-CRP ($p < 0.001$) and NT-proBNP ($p < 0.001$) than patients in the control group.

The cause of AS in test group patients was calcification of a trileaflet valve ($n = 39$), presence of a bicuspid aortic valve ($n = 6$), rheumatic disease ($n = 4$), or undetermined ($n = 3$). 47 (90%) patients with AS were symptomatic. LVEF was preserved in most test group patients ($n = 38$; 73%). Indexed LVM was increased $\geq 92\ g/m^2$ in 28 patients (53.8%) and reduced LAS < −18% was documented in 20 patients with AS (38.4%). LGE was found in 30 patients with AS (57.7%). LGE was distributed mid-wall in 12 patients (23%), in the sub-epicardial myocardium in 5 patients (9.6%), was focal in 10 patients (19.2%), and diffuse in 3 patients (5.7%).

3.2. Reproducibility of CMR Measurements

CMR measurements were repeatedly performed on the same set of images, acquired from all patients in the study group. Intra- and inter-observer reproducibility of LVEF and LAS measurements, and the assessment of LGE by CMR were excellent. The kappa coefficients of agreement were 0.89 (inter-reader) and 0.91 (intra-reader) for the assessment of LGE, and 0.93 (inter-reader) and 0.96 (intra-reader) for LAS (Table 2).

Table 2. Reproducibility inter and intra-reader agreement of CMR measurements.

Parameter	Coefficient Kappa	95% Confidence Interval	Standard Error
Inter-reader			
LVEF	0.95	0.907 to 0.974	0.023
LAS	0.93	0.912 to 0.962	0.027
LGE	0.89	0.795 to 0.940	0.078
Intra-reader			
LVEF	0.99	0.989 to 0.998	0.002
LAS	0.96	0.953 to 0.985	0.014
LGE	0.91	0.905 to 0.942	0.033

Abbreviations: LAS, left ventricular longitudinal-axis strain; LGE, left ventricular late gadolinium enhancement; LVEF, left ventricular ejection fraction.

3.3. Survival Analysis

All patients underwent surgery and aortic valve replacement was performed. During a median follow-up period of 386 (60 to 730) days, 22 patients (42.3%) had MACEs: non-fatal myocardial infarction ($n = 2$), sustained ventricular arrhythmias ($n = 2$), third-degree atrioventricular block ($n = 3$) and hospitalization for heart failure ($n = 15$). In three patients, MACEs (ventricular tachycardia and hospitalization for heart failure, respectively) occurred before surgery. One patient developed third degree atrio-ventricular block during surgery and required permanent pacing. Nineteen other patients experienced MACEs after aortic valve replacement. Most patients ($n = 17$, 77.2%) with LGE on CMR imaging had MACEs during follow-up.

The discriminative performance of additional markers for MACEs was calculated by receiver operating characteristic curve analysis for the combined end-point: LVEF (optimized cut-off value, <50%; AUC, 0.759; $p < 0.01$) and LAS (optimized cut-off value, $<-18\%$; AUC, 0.883; $p < 0.0001$) (Table 3). Interestingly, the biomarkers for enhanced collagen turnover had no discriminative ability for MACEs in severe AS patients.

Table 3. Predictive ability of biological markers and imaging parameters for outcomes in severe AS patients considered for aortic valve replacement surgery.

Variables	Sensibility	Specificity	PPV	NPV	ROC Threshold	AUC
LVEF	0.67	0.90	0.87	0.73	<50	0.759
LGE	0.75	0.68	0.66	0.76	+	0.717
LAS	0.77	0.90	0.85	0.84	<-18	0.883
PICP	0.56	0.73	0.64	0.67	>0.84	0.535
PIIINP	0.50	0.79	0.67	0.65	>16.1	0.572

Abbreviations: PICP, procollagen type I C-terminal propeptide; PIIINP, procollagen type III N-terminal propeptide; LAS, left ventricular longitudinal axis strain; LGE, left ventricular late gadolinium enhancement; LVEF, left ventricular ejection fraction.

Kaplan–Meier curves for event-free survival showed a significantly higher rate of MACEs in patients with LGE ($p < 0.01$) and decreased LAS ($p < 0.001$) at CMR imaging (Figure 3).

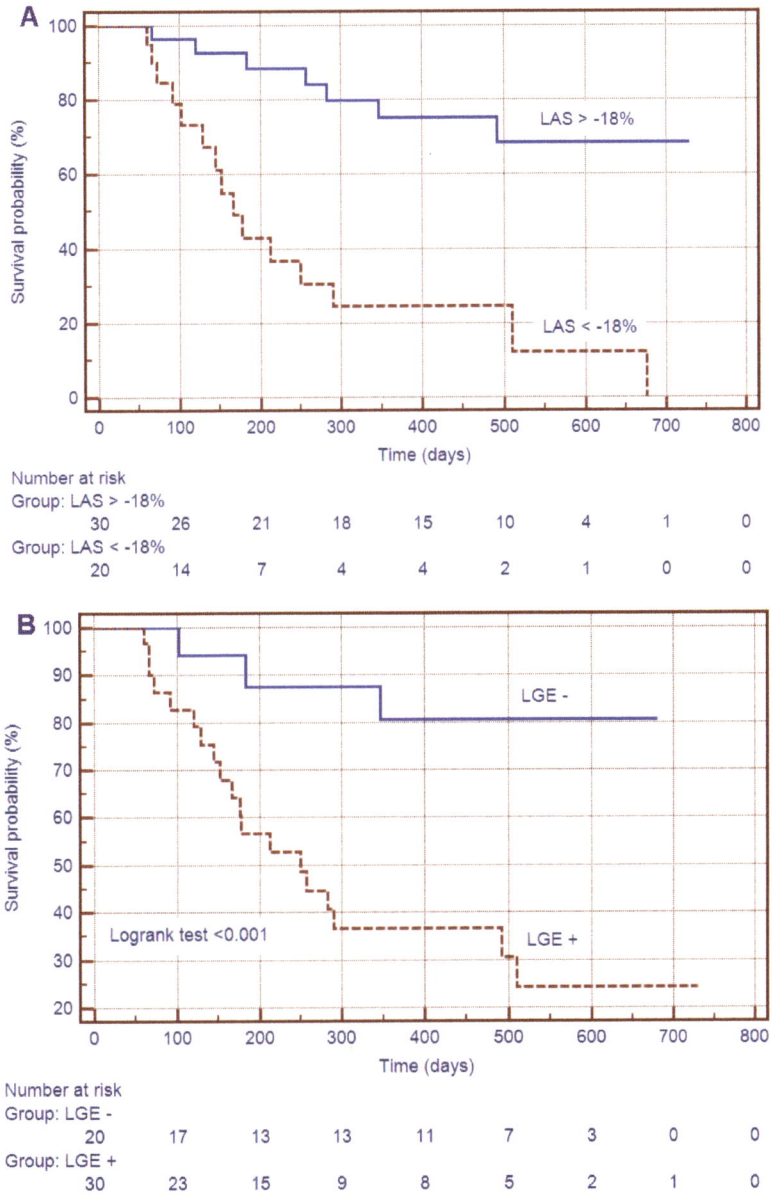

Figure 3. Kaplan–Meier curves for event-free survival for (**A**) Longitudinal Axis Strain (LAS); (**B**) late gadolinium enhancement (LGE).

3.4. Uni- and Multivariate Analysis

Several clinical parameters were predictors for the combined end-point in univariate analysis: the 6MWD, E/E′ ratio, LVEDV indexed, LVESV indexed, LVEF, LGE and LAS (Table 3).

In multivariate Cox regression analysis, only LGE and LAS (adjusted HR = 9.86, 95% CI 1.77 to 54.0, $p < 0.01$, respectively, HR = 1.32, 95% CI 1.01–1.71, $p < 0.01$) remained independent predictors for MACEs (Table 4).

Table 4. Univariate and Multivariate Cox Analysis testing between studied parameters and major cardiovascular events (MACEs).

	No Events $n = 30$	Events $n = 22$	Univariate Analysis		Multivariate Analysis	
			Unadjusted HR (95% CI)	p Value	Adjusted HR (95% CI)	p Value
Age, years	66 (10.1)	68 (7.1)	1.02 (0.95–1.09)	NS		
Male gender, n, %	14 (46.6)	15 (68.1)	0.40 (0.12–1.28)	NS		
Body surface area, m^2	1.91 (0.27)	1.89 (0.20)	0.76 (0.08–7.20)	NS		
Systolic blood pressure	131 (10.5)	133 (15.2)	1.00 (0.97–1.03)	NS		
PICP, ng/mL, IQR	1.2 (0.37–5.0)	0.81 (0.38–7.3)	1.06 (0.76–1.49)	NS		
PIIINP, ng/mL, IQR	10.5 (6.4–68.3)	14.1 (2.5–56.8)	1.01 (0.97–1.06)	NS		
hs-CRP, pg/mL	1.1 (0.49–1.9)	0.94 (0.51–1.8)	0.18 (0.03–0.95)	NS		
NT-proBNP, pg/mL	2206 (170–6735)	2734 (234–9893)	1.00 (0.99–1.01)	NS		
eGFR, ml/min/1.73 m^2	91.9 (25.4)	88.5 (22.6)	0.99 (0.97–1.01)	NS		
6MWD, m	455 (129)	340 (122)	0.99 (0.98–1.00)	0.001	0.99 (0.98–1.00)	NS
LVEDV index, mL/m^2	75.3 (20.9)	92.1 (18.8)	1.02 (0.99–1.06)	<0.05		
LVESV index, mL/m^2	29.9 (13.3)	43.6 (17.8)	1.04 (1.01–1.08)	<0.05		
LVM index, g/m^2	93.2 (25.4)	100.3 (22.5)	1.01 (0.98–1.03)	NS		
LVEF, %	61.6 (7.9)	54.1 (10.5)	0.93 (0.87–0.99)	<0.01	0.97 (0.88–1.07)	NS
LAV index, mL/m^2	49.8 (11.8)	48.2 (11.6)	0.98 (0.94–1.03)	NS		
LVM/LVEDV, g/mL	1.29 (0.36)	1.12 (0.31)	0.23 (0.04–1.27)	NS		
LGE, n (%)	12 (40)	17 (77.2)	5.55 (1.50–20.5)	<0.001	9.86 (1.77–54.0)	<0.01
LAS (%)	−19.6 (3.1)	−15.1 (3.3)	1.29 (1.07–1.55)	<0.001	1.32 (1.01–1.71)	<0.01
TAPSE, mm	19.3 (3.1)	20.4 (4.3)	1.08 (0.93–1.26)	NS		
E/E' ratio	8.9 (1.9)	11.1 (4.1)	1.25 (1.02–1.53)	<0.01	1.36 (0.98–1.88)	NS
Peak aortic velocity, m/s	4.35 (0.33)	4.59 (0.59)	3.18 (0.84–11.9)	NS		
Peak aortic gradient, mmHg	78.7 (12.9)	86.9 (22.6)	1.02 (0.99–1.06)	NS		
Mean aortic gradient, mmHg	51.5 (12.5)	54.7 (17.4)	1.01 (0.97–1.05)	NS		
AVA index, cm^2/m^2	0.52 (0.08)	0.51 (0.08)	0.17 (0.08–0.98)	NS		

Abbreviations: n, number of patients; NT-proBNP, N-terminal pro-Brain Natriuretic Peptide; hs-CRP, high sensitive C reactive protein; eGFR, estimated glomerular filtration rate; PICP, procollagen type I C-terminalpropeptide; PIIINP, procollagen type III N-terminal propeptide; LAS, left ventricular longitudinal-axis strain; LGE, left ventricular late gadolinium enhancement; LVEDV, left ventricular end-diastolic volume; LVESV, left ventricular end-systolic volume; LVM, left ventricular mass; LVEF, left ventricular ejection fraction; LAV, left atrial volume; E, peak mitral flow velocity; E', peak myocardial velocity at the mitral valve annulus; DT, early diastolic filling deceleration time; sPAP, systolic pulmonary artery pressure; TAPSE, tricuspid annular plane systolic excursion; AVA, aortic valve area; 6MWD, six minute walk distance.

Subsequently, a stepwise multivariate Cox regression model was constructed, including age, 6MWD, E/E′ratio, LVEF, LAS and the presence of LGE. Only reduced LAS (HR 1.33 (95% CI 1.01–1.74; chi-square: 15.1, $p < 0.001$) and LGE (HR 11.3 (95% CI 1.82–70.2); chi-square: 24.3, $p < 0.001$) were independent predictors for the combined end-point (Table 5).

Table 5. Stepwise Multivariate Proportional Hazard Model for the Combined End Point.

Variables	Model 1 HR 95%	Model 2 HR 95%	Model 3 HR 95%	Model 4 HR 95%	Model 5 HR 95%	Model 6 HR 95%
Age	1.01 (0.95–1.08)	0.96 (0.89–1.03)	1.01 (0.95–1.08)	1.00 (0.95–1.06)	1.00 (0.95–1.06)	1.01 (0.96–1.07)
6MWD		0.99 (0.98–1.00)				
E/E′			1.24 (1.01–1.54) **			
LVEF				0.94 (0.88–1.01)		
LAS					1.33 (1.01–1.74) **	
LGE						11.3 (1.82–70.2) *

Abbreviations: 6MWD, six minute walk distance; E, peak mitral flow velocity; E′, peak myocardial velocity at the mitral valve annulus; LAS, left ventricular longitudinal-axis strain; LGE, left ventricular late gadolinium enhancement; LVEF, left ventricular ejection fraction. * $p < 0.001$; ** $p < 0.01$.

3.5. Incremental Predictive Value for the Combined End-Point

Sequential Cox proportional-hazards models yielded significantly increased predictive power for the combined end-point of MACEs when both LGE and LAS were used in addition to LVEF (chi-square = 19.74, one degree of freedom). Neither LGE, nor LAS provided incremental predictive power when used alone, in addition to LVEF (Figure 4).

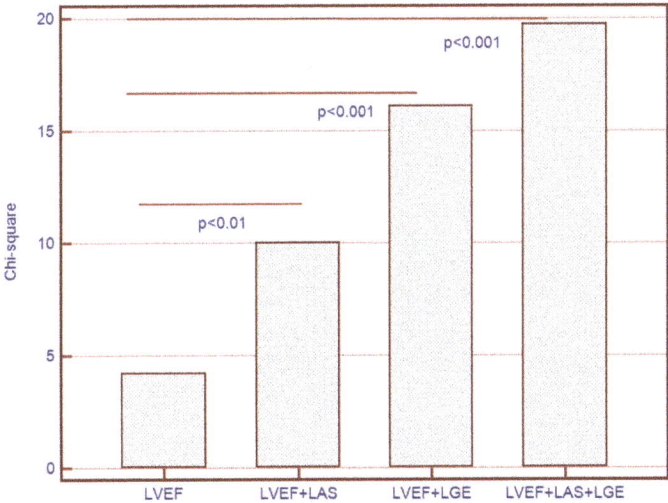

Figure 4. Incremental predictive value of longitudinal axis strain (LAS) and late gadolinium enhancement (LGE) added to left ventricular ejection fraction (LVEF) for the combined end-point in AS patients.

4. Discussion

In this prospective pilot study, we aimed to establish whether advanced CMR imaging techniques provide additional value in identifying patients with severe AS at risk for MACEs.

We have shown that both LAS and the presence of LGE are more reliable than LVEF for predicting MACEs in patients with severe AS, and that their combined use, in addition to LVEF, provided incremental value to any marker used alone.

Earlier echocardiography-based studies have demonstrated that global longitudinal strain is a reliable marker of cardiovascular events in different categories of patients [25,26] and is superior to traditional measurements of LVEF for predicting MACEs in patients with cardiovascular diseases [27].

Two relatively recent studies confirmed that CMR feature tracking with SSFP is a robust method for assessing LV mechanics and compares well to global longitudinal strain assessed by echocardiography [28,29]. Also, studies have recently emerged showing that impaired myocardial strain at CMR identifies ventricular function impairment in preclinical arrhythmogenic right ventricular dysplasia [30] and light chain amyloidosis, even if LVEF is preserved [31]. Considering these findings, myocardial strain assessment by CMR might become a valuable tool for the early identification of myocardial impairment.

Currently, data on the use of strain assessment by CMR in patients with AS is scarce. Al Musa et al. reported that strain by CMR is significantly decreased in patients with severe AS and preserved LVEF by comparison with healthy volunteers, and is even more impaired if patients are symptomatic [32]. To our knowledge, there is currently no other published data on the prognostic use of LAS in such patients, and our research is the first to address the relation with cardiovascular events.

By contrast, the presence of LGE has already been validated by previous studies as a marker of poor prognosis in severe AS. The presence of LGE was associated with poorer outcomes after aortic valve replacement, including the lack of improvement in symptoms and increased mortality [12,33]. Moreover, in the study by Dweck et al., LGE provided incremental value to LVEF for survival in patients with moderate to severe AS [10]. The quantitative assessment of LGE also seems useful for predicting functional improvement and all-cause mortality after aortic valve replacement [10].

Although LGE assessment is obviously a valuable tool for risk stratification, in our study the predictive power for MACEs was increased when LAS was added to the model. By contrast, PICP and PIIINP did not contribute at all, which is consistent with previously published research [34]. Considering the results of our research and previously published data, LAS might become an important part of LV function assessment at CMR, particularly considering that it does not require contrast administration. Further research is needed to validate this hypothesis.

Firstly, the study was conducted in a single institution and has the inherent limitations of that approach. Secondly, endomyocardial biopsies were not performed during surgery to assess the presence or absence of myocardial fibrosis in AS patients. Also, we were unable to acquire T1 mapping sequences, and therefore extracellular volume and diffuse myocardial fibrosis could not be quantified.

Finally, LAS, as a marker of longitudinal contractile function, is an independent predictor of outcomes in patients with AS and provides incremental value beyond the assessment of LVEF and the presence of LGE.

We hypothesise that, if more data is collected to endorse it, LGE and LAS at CMR should provide incremental value to current risk scores for stratifying prognosis in patients undergoing surgical aortic valve replacement.

Author Contributions: L.A.-C. and D.F.-conceived and designed the study; L.A.-C.-acquisition, analysis and interpretation of data; statistical methods and statistical interpretation of results; drafting of the manuscript; agreement to be accountable for all aspects of the work in ensuring that questions related to the accuracy or integrity of any part of the work are appropriately investigated and resolved; project administration. K.B., C.C.; C.P., L.S. and C.O.-acquisition, analysis and interpretation of data; critical revision of the manuscript for intellectual content. S.L.-analysis and interpretation of data; original draft preparation; critical revision of the manuscript for intellectual content. T.M.-analysis and interpretation of data; statistical methods and statistical interpretation of results; critical revision of the manuscript for intellectual content; final approval of the version to be published. All authors read and approved the manuscript.

Acknowledgments: This work was supported by internal institutional grant no. 4994/1/2016 from the Iuliu Hatieganu University of Medicine and Pharmacy of Cluj-Napoca.

Conflicts of Interest: The authors declare no conflict of interest.

References

1. Thaden, J.J.; Nkomo, V.T.; Enriquez-Sarano, M. The global burden of aortic stenosis. *Prog. Cardiovasc. Dis.* **2014**, *56*, 565–571. [CrossRef] [PubMed]
2. Ng, A.C.; Delgado, V.; Bertini, M.; Antoni, M.L.; van Bommel, R.J.; van Rijnsoever, E.P.; van der Kley, F.; Ewe, S.H.; Witkowski, T.; Auger, D.; et al. Alterations in multidirectional myocardial functions in patients with aortic stenosis and preserved ejection fraction: A two-dimensional speckle tracking analysis. *Eur. Heart J.* **2011**, *32*, 1542–1550. [CrossRef] [PubMed]
3. Nucifora, G.; Tantiongco, J.P.; Crouch, G.; Bennetts, J.; Sinhal, A.; Tully, P.J.; Bradbrook, C.; Baker, R.A.; Selvanayagam, J.B. Changes of left ventricular mechanics after trans-catheter aortic valve implantation and surgical aortic valve replacement for severe aortic stenosis: A tissue-tracking cardiac magnetic resonance study. *Int. J. Cardiol.* **2017**, *228*, 184–190. [CrossRef]
4. Kupari, M.; Turto, H.; Lommi, J. Left ventricular hypertrophy in aortic valve stenosis: Preventive or promotive of systolic dysfunction and heart failure? *Eur. Heart J.* **2005**, *26*, 1790–1796. [CrossRef] [PubMed]
5. Cioffi, G.; Faggiano, P.; Vizzardi, E.; Tarantini, L.; Cramariuc, D.; Gerdts, E.; de Simone, G. Prognostic effect of inappropriately high left ventricular mass in asymptomatic severe aortic stenosis. *Heart* **2011**, *97*, 301–307. [CrossRef]
6. Natarajan, D.; Prendergast, B. Aortic stenosis—Pathogenesis, prediction of progression, and percutaneous intervention. *J. R. Coll. Physicians Edinb.* **2017**, *47*, 172–175. [CrossRef]
7. Gallego, I.; Beaumont, J.; López, B.; Ravassa, S.; Gómez-Doblas, J.J.; Moreno, M.U.; Valencia, F.; de Teresa, E.; Díez, J.; González, A. Potential role of microRNA-10b down-regulation in cardiomyocyte apoptosis in aortic stenosis patients. *Clin. Sci.* **2016**, *130*, 2139–2149. [CrossRef] [PubMed]
8. Alvarez-Llamas, G.; Martín-Rojas, T.; de la Cuesta, F.; Calvo, E.; Gil-Dones, F.; Dardé, V.M.; Lopez-Almodovar, L.F.; Padial, L.R.; Lopez, J.A.; Vivanco, F.; et al. Modification of the secretion pattern of proteases, inflammatory mediators, and extracellular matrix proteins by human aortic valve is key in severe aortic stenosis. *Mol. Cell. Proteom.* **2013**, *12*, 2426–2439. [CrossRef]
9. Kamimura, D.; Suzuki, T.; Fox, E.R.; Skelton, T.N.; Winniford, M.D.; Hall, M.E. Increased left ventricular diastolic stiffness is associated with heart failure symptoms in aortic stenosis patients with preserved ejection fraction. *J. Card. Fail.* **2017**, *23*, 81–88. [CrossRef]
10. Dweck, M.R.; Joshi, S.; Murigu, T.; Alpendurada, F.; Jabbour, A.; Melina, G.; Banya, W.; Gulati, A.; Roussin, I.; Raza, S.; et al. Midwall fibrosis is an independent predictor of mortality in patients with aortic stenosis. *J. Am. Coll. Cardiol.* **2011**, *58*, 1271–1279. [CrossRef]
11. Barone-Rochette, G.; Piérard, S.; De Meester de Ravenstein, C.; Seldrum, S.; Melchior, J.; Maes, F.; Pouleur, A.C.; Vancraeynest, D.; Pasquet, A.; Vanoverschelde, J.L.; et al. Prognostic significance of LGE by CMR in aortic stenosis patients undergoing valve replacement. *J. Am. Coll. Cardiol.* **2014**, *64*, 144–154. [CrossRef] [PubMed]
12. Milano, A.D.; Faggian, G.; Dodonov, M.; Golia, G.; Tomezzoli, A.; Bortolotti, U.; Mazzucco, A. Prognostic value of myocardial fibrosis in patients with severe aortic valve stenosis. *J. Thorac. Cardiovasc. Surg.* **2012**, *144*, 830–837. [CrossRef] [PubMed]
13. Thavendiranathan, P.; Grant, A.D.; Negishi, T.; Plana, J.C.; Popović, Z.B.; Marwick, T.H. Reproducibility of echocardiographic techniques for sequential assessment of left ventricular ejection fraction and volumes: Application to patients undergoing cancer chemotherapy. *J. Am. Coll. Cardiol.* **2013**, *61*, 77–84. [CrossRef] [PubMed]
14. Thavendiranathan, P.; Popović, Z.B.; Flamm, S.D.; Dahiya, A.; Grimm, R.A.; Marwick, T.H. Improved interobserver variability and accuracy of echocardiographic visual left ventricular ejection fraction assessment through a self directed learning program using cardic magnetic resonance images. *J. Am. Soc. Echocardiogr.* **2013**, *26*, 1267–1273. [CrossRef] [PubMed]
15. Delgado, V.; Tops, L.F.; van Bommel, R.J.; van der Kley, F.; Marsan, N.A.; Klautz, R.J.; Versteegh, M.I.; Holman, E.R.; Schalij, M.J.; Bax, J.J. Strain analysis in patients with severe aortic stenosis and preserved left ventricular ejection fraction undergoing surgical valve replacement. *Eur. Heart J.* **2009**, *30*, 3037–3047. [CrossRef] [PubMed]

16. Naji, P.; Shah, S.; Svensson, L.G.; Gillinov, A.M.; Johnston, D.R.; Rodriguez, L.L.; Grimm, R.A.; Griffin, B.P.; Desai, M.Y. Incremental prognostic use of left ventricular global longitudinal strain in asymptomatic/minimally symptomatic patients with severe bioprosthetic aortic stenosis undergoing redo aortic valve replacement. *Circ. Cardiovasc. Imaging* **2017**, *10*, e005942. [CrossRef] [PubMed]
17. Azevedo, C.F.; Nigri, M.; Higuchi, M.L.; Pomerantzeff, P.M.; Spina, G.S.; Sampaio, R.O.; Tarasoutchi, F.; Grinberg, M.; Rochitte, C.E. Prognostic significance of myocardial fibrosis quantification by histopathology and magnetic resonance imaging in patients with severe aortic valve disease. *J. Am. Coll. Cardiol.* **2010**, *56*, 278–287. [CrossRef]
18. Arenja, N.; Riffel, J.H.; Fritz, T.; André, F.; Aus dem Siepen, F.; Mueller-Hennessen, M.; Giannitsis, E.; Katus, H.A.; Friedrich, M.G.; Buss, S.J. Diagnostic and prognostic value of long axis strain and myocardial contraction fraction using standard cardiovascular MR Imaging in patients with nonischemic dilated cardiomyopathies. *Radiology* **2017**, *283*, 681–691. [CrossRef]
19. Nishimura, R.A.; Otto, C.M.; Bonow, R.O.; Carabello, B.A.; Erwin, J.P., III; Guyton, R.A.; O'Gara, P.T.; Ruiz, C.E.; Skubas, N.J.; Sorajja, P.; et al. 2014 AHA/ACC Guideline for the management of patients with valvular heart disease: Executive summary: A report of the American College of Cardiology/American Heart Association Task Force on Practice Guidelines. *Circulation* **2014**, *129*, 2440–2492. [CrossRef]
20. Baumgartner, H.; Falk, V.; Bax, J.J.; De Bonis, M.; Hamm, C.; Holm, P.J.; Iung, B.; Lancellotti, P.; Lansac, E.; Muñoz, D.R.; et al. 2017 ESC/EACTS Guidelines for the management of valvular heart disease: The Task Force for the management of valvular heart disease of the European Society of Cardiology (ESC) and the European Association for cardio-Thoracic Surgery (EACTS). *Eur. Heart J.* **2017**, *38*, 2739–2791. [CrossRef]
21. Paparella, D.; Guida, P.; Di Eusanio, G.; Caparrotti, S.; Gregorini, R.; Cassese, M.; Fanelli, V.; Speziale, G.; Mazzei, V.; Zaccaria, S.; et al. Risk stratification for in-hospital mortality after cardiac surgery: External validation of EuroSCORE II in a prospective regional registry. *Eur. J. Cardiothorac. Surg.* **2014**, *46*, 840–888. [CrossRef] [PubMed]
22. Nagueh, S.F.; Smiseth, O.A.; Appleton, C.P.; Byrd, B.F., III; Dokainish, H.; Edvardsen, T.; Flachskampf, F.A.; Gillebert, T.C.; Klein, A.L.; Lancellotti, P.; et al. Recommendations for the evaluation of left ventricular diastolic function by echocardiography: An update from the American Society of Echocardiography and the European Association of Cardiovascular Imaging. *J. Am. Soc. Echocardiogr.* **2016**, *29*, 277–314. [CrossRef] [PubMed]
23. Lang, R.M.; Badano, L.P.; Mor-Avi, V.; Afilalo, J.; Armstrong, A.; Ernande, L.; Flachskampf, F.A.; Foster, E.; Goldstein, S.A.; Kuznetsova, T.; et al. Recommendations for cardiac chamber quantification by echocardiography in adults: An update from the American Society of Echocardiography and the European Association of Cardiovascular Imaging. *J. Am. Soc. Echocardiogr.* **2015**, *28*, 1–39. [CrossRef]
24. American Heart Association Writing Group on Myocardial Segmentation and Registration for Cardiac Imaging; Cerqueira, M.D.; Weissman, N.J.; Dilsizian, V.; Jacobs, A.K.; Kaul, S.; Laskey, W.K.; Pennell, D.J.; Rumberger, J.A.; Ryan, T.; et al. Standardized myocardial segmentation and nomenclature for tomographic imaging of the heart. A statement for healthcare professionals from the Cardiac Imaging Committee of the Council on Clinical Cardiology of the American Heart Association. *Circulation* **2002**, *105*, 539–542. [PubMed]
25. Motoki, H.; Borowski, A.G.; Shrestha, K.; Troughton, R.W.; Tang, W.H.; Thomas, J.D.; Klein, A.L. Incremental prognostic value of assessing left ventricular myocardial mechanics in patients with chronic systolic heart failure. *J. Am. Coll. Cardiol.* **2012**, *60*, 2074–2081. [CrossRef] [PubMed]
26. Stanton, T.; Leano, R.; Marwick, T.H. Prediction of all-cause mortality from global longitudinal speckle strain: Comparison with ejection fraction and wall motion scoring. *Circ. Cardiovasc. Imaging* **2009**, *2*, 356–364. [CrossRef] [PubMed]
27. Kalam, K.; Otahal, P.; Marwick, T.H. Prognostic implications of global LV dysfunction: A systematic review and meta-analysis of global longitudinal strain and ejection fraction. *Heart* **2014**, *100*, 1673–1680. [CrossRef]
28. Obokata, M.; Nagata, Y.; Wu, V.C.; Kado, Y.; Kurabayashi, M.; Otsuji, Y.; Takeuchi, M. Direct comparison of cardiac magnetic resonance feature tracking and 2D/3D echocardiography speckle tracking for evaluation of global left ventricular strain. *Eur. Heart J. Cardiovasc. Imaging* **2016**, *17*, 525–532. [CrossRef]
29. Onishi, T.; Saha, S.K.; Delgado-Montero, A.; Ludwig, D.R.; Onishi, T.; Schelbert, E.B.; Schwartzman, D.; Gorcsan, J., III. Global longitudinal strain and global circumferential strain by speckle-tracking echocardiography and feature-tracking cardiac magnetic resonance imaging: Comparison with left ventricular ejection fraction. *J. Am. Soc. Echocardiogr.* **2015**, *28*, 587–596. [CrossRef]

30. Bourfiss, M.; Vigneault, D.M.; Aliyari Ghasebeh, M.; Murray, B.; James, C.A.; Tichnell, C.; Hoesein, F.A.; Zimmerman, S.L.; Kamel, I.R.; Calkins, H.; et al. Feature tracking CMR reveals abnormal strain in preclinical arrhythmogenic right ventricular dysplasia, cardiomyopathy: A multisoftware feasibility and clinical implementation study. *J. Cardiovasc. Magn. Reson.* **2017**, *19*, 66. [CrossRef]
31. Li, R.; Yang, Z.G.; Xu, H.Y.; Shi, K.; Liu, X.; Diao, K.Y.; Guo, Y.K. Myocardial deformation in cardiac amyloid light-chain amyloidosis: Assessed with 3T cardiovascular magnetic resonance feature tracking. *Sci. Rep.* **2017**, *7*, 3794. [CrossRef] [PubMed]
32. Al Musa, T.; Uddin, A.; Swoboda, P.P.; Garg, P.; Fairbairn, T.A.; Dobson, L.E.; Steadman, C.D.; Singh, A.; Erhayiem, B.; Plein, S.; et al. Myocardial strain and symptom severity in severe aortic stenosis: Insights from cardiovascular magnetic resonance. *Quant. Imaging Med. Surg.* **2017**, *7*, 38–47. [CrossRef] [PubMed]
33. Weidemann, F.; Herrmann, S.; Störk, S.; Niemann, M.; Frantz, S.; Lange, V.; Beer, M.; Gattenlöhner, S.; Voelker, W.; Ertl, G.; et al. Impact of myocardial fibrosis in patients with symptomatic severe aortic stenosis. *Circulation* **2009**, *120*, 577–584. [CrossRef] [PubMed]
34. Kupari, M.; Laine, M.; Turto, H.; Lommi, J.; Werkkala, K. Circulating collagen metabolites, myocardial fibrosis and heart failure in aortic valve stenosis. *J. Heart Valve Dis.* **2013**, *22*, 166–176. [PubMed]

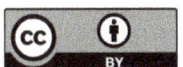

© 2019 by the authors. Licensee MDPI, Basel, Switzerland. This article is an open access article distributed under the terms and conditions of the Creative Commons Attribution (CC BY) license (http://creativecommons.org/licenses/by/4.0/).

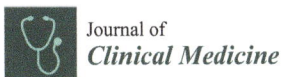

Article

Coronary Artery Bypass in Young Patients—On or Off-Pump?

Ryoi Okano [1,2], Yi-Jia Liou [3], Hsi-Yu Yu [1], I-Hui Wu [1], Nai-Kuan Chou [1], Yih-Sharng Chen [1] and Nai-Hsin Chi [1,*]

1. Department of Surgery, National Taiwan University Hospital and National Taiwan University College of Medicine, Taipei 10002, Taiwan; ryoi.okano@gmail.com (R.O.); hsiyuyu@gmail.com (H.-Y.Y.); aaronihuiwu@gmail.com (I-H.W.); nickchou@ntu.edu.tw (N.-K.C.); yschen1234@gmail.com (Y.-S.C.)
2. Department of Cardiovascular Surgery, Ageo Central General Hospital, Saitama 362-8588, Japan
3. Department of Life Science, National Dong Hwa University, Hualien 97401, Taiwan; conlyc7779@gmail.com
* Correspondence: chinaihsin@gmail.com; Tel.: +886-972-653-203

Received: 24 December 2018; Accepted: 20 January 2019; Published: 22 January 2019

Abstract: A definitive conclusion regarding whether on-pump or off-pump coronary artery bypass is preferable in young patients is lacking. The aim of our study was to perform a long-term comparison of the two approaches in young patients. We analyzed the National Health Insurance Research Database, using data for patients between 18 and 45 years of age who had undergone isolated coronary artery bypass between 2001 and 2011. The study endpoints were: all-cause death, major adverse cardiac and cerebrovascular events, and repeat revascularization within 30 days, 1 year, 5 years, and the entire 10-year follow-up period. A total of 344 patients received off-pump surgery and 741 patients received on-pump surgery. Preoperative characteristics and comorbidities were similar in both groups, and all-cause mortality was almost equal ($p = 0.716$). The 5-year survival rates were 93.9% and 92.2% in the off-pump and on-pump groups, respectively, and the 10-year survival rates were 86.3% and 82.1%, respectively. The repeat revascularization rate was significantly lower in the on-pump group ($p = 0.0407$). Both the on-pump and off-pump methods offer equally good long-term outcomes in terms of mortality and major adverse cardiac and cerebrovascular events. However, the need for repeat revascularization is a concern in the long term after off-pump surgery.

Keywords: coronary artery bypass; on-pump coronary artery bypass; off-pump coronary artery bypass; young patients

1. Introduction

The efficacy and appropriate indications for off-pump coronary artery bypass grafting (CABG) have been a source of contention since its enthusiastic re-emergence in the 1990s [1]. Recently, several large randomized trials have compared on-pump with off-pump CABG [2–6]. They showed the superiority, or at least non-inferiority, of on-pump CABG to off-pump CABG for most patients and in the hands of most surgeons [7]. However, the main participants in these trials were elderly patients. In most of the trials the average age was approximately 60 years, and in some trials patients under 45 years were even excluded [2–6].

Young patients account for 3% of all patients with coronary artery disease (CAD) and have a different background and propensity to elderly patients [8]. They are more likely to be male, smokers, obese, have a family history, and some of them have non-atherosclerotic diseases [8–17]. Although the appropriateness of CABG in young patients is currently being considered [8–14,16], there is insufficient data to form a definitive conclusion. In particular, there have been no studies comparing long-term outcomes between on-pump and off-pump CABG in young patients.

The aim of our study was to perform the first long-term, high-volume comparison of on-pump versus off-pump CABG in young patients using the Taiwan Nationwide Database.

2. Experimental Section

2.1. Materials and Methods

The Taiwanese National Health Insurance (NHI) program has been operating since 1995. By 2014, approximately 99.9% of the Taiwanese population was enrolled in the NHI program [18]. For the current analysis, we used a data subset of the NHI Research Database, namely the registry for patients with catastrophic illness, which contains the records of all prevalent cases of patients who have major illnesses.

From the database, we included patients between 18 and 45 years of age who had undergone isolated on-pump or off-pump CABG between 2001 and 2011, as shown in Figure 1. We searched the database to determine the presence of comorbidities such as hypertension, diabetes mellitus, peripheral vascular disease, chronic obstructive pulmonary disease stroke, myocardial infarction (MI), implanted cardiac pacemaker, or atrial fibrillation. The extent of CAD (single, double, or triple vessel disease) and renal function were also compared. The study endpoints were all-cause death, major adverse cardiac and cerebrovascular events (MACCE; defined as all-cause death, MI, and stroke); and repeat revascularization within 30 days, 1 year, 5 years, and over the entire follow-up period.

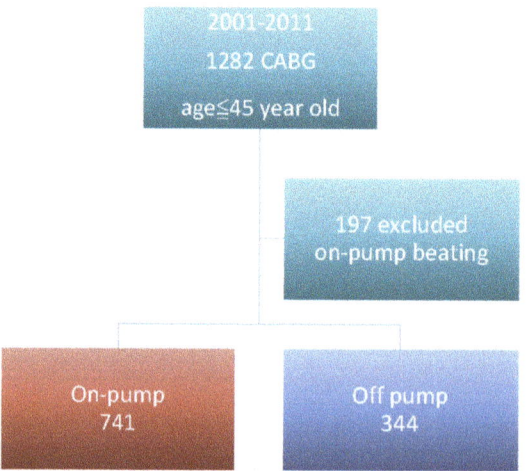

Figure 1. Flowchart of patient enrollment. We included 1282 patients, who were 45 years old or younger, and had isolated on-pump arrest or off-pump coronary artery bypass grafting (CABG). Among them, 197 patients were excluded for the surgeons' adopted on-pump beating techniques. Mean follow up time was 5.53 years and longest follow up time was 16 years, with 100% complete follow up.

2.2. Statistical Analysis

The characteristics of patients were analyzed using the chi-square test for categorical variables and *t*-tests for continuous variables to identify potential differences between the two groups. We used standardized difference to measure the balance of covariates, whereby an absolute standardized difference of greater than 10% represented meaningful imbalance.

The survival was compared between the groups of patients using Kaplan–Meier survival curves and log-rank tests. The factors affecting survival were analyzed by univariate and multivariate Cox's proportional hazard models to estimate the hazard ratio (HR) with a 95% confidence interval

(95% CI). All the analyses were performed with SAS 9.3 software (SAS Institute Inc, Cary, NC, USA). A *p*-value <0.05 was considered statistically significant.

3. Results

There were 31,448 patients that had undergone CABG in the database. From these, we included 1282 patients who were 45 years old or younger and had isolated on-pump or off-pump CABG. Among these, 197 patients were excluded due the use of an on-pump beating heart technique, as shown in Figure 1. The average overall follow-up time was 5.3 years and the longest was 16 years, with 100% complete follow up. The mean follow-up times were 4.79 years for off-pump CABG and 5.53 years for on-pump CABG.

A total of 344 patients received off-pump surgery and 741 patients received on-pump surgery, as shown in Table 1. Both groups were comprised of predominantly male patients, and mean age was similar in both groups (approximately 41 years in both; $p = 0.18$). The distribution of one-vessel disease was greater in the off-pump group (15.99% off-pump vs. 6.34% on-pump). Before the operation, both groups had a similar incidence of diabetes mellitus, hyperlipidemia, familial hypercholesterolemia, chronic obstructive pulmonary disease, stroke, peripheral vascular disease, hypertension, previous myocardial infarction, atrial fibrillation, implanted pacemaker, and presence of renal dysfunction, as shown in Table 1. In the off-pump group, there were 28.19% of them that received previous percutaneous coronary intervention and in the on-pump group it was 26.85% ($p = 0.63$). The emergent operations of both groups were similar; they accounted for 13.95% in the off-pump and 13.76% in the on-pump group ($p = 0.41$).

Regarding the completeness of revascularization, we used graft number/disease vessels as a marker; if the number is more than 1, we deem this as complete revascularization in our database. By doing so, the completeness of revascularization in one vessel disease was 100% in both groups. The completeness of revascularization in two-vessel disease was 93% in the off-pump group and 95% in the on-pump group. The completeness of revascularization in three-vessel disease was 91% in the off-pump group and 92% in the on-pump group.

Table 1. Baseline characteristics of the patients.

Characteristic	Age ≤ 45 Year (N = 1282)					
	Off-Pump CABG		On-Pump CABG		P Value	Standardized Difference (%)
	N	%	N	%		
Patients, total No.—no. (%)	344		741			
Female sex	34	9.88	94	12.69	0.18	8.86
Age—year Mean/Std. Dev.	41.04 ± 4.15		40.95 ± 4.13			2.17
Extent of coronary artery disease						
One-vessel disease	55	15.99	47	6.34	<0.0001	30.99
Two-vessel disease	72	20.93	113	15.25		14.80
Three-vessel disease	217	63.08	581	78.41		34.18
Number of grafting						
1	57	16.56	45	6.07	<0.0001	25.14
2	42	12.20	61	8.23		9.63
3 and >3	245	71.22	635	85.69		8.14
Comorbidity						
Diabetes Mellitus	116	33.72	236	31.85	0.54	3.99
Hyperlipidemia	65	18.89	131	17.67	0.62	4.21
Familial hypercholesterolemia	6	1.74	15	2.02	0.31	5.11
Insulin-dependent diabetes mellitus	8	2.33	7	0.94	0.07	10.90
Chronic obstructive pulmonary disease	8	2.33	16	2.16	0.86	1.12

Table 1. Cont.

Characteristic	Age ≤ 45 Year (N = 1282)				P Value	Standardized Difference (%)
	Off-Pump CABG		On-Pump CABG			
	N	%	N	%		
Previous stroke	23	6.69	45	6.07	0.70	2.51
Peripheral vascular disease	9	2.62	19	2.56	0.96	0.33
Hypertension	195	56.69	400	53.98	0.40	5.44
History of myocardial infarction	107	31.10	214	28.88	0.45	4.86
History of atrial fibrillation	5	1.45	6	0.81	0.32	6.09
Implanted pacemaker	7	2.03	8	1.08	0.21	7.72
Normal renal function	322	93.60	698	94.20	0.70	2.48
Chronic kidney disease	5	1.45	8	1.08	0.60	3.34
Renal-replacement therapy	17	4.94	36	4.86	0.95	0.39
Prior percutaneous coronary intervention	97	28.19	199	26.85	0.63	5.23
Surgical Timing—emergency	48	13.95	102	13.76	0.91	0.41

CABG: coronary artery bypass grafting; Std. Dev.: Standard Deviation.

The 30-day outcomes, as shown in Table 2, and the 1-year outcomes, as shown in Table 3, in terms of death, myocardial infarction, and stroke were not different between the groups. The operative outcome, as shown in Table 2, including transfusion amount, post-operative atrial fibrillation, ICU (intensive care unit) stay, and hospital stay were no different. The incidence of post-operative atrial fibrillation was 10.46% in the off-pump and 13.76% in the on-pump groups ($p = 0.535$). Further, at 5 years and 10 years, there were no differences in death, MI, stroke, and MACCE, as shown in Tables 4 and 5. The Kaplan–Meier curve shows that the rates of all-cause mortality were almost equal in both groups ($p = 0.716$), as shown in Figure 2A. The 5-year survival rate was 93.9% in the off-pump group and 92.2% in the on-pump group and the 10-year survival rates were 86.3% and 82.1%, respectively. There was no significant difference in freedom from MACCE at 5 and 10 years in patients receiving on-pump versus off-pump surgery (79.1% vs. 81.8% and 64.8% vs. 70.0%, respectively; $p = 0.3310$), as shown in Figure 2B.

Table 2. Outcomes at 30 days.

Outcome	Off-Pump CABG	On-Pump CABG	Adjusted Gender and Age and Other Variables (with Stepwise Selection)			
			Hazard Ratio (On:off)			
			HR	95% C.I.		P Value
				Low	Up	
Operative outcome						
Transfusion—pRBC (unit)	2.56 ± 1.45	3.12 ± 1.63	0.93	0.34	2.42	0.672
Post-OP atrial fibrillation—no. (%)	36 (10.46)	102 (13.76)	1.32	0.41	2.16	0.535
ICU stay (days)	1.4 ± 0.82	1.5 ± 0.93	1.02	0.81	1.32	0.812
Hospital stay (days)	8.2 ± 3.58	9.1 ± 4.21	1.15	0.36	4.21	0.781
Components of primary outcome—no. (%)						
Death	2 (0.58%)	3 (0.4%)	1.43	0.15	13.75	0.7581
Myocardial infarction	4 (0.11%)	7 (0.94%)	0.84	0.25	2.87	0.7805
Stroke	2 (0.58%)	2 (0.28%)	0.41	0.03	6.63	0.5266
New renal failure requiring dialysis	5 (1.45%)	12 (1.62%)	1.10	0.39	3.14	0.8596
Other specified outcomes—no. (%)						
Cardiovascular-related death	1 (0.29%)	1 (0.13%)	0.46	0.03	7.29	0.5781

pRBC: Red blood cell; ICU: intensive care unit; CABG: coronary artery bypass grafting; HR: hazard ratio; C.I.: confidence interval.

Table 3. Outcomes at 1 year.

Outcome	Off-Pump CABG	On-Pump CABG	Adjusted Gender and Age and Other Variables (with Stepwise Selection)			
			Hazard Ratio (On:off)			P Value
			HR	95% C.I. Low	95% C.I. Up	
Components of primary outcome—no. (%)						
Death	7 (2.03%)	12 (1.62%)	0.80	0.32	2.03	0.6392
Myocardial infarction	11 (3.2%)	36 (4.86%)	1.46	0.73	2.89	0.2819
Stroke	6 (1.74%)	11 (1.48%)	0.87	0.31	2.41	0.7879
New renal failure requiring dialysis	13 (3.78%)	35 (4.72%)	1.59	0.83	3.05	0.1622
Other specified outcomes—no. (%)						
Cardiovascular-related death	13 (3.78%)	11 (1.48%)	0.98	0.23	4.22	0.9738

Table 4. Outcomes at 5 years.

Outcome	Off-Pump CABG	On-Pump CABG	Adjusted Gender and Age and Other Variables (with Stepwise Selection)			
			Hazard Ratio (On:off)			P Value
			HR	95% C.I. Low	95% C.I. Up	
Components of primary outcome—no. (%)						
Death	16 (4.65%)	45 (6.07%)	1.27	0.72	2.25	0.4109
Myocardial infarction	28 (8.14%)	67 (9.04%)	1.11	0.71	1.74	0.6420
Stroke	18 (5.23%)	37 (4.99%)	1.00	0.56	1.77	0.9909
New renal failure requiring dialysis	29 (8.43%)	68 (9.18%)	1.18	0.76	1.84	0.4650
Other specified outcomes—no. (%)						
Cardiovascular-related death	5 (1.45%)	13 (1.75%)	1.14	0.41	3.21	0.7996
Cerebrovascular disease death	2 (0.58%)	2 (0.27%)	1.18	0.10	13.64	0.8945

Table 5. Outcomes followed by death.

Outcome	Off-Pump CABG	On-Pump CABG	Adjusted Gender and Age and other Variables (with Stepwise Selection)			
			Hazard Ratio (On:off)			P Value
			HR	95% C.I. Low	95% C.I. Up	
Components of primary outcome—no. (%)						
Death	25 (7.27%)	70 (9.45%)	1.15	0.73	1.83	0.5492
Myocardial infarction	35 (10.17%)	90 (12.15%)	1.12	0.75	1.67	0.5737
Stroke	22 (6.4%)	48 (6.48%)	0.99	0.60	1.65	0.9731
New renal failure requiring dialysis	32 (9.3%)	79 (10.66%)	1.14	0.75	1.72	0.5533
Other specified outcomes—no. (%)						
Cardiovascular-related death	5 (1.45%)	15 (2.02%)	1.30	0.47	3.58	0.6113
Cerebrovascular disease death	2 (0.58%)	2 (0.27%)	1.18	0.10	13.64	0.8945

Repeat revascularization was defined by further admission intervention of coronary artery or repeat coronary artery bypass surgery 6 months after first operation. The reason we defined repeat revisualization by 6 months after first operation was to eliminate the scheduled hybrid procedures, because most of the hybrid procedures were performed within 3 months.

The repeat revascularization rate was significantly lower in the on-pump group ($p = 0.0407$), as shown in Figure 2C. Freedom from revascularization at 5 years was 86.2% in the on-pump versus 80.8% in the off-pump group, and at 10 years was 76.1% versus 65.9%, respectively.

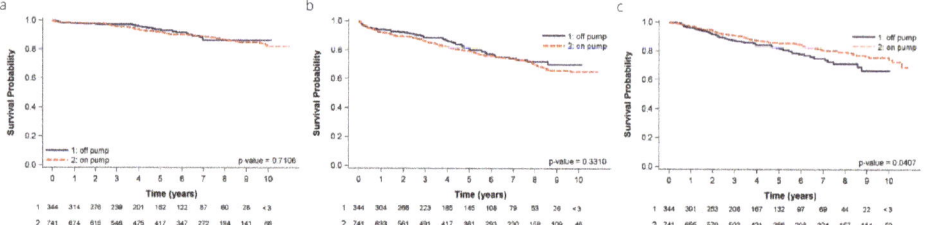

Figure 2. Kaplan–Meier survival curve. (**a**) All cause of death in both groups. The 5-year survival rate was 93.9% in the off-pump and 92.2% in on-pump groups; the 10-year survival rate was 86.3% in the off-pump and 82.1% in the on-pump groups. (**b**) Major cardiac and cerebrovascular events (death, myocardial infarction, and stoke). The 5-year free from major adverse cardiac and cerebrovascular events (MACCE) rate was 79.1% in the off-pump and 81.8% in the on-pump groups; the 10-year free from MACCE rate was 64.8% in the off-pump and 70.0% in the on-pump groups. (**c**) Kaplan–Meier survival curve of repeat revascularization. Off-pump carries concern of repeat revascularization in the long term. Free from revascularization at 5 years was 86.2% in on-pump vs. 80.8% in off-pump, and at 10 years, 76.1% vs. 65.9%, respectively.

4. Discussion

In our study, we compared the outcomes of on-pump and off-pump CABG in 1085 young patients. There was no difference in the 30-day, 1-year, and 5-year outcomes in terms of death, MI, stroke, and new renal failure. Kaplan–Meier and long-rank analysis showed that all-cause mortality and MACCE were not significantly different. Off-pump surgery was not inferior to on-pump surgery in terms of death, MI, and MACCE. However, the repeat revascularization rate was significantly higher in the off-pump group. The long-term survival was excellent in both groups.

For young coronary artery bypass patients, the long-term durability of the vascular graft and the long-term survival benefit are the major concerns. Young patients have less comorbidities than older patients. They have better renal function, less incidence of diabetes, and less renal impairment compared with older patients. Therefore, in both groups, young patients have less surgical risk [19].

The characteristics of coronary artery disease in young patients are different from older patients: 80% is atherosclerotic and 20% is non-atherosclerotic (e.g., coronary embolism, thrombosis, congenital anomalies, vessel inflammation, spasm) [9–17].

Compared with older patients, coronary heart disease in young patients is more closely associated with male sex, smoking, obesity, and family history. Conversely, the proportion of patients with diabetes mellitus and hypertension is smaller [8–13,17]. In our patients, the prevalence of diabetes was 33.72% and 31.85% in the off-pump and on-pump groups, respectively; in contrast, in our previous nationwide study where the mean age of patients was 62 years, the incidence was approximately 70% [19]. The overall prevalence of hypertension was 55%, and 90% of the cohort were males.

Young patients with coronary artery disease have fewer comorbidities than older patients [10,12]. In our study, the incidence of stroke, peripheral vascular disease, chronic obstructive pulmonary disease, and atrial fibrillation were low, and renal function was preserved in most patients.

Triple vessel disease was the predominant pathology in our cohort, in accordance with similar findings reported recently by Saraiva et al. [10].

Kaplan–Meier analysis in this study revealed excellent survival in young patients, and there were no significant differences between on-pump and off-pump CABG. However, the repeat revascularization rate was significantly higher after off-pump CABG. As recognized in the European Society of Cardiology/European Association for Cardiothoracic Surgery 2014 guidelines, there is substantial evidence indicating that on-pump CABG provides superior or equal short-and-long term outcomes compared with off-pump CABG in elderly patients [2–7]. However, the more frequent need for revascularization may be a major concern when treating younger patients who would be expected to live longer, and their rates of revascularization may keep rising in parallel to their follow-up.

Previous studies had suggested that the higher rate of repeat revascularization in off-pump CABG patients was related to incomplete revascularization and the surgeon's experience [20]. In addition, the rapid progression of atherosclerosis in young patients [15] might also have precipitated the high rate of repeat revascularization in our study. Regarding the completeness of revascularization, we used graft number/disease vessels as a marker; if the number is more than 1, we deem this is complete revascularization in our database. By doing so, the completeness of revascularization in one vessel disease was 100% in both groups. The completeness of revascularization in two-vessel disease was 93% in the off-pump group and 95% in the on-pump group. The completeness of revascularization in three-vessel disease was 91% in the off-pump group and 92% in the on-pump group. In our national database, the completeness of revascularization in coronary artery patients was more than 91% in all, and there were no differences in both groups. However, we cannot trace specific surgeon's experience in the registry database. Presuming that both groups have an equal completeness revascularization rate, we could say that the repeat revascularization was not due to incomplete surgery at the first operation. The differences might come from the procedure itself.

Actually, both methods offer good immediate results and provide also good long-term outcomes in terms of death, myocardial infarction, and stroke. We thought the choice of off-pump and on-pump procedures in the young patient should be decided by the patient's lesion anatomy, and the surgeon's experience and preference.

Several possible limitations to our study must be addressed. Because the study analysis was retrospective and only clinical events and services regulated by reimbursement were recorded, factors such as the extension of diseased coronary arteries and the completeness of revascularization, left ventricular ejection fraction or patients' functional capacity, choice of conduit (percentage of bilateral internal mammary arteries or total arterial grafting), conversion between on-pump and off-pump, and surgeon experience were not evaluated. The decision to perform off-pump versus on-pump CABG was dependent on the patients' clinical characteristics and the surgeons' preferences. Unmeasured confounders or detection bias may thus have affected our results.

5. Conclusions

We compared on-pump and off-pump CABG in young patients using a nationwide database. There was no significant difference in short-and-long term outcomes in terms of death and MACCE. However, the need for repeat revascularization might be a concern over the long term after off-pump surgery.

Author Contributions: Conceptualization, R.O., Y.-S.C., and N.-H.C.; Formal analysis, H.-Y.Y. and N.-H.C.; Investigation, N.-H.C.; Methodology, R.O. and N.-H.C.; Resources, I-H.W., N.-K.C., and Y.-S.C.; Supervision, N.-H.C.; Validation, R.O.; Visualization, Y.-J.L.; Writing—original draft, R.O.; Writing—review & editing, N.-H.C.

Funding: This research received no external funding.

Acknowledgments: The authors thank the staff at the Seventh Core Laboratory, Department of Medical Research, National Taiwan University Hospital for their technical support. We thank members of the Department of Medical Research at National Taiwan University Hospital for helpful discussions during manuscript preparation. We would especially like to thank Yi-Jia Liou for preparing the figures. The authors would also like to acknowledge the statistical assistance provided by the Taiwan Clinical Trial Statistical Center, Training Center, and Pharmacogenomics Laboratory (founded by the National Research Program for Biopharmaceuticals) at the Ministry of Science and Technology of Taiwan. (MOST 104-2325-B-002-032, MOST 105-2314-B-002-128).

Conflicts of Interest: The authors declare no conflict of interest.

References

1. Benetti, F.J.; Naselli, G.; Wood, M.; Geffner, L. Direct Myocardial Revascularization without Extracorporeal Circulation: Experience in 700 Patients. *Chest* **1991**, *100*, 312–316. [CrossRef] [PubMed]
2. Lamy, A.; Devereaux, P.J.; Prabhakaran, D.; Taggart, D.P.; Hu, S.; Paolasso, E.; Straka, Z.; Piegas, L.S.; Akar, A.R.; Jain, A.R.; et al. Effects of Off-Pump and On-Pump Coronary-Artery Bypass Grafting at 1 Year. *N. Engl. J. Med.* **2013**, *368*, 1179–1188. [CrossRef] [PubMed]
3. Lamy, A.; Devereaux, P.J.; Prabhakaran, D.; Taggart, D.P.; Hu, S.; Straka, Z.; Piegas, L.S.; Avezum, A.; Akar, A.R.; Lanas Zanetti, F.; et al. Five-Year Outcomes after Off-Pump or On-Pump Coronary-Artery Bypass Grafting. *N. Engl. J. Med.* **2016**, *375*, 2359–2368. [CrossRef] [PubMed]
4. Shroyer, A.L.; Hattler, B.; Wagner, T.H.; Collins, J.F.; Baltz, J.H.; Quin, J.A.; Almassi, G.H.; Kozora, E.; Bakaeen, F.; Cleveland, J.C., Jr.; et al. Five-Year Outcomes after On-Pump and Off-Pump Coronary-Artery Bypass. *N. Engl. J. Med.* **2017**, *377*, 623–632. [CrossRef] [PubMed]
5. Diegeler, A.; Börgermann, J.; Kappert, U.; Breuer, M.; Böning, A.; Ursulescu, A.; Rastan, A.; Holzhey, D.; Treede, H.; Rieß, F.C.; et al. Off-Pump versus On-Pump Coronary-Artery Bypass Grafting in Elderly Patients. *N. Engl. J. Med.* **2013**, *368*, 1189–1198. [CrossRef] [PubMed]
6. Houlind, K.; Kjeldsen, B.J.; Madsen, S.N.; Rasmussen, B.S.; Holme, S.J.; Nielsen, P.H.; Mortensen, P.E.; DOORS Study, Group. On-pump versus off-pump coronary artery bypass surgery in elderly patients: results from the Danish on-pump versus off-pump randomization study. *Circulation* **2012**, *125*, 2431–2439. [CrossRef] [PubMed]
7. Windecker, S.; Kolh, P.; Alfonso, F.; Collet, J.-P.; Cremer, J.; Falk, V.; Filippatos, G.; Hamm, C.; Head, S.J.; Jüni, P.; et al. 2014 ESC/EACTS Guidelines on myocardial revascularization: The Task Force on Myocardial Revascularization of the European Society of Cardiology (ESC) and the European Association for Cardio-Thoracic Surgery (EACTS) Developed with the special contribution of the European Association of Percutaneous Cardiovascular Interventions (EAPCI). *Eur. Heart J.* **2014**, *35*, 2541–2619. [CrossRef] [PubMed]
8. Alkhawam, H.; Zaiem, F.; Sogomonian, R.; El-Hunjul, M.; Al-kateb, M.; Umair Bakhsh, M.; Madanieh, R. Coronary Artery Disease in Young Adults. *Am. J. Med. Sci.* **2015**, *350*, 479–483. [CrossRef] [PubMed]
9. Rubin, J.B.; Borden, W.B. Coronary Heart Disease in Young Adults. *Curr. Atheroscler. Rep.* **2012**, *14*, 140–149. [CrossRef] [PubMed]
10. Saraiva, J.; Antunes, P.E.; Antunes, M.J. Coronary artery bypass surgery in young adults: excellent perioperative results and long-term survival. *Interact. Cardiovasc. Thorac. Surg.* **2017**, *24*, 691–695. [CrossRef] [PubMed]
11. Furukawa, Y.; Ehara, N.; Kita, T.; Kimura, T. Abstract: P1356 CORONARY RISK FACTOR PROFILE AND PROGNOSTIC FACTORS FOR YOUNG JAPANESE PATIENTS UNDERGOING CORONARY REVASCULARIZATION. *Atheroscler. Suppl.* **2009**, *10*, e325. [CrossRef]
12. Trzeciak, P.; Karolak, W.; Gąsior, M.; Zembala, M. In-hospital and long-term outcomes of coronary artery bypass graft surgery in patients ≤ 45 years of age and older (from the KROK registry). *Kardiol. Pol.* **2017**, *75*, 884–892. [CrossRef] [PubMed]
13. Tini, G.; Proietti, G.; Casenghi, M.; Colopi, M.; Bontempi, K.; Autore, C.; Volpe, M.; Musumeci, B. Long-Term Outcome of Acute Coronary Syndromes in Young Patients. *High Blood Press. Cardiovasc. Prev.* **2017**, *24*, 77–84. [CrossRef] [PubMed]
14. Fleissner, F.; Warnecke, G.; Cebotari, S.; Rustum, S.; Haverich, A.; Ismail, I. Coronary artery bypass grafting in young patients—insights into a distinct entity. *J. Cardiothorac. Surg.* **2015**, *10*, 65. [CrossRef] [PubMed]
15. Rohrer-Gubler, I.; Niederhauser, U.; Turina, M.I. Late outcome of coronary artery bypass grafting in young versus older patients. *Ann. Thorac. Surg.* **1998**, *65*, 377–382. [CrossRef]
16. Cole, J.H.; Miller, J.I.; Sperling, L.S.; Weintraub, W.S. Long-term follow-up of coronary artery disease presenting in young adults. *J. Am. Coll. Cardiol.* **2003**, *41*, 521–528. [CrossRef]
17. Choudhury, L.; Marsh, J.D. Myocardial infarction in young patients. *Am. J. Med.* **1999**, *107*, 254–261. [CrossRef]
18. National Health Insurance Annual Report 2014–2015. Ministry of Health and Welfare: Taiwan, R.O.C., 2014. Available online: https://goo.gl/xrKWwj (accessed on 12 December 2013).

19. Chen, J.-J.; Lin, L.-Y.; Yang, Y.-H.; Hwang, J.-J.; Chen, P.-C.; Lin, J.-L.; Chi, N.-H. On pump versus off pump coronary artery bypass grafting in patients with end-stage renal disease and coronary artery disease—A nation-wide, propensity score matched database analyses. *Int. J. Cardiol.* **2017**, *227*, 529–534. [CrossRef] [PubMed]
20. Puskas, J.D.; Mack, M.J.; Smith, C.R. On-pump versus off-pump CABG. *N. Engl. J. Med.* **2010**, *362*, 851–854. [CrossRef] [PubMed]

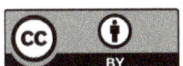

© 2019 by the authors. Licensee MDPI, Basel, Switzerland. This article is an open access article distributed under the terms and conditions of the Creative Commons Attribution (CC BY) license (http://creativecommons.org/licenses/by/4.0/).

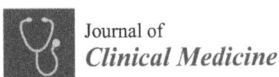

Review

Bioresorbable Vascular Scaffolds—Dead End or Still a Rough Diamond?

Mateusz P. Jeżewski [1], Michał J. Kubisa [1], Ceren Eyileten [1], Salvatore De Rosa [2], Günter Christ [3], Maciej Lesiak [4], Ciro Indolfi [2], Aurel Toma [5], Jolanta M. Siller-Matula [1,5,*] and Marek Postuła [1]

1. Department of Experimental and Clinical Pharmacology, Centre for Preclinical Research and Technology, Medical University of Warsaw, 02091 Warsaw, Poland; matjezewski@wp.pl (M.P.J.); kubisa.michal@gmail.com (M.J.K.); cereneyileten@gmail.com (C.E.); mpostula@wum.edu.pl (M.P.)
2. Department of Medical and Surgical Sciences, Division of Cardiology, "Magna Graecia" University, 88100 Catanzaro, Italy; saderosa@unicz.it (S.D.R.); indolfi@hotmail.com (C.I.)
3. Department of Cardiology, 5th Medical Department with Cardiology, Kaiser Franz Josef Hospital, 31100 Vienna, Austria; guenter.christ@wienkav.at
4. 1st Department of Cardiology, Poznan University of Medical Sciences, 1061701 Poznań, Poland; maciej.lesiak@skpp.edu.pl
5. Department of Internal Medicine II, Division of Cardiology, Medical University of Vienna, 231090 Vienna, Austria; aurel.toma@meduniwien.ac.at
* Correspondence: jolanta.siller-matula@meduniwien.ac.at; Tel.: +43-140-4004-6140

Received: 11 November 2019; Accepted: 4 December 2019; Published: 7 December 2019

Abstract: Percutaneous coronary interventions with stent-based restorations of vessel patency have become the gold standard in the treatment of acute coronary states. Bioresorbable vascular scaffolds (BVS) have been designed to combine the efficiency of drug-eluting stents (DES) at the time of implantation and the advantages of a lack of foreign body afterwards. Complete resolution of the scaffold was intended to enable the restoration of vasomotor function and reduce the risk of device thrombosis. While early reports demonstrated superiority of BVS over DES, larger-scale application and longer observation exposed major concerns about their use, including lower radial strength and higher risk of thrombosis resulting in higher rate of major adverse cardiac events. Further focus on procedural details and research on the second generation of BVS with novel properties did not allow to unequivocally challenge position of DES. Nevertheless, BVS still have a chance to present superiority in distinctive indications. This review presents an outlook on the available first and second generation BVS and a summary of results of clinical trials on their use. It discusses explanations for unfavorable outcomes, proposed enhancement techniques and a potential niche for the use of BVS.

Keywords: bioresorbable vascular scaffold; drug-eluting stent; percutaneous coronary intervention; angioplasty; acute coronary syndrome

1. Introduction

Cardiovascular disease is the most common cause of death, and by the year 2030, up to 44% of the adult US population is projected to suffer from some form of it, including ischaemic heart disease and acute coronary syndromes [1]. The effective restoration and maintenance of coronary vessel patency is a major problem requiring evaluation [2]. The idea of vascular restoration after the implantation of coronary stents has projected the development of bioresorbable vascular scaffolds (BVS) at the forefront of technological advancement in the field of coronary devices [3–6]. The design of BVS was prompted in an attempt to solve the limitations of durable drug eluting stents (DES), including (i) the occurrence of very late stent thrombosis (VLST), (ii) late expansive and adaptive vessel remodelling, (iii) anatomical limitations in case of surgical revascularization and (iv) impairment of computer tomography imaging [7,8]. After the initial excessive enthusiasm around BVS, the community was overly disappointed by the results of clinical trials. Complete resorption and improved vasomotor response of first generation of BVS which were believed to result in a reduced risk of target lesion failure (TLF) and stent thrombosis (ST) have been largely questioned [9–13]. In particular, the resorption time for the first commercially available BVS, ABSORB, has turned out to be substantially longer than initially thought. Therefore, it has been hypothesized that the resorption process itself or its delay can trigger complications [14–16]. A poor safety profile, especially in terms of target vessel myocardial infarction (TVMI) and an ST of 3 year follow up in ABSORB, as well as the negative results of the Amsterdam Investigator-Initiated ABSORB Strategy All-Comers Trial (AIDA) induced the manufacturer, Abbott Vascular, to halt the commercialization of ABSORB BVS [17–19]. Similarly, despite good outcomes of the BIOSOLVE I trial, the DREAMS BVS is still not ready for clinical use as the sparse data available stem from a small number of nonrandomized studies, conducted on a small number of patients [20–23]. Nevertheless, thanks to the encouraging results from the BIOSOLVE II and III studies which report very good outcomes in the 184 patients enrolled, with a more complex anatomical setting, we are facing a steady rise in the clinical use of the Magmaris stent within the ongoing prospective registry BIOSOLVE IV [24,25].

Overall, BVS appear to be a 'critical' development phase, and the currently clinically available BVS were given a class III indication for clinical use outside of studies in the current European Society of Cardiology (ESC) guidelines [26]. However, the disappointing outcomes mentioned above derive from studies in which optimal implantation strategies, proper imaging and long and potent platelet inhibition have not been extensively applied. On the contrary, it is proved that proper assessment of the target vessel segment with intravascular ultrasonography (IVUS) or optical coherence tomography (OCT) together with pre- and/or post-dilation can efficiently improve safety profile of BVS [27–29]. Thus, it is highly possible that refined second generation scaffolds with optimized implantation technique and proper imaging may restore the position of BVS and be competitive towards DES.

Our systematic review discusses the hypothetical advantages of BVS in the light of disappointing results obtained so far in clinical trials. Additionally, we aimed to explore possible methods to improve BVS performance starting from the design of next generation BVS and ending with procedural and pharmacological highlights.

2. Potential Advantages of BVS over Current Generation DES

Fully bioresorbable stents consist of synthetic biodegradable polymers that are intended to initially display functions similar to DES, and then dissolve within months after implantation, which may lead to the restoration of vasomotor function. In order to hold their promise, BVS should provide all potential advantages without sacrificing too much in terms of performance in comparison to DES. Another noticeable phenomenon (unrealistic using a solid metal stent) is the restoration of endothelial function with secondary reduction of atherosclerotic plaque [30,31]. After dissolving, it allows to maintain the integrity of the artery and return to its physiological properties (systolic and diastolic), thereby facilitating a beneficial remodeling and, consequently, causing a reduced passage for persistent inflammation (Figure 1) [31,32]. Therefore, a hypothesis has been put forward regarding the benefits of BVS, especially in younger patients or those with acute coronary syndromes, in which the metal stain is less likely to heal [33]. Among other features, the unfailing of the covered side branches after resorption, as well as avoiding the effect of a 'full metal coat', especially during diffuse disease, were also foreseen, providing early treatment of restenosis in the stent without additional layers of metal stents occupying the space [34]. BVS also give the possibility of a surgical revascularization procedure [31]. Moreover, this new technology also has significant benefits in the patient's personal preferences to avoid having a permanent foreign body [32]. However, data available so far show us that most promises associated with the advantage of resorption had been overestimated. In fact, an ultimate demonstration of most potential advantages of BVS, such as restoration of the physiological function of vessels and endothelium, and the possibility of future surgical interventions within the same lesion, are still lacking [35].

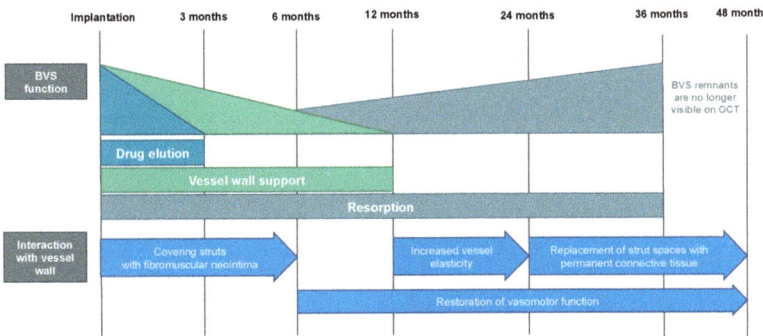

Figure 1. Timeline of bioresorbable vascular scaffolds (BVS) resorption and its interactions with vessel wall [6,16]. Presented course of phases and events is a generalization for available BVS. Certain time points are specific for ABSORB BVS-see Table 1. Abbreviations: BVS, bioresorbable vascular scaffold; OCT, optical coherence tomography.

3. Overview of First and Second Generation BVS

The first generation of BVS was initiated by ABSORB and DESolve scaffolds based on poly-L-lactic acid (PLLA) and DREAMS G1 scaffold based on magnesium [36,37]. Second generation of BVS embraces constantly expanding variety of scaffolds with enhanced properties and novel features. PLLA-based ART (Terumo, Tokyo, Japan) and DESolve Cx plus, the tyrosine analogue-based Fantom (REVA Medical, Inc., San Diego, CA, USA) and the magnesium-based Magmaris (Biotronik, Berlin, Germany) were introduced to clinical practice. The general characteristics of BVS are presented in Table 1. Yet, the variety of other devices based on polymers, metallic alloys or their combination remains in development [38,39]. Their development originates from an attempt to arrange a scaffold with thinner struts. The diameter of struts may not exceed 100 μm, whereas in the first generation it ranged from 150 μm [40]. The reduced thickness is believed to cause less blood flow disturbances and therefore to be associated with a lower risk of in-ST and a shorter requirement of dual antiplatelet therapy (DAPT). Additionally, tiny meshes become covered with a thinner layer of neointima and protected from the narrowing of the vessel lumen [41]. The newest devices are made of either magnesium alloy or polymers, including derivatives of PLLA and deaminotyrosine polycarbonate. These materials ensure greater resistance to fractures during post-implantation dilation and attain mechanical properties comparable to ordinary DES [30,42–44].

The ABSORB stent has a PLLA backbone, strut thickness is about 150 μm, with a bioresorbable coating of poly-D,L-lactic (PDLLA) with a thickness of 7 μm, secreting everolimus with a similar pharmacokinetics to the Xience DES [31,34,35,45–49]. Due to the presence of ester bonds between the PLLA and PDLLA monomers, degradation occurs by stepwise hydrolysis. In the final stage, either PLLA or PDLLA particles degrade entirely to lactic acid, or remnants smaller than 2 μm are phagocytized by macrophages [31,50]. Degradation is a mild, progressive process with minimal inflammatory reaction [51]. In order to obtain the appropriate mechanical framework of these stents, it became necessary to increase the thickness of the strut, because of lower tensile strength, reduced stiffness and the chance of deformation [35,52]. Studies have shown that in order to avoid strut rupture or abnormal decomposition, ABSORB stents require accurate lesion, judicious patient selection and an appropriate implantation technique, as they are able to stretch up to 0.7 mm beyond the nominal diameter [36,53]. ABSORB stents are radiolucent and therefore may not be visualized in fluoroscopy. For this reason, the stent at both ends was provided with two platinum markers, present to allow radiographic recognition. However, due to their tiny dimensions they identification requires high quality fluoroscopic imaging [52].

Table 1. Summary of efficacy and safety of the bioresorbable vascular scaffolds in clinical trials. Poly-L-lactic acid, PLLA; poly-D,L-lactic, PDLA.

Device	Material	Year of Receiving CE Marking	Drug Eluted	Strut Thickness (µm)	Minimal Resolution Time (months)
First generation					
ABSORB	PLLA	2012	everolimus	156	>36
DESolve	PLLA	2014	novolimus	150	<24
DESolve Cx plus	PLLA	2017	novolimus	120	<24
DREAMS 1G	Magnesium alloy	2015	paclitaxel	120	9–12
Second generation					
Magmaris (DREAMS 2G)	Magnesium alloy	2016	sirolimus	120	9–12
Fantom	Tyrosine polycarbonate	2017	sirolimus	125	36
ART	PDLLA	2015	none	170	6

DESolve has a similar strut thickness (150 µm in the first generation), is composed of a PLLA-based scaffold and equipped with two platinum-iridium markers to enable radiographic visualization. The second generation, DESolve Cx plus, has a strut thickness of 120 µm, with a length of 14 to 28 mm and a diameter of 2.5 to 4.0 mm [54]. In the initial version, it eluted novelists at a rate of 80% during a month after implantation [55–57]. High flexibility enables extension up to 5 mm, without risk of breakage and provides greater radial strength in the vessel during the critical period of up to 4 months after implantation. In addition, DESolve scaffolds presents were observed of passively expand within 1 h after implantation, whereas ABSORB stents present a tendency to recoil [56,57]. However, under experimental conditions it was noticed that this 'autocorrect' feature is able to generate only small radial forces, so that it improves stent positioning, but does not exert a relevant impact on the vessel wall [58]. It has been hypothesized that it may either contribute to the reduced risk of malfunction of the stent immediately after implantation or may prove to be a beneficial feature in acute myocardial infarction, where the stent may be undersized. However, there is no data to support this concept [54]. The new model also promises biodegradation in the first year by as much as 95% with the assumption of full resorption of the stent up to 2 years [54,56,59]. After this period, the polymer is replaced with a loose net mainly composed of proteoglycan, followed by a new connective tissue [54]. DESolve scaffolds differ, therefore, from ABSORB stents due to the properties of self-expansion and increased tolerance to excessive stretching.

DREAMS G1 stent is based on a frame made of absorbable magnesium alloy. Magnesium attains better mechanical properties such as a higher capacity of elongation and an increased tensile strength, allowing to use a thinner strut structure [54,60]. Due to the intrinsic radiolucency of magnesium and lack of markers mounted, the first generation stents are not visible in conventional imaging, but at the same time they are compatible with magnetic resonance imaging (MRI). These stents have bioresorbable coating of poly-lactic-co-glycolic acid (PLGA) eluting paclitaxel, and decompose in approximately 3–4 months [20,22,61–63]. The absorption of the magnesium alloy is a two-stage process, starting on the luminal surface of the scaffold, progressing towards the layers, until only the trace of hydroxyapatite remains at the site of implantation. In addition, magnesium reacts with water to form magnesium hydroxide, which starts the corrosion process [56]. Corrosion, however, does not proceed to the same extent on all sides, preferring the lateral surfaces of the struts. The initial crystal structure of magnesium hydroxide is gradually transformed into an amorphous body with a high-water content. After a time, the material is absorbed again through the core-infiltration of the cells [20]. In addition, some in vitro studies have shown that elevated magnesium concentrations in the coronary arteries per se reduce smooth muscle cell proliferation and increased endothelial cell proliferation [60,64]. Another advantage of these devices was the evidence of lower thrombogenicity in animal studies [60]. Despite the anti-arrhythmic properties of magnesium and its inhibitory effect on the release of endothelin-1, no adverse effects have been observed due to stent degradation [20,65]. The next generation, DREAMS

2 BVS (Magmaris), was enhanced in following ways: (i) its coating was thickened from 1 µm to 7 µm and converted from PLGA to PLLA, (ii) paclitaxel was substituted with sirolimus with greater elution (1.4 µg/mm^2), and (iii) the strut thickness increased to 150 µm × 140 µm [61].

The main highlight of the Fantom scaffold is its intrinsic radio-opacity. The presence of iodinated tyrosine analogue polymer enables more precise deployment and non-invasive radiological assessment throughout the whole degradation time. The content of iodine in a single device is negligible in comparison with the amount administered in a contrast media [38].

4. Real-World BVS Performance—Outcomes and Evaluation

The safety and efficacy of BVS devices in clinical trials are presented in Figure 2 and Table 2. As for now, the superiority of any BVS over DES has not been shown in a randomized trial.

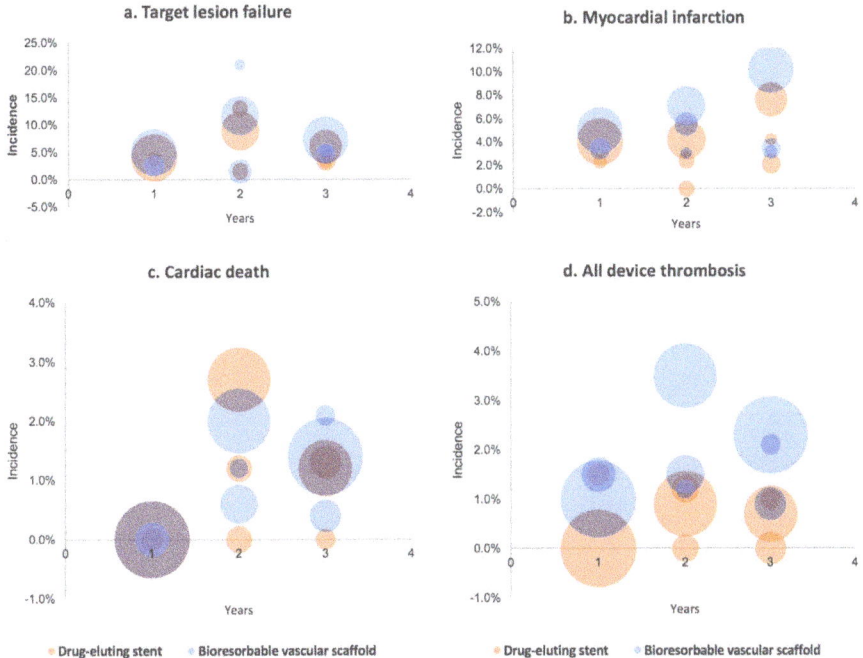

Figure 2. Comparison of incidence rate of major adverse events in randomized trials: (**a**) target lesion failure, (**b**) myocardial infarction, (**c**) cardiac death and (**d**) all device thrombosis. Figure presents data from ABSORB, AIDA, EVERBIO II and TROFI II trials. The circle diameter represents the number of patients in respective trials [17,19,66–70].

Table 2. Summary of the efficacy and safety of the bioresorbable vascular scaffolds in clinical trials. Target lesion failure, TLF; Target lesion revascularization TLR.

Study/Publication Date	Study Type	Follow-Up Time	No of Patients	No of Devices per Patient	Length of Devices (mm)	TLF (%)	ScT Definite/ Probable (%)	MI (%)	TLR (%)	Cardiac Death (%)	Commercial Funcing
ABSORB (Abbott, Lake County, IL, USA)											
ABSORB Cohort A [31]/Mar 2008	Observational	5 years	30	1	12 or 18	3.4	0/0	3.4	10.3	0	Abbott Vascular
ABSORB Japan [71]/Dec 2015	Randomized	1 year	400	1–2	8, 12 or 18	4.2	1.5/1.5	3.4	2.6	0	Abbott Vascular
ABSORB Cohort B [72]/Feb 2016	Observational	5 years	101	1	18	14.0	0/0	3.0	11.0	0	Abbott Vascular
PRAGUE-19 [73]/May 2016	Observational	3 years	113	1	<24	11.5	1.8/0.9	1.8	3.5	1.8	Abbott Vascular
ABSORB II [17]/Nov 2016	Randomized	3 years	335	1–2	<48	10	3.0/3.0	8.0	7.0	1.0	Abbott Vascular
ABSORB China [74]/Oct 2017	Randomized	3 years	238	1–2	<24	6.8	0.4/0.4	3.4	4.7	0.4	Abbott Vascular
ABSORB III [67]/Oct 2017	Randomized	2 years	1322	1–2	<24	3.7	1.9	1.3	2.6	0.5	Abbott Vascular
ABSORB IV [68]/Oct 2018	Randomized	3 years	1322	1–3	<24	13.4	2.3	4.2	7.3	0.9	Abbott Vascular
AIDA [19]/Jun 2017	Randomized	1 year	1296	1–2	>24	5	1	5	2	0	Abbott Vascular
EVERBIO II [69]/Sep 2017	Randomized	2 years	924	1–2	N/A	11.7	3.1/0.4	7.1	7	2	Abbott Vascular
EVERBIO II [69]/Sep 2017	Randomized	2 years	78	N/A	N/A	21	1.2	3	23	1.2	Abbott Vascular, Biosensors International, Boston Scientific
TROFI II [70]/Nov 2018	Randomized	3 years	95	1	8, 12, 18 or 28	5.3	2.1	3.2	4.2	2.1	Abbott Vascular, Terumo
ISAR- ABSORB MI [75]/Dec 2018	Randomized	1 year	173	1	1	7.0	1.2/0.6	0.6	4.8	2.3	Abbott Vascular
DESolve NX (Elixir Medical Corporation, Milpitas, CA, USA)											
DESolve First-in-Man trial [59]/Jan 2014	Observational	1 year	15	1–2	14 or 18	6.7	0.8	6.7	6.7	6.7	Elixir Medical
DESolve 2 years [56]/Mar 2016	Observational	2 years	122	1	14 or 18	7.4	0.8	1.6	4.0	3.2	Elixir Medical
DESolve Cx [76]/Oct 2017	Observational	6 months	50	1	14, 18, 13 or 28	0	0	0	0	0	Elixir Medical
DESolve PCMF Study [77]/Nov 2018	Observational	12 months	102	1–2	14, 18 or 28	2.0	1.0/0	1.0	1.0	0	Elixir Medical
DREAMS (Biotronik, Berlin, Germany)											
BIOSOLVE-I [23]/Jun 2016	Observational	3 years	46	1	16	6.6	0	2.2	4.3	0	Biotronik AG
BIOSOLVE-II [22,24]/Sep 2016	Observational	2 years	118	1–2	≤21	5.9	0	0.9	3.4	1.7	Biotronik AG
BIOSOLVE-II and BIOSOLVE-III [24]/Jul 2017	Observational	6 months	184	1–2	≤21	3.3	0	0.6	1.7	1.1	Biotronik AG
Fantom (REVA Medical Inc., San Diego, CA, USA)											
Fantom I [78]/Apr 2016	Observational	4 months	7	1	18		0			0	N/A
Fantom II [79]/Sep 2017	Observational	6 months	117	1	18 or 24	2.6	0.9	1.7	1.7	0	REVA Medical

The first data describing BVS performance stems from a single arm ABSORB I study comprising of a 5 year observation of 130 patients in total. Safety and efficacy were assessed by observing events of ST and occurrence of major adverse cardiac effects (MACE). MACE was defined as nonfatal stroke, nonfatal myocardial infarction and cardiovascular death. The 5 year results were promising, inasmuch as in both cohorts no ST was observed, and the MACE rate ranged from 3.4% to 11% in cohorts A and B, respectively. It indicated that ABSORB BVS has a potential to overtake DES in the terms of safety profile and led to trials directly comparing ABSORB BVS with Xience V DES [31,72]. ABSORB II and ABSORB III studies were prospective, randomized, single-blind, multi-center trials which aimed on proving the non-inferiority of ABSORB BVS versus drug eluting Xience V DES. The primary endpoints of the study enclosed comparison of cardiac death (CD), TVMI and target lesion revascularization (TLR) rates one year after implantation, while secondary endpoints included the assessment of primary endpoint parameters at 2–5 years' time and the assessment of ST, VLST and cost-related data.

The ABSORB II trial was the first to report inferiority of ABSORB BVS. 3 year follow-up was associated with a two-fold greater risk of TLF in comparison with Xience V (10% vs. 5%; $p = 0.0425$) [17,80]. Later, 2 year and 3 year observations in ABSORB III trials demonstrated ABSORB BVS inferiority in terms of overall ST and TLF driven mainly by TVMI [66,67]. Finally, the preliminary 30 day results of the most up to date and most populous ABSORB IV study revealed lower acute device success rate (94.6% vs. 99.0% ($P < 0.0001$)), greater risk of TLF (5.0% vs. 3.7%; $p = 0.02$) and greater ischemia-driven target vessel revascularization rate (ID-TVR) (1.2% vs. 0.2%; $p = 0.003$) [68]. Simultaneously, cumulative meta-analyses embracing ABSORB II, III, AIDA, EVERBIO II and TROFI II trials indicated the superiority of DES in the terms of both TLF and overall ST [9,10,69,70]. So far, only two country-specific trials (ABSORB JAPAN and ABSORB CHINA) demonstrated superiority of ABSORB BVS over Xience V DES [71,74]. The published meta-analyses and the results of the ABSORB IV trial formed the basis of the decision to cease production of ABSORB BVS in late 2017.

DREAMS G1 performance was assessed in 1 and 3 years' long observation in the course of the BIOSOLVE I study [21,23]. The BIOSOLVE I trial included 46 patients with silent ischemia, stable or unstable angina and assessed angiographic and IVUS follow-up at 6 and 12 months together with 3 years' clinical follow-up. In opposition to ABSORB trials, proper implantation strategy elements such as pre-dilatation were compulsory [20]. TLF occurrence at 6 months and 12 months is presented in Table 3. While no cardiac deaths or ST events were observed, the final results available in 3 year follow-up indicated 6.6% of TLF, 4.3% ischemia driven target lesion revascularization (ID-TLR) and 2.2% TVMI. Based on the angiographic results, it was assumed that DREAMS still could not compete with the 3rd generation of DES. BIOSOLVE-II and BIOSOLVE-III trials have been designed to observe its performance 3 years after implantation. As for now, data is available for 184 patients with single and multiple lesions in up to 2 years' follow-up. Pooled analysis concluded with no trace of thrombosis, and TLF occurred in 3.3% and 5.9% of patients in the BIOSOLVE-II and BIOSOLVE-III groups respectively. It is worth noting that four cardiac deaths were observed among both groups [22,24].

Table 3. Summary of incidence of primary endpoints in randomized studies comparing BVS and drug-eluting stents (DES).

Study	Compared Devices (No of Patients in Groups)	TVF RR/HR (95% CI)	Ischemia Driven TLR RR/HR (95% CI)	Cardiac Death RR/HR (95% CI)	TVMI RR/HR (95% CI)	Device Thrombosis Probable/Definitive RR/HR (95% CI)
ABSORB Japan [71]	ABSORB BVS vs. Xience DES (266/134)	1.15 [0.48, 2.72] p = 0.75	1.17 [0.31, 4.46] p = 1.00	N/A	1.51 [0.41, 5.47] p = 0.76	1.02 [0.19, 5.47] p = 1.00
ABSORB II [17]	ABSORB BVS vs. Xience DES (335/166)	2.11 [1.00, 4.44] p = 0.0425	1.65 [0.46, 5.92] p = 0.56	0.50 [0.10, 2.43] p = 0.56	5.70 [1.36, 23.87] p = 0.0061	N/A p = 0.0331
ABSORB China [74]	ABSORB BVS vs. Xience DES (236/235)	1.00 [0.51, 1.94] p = 0.99	1.66 [0.61, 4.49] p = 0.31	0.33 [0.03, 3.17] p = 0.37	2.99 [0.61, 14.65] p = 0.28	N/A P = 0.50
ABSORB III [66]	ABSORB BVS vs. Xience DES (1322/686)	1.41 [1.10, 1.81] p = 0.006	1.23 [0.85, 1.79] p = 0.27	1.17 [0.51, 2.69] p = 0.71	1.47 [1.02, 2.11] p = 0.03	3.12 [1.21, 8.05] p = 0.01
ABSORB IV [68]	ABSORB BVS vs. Xience DES (1296/1308)	1.35 [0.93, 1.97] p = 0.11	2.28 [0.99, 5.25] p = 0.0457	N/A	1.23 [0.84, 1.81] p = 0.29	4.05 [0.86, 19.06] p = 0.06
AIDA [19]	ABSORB BVS vs. Xience DES (924/921)	1.12 [0.85, 1.48] p = 0.43	1.60 [0.86, 1.58] p = 0.31	0.78 [0.42, 1.44] p = 0.43	1.60 [1.01, 2.53] p = 0.04	3.87 [1.78, 8.42] P < 0.001
EVERBIO II [81]	ABSORB BVS vs. Promus Element and Biomatrix Flex DES (78/160)	p = 0.12	p = 0.23	p = 0.55	p = 0.11	N/A
TROFI II [70]	ABSORB BVS vs. Xience DES (95/96)	p = 0.465	p = 0.678	N/A	p = 0.327	p = 0.55
ISAR-Absorb II [75]	ABSORB BVS vs. EES (173/89)	1.04 [0.39, 2.78]	0.84 [0.27, 2.57]	1.02 [0.19, 5.58]	0.51 [0.03, 8.20]	0.51 [0.07, 3.62]

BIOSOLVE-IV—a prospective, observational trial—is currently ongoing and aims at enrolling 2054 patients to be followed-up for 5 years. First year outcomes for the first 400 patients were recently published [25]. Procedural success was achieved in all but three patients. Target lesion failure (TLF) (primary endpoint) was registered in 4.3% of patients, and was exclusively composed of target lesion revascularizations. The rate of target vessel myocardial infarction was 0.88% and a single definite scaffold thrombosis was reported (0.3%) 10 days after implantation in a calcified lesion after a 5 day interruption of DAPT to perform a surgical minimally invasive revascularization of a non-target vessel.

Despite DESolve's greater self-expansion properties and its unique self-correction property, which helps to avoid malapposition, no study proved its superiority over DES [54]. In addition, recent observational studies indicated propitious results [76,77]. Nevertheless, a non-complete follow-up represents the study's limitations in long-term DESolve performance and the risk of late complications, e.g., VLST has not been properly investigated yet. As a consequence, the first generation of DESolve did not find application on the market. As such, the next generation, DESolve CX plus, has been halted.

The performance of Fantom scaffolds has been examined in two studies: Fantom I and Fantom II, including 7 and 117 patients respectively. The Fantom I pilot trial resulted in preserved patency in target vessels observed in IVUS after four months and no cardiac events after six months [78]. The multi-centre Fantom II trial observed short-term procedural success in 99.1% of cases, a 2.8% rate of MACE and one event of in-ST after six months. Investigators and commenters find these results comparable with other BVS. More encouraging results are anticipated from Cohort B of the Fantom II study, including 240 patients and nine month follow-up [79,82].

5. Anatomy of Failure: Explanation for Unfavorable Outcomes

As for now, the superiority of BVS over DES has not been shown in a randomized trial. A series of large-scale, post-registration studies showed long-term performance to be influenced by factors on every step of application of BVS, i.e., from device design to procedural specifics and vascular properties at the site of implantation (Figure 3) [83,84]. Optical analysis of intraluminal changes brings closer an explanation of the inferiority of BVS in clinical trials. Firstly, BVS implantation correlates with a greater asymmetry index (AI) and eccentricity index (EI) of the vessel in long term follow-up [85]. EI is defined as the ratio of minimum and maximum scaffold/stent diameter per cross section, while AI is defined as the ratio of minimal to maximal device diameter [85]. The greater the AI and EI value, the less symmetric the vessel section. Greater AI and EI were the consequence of the fact that ABSORB BVS is 'less forgiving' in case of inadequate deployment technique. Improper implantation, and consequently greater AI and EI, was determined to have a direct and significant impact on TLF occurrence in the ABSORB group [85,86]. Additionally, in numerous trials, the implantation of ABSORB correlated with lower minimal lumen diameter than Xience V, more extensive vessel remodeling, greater late luminal loss and decreased mean lumen area [17,87,88].

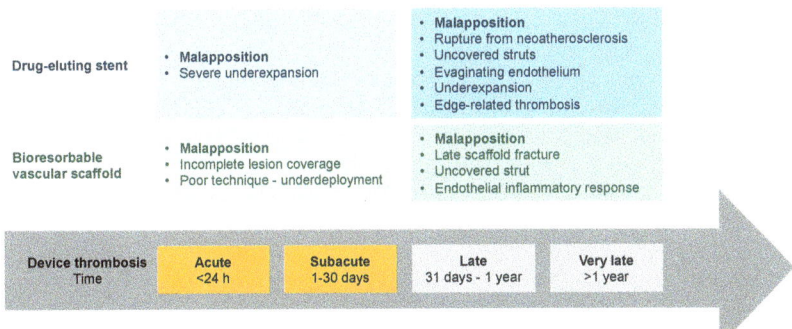

Figure 3. Comparison of the causes of device thrombosis in drug eluting stents (DES) and bioresorbable vascular scaffolds (BVS) [12].

Furthermore, as shown by randomized studies, after the implantation of bioresorbable stents, a lower minimal diameter of the vessel lumen significantly increased initial stenosis which results in a greater risk of recoil in vivo [53,81,89]. The mentioned phenomena were caused by an increased strut thickness, greater than in DES; bulky, discontinuous, malapposed struts; structural disruption; and finally, incomplete resorption (even in 3 year observation time (the PRAGUE-19 trial)) [73,86]. Mentioned factors led to greater neointimal hyperplasia, greater volume of intraluminal masses and eventually greater coronary artery lumen narrowing, resulting in device failure [90,91]. Thus, it is highly probable that the failure of ABSORB was caused by a combination of faulty device design and a far from optimal implantation technique.

BVS are much more demanding in terms of the implantation technique and require specific protocol called the 'PSP technique' (Prepare the lesion, Size adequately, Post-dilate). Prior to implantation, it is necessary to perform an in-depth target segment imaging, in order to accurately assess the dimensions of the vessel and detect the presence of possible calcification [20,32,35,92,93]. Recent studies and reconsideration of the results of five ABSORB studies correlate with accurate adjustment of a scaffold and optimal post-dilation with a lower risk of TLF, and excessive pre-dilation with a lower risk of ST [94–96]. Therefore, BVS should not be implanted in places which cannot be accessed with a pre-dilating balloon. In next step, the scaffold should be expanded gradually by means of a five second pressure increase by two atmospheres, and the target pressure should be maintained for 30 s [32]. On the contrary, proper positioning of DES is a one-step procedure with limited time of ischemia [20]. However, prolonged ischemia appears not to impact BVS efficacy, and their use may be warranted even in chronic total coronary occlusions [97].

Recent studies have identified clinical scenarios which require particular attention. Desirable post-dilation steps cannot be performed safely on scaffolds longer than 28 mm, due to the risk of breakage. Therefore, long lesions demand a specific 'scaffold to scaffold' technique to avoid overlapping, resulting in impaired radial strength [98]. The use of BVS in lesions located on vessel bifurcations is associated with an acceptable risk of TLR, however, still greater than in use of DES [99]. Eventually, BVS are contraindicated in aorto-ostial lesions [100]. Acute coronary syndromes seemed to be a propitious target for BVS due to feature of restoration of the native vessel lumen and vasomotor function. This indication is supported by the results of randomized TROFI II and ISAR- ABSORB MI trials on STEMI patients treated with either ABSORB BVS or DES, which concluded with a comparable healing score and risk of adverse events [70,75].

The first-generation BVS ABSORB seems to increase the risk of ST and TVMI as shown by recent meta-analyses [101–105]. Furthermore, analysis of the data collected by several registries shows that this BVS associates with a high rate of early (within 30 days) definite or probable ST of 1.3–1.5% [106,107]. Moreover, 1 year after implantation, the definite or probable ST rates are markedly higher (up to 3.1%) than the rates detected by the randomized trials [108–114]. This apparently higher thrombogenicity may be caused by two major limitations of the first-generation thick-strut poly-lactic acid BVS. First, mechanical limitations of the BVS demand a more elaborate percutaneous coronary intervention (PCI) technique [115]. This may increase the risk of suboptimal scaffold implantation. Second, structural limitations of the BVS lead to the creation of laminar flow disruptions [116]. This may serve as a nidus for inter-strut thrombus formation.

The mean number and length of BVS implantation and its relation to the incidence of ST is illustrated in Figure 3, based on data from randomized controlled trials and registries with ≥100 patients that report a 6–12 month follow-up and BVS details [81,101–104,106–114,117–123]. Only the ASSURE registry, which included 183 patients, reported no cases of ST at 1 year follow-up [119]. However, the mean number and length of the implanted BVS in the ASSURE registry were comparable to those in the selected patient populations of the randomized controlled trials. Thus, it suggests that the cohort of the ASSURE registry was rather a low risk population and that this may account for the low event rate that has been observed [102]. Figure 4 illustrates that there is a trend toward an association between the stent length/number of implanted stents per patient and the incidence of ST. Since late ST is a crucial concern in the use of BVS, a long-term (at least 3–5 years) observation period should be warranted in upcoming trials.

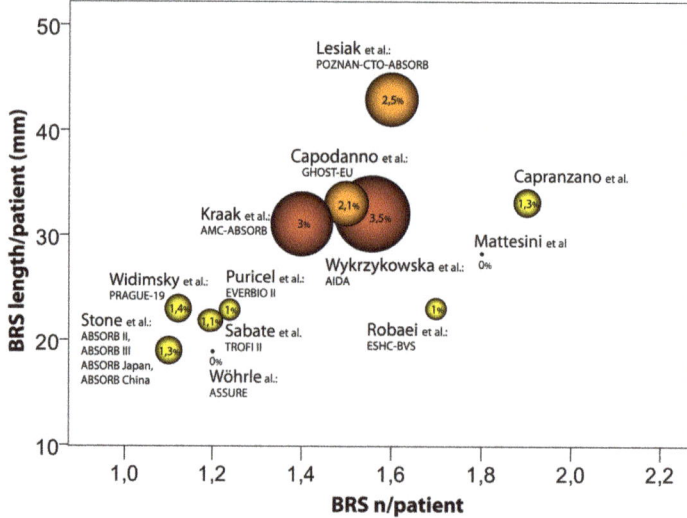

Figure 4. Bubble graph showing the relationship between the mean number and length of the implanted scaffolds and the incidence of scaffold thrombosis at the 6–12 month follow-up. Only randomized controlled trials, or registries with ≥100 patients that reported the required scaffold implantation details and had a follow-up duration of 6–12 months were included. The circle diameter indicates the reported percentage of definite or probable scaffold thrombosis [19,80,81,102,107,112–114,117,119,120,124].

6. Niche for BVS and Optimization of BVS Action

The excellent performance of DES makes them a tough benchmark to beat. The current generation of DES provides a very good vascular scaffolding with excellent radial strength. In fact, their use is associated with low rates of restenosis, ST or MACE [125–128]. Nevertheless, there are still concerns about their use [20,43,129]. The constant presence of a durable metallic prosthesis impairs vasomotor response vasodilation and causes a prolonged inflammatory reaction, which may eventually manifest in clinical observation [71,130–133]. Hence, BVS are believed to be distinctively beneficial in younger patients [73]. BVS may also serve patients' personal preferences to avoid carrying a permanent foreign body [32]. BVS theoretically enable surgical revascularization at the site of implantation, however this concept has not been yet appraised in a clinical trial [31]. On the other hand, the group of preferred candidates is limited to those who clearly take advantage of the resolution of the scaffold. BVS are still discouraged in patients with limited life expectancy, inasmuch as a still uncertain safety profile prevails over the possible benefits associated with biodegradation [60].

The next generations of BVS resolving without antiproliferative drugs may overcome recent concerns about the use of DES in the management of peripheral artery disease. After years of satisfactory performance, the elution of paclitaxel is currently suspected to increase late mortality [134]. Despite the lack of an exact mechanism linking the action of an antiproliferative drug and all-cause mortality, the Vascular Leaders Forum convened by physicians, manufacturers and the Food and Drug Administration (FDA) in March, 2019 recommends cautious monitoring and reconsideration of alternative treatment options [135]. These circumstances may facilitate further development and show new indications for BVS.

The importance of routine pre-procedural imaging and strict compliance to the PSP technique should be highlighted [136,137]. The PSP technique is distinctively beneficial in the case of aggravated risk of thrombosis, e.g., in diabetic patients [124,138]. In line with this concept, the use of a longer inflation time, as suggested by the producer, allows better for device expansion and a more homogeneous apposition [53]. In order to select the proper size of BVS, the measurement of the target's diameter was observed to be equally accurate under the guidance of either angiography or OCT [139]. Eventually, MRI enables non-invasive and non-radiative assessment of BVS patency after implantation and may be an alternative for patients with recurrent angina after angioplasty [140]. Despite the design of comparable radial strength of BVS to DES, it was noted that excessive stretching decreases its radial strength and elasticity and consequently leads to breakage [32,115,141]. This observation was confirmed in an experiment performed on a computational model. An arrangement of a mesh and the dimensions of a single strut determine the specific post-dilation size of a scaffold at which optimal mechanical and drug release properties are attained [142]. It is worth noting that available BVS devices are not equal in terms of their mechanical properties. PLLA-based scaffolds attain greater bending stiffness but lower radial strength, and tend more to recoil than magnesium-based scaffolds [58]. Among polymer-based scaffolds, the DESolve device attains greater flexibility and adapts better adaptation to the shape of the vessel [57,143]. These features are likely to contribute to upcoming studies as specific indications for certain devices. Greater radial strength may be utilizable in large vessels, while greater elasticity in tortuous vessels.

Another important issue is the residual high platelet reactivity (HPR) under DAPT, which represents one of the major determinants for worse outcomes of patients after PCI [144–147]. Therefore, the existence of a therapeutic window of platelet reactivity for $P2Y_{12}$ pathway inhibition was proposed [148]. Indeed, it has been shown previously in an all-comer PCI population that if both the $P2Y_{12}$ and cyclooxygenase-1 pathway inhibition of DAPT are personalized using Multiplate (a "point of care" platelet function assay which determines multiple electrode platelet aggregometry), HPR rates improve along with the clinical outcomes of patients [149–151]. Therefore, it would be interesting to know whether personalizing DAPT, by intensifying the treatment in the case of HPR to $P2Y_{12}$ receptor blocker and/or aspirin, would have an impact on the rates of ST after BVS implantation. Personalization of DAPT remains a controversial issue because the randomized trials on this subject had considerable shortcomings [152,153]. Nevertheless, it has been already shown that strict peri- and post-interventional optimization of platelet reactivity improves patient outcomes at 30 days in an all-comers PCI population who underwent metallic stent implantation [149–151]. It might be that optimizing platelet reactivity may be of even greater importance in BVS implantation, primarily because the thicker struts of the first-generation scaffold disrupt laminar flow and thereby increase the risk of thrombus formation [116]. In our opinion, not even the best implantation technique is capable of completely counteracting this inherent limitation of the current BVS. This suggests that to improve patient outcomes after PCI with this BVS, it might be necessary to optimize the platelet reactivity. Several catheterization laboratories intensify platelet inhibition through the routine prescription of the newer potent $P2Y_{12}$ receptor blockers for a longer duration (up to 3 years) to reduce the rates of ST after BVS implantation. A currently ongoing study on the administration of ticagrelor after the use of BVS in coronary vessels is believed to elucidate this matter [154,155].

7. Conclusions

After the initial excessive enthusiasm around BVS stemming from the dream of disappearing stents, clinical trials brought a great disillusionment. Existing DES devices still remain first choice in majority of cases and at the moment it is hard to believe that the current BVS could jeopardize their position. The next generations of BVS are anticipated to overcome the limitations which emerged in the initial clinical experiences. In particular, the procedural complexity and higher than expected restenosis and thrombosis represent major limitations. In fact, both technological advances and clinical expertise are about to shed new light on application of BVS devices.

Author Contributions: Writing—original draft preparation, M.P.J., M.J.K., C.E., A.T. and J.M.S.-M.; writing-review and editing, M.P.J., M.J.K., C.E., S.D.R., G.C., M.L., C.I., A.T., J.M.S.-M and M.P.; visualization, M.P.J., C.E., M.L. and J.M.S.-M.; supervision, S.D.R., G.C., M.L., C.I., J.M.S.-M and M.P.

Funding: This work was implemented with CEPT infrastructure financed by the European Union-the European Regional Development Fund within the Operational Program "Innovative economy" for 2007–2013.

Conflicts of Interest: The authors declare no conflict of interest.

References

1. Townsend, N.; Nichols, M.; Scarborough, P.; Rayner, M. Cardiovascular disease in Europe—Epidemiological update 2015. *Eur. Heart J.* **2015**, *36*, 2696–2705. [CrossRef]
2. Benjamin, E.J.; Blaha, M.J.; Chiuve, S.E.; Cushman, M.; Das, S.R.; Deo, R. Heart Disease and Stroke Statistics-2017 Update: A Report from the American Heart Association. *Circulation* **2017**, *135*, e146–e603. [CrossRef]
3. Schmidt, T.; Abbott, J.D. Coronary Stents: History, Design, and Construction. *J. Clin. Med.* **2018**, *7*, 126. [CrossRef] [PubMed]
4. Vahl, T.P.; Gasior, P.; Gongora, C.A.; Ramzipoor, K.; Lee, C.; Cheng, Y. Four-year polymer biocompatibility and vascular healing profile of a novel ultrahigh molecular weight amorphous PLLA bioresorbable vascular scaffold: An OCT study in healthy porcine coronary arteries. *EuroIntervention* **2016**, *12*, 1510–1518. [CrossRef] [PubMed]
5. Gonzalo, N.; Otaegui, I.; Rumoroso, J.R.; Gutiérrez, H.; Alfonso, F.; Marti, G. Device specificity of vascular healing following implantation of bioresorbable vascular scaffolds and bioabsorbable polymer metallic drug-eluting stents in human coronary arteries: The ESTROFA OCT BVS vs. BP-DES study. *EuroIntervention* **2018**, *14*, e1295–e1303. [CrossRef]
6. Kereiakes, D.J.; Onuma, Y.; Serruys, P.W.; Stone, G.W. Bioresorbable Vascular Scaffolds for Coronary Revascularization. *Circulation* **2016**, *134*, 168–182. [CrossRef]
7. Serruys, P.W.; Ormiston, J.A.; Onuma, Y.; Regar, E.; Gonzalo, N.; Garcia-Garcia, H.M. A bioabsorbable everolimus-eluting coronary stent system (ABSORB): 2-year outcomes and results from multiple imaging methods. *Lancet* **2009**, *373*, 897–910. [CrossRef]
8. Tesfamariam, B. Bioresorbable vascular scaffolds: Biodegradation, drug delivery and vascular remodeling. *Pharm. Res.* **2016**, *107*, 163–171. [CrossRef]

9. Montone, R.A.; Niccoli, G.; De Marco, F.; Minelli, S.; D'Ascenzo, F.; Testa, L. Temporal Trends in Adverse Events After Everolimus-Eluting Bioresorbable Vascular Scaffold Versus Everolimus-Eluting Metallic Stent Implantation: A Meta-Analysis of Randomized Controlled Trials. *Circulation* **2017**, *135*, 2145–2154. [CrossRef]
10. Zhang, X.L.; Zhu, Q.Q.; Kang, L.N.; Li, X.L.; Xu, B. Mid- and Long-Term Outcome Comparisons of Everolimus-Eluting Bioresorbable Scaffolds Versus Everolimus-Eluting Metallic Stents: A Systematic Review and Meta-analysis. *Ann. Intern. Med.* **2017**, *167*, 642–654. [CrossRef]
11. Gheorghe, L.; Millán, X.; Jimenez-Kockar, M.; Gomez-Lara, J.; Arzamendi, D.; Danduch, L.; Agudelo, V.; Serra, A. Bioresorbable vascular scaffolds in coronary chronic total occlusions: Clinical, vasomotor and optical coherence tomography findings at three-year follow-up (ABSORB-CTO study). *EuroIntervention* **2019**, *15*, 99–107. [CrossRef] [PubMed]
12. Mori, H.; Virmani, R.; Finn, A.V. Bioresorbable vascular scaffolds: Implication of very late scaffold thrombosis. *Coron. Artery Dis.* **2017**, *28*, 533–538. [CrossRef] [PubMed]
13. Alfonso, F.; Cuesta, J. Bioresorbable Vascular Scaffolds Restenosis: Pathophysiology and Predictors. *JACC Cardiovasc. Interv.* **2017**, *10*, 1828–1831. [CrossRef] [PubMed]
14. De Rosa, S.; Indolfi, C. Letter by De Rosa and Indolfi regarding article, "Clinical presentation and outcomes of coronary in-stent restenosis across 3-stent generations". *Circ. Cardiovasc. Interv.* **2015**, *8*. [CrossRef]
15. Indolfi, C.; Mongiardo, A.; Spaccarotella, C.; Caiazzo, G.; Torella, D.; De Rosa, S. Neointimal proliferation is associated with clinical restenosis 2 years after fully bioresorbable vascular scaffold implantation. *Circ. Cardiovasc. Imaging* **2014**, *7*, 755–757. [CrossRef]
16. Serruys, P.W.; Onuma, Y.; Garcia-Garcia, H.M.; Muramatsu, T.; Dudek, D.; Thuesen, L. Dynamics of vessel wall changes following the implantation of the absorb everolimus-eluting bioresorbable vascular scaffold: A multi-imaging modality study at 6, 12, 24 and 36 months. *EuroIntervention* **2014**, *9*, 1271–1284. [CrossRef]
17. Serruys, P.W.; Chevalier, B.; Sotomi, Y.; Cequier, A.; Carrié, D.; Piek, J.J.; Van Boven, J.; Marcello, D.; Dariusz, D.; McClean, D.; et al. Comparison of an everolimus-eluting bioresorbable scaffold with an everolimus-eluting metallic stent for the treatment of coronary artery stenosis (ABSORB II): A 3 year, randomised, controlled, single-blind, multicentre clinical trial. *Lancet* **2016**, *388*, 2479–2491. [CrossRef]
18. Chevalier, B.; Cequier, A.; Dudek, D.; Haude, M.; Carrie, D.; Sabaté, M.; Windecker, S.; Reith, S.; de Sousa Almeida, M.; Campo, G.; et al. Four-year follow-up of the randomised comparison between an everolimus-eluting bioresorbable scaffold and an everolimus-eluting metallic stent for the treatment of coronary artery stenosis (ABSORB II Trial). *EuroIntervention* **2018**, *13*, 1561–1564. [CrossRef]
19. Wykrzykowska, J.J.; Kraak, R.P.; Hofma, S.H.; van der Schaaf, R.J.; Arkenbout, E.K.; IJsselmuiden, A.J.; Joëlle, E.; Ivo, M.; Ruben, Y.G.; Karel, T.K.; et al. Bioresorbable Scaffolds versus Metallic Stents in Routine PCI. *N. Engl. J. Med.* **2017**, *376*, 2319–2328. [CrossRef]
20. Rapetto, C.; Leoncini, M. Magmaris: A new generation metallic sirolimus-eluting fully bioresorbable scaffold: Present status and future perspectives. *J. Thorac. Dis.* **2017**, *9* (Suppl. S9), 903–913. [CrossRef]
21. Haude, M.; Erbel, R.; Erne, P.; Verheye, S.; Degen, H.; Böse, D. Safety and performance of the drug-eluting absorbable metal scaffold (DREAMS) in patients with de-novo coronary lesions: 12 month results of the prospective, multicentre, first-in-man BIOSOLVE-I trial. *Lancet* **2013**, *381*, 836–844. [CrossRef]
22. Haude, M.; Ince, H.; Abizaid, A.; Toelg, R.; Lemos, P.A.; von Birgelen, C.; Evald, H.C.; William, W.; Franz-Josef, N.; Christoph, K.; et al. Sustained safety and performance of the second-generation drug-eluting absorbable metal scaffold in patients with de novo coronary lesions: 12-month clinical results and angiographic findings of the BIOSOLVE-II first-in-man trial. *Eur. Heart J.* **2016**, *37*, 2701–2709. [CrossRef]
23. Haude, M.; Erbel, R.; Erne, P.; Verheye, S.; Degen, H.; Vermeersch, P. Safety and performance of the DRug-Eluting Absorbable Metal Scaffold (DREAMS) in patients with de novo coronary lesions: 3-year results of the prospective, multicentre, first-in-man BIOSOLVE-I trial. *EuroIntervention* **2016**, *12*, e160–e166. [CrossRef] [PubMed]
24. Haude, M.; Ince, H.; Kische, S.; Abizaid, A.; Tölg, R.; Alves, L.P. Sustained safety and clinical performance of a drug-eluting absorbable metal scaffold up to 24 months: Pooled outcomes of BIOSOLVE-II and BIOSOLVE-III. *EuroIntervention* **2017**, *13*, 432–439. [CrossRef] [PubMed]
25. Verheye, S.; Wlodarczak, A.; Montorsi, P.; Bennett, J.; Torzewski, J.; Haude, M. Safety and performance of a resorbable magnesium scaffold under real-world conditions: 12-month outcomes of the first 400 patients enrolled in the BIOSOLVE-IV registry. *EuroIntervention* **2019**. [CrossRef]

26. Neumann, F.J.; Sousa-Uva, M. 2018 ESC/EACTS Guidelines on myocardial revascularization. *Eur. Heart J.* **2019**, *40*, 87–165. [CrossRef] [PubMed]
27. Cortese, B.; di Palma, G.; Cerrato, E.; Latini, R.A.; Elwany, M.; Orrego, P.S.; Seregni, R.G. Clinical and angiographic outcome of a single center, real world population treated with a dedicated technique of implantation for bioresorbable vascular scaffolds. The FAtebenefratelli Bioresorbable Vascular Scaffold (FABS) registry. *J. Interv. Cardiol.* **2017**, *30*, 427–432. [CrossRef]
28. Li, H.; Rha, S.W.; Choi, C.U.; Oh, D.J. Optical Coherence Tomography and Stent Boost Imaging Guided Bioresorbable Vascular Scaffold Overlapping for Coronary Chronic Total Occlusion Lesion. *Yonsei Med. J.* **2017**, *58*, 1071–1074. [CrossRef]
29. Caiazzo, G.; Longo, G.; Giavarini, A.; Kilic, I.D.; Fabris, E.; Serdoz, R.; Alessio, M.; Nicolas, F.; Gioel, G.; Seccob, S.; et al. Optical coherence tomography guidance for percutaneous coronary intervention with bioresorbable scaffolds. *Int. J. Cardiol.* **2016**, *221*, 352–358. [CrossRef]
30. Caiazzo, G.; Kilic, I.D.; Fabris, E.; Serdoz, R.; Mattesini, A.; Foin, N. Absorb bioresorbable vascular scaffold: What have we learned after 5 years of clinical experience? *Int. J. Cardiol.* **2015**, *201*, 129–136. [CrossRef]
31. Onuma, Y.; Dudek, D.; Thuesen, L.; Webster, M.; Nieman, K.; Garcia-Garcia, H.M. Five-year clinical and functional multislice computed tomography angiographic results after coronary implantation of the fully resorbable polymeric everolimus-eluting scaffold in patients with de novo coronary artery disease: The ABSORB cohort A trial. *JACC Cardiovasc. Interv.* **2013**, *6*, 999–1009. [CrossRef] [PubMed]
32. Khamis, H.; Sanad, O.; Elrabbat, K.; Attia, A.; Adel, M.; Alkady, H.; Masoud, A. Bioresorbable vascular scaffold (BVS) for the treatment of native coronary artery stenosis: One year outcome. *Egypt. Heart J.* **2016**, *68*, 253–259. [CrossRef]
33. Otsuka, F.; Vorpahl, M.; Nakano, M.; Foerst, J.; Newell, J.B.; Sakakura, K.; Robert, K.; Elena, L.; Aloke, V.F.; Frank, D.K.; et al. Pathology of second-generation everolimus-eluting stents versus first-generation sirolimus- and paclitaxel-eluting stents in humans. *Circulation* **2014**, *129*, 211–223. [CrossRef] [PubMed]
34. Yamaji, K.; Kimura, T.; Morimoto, T.; Nakagawa, Y.; Inoue, K.; Soga, Y. Very long-term (15 to 20 years) clinical and angiographic outcome after coronary bare metal stent implantation. *Circ. Cardiovasc. Interv.* **2010**, *3*, 468–475. [CrossRef]
35. Pavasini, R.; Serenelli, M.; Gallo, F.; Bugani, G.; Geraci, S.; Vicinelli, P.; Campo, G. Effectiveness and safety of the ABSORB bioresorbable vascular scaffold for the treatment of coronary artery disease: Systematic review and meta-analysis of randomized clinical trials. *J. Thorac. Dis.* **2017**, *9* (Suppl. S9), 887–897. [CrossRef]
36. Onuma, Y.; Serruys, P.W. Bioresorbable scaffold: The advent of a new era in percutaneous coronary and peripheral revascularization? *Circulation* **2011**, *123*, 779–797. [CrossRef]
37. Campos, C.M.; Muramatsu, T.; Iqbal, J.; Zhang, Y.J.; Onuma, Y.; Garcia-Garcia, H.M. Bioresorbable drug-eluting magnesium-alloy scaffold for treatment of coronary artery disease. *Int. J. Mol. Sci.* **2013**, *14*, 24492–24500. [CrossRef]
38. Regazzoli, D.; Leone, P.P.; Colombo, A.; Latib, A. New generation bioresorbable scaffold technologies: An update on novel devices and clinical results. *J. Thorac. Dis.* **2017**, *9* (Suppl. S9), 979–985. [CrossRef]
39. Waksman, R.; Zumstein, P.; Pritsch, M.; Wittchow, E.; Haude, M.; Lapointe-Corriveau, C. Second-generation magnesium scaffold Magmaris: Device design and preclinical evaluation in a porcine coronary artery model. *EuroIntervention* **2017**, *13*, 440–449. [CrossRef]
40. Giacchi, G.; Ortega-Paz, L.; Brugaletta, S.; Ishida, K.; Sabaté, M. Bioresorbable vascular scaffolds technology: Current use and future developments. *Med. Devices* **2016**, *9*, 185–198. [CrossRef]
41. Foin, N.; Lee, R.D.; Torii, R.; Guitierrez-Chico, J.L.; Mattesini, A.; Nijjer, S. Impact of stent strut design in metallic stents and biodegradable scaffolds. *Int. J. Cardiol.* **2014**, *177*, 800–808. [CrossRef] [PubMed]
42. Bil, J.; Gil, R.J. Bioresorbable vascular scaffolds—What does the future bring? *J. Thorac. Dis.* **2016**, *8*, E741–E745. [CrossRef] [PubMed]
43. Katagiri, Y.; Stone, G.W.; Onuma, Y.; Serruys, P.W. State of the art: The inception, advent and future of fully bioresorbable scaffolds. *EuroIntervention* **2017**, *13*, 734–750. [CrossRef] [PubMed]
44. Joner, M.; Ruppelt, P.; Zumstein, P.; Lapointe-Corriveau, C.; Leclerc, G.; Bulin, A. Preclinical evaluation of degradation kinetics and elemental mapping of first- and second-generation bioresorbable magnesium scaffolds. *EuroIntervention* **2018**, *14*, e1040–e1048. [CrossRef] [PubMed]

45. Bangalore, S.; Kumar, S.; Fusaro, M.; Amoroso, N.; Attubato, M.J.; Feit, F. Short- and long-term outcomes with drug-eluting and bare-metal coronary stents: A mixed-treatment comparison analysis of 117 762 patient-years of follow-up from randomized trials. *Circulation* **2012**, *125*, 2873–2891. [CrossRef] [PubMed]
46. Cassese, S.; Katagiri, Y.; Byrne, R.A.; Brugaletta, S.; Alfonso, F.; Räber, L. Angiographic and clinical outcomes of STEMI patients treated with bioresorbable or metallic everolimus-eluting stents. A pooled analysis of individual patient data from 2 randomized trials. *EuroIntervention* **2019**. [CrossRef]
47. La Manna, A.; Chisari, A.; Giacchi, G.; Capodanno, D.; Longo, G.; Di Silvestro, M. Everolimus-eluting bioresorbable vascular scaffolds for treatment of complex chronic total occlusions. *EuroIntervention* **2017**, *13*, 355–363. [CrossRef]
48. La Manna, A.; Chisari, A.; Giacchi, G.; Capodanno, D.; Longo, G.; Di Silvestro, M. Systemic Pharmacokinetics of Everolimus Eluted from the Absorb Bioresorbable Vascular Scaffold: An ABSORB III Substudy. *J. Am. Coll. Cardiol.* **2015**, *66*, 2467–2469. [CrossRef]
49. Tanabe, K.; Popma, J.J.; Kozuma, K.; Saito, S.; Muramatsu, T.; Nakamura, S. Multislice computed tomography assessment of everolimus-eluting Absorb bioresorbable scaffolds in comparison with metallic drug-eluting stents from the ABSORB Japan randomised trial. *EuroIntervention* **2018**, *14*, e1020–e1028. [CrossRef]
50. Ang, H.Y.; Bulluck, H.; Wong, P.; Venkatraman, S.S.; Huang, Y.; Foin, N. Bioresorbable stents: Current and upcoming bioresorbable technologies. *Int. J. Cardiol.* **2017**, *228*, 931–939. [CrossRef]
51. Ali, Z.A.; Serruys, P.W.; Kimura, T.; Gao, R.; Ellis, S.G.; Kereiakes, D.J. 2-year outcomes with the Absorb bioresorbable scaffold for treatment of coronary artery disease: A systematic review and meta-analysis of seven randomised trials with an individual patient data substudy. *Lancet* **2017**, *390*, 760–772. [CrossRef]
52. Varcoe, R.L.; Thomas, S.D.; Rapoza, R.J.; Kum, S. Lessons Learned Regarding Handling and Deployment of the Absorb Bioresorbable Vascular Scaffold in Infrapopliteal Arteries. *J. Endovasc. Ther.* **2017**, *24*, 337–341. [CrossRef] [PubMed]
53. Sorrentino, S.; De Rosa, S.; Ambrosio, G.; Mongiardo, A.; Spaccarotella, C.; Polimeni, A.; Jolanda, S.; Daniele, T.; Gianluca, C.; Ciro, I. The duration of balloon inflation affects the luminal diameter of coronary segments after bioresorbable vascular scaffolds deployment. *BMC Cardiovasc. Disord.* **2015**, *15*, 169. [CrossRef] [PubMed]
54. Mattesini, A.; Bartolini, S.; Dini, C.S.; Valente, S.; Parodi, G.; Stolcova, M.; Di Mario, C. The DESolve novolimus bioresorbable Scaffold: From bench to bedside. *J. Thorac. Dis.* **2017**, *9* (Suppl. S9), 950–958. [CrossRef] [PubMed]
55. Nef, H.M.; Wiebe, J.; Foin, N.; Blachutzik, F.; Dörr, O.; Toyloy, S.; Hamm, C.W. A new novolimus-eluting bioresorbable coronary scaffold: Present status and future clinical perspectives. *Int. J. Cardiol.* **2017**, *227*, 127–133. [CrossRef]
56. Abizaid, A.; Costa, R.A.; Schofer, J.; Ormiston, J.; Maeng, M.; Witzenbichler, B. Serial Multimodality Imaging and 2-Year Clinical Outcomes of the Novel DESolve Novolimus-Eluting Bioresorbable Coronary Scaffold System for the Treatment of Single De Novo Coronary Lesions. *JACC Cardiovasc. Interv.* **2016**, *9*, 565–574. [CrossRef]
57. Ormiston, J.A.; Webber, B.; Ubod, B.; Darremont, O.; Webster, M.W. An independent bench comparison of two bioresorbable drug-eluting coronary scaffolds (Absorb and DESolve) with a durable metallic drug-eluting stent (ML8/Xpedition). *EuroIntervention* **2015**, *11*, 60–67. [CrossRef]
58. Schmidt, W.; Behrens, P.; Brandt-Wunderlich, C.; Siewert, S.; Grabow, N.; Schmitz, K.P. In vitro performance investigation of bioresorbable scaffolds - Standard tests for vascular stents and beyond. *Cardiovasc. Revasc. Med.* **2016**, *17*, 375–383. [CrossRef]
59. Verheye, S.; Ormiston, J.A.; Stewart, J.; Webster, M.; Sanidas, E.; Costa, R.; Ribamar, C., Jr.; Daniel, C.; Andrea, S.A.; Ibraim, P.; et al. A next-generation bioresorbable coronary scaffold system: From bench to first clinical evaluation: 6- and 12-month clinical and multimodality imaging results. *JACC Cardiovasc. Interv.* **2014**, *7*, 89–99. [CrossRef]
60. de Pommereau, A.; de Hemptinne, Q.; Varenne, O.; Picard, F. Bioresorbable vascular scaffolds: Time to absorb past lessons or fade away? *Arch. Cardiovasc. Dis.* **2018**. [CrossRef]
61. Haude, M.; Ince, H.; Abizaid, A.; Toelg, R.; Lemos, P.A.; von Birgelen, C. Safety and performance of the second-generation drug-eluting absorbable metal scaffold in patients with de-novo coronary artery lesions (BIOSOLVE-II): 6 month results of a prospective, multicentre, non-randomised, first-in-man trial. *Lancet* **2016**, *387*, 31–39. [CrossRef]

62. Ghimire, G.; Spiro, J.; Kharbanda, R.; Roughton, M.; Barlis, P.; Mason, M. Initial evidence for the return of coronary vasoreactivity following the absorption of bioabsorbable magnesium alloy coronary stents. *EuroIntervention* **2009**, *4*, 481–484. [CrossRef] [PubMed]
63. Varenhorst, C.; Lindholm, M.; Sarno, G.; Olivecrona, G.; Jensen, U.; Nilsson, J.; Jörg, C.; Stefan, J.; Bo, L. Stent thrombosis rates the first year and beyond with new- and old-generation drug-eluting stents compared to bare metal stents. *Clin. Res. Cardiol.* **2018**, *107*, 816–823. [CrossRef] [PubMed]
64. Sternberg, K.; Gratz, M.; Koeck, K.; Mostertz, J.; Begunk, R.; Loebler, M.; Beatrice, S.; Anne, S.; Petra, H.; Georg, H.; et al. Magnesium used in bioabsorbable stents controls smooth muscle cell proliferation and stimulates endothelial cells in vitro. *J. Biomed. Mater. Res. B Appl. Biomater.* **2012**, *100*, 41–50. [CrossRef] [PubMed]
65. Berthon, N.; Laurant, P.; Fellmann, D.; Berthelot, A. Effect of magnesium on mRNA expression and production of endothelin-1 in DOCA-salt hypertensive rats. *J. Cardiovasc. Pharmacol.* **2003**, *42*, 24–31. [CrossRef] [PubMed]
66. Kereiakes, D.J.; Ellis, S.G. 3-Year Clinical Outcomes with Everolimus-Eluting Bioresorbable Coronary Scaffolds: The ABSORB III Trial. *J. Am. Coll. Cardiol.* **2017**. [CrossRef]
67. Ellis, S.G.; Kereiakes, D.J. *Everolimus-Eluting Bioresorbable Vascular Scaffolds in Patients with Coronary Artery Disease: ABSORB III Trial 2-Year Results*; American College of Cardiology Annual Scientific Session: Washington, DC, USA, 2017.
68. Stone, G.W.; Ellis, S.G.; Gori, T.; Metzger, D.C.; Stein, B.; Erickson, M. Blinded outcomes and angina assessment of coronary bioresorbable scaffolds: 30-day and 1-year results from the ABSORB IV randomised trial. *Lancet* **2018**, *392*, 1530–1540. [CrossRef]
69. Arroyo, D.; Gendre, G.; Schukraft, S.; Kallinikou, Z.; Müller, O.; Baeriswyl, G.; Stauffera, J.C.; Goya, J.J.; Tognia, M.; Cooka, S.; et al. Comparison of everolimus- and biolimus-eluting coronary stents with everolimus-eluting bioresorbable vascular scaffolds: Two-year clinical outcomes of the EVERBIO II trial. *Int. J. Cardiol.* **2017**, *243*, 121–125. [CrossRef]
70. Katagiri, Y.; Onuma, Y. Three-year follow-up of the randomised comparison between an everolimus-eluting bioresorbable scaffold and a durable polymer everolimus-eluting metallic stent in patients with ST-segment elevation myocardial infarction (TROFI II trial). *EuroIntervention* **2018**, *14*, e1224–e1226. [CrossRef]
71. Kimura, T.; Kozuma, K.; Tanabe, K.; Nakamura, S.; Yamane, M.; Muramatsu, T. A randomized trial evaluating everolimus-eluting Absorb bioresorbable scaffolds vs. everolimus-eluting metallic stents in patients with coronary artery disease: ABSORB Japan. *Eur. Heart J.* **2015**, *36*, 3332–3342. [CrossRef]
72. Serruys, P.W.; Ormiston, J.; van Geuns, R.J.; de Bruyne, B.; Dudek, D.; Christiansen, E.; Bernard, C.; Pieter, S.; Dougal, M.; Jacques, K.; et al. A Polylactide Bioresorbable Scaffold Eluting Everolimus for Treatment of Coronary Stenosis: 5-Year Follow-Up. *J. Am. Coll. Cardiol.* **2016**, *67*, 766–776. [CrossRef] [PubMed]
73. Toušek, P.; Kočka, V.; Malý, M.; Kozel, M.; Petr, R.; Hajsl, M. Long-term follow-up after bioresorbable vascular scaffold implantation in STEMI patients: PRAGUE-19 study update. *EuroIntervention* **2016**, *12*, 23–29. [CrossRef] [PubMed]
74. Xu, B.; Yang, Y.; Han, Y.; Huo, Y.; Wang, L.; Qi, X. Comparison of everolimus-eluting bioresorbable vascular scaffolds and metallic stents: Three-year clinical outcomes from the ABSORB China randomised trial. *EuroIntervention* **2018**, *14*, e554–e561. [CrossRef] [PubMed]
75. Byrne, R.A.; Alfonso, F.; Schneider, S.; Maeng, M.; Wiebe, J.; Kretov, E. Prospective, randomized trial of bioresorbable scaffolds vs. everolimus-eluting stents in patients undergoing coronary stenting for myocardial infarction: The Intracoronary Scaffold Assessment a Randomized evaluation of Absorb in Myocardial Infarction (ISAR-Absorb MI) trial. *Eur. Heart J.* **2019**, *40*, 167–176. [CrossRef] [PubMed]
76. Abizaid, A.; Vrolix, M.; Costa, J.R.; Chamie, D.; Abizaid, A.; Castro, J. TCT-330 Multi-Center Evaluation of a Novel 120 μm Novolimus-Eluting, Fully Bioresorbable Coronary Scaffold: First Report of 6-month Imaging and 12-Month Clinical Results. *J. Am. Coll. Cardiol.* **2017**, *70*, 135–136. [CrossRef]
77. Nef, H.; Wiebe, J.; Boeder, N.; Dörr, O.; Bauer, T.; Hauptmann, K.E. A multicenter post-marketing evaluation of the Elixir DESolve((R)) Novolimus-eluting bioresorbable coronary scaffold system: First results from the DESolve PMCF study. *Catheter. Cardiovasc. Interv.* **2018**, *92*, 1021–1027. [CrossRef]
78. de Ribamar Costa, J.; Abizaid, A.; Chamie, D.; Lansky, A.; Kochman, J.; Koltowski, L. Initial results of the fantom 1 trial: A first-in-man evaluation of a novel, radiopaque sirolimus-eluting bioresorbable vascular scaffold. *J. Am. Coll. Cardiol.* **2016**, *67*, 232. [CrossRef]

79. Abizaid, A.; Carrié, D.; Frey, N.; Lutz, M.; Weber-Albers, J.; Dudek, D. 6-Month Clinical and Angiographic Outcomes of a Novel Radiopaque Sirolimus-Eluting Bioresorbable Vascular Scaffold: The FANTOM II Study. *JACC Cardiovasc. Interv.* **2017**, *10*, 1832–1838. [CrossRef]
80. Kraak, R.P.; Grundeken, M.J.; Hassell, M.E.; Elias, J.; Koch, K.T.; Henriques, J.P. Two-year clinical outcomes of Absorb bioresorbable vascular scaffold implantation in complex coronary artery disease patients stratified by SYNTAX score and ABSORB II study enrolment criteria. *EuroIntervention* **2016**, *12*, e557–e565. [CrossRef]
81. Puricel, S.; Arroyo, D.; Corpataux, N.; Baeriswyl, G.; Lehmann, S.; Kallinikou, Z. Comparison of everolimus- and biolimus-eluting coronary stents with everolimus-eluting bioresorbable vascular scaffolds. *J. Am. Coll. Cardiol.* **2015**, *65*, 791–801. [CrossRef]
82. Ellis, S.G. Fantom Bioresorbable Scaffold: Verse, But Not Yet Chorus (An Incomplete Composition). *JACC Cardiovasc. Interv.* **2017**, *10*, 1839–1840. [CrossRef] [PubMed]
83. Ellis, S.G.; Gori, T.; Serruys, P.W.; Nef, H.; Steffenino, G.; Brugaletta, S. Clinical, Angiographic, and Procedural Correlates of Very Late Absorb Scaffold Thrombosis: Multistudy Registry Results. *JACC Cardiovasc. Interv.* **2018**, *11*, 638–644. [CrossRef] [PubMed]
84. Mahmud, E.; Reeves, R.R. Bioresorbable Vascular Scaffolds: Back to the Drawing Board. *JACC Cardiovasc. Interv.* **2018**, *11*, 645–647. [CrossRef]
85. Suwannasom, P.; Sotomi, Y.; Ishibashi, Y.; Cavalcante, R.; Albuquerque, F.N.; Macaya, C. The Impact of Post-Procedural Asymmetry, Expansion, and Eccentricity of Bioresorbable Everolimus-Eluting Scaffold and Metallic Everolimus-Eluting Stent on Clinical Outcomes in the ABSORB II Trial. *JACC Cardiovasc. Interv.* **2016**, *9*, 1231–1242. [CrossRef]
86. Costa, J.R.; Abizaid, A. Bioresorbable Coronary Scaffolds: Deployment Tips and Tricks and the Future of the Technology. *Methodist DeBakey Cardiovasc. J.* **2018**, *14*, 42–49. [CrossRef]
87. Zhang, Y.J.; Bourantas, C.V.; Muramatsu, T.; Iqbal, J.; Farooq, V.; Diletti, R. Comparison of acute gain and late lumen loss after PCI with bioresorbable vascular scaffolds versus everolimus-eluting stents: An exploratory observational study prior to a randomised trial. *EuroIntervention* **2014**, *10*, 672–680. [CrossRef]
88. Serruys, P.W.; Katagiri, Y.; Sotomi, Y.; Zeng, Y.; Chevalier, B.; van der Schaaf, R.J. Arterial Remodeling After Bioresorbable Scaffolds and Metallic Stents. *J. Am. Coll. Cardiol.* **2017**, *70*, 60–74. [CrossRef]
89. Danzi, G.B.; Sesana, M.; Arieti, M.; Villa, G.; Rutigliano, S.; Aprile, A. Does optimal lesion preparation reduce the amount of acute recoil of the Absorbe BVS? Insights from a real-world population. *Catheter. Cardiovasc. Interv.* **2015**, *86*, 984–991. [CrossRef]
90. Onuma, Y.; Sotomi, Y.; Shiomi, H.; Ozaki, Y.; Namiki, A.; Yasuda, S. Two-year clinical, angiographic, and serial optical coherence tomographic follow-up after implantation of an everolimus-eluting bioresorbable scaffold and an everolimus-eluting metallic stent: Insights from the randomised ABSORB Japan trial. *EuroIntervention* **2016**, *12*, 1090–1101. [CrossRef]
91. Kochman, J.; Tomaniak, M.; Jąkała, J.; Proniewska, K.; Legutko, J.; Roleder, T. First serial optical coherence tomography assessment at baseline, 12 and 24 months in STEMI patients treated with the second generation ABSORB bioresorbable vascular scaffold. *EuroIntervention* **2017**. [CrossRef]
92. Oberhauser, J.P.; Hossainy, S.; Rapoza, R.J. Design principles and performance of bioresorbable polymeric vascular scaffolds. *EuroIntervention* **2009**, *5*, 15–22. [CrossRef] [PubMed]
93. Ortega-Paz, L.; Brugaletta, S.; Sabaté, M. Impact of PSP Technique on Clinical Outcomes Following Bioresorbable Scaffolds Implantation. *J. Clin. Med.* **2018**, *7*, 27. [CrossRef] [PubMed]
94. Imori, Y.; D'Ascenzo, F.; Gori, T.; Münzel, T.; Ugo, F.; Campo, G. Impact of postdilatation on performance of bioresorbable vascular scaffolds in patients with acute coronary syndrome compared with everolimus-eluting stents: A propensity score-matched analysis from a multicenter "real-world" registry. *Cardiol. J.* **2016**, *23*, 374–383. [CrossRef] [PubMed]
95. Yamaji, K.; Brugaletta, S.; Sabaté, M.; Iñiguez, A.; Jensen, L.O.; Cequier, A. Effect of Post-Dilatation Following Primary PCI With Everolimus-Eluting Bioresorbable Scaffold Versus Everolimus-Eluting Metallic Stent Implantation: An Angiographic and Optical Coherence Tomography TROFI II Substudy. *JACC Cardiovasc. Interv.* **2017**, *10*, 1867–1877. [CrossRef]
96. Stone, G.W.; Abizaid, A.; Onuma, Y.; Seth, A.; Gao, R.; Ormiston, J. Effect of Technique on Outcomes Following Bioresorbable Vascular Scaffold Implantation: Analysis from the ABSORB Trials. *J. Am. Coll. Cardiol.* **2017**, *70*, 2863–2874. [CrossRef]

97. Polimeni, A.; Anadol, R.; Münzel, T.; Geyer, M.; De Rosa, S.; Indolfi, C.; Gori, T. Bioresorbable vascular scaffolds for percutaneous treatment of chronic total coronary occlusions: A meta-analysis. *BMC Cardiovasc. Disord.* **2019**, *19*, 59. [CrossRef]
98. Abizaid, A.; Ribamar Costa, J., Jr. Bioresorbable Scaffolds for Coronary Stenosis: When and How Based Upon Current Studies. *Curr. Cardiol. Rep.* **2017**, *19*, 27. [CrossRef]
99. Geraci, S.; Kawamoto, H.; Caramanno, G.; Ruparelia, N.; Capodanno, D.; Brugaletta, S. Bioresorbable Everolimus-Eluting Vascular Scaffold for Long Coronary Lesions: A Subanalysis of the International, Multicenter GHOST-EU Registry. *JACC Cardiovasc. Interv.* **2017**, *10*, 560–568. [CrossRef]
100. Gori, T.; Wiebe, J.; Capodanno, D.; Latib, A.; Lesiak, M.; Pyxaras, S.A. Early and midterm outcomes of bioresorbable vascular scaffolds for ostial coronary lesions: Insights from the GHOST-EU registry. *EuroIntervention* **2016**, *12*, e550–e556. [CrossRef]
101. Cassese, S.; Byrne, R.A.; Ndrepepa, G.; Kufner, S.; Wiebe, J. Everolimus-eluting bioresorbable vascular scaffolds versus everolimus-eluting metallic stents: A meta-analysis of randomised controlled trials. *Lancet* **2016**, *387*, 537–544. [CrossRef]
102. Stone, G.W.; Gao, R.; Kimura, T.; Kereiakes, D.J.; Ellis, S.G.; Onuma, Y. 1-year outcomes with the Absorb bioresorbable scaffold in patients with coronary artery disease: A patient-level, pooled meta-analysis. *Lancet* **2016**, *387*, 1277–1289. [CrossRef]
103. MiYaZaKi, Y.; Zeng, Y.; TUMMala, K.; STaneTiC, B.; TiJSSen, J. Early, late and very late incidence of bioresorbable scaffold thrombosis: A systematic review and meta-analysis of randomized clinical trials and observational studies. *Minerva Cardioangiol.* **2017**, *65*, 32–51. [CrossRef]
104. Lipinski, M.J.; Escarcega, R.O.; Baker, N.C.; Benn, H.A.; Gaglia, M.A.; Torguson, R.; Waksman, R. Scaffold Thrombosis After Percutaneous Coronary Intervention with ABSORB Bioresorbable Vascular Scaffold: A Systematic Review and Meta-Analysis. *JACC Cardiovasc. Interv.* **2016**, *9*, 12–24. [CrossRef] [PubMed]
105. Kang, S.H.; Gogas, B.D.; Jeon, K.H.; Park, J.S.; Lee, W.; Yoon, C.H. Long-term safety of bioresorbable scaffolds: Insights from a network meta-analysis including 91 trials. *EuroIntervention* **2018**, *13*, 1904–1913. [CrossRef] [PubMed]
106. Capranzano, P.; Longo, G.; Tamburino, C.I.; Gargiulo, G.; Ohno, Y. One-year outcomes after Absorb bioresorbable vascular scaffold implantation in routine clinical practice. *EuroIntervention* **2016**, *12*, e152–e159. [CrossRef]
107. Capodanno, D.; Gori, T.; Nef, H.; Latib, A.; Mehilli, J.; Lesiak, M. Percutaneous coronary intervention with everolimus-eluting bioresorbable vascular scaffolds in routine clinical practice: Early and midterm outcomes from the European multicentre GHOST-EU registry. *EuroIntervention* **2015**, *10*, 1144–1153. [CrossRef]
108. Hoppmann, P.; Kufner, S.; Cassese, S.; Wiebe, J.; Schneider, S.; Pinieck, S.; Laugwitz, K.L. Angiographic and clinical outcomes of patients treated with everolimus-eluting bioresorbable stents in routine clinical practice: Results of the ISAR-ABSORB registry. *Catheter. Cardiovasc. Interv.* **2016**, *87*, 822–829. [CrossRef]
109. Tröbs, M.; Achenbach, S.; Röther, J.; Klinghammer, L.; Schlundt, C. Bioresorbable vascular scaffold thrombosis in a consecutive cohort of 550 patients. *Catheter. Cardiovasc. Interv.* **2016**, *88*, 872–880. [CrossRef]
110. Gori, T.; Schulz, E.; Hink, U.; Kress, M.; Weiers, N.; Weissner, M.; Münzel, T. Clinical, Angiographic, Functional, and Imaging Outcomes 12 Months After Implantation of Drug-Eluting Bioresorbable Vascular Scaffolds in Acute Coronary Syndromes. *JACC Cardiovasc. Interv.* **2015**, *8*, 770–777. [CrossRef]
111. Kraak, R.P.; Hassell, M.E.; Grundeken, M.J.; Koch, K.T.; Henriques, J.P.; Piek, J.J. Initial experience and clinical evaluation of the Absorb bioresorbable vascular scaffold (BVS) in real-world practice: The AMC Single Centre Real World PCI Registry. *EuroIntervention* **2015**, *10*, 1160–1168. [CrossRef]
112. Widimsky, P.; Petr, R.; Tousek, P.; Maly, M.; Linkova, H.; Vrana, J.; Kocka, V. One-Year Clinical and Computed Tomography Angiographic Outcomes After Bioresorbable Vascular Scaffold Implantation During Primary Percutaneous Coronary Intervention for ST-Segment-Elevation Myocardial Infarction: The PRAGUE-19 Study. *Circ. Cardiovasc. Interv.* **2015**, *8*, e002933. [CrossRef] [PubMed]
113. Hoye, A.; van Domburg, R.T.; Sonnenschein, K.; Serruys, P.W. Percutaneous coronary intervention for chronic total occlusion of the coronary artery with the implantation of bioresorbable everolimus-eluting scaffolds. Poznan CTO-Absorb Pilot Registry. *EuroIntervention* **2016**, *12*, e144–e151. [CrossRef]
114. Robaei, D.; Back, L.; Ooi, S.Y.; Pitney, M.; Jepson, N. Twelve-Month Outcomes with a Bioresorbable Everolimus-Eluting Scaffold: Results of the ESHC-BVS Registry at Two Australian Centers. *J. Invasive Cardiol.* **2016**, *28*, 316–322. [PubMed]

115. Tamburino, C.; Latib, A.; Sabate, M.; Mehilli, J.; Gori, T.; Achenbach, S. Contemporary practice and technical aspects in coronary intervention with bioresorbable scaffolds: A European perspective. *EuroIntervention* **2015**, *11*, 45–52. [CrossRef]
116. Tenekecioglu, E.; Poon, E.K.; Collet, C.; Thondapu, V.; Torii, R.; Bourantas, C.V. The Nidus for Possible Thrombus Formation: Insight from the Microenvironment of Bioresorbable Vascular Scaffold. *JACC Cardiovasc. Interv.* **2016**, *9*, 2167–2168. [CrossRef]
117. Mattesini, A.; Secco, G.G.; Dall'Ara, G.; Ghione, M.; Rama-Merchan, J.C.; Lupi, A. ABSORB biodegradable stents versus second-generation metal stents: A comparison study of 100 complex lesions treated under OCT guidance. *JACC Cardiovasc. Interv.* **2014**, *7*, 741–750. [CrossRef]
118. Brugaletta, S.; Gori, T.; Low, A.F.; Tousek, P.; Pinar, E.; Gomez-Lara, J. Absorb bioresorbable vascular scaffold versus everolimus-eluting metallic stent in ST-segment elevation myocardial infarction: 1-year results of a propensity score matching comparison: The BVS-EXAMINATION Study (bioresorbable vascular scaffold-a clinical evaluation of everolimus eluting coronary stents in the treatment of patients with ST-segment elevation myocardial infarction). *JACC Cardiovasc. Interv.* **2015**, *8*, 189–197. [CrossRef]
119. Wöhrle, J.; Naber, C.; Schmitz, T.; Schwencke, C.; Frey, N.; Butter, C.; Mathey, D.G. Beyond the early stages: Insights from the ASSURE registry on bioresorbable vascular scaffolds. *EuroIntervention* **2015**, *11*, 149–156. [CrossRef]
120. Sabaté, M.; Windecker, S.; Iñiguez, A.; Okkels-Jensen, L.; Cequier, A.; Brugaletta, S.; Pilgrim, T. Everolimus-eluting bioresorbable stent vs. durable polymer everolimus-eluting metallic stent in patients with ST-segment elevation myocardial infarction: Results of the randomized ABSORB ST-segment elevation myocardial infarction-TROFI II trial. *Eur. Heart J.* **2016**, *37*, 229–240. [CrossRef]
121. Christ, G.; Hafner, T.; Siller-Matula, J.M.; Francesconi, M.; Grohs, K.; Wilhelm, E.; Podczeck-Schweighofer, A. Platelet inhibition by abciximab bolus-only administration and oral ADP receptor antagonist loading in acute coronary syndrome patients: The blocking and bridging strategy. *Thromb. Res.* **2013**, *132*, e36–e41. [CrossRef]
122. Vaquerizo, B.; Barros, A.; Pujadas, S.; Bajo, E.; Jiménez, M.; Gomez-Lara, J.; Serra, A. One-Year Results of Bioresorbable Vascular Scaffolds for Coronary Chronic Total Occlusions. *Am. J. Cardiol.* **2016**, *117*, 906–917. [CrossRef] [PubMed]
123. Ojeda, S.; Pan, M.; Romero, M.; de Lezo, J.S.; Mazuelos, F.; Segura, J.; Medina, A. Outcomes and computed tomography scan follow-up of bioresorbable vascular scaffold for the percutaneous treatment of chronic total coronary artery occlusion. *Am. J. Cardiol.* **2015**, *115*, 1487–1493. [CrossRef] [PubMed]
124. Capranzano, P.; Capodanno, D.; Brugaletta, S.; Latib, A.; Mehilli, J.; Nef, H.; Mattesini, A. Clinical outcomes of patients with diabetes mellitus treated with Absorb bioresorbable vascular scaffolds: A subanalysis of the European Multicentre GHOST-EU Registry. *Catheter. Cardiovasc. Interv.* **2018**, *91*, 444–453. [CrossRef] [PubMed]
125. Palmerini, T.; Kirtane, A.J.; Serruys, P.W.; Smits, P.C.; Kedhi, E.; Kereiakes, D.; De Waha, A. Stent thrombosis with everolimus-eluting stents: Meta-analysis of comparative randomized controlled trials. *Circ. Cardiovasc. Interv.* **2012**, *5*, 357–364. [CrossRef] [PubMed]
126. Authors/Task Force members; Windecker, S.; Kolh, P.; Alfonso, F.; Collet, J.P.; Cremer, J.; Jüni, P. 2014 ESC/EACTS Guidelines on myocardial revascularization: The Task Force on Myocardial Revascularization of the European Society of Cardiology (ESC) and the European Association for Cardio-Thoracic Surgery (EACTS)Developed with the special contribution of the European Association of Percutaneous Cardiovascular Interventions (EAPCI). *Eur. Heart J.* **2014**, *35*, 2541–2619. [CrossRef] [PubMed]
127. Iqbal, J.; Serruys, P.W.; Silber, S.; Kelbaek, H.; Richardt, G.; Morel, M.A.; Windecker, S. Comparison of zotarolimus- and everolimus-eluting coronary stents: Final 5-year report of the RESOLUTE all-comers trial. *Circ. Cardiovasc. Interv.* **2015**, *8*, e002230. [CrossRef]
128. Fallesen, C.O.; Antonsen, L.; Thayssen, P.; Jensen, L.O.; Lee, P.H.; Lee, S.W.; Brugaletta, S. How should I treat a bioresorbable vascular scaffold edge restenosis and intra-scaffold dissection? *EuroIntervention* **2018**, *13*, 1730–1734. [CrossRef]
129. Colombo, A.; Azzalini, L. Bioresorbable scaffolds: Reflections after a setback—Losing a battle does not mean losing the war! *EuroIntervention* **2017**, *13*, 785–786. [CrossRef]

130. Stettler, C.; Wandel, S.; Allemann, S.; Kastrati, A.; Morice, M.C.; Schömig, A.; Goy, J.J. Outcomes associated with drug-eluting and bare-metal stents: A collaborative network meta-analysis. *Lancet* **2007**, *370*, 937–948. [CrossRef]

131. FinnAV, J.; NakazawaG, K.; NewellJ, J. Pathological correlates of late drug-eluting stent thrombosis: Strut coverage as a marker of endothelialization. *Circulation* **2007**, *115*, 2435–2441. [CrossRef]

132. Finn, A.V.; Nakazawa, G.; Joner, M.; Kolodgie, F.D.; Mont, E.K.; Gold, H.K.; Virmani, R. Vascular responses to drug eluting stents: Importance of delayed healing. *Arter. Thromb. Vasc. Biol.* **2007**, *27*, 1500–1510. [CrossRef] [PubMed]

133. Joner, M.; Finn, A.V.; Farb, A.; Mont, E.K.; Kolodgie, F.D.; Ladich, E.; Virmani, R. Pathology of drug-eluting stents in humans: Delayed healing and late thrombotic risk. *J. Am. Coll. Cardiol.* **2006**, *48*, 193–202. [CrossRef] [PubMed]

134. Katsanos, K.; Spiliopoulos, S.; Kitrou, P.; Krokidis, M.; Karnabatidis, D. Risk of Death Following Application of Paclitaxel-Coated Balloons and Stents in the Femoropopliteal Artery of the Leg: A Systematic Review and Meta-Analysis of Randomized Controlled Trials. *J. Am. Heart Assoc.* **2018**, *7*, e011245. [CrossRef] [PubMed]

135. Beckman, J.A.; White, C.J. Paclitaxel-Coated Balloons and Eluting Stents: Is There a Mortality Risk in Patients with Peripheral Artery Disease? *Circulation* **2019**. [CrossRef]

136. Ali, Z.A.; Karimi Galougahi, K.; Shlofmitz, R.; Maehara, A.; Mintz, G.S.; Abizaid, A.; Stone, G.W. Imaging-guided pre-dilatation, stenting, post-dilatation: A protocolized approach highlighting the importance of intravascular imaging for implantation of bioresorbable scaffolds. *Expert Rev. Cardiovasc. Ther.* **2018**, *16*, 431–440. [CrossRef]

137. Ortega-Paz, L.; Capodanno, D.; Gori, T.; Nef, H.; Latib, A.; Caramanno, G.; Wiebe, J. Predilation, sizing and post-dilation scoring in patients undergoing everolimus-eluting bioresorbable scaffold implantation for prediction of cardiac adverse events: Development and internal validation of the PSP score. *EuroIntervention* **2017**, *12*, 2110–2117. [CrossRef]

138. Markovic, S.; Kugler, C.; Rottbauer, W.; Wöhrle, J. Long-term clinical results of bioresorbable absorb scaffolds using the PSP-technique in patients with and without diabetes. *J. Interv. Cardiol.* **2017**, *30*, 325–330. [CrossRef]

139. Heeger, C.H.; Schedifka, A.S.; Meincke, F.; Spangenberg, T.; Wienemann, H.; Kreidel, F. Optical coherence tomography-guided versus angiography-guided implantation of everolimus-eluting bioresorbable vascular scaffolds: Comparison of coverage, apposition and clinical outcome. The ALSTER-OCT ABSORB registry. *Cardiol. J.* **2018**. [CrossRef]

140. von Zur Mühlen, C.; Reiss, S.; Krafft, A.J.; Besch, L.; Menza, M.; Zehender, M.; Reinöhl, J. Coronary magnetic resonance imaging after routine implantation of bioresorbable vascular scaffolds allows non-invasive evaluation of vascular patency. *PLoS ONE* **2018**, *13*, e0191413. [CrossRef]

141. Capodanno, D. Bioresorbable Scaffolds in Coronary Intervention: Unmet Needs and Evolution. *Korean Circ. J.* **2018**, *48*, 24–35. [CrossRef]

142. Ferdous, J.; Kolachalama, V.B.; Kolandaivelu, K.; Shazly, T. Degree of bioresorbable vascular scaffold expansion modulates loss of essential function. *Acta Biomater.* **2015**, *26*, 195–204. [CrossRef] [PubMed]

143. Mattesini, A.; Boeder, N.; Valente, S.; Löblich, K.; Dörr, O.; Secco, G.G. Absorb vs. DESolve: An optical coherence tomography comparison of acute mechanical performances. *EuroIntervention* **2016**, *12*, e566–e573. [CrossRef] [PubMed]

144. Stone, G.W.; Witzenbichler, B.; Weisz, G.; Rinaldi, M.J.; Neumann, F.J. Platelet reactivity and clinical outcomes after coronary artery implantation of drug-eluting stents (ADAPT-DES): A prospective multicentre registry study. *Lancet* **2013**, *382*, 614–623. [CrossRef]

145. Siller-Matula, J.M.; Trenk, D.; Schrör, K.; Gawaz, M.; Kristensen, S.D.; Storey, R.F.; Huber, K. Response variability to P2Y12 receptor inhibitors: Expectations and reality. *JACC Cardiovasc. Interv.* **2013**, *6*, 1111–1128. [CrossRef]

146. Mangiacapra, F.; Patti, G.; Barbato, E.; Peace, A.J.; Ricottini, E.; Vizzi, V. A therapeutic window for platelet reactivity for patients undergoing elective percutaneous coronary intervention: Results of the ARMYDA-PROVE (Antiplatelet therapy for Reduction of MYocardial Damage during Angioplasty-Platelet Reactivity for Outcome Validation Effort) study. *JACC Cardiovasc. Interv.* **2012**, *5*, 281–289. [CrossRef]

147. Byrne, R.A.; Stefanini, G.G.; Capodanno, D.; Onuma, Y.; Baumbach, A.; Escaned, J. Report of an ESC-EAPCI Task Force on the evaluation and use of bioresorbable scaffolds for percutaneous coronary intervention: Executive summary. *Eur. Heart J.* **2018**, *39*, 1591–1601. [CrossRef]

148. Tantry, U.S.; Bonello, L.; Aradi, D.; Price, M.J.; Jeong, Y.H.; Angiolillo, D.J. Consensus and update on the definition of on-treatment platelet reactivity to adenosine diphosphate associated with ischemia and bleeding. *J. Am. Coll. Cardiol.* **2013**, *62*, 2261–2273. [CrossRef]
149. Christ, G.; Siller-Matula, J.M.; Francesconi, M.; Dechant, C.; Grohs, K.; Podczeck-Schweighofer, A. Individualising dual antiplatelet therapy after percutaneous coronary intervention: The IDEAL-PCI registry. *BMJ Open* **2014**, *4*, e005781. [CrossRef]
150. Siller-Matula, J.M.; Gruber, C.; Francesconi, M.; Dechant, C.; Jilma, B.; Delle-Karth, G. The net clinical benefit of personalized antiplatelet therapy in patients undergoing percutaneous coronary intervention. *Clin. Sci.* **2015**, *128*, 121–130. [CrossRef]
151. Siller-Matula, J.M.; Francesconi, M.; Dechant, C.; Jilma, B.; Maurer, G. Personalized antiplatelet treatment after percutaneous coronary intervention: The MADONNA study. *Int. J. Cardiol.* **2013**, *167*, 2018–2023. [CrossRef]
152. Siller-Matula, J.M.; Hintermeier, A.; Kastner, J.; Kreiner, G.; Maurer, G.; Kratochwil, C. Distribution of clinical events across platelet aggregation values in all-comers treated with prasugrel and ticagrelor. *Vascul. Pharmacol.* **2016**, *79*, 6–10. [CrossRef] [PubMed]
153. Siller-Matula, J.M.; Jilma, B. Why have studies of tailored anti-platelet therapy failed so far? *Thromb. Haemost.* **2013**, *110*, 628–631. [CrossRef] [PubMed]
154. Kubisa, M.J.; Jezewski, M.P.; Gasecka, A.; Siller-Matula, J.M.; Postuła, M. Ticagrelor—Toward more efficient platelet inhibition and beyond. *Ther. Clin. Risk Manag.* **2018**, *14*, 129–140. [CrossRef] [PubMed]
155. Brugaletta, S.; Gomez-Lara, J.; Caballero, J.; Ortega-Paz, L.; Teruel, L. TIcaGrEloR and Absorb bioresorbable vascular scaffold implantation for recovery of vascular function after successful chronic total occlusion recanalization (TIGER-BVS trial): Rationale and study design. *Catheter. Cardiovasc. Interv.* **2018**, *91*, 1–6. [CrossRef]

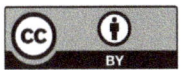

© 2019 by the authors. Licensee MDPI, Basel, Switzerland. This article is an open access article distributed under the terms and conditions of the Creative Commons Attribution (CC BY) license (http://creativecommons.org/licenses/by/4.0/).

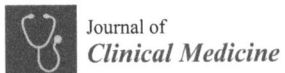

Review

Antithrombotic Therapy for Percutaneous Cardiovascular Interventions: From Coronary Artery Disease to Structural Heart Interventions

Alessandro Caracciolo [1], Paolo Mazzone [1], Giulia Laterra [1], Victoria Garcia-Ruiz [2], Alberto Polimeni [3], Salvatore Galasso [1], Francesco Saporito [1], Scipione Carerj [1], Fabrizio D'Ascenzo [4], Guillaume Marquis-Gravel [5,6], Gennaro Giustino [7,8] and Francesco Costa [1,*]

1. Department of Clinical and Experimental Medicine, Policlinic "G. Martino", University of Messina, 98100 Messina, Italy; caracciolo.alessandro.ac@gmail.com (A.C.); mazzonepaolo89@gmail.com (P.M.); giulia.laterra1990@gmail.com (G.L.); sgalasso@gmail.com (S.G.); fsaporito@unime.it (F.S.); scarerj@unime.it (S.C.)
2. UGC del Corazón, Servicio de Cardiología, Hospital Clínico Universitario Virgen de la Victoria, 29010 Málaga, Spain; mavigaru@gmail.com
3. Division of Cardiology, Department of Medical and Surgical Sciences, Magna Graecia University, 88100 Catanzaro, Italy; polimeni@unicz.it
4. Division of Cardiology, Department of Medical Sciences, Città della Salute e della Scienza, University of Turin, 10124 Turin, Italy; fabrizio.dascenzo@gmail.com
5. Duke Clinical Research Institute, Durham, NC 27708, USA; guillaume.marquis.gravel@duke.edu
6. Montreal Heart Institute, Montreal, QC H1T 1C8, Canada
7. The Zena and Michael A. Wiener Cardiovascular Institute, Icahn School of Medicine at Mount Sinai, New York, NY 10029-6574, USA; gennaro.giustino@mountsinai.org
8. Department of Population Health Science and Policy, Icahn School of Medicine at Mount Sinai, New York, NY 10029-6574, USA
* Correspondence: dottfrancescocosta@gmail.com; Tel.: +39-090-221-23-41; Fax: +39-090-221-23-81

Received: 9 October 2019; Accepted: 15 November 2019; Published: 19 November 2019

Abstract: Percutaneous cardiovascular interventions have changed dramatically in recent years, and the impetus given by the rapid implementation of novel techniques and devices have been mirrored by a refinement of antithrombotic strategies for secondary prevention, which have been supported by a significant burden of evidence from clinical studies. In the current manuscript, we aim to provide a comprehensive, yet pragmatic, revision of the current available evidence regarding antithrombotic strategies in the domain of percutaneous cardiovascular interventions. We revise the evidence regarding antithrombotic therapy for secondary prevention in coronary artery disease and stent implantation, the complex interrelation between antiplatelet and anticoagulant therapy in patients undergoing percutaneous coronary intervention with concomitant atrial fibrillation, and finally focus on the novel developments in the secondary prevention after structural heart disease intervention. A special focus on treatment individualization is included to emphasize risk and benefits of each therapeutic strategy.

Keywords: dual antiplatelet therapy; antiplatelet; coronary artery disease; structural heart disease

1. Introduction

The link between percutaneous cardiovascular intervention and antithrombotic therapy begins right at the time of the first coronary angioplasties performed by Andreas Grüntzig. After the introduction of this technique in 1977, post-procedural warfarin therapy was initiated for 6–9 months after intervention to reduce the risk of post-procedural ischemic complications [1]. A few years later, the same group tested whether aspirin (ASA), with its secondary inhibition capacity of platelet's thromboxane A2 pathway, was superior to the oral anticoagulation in decreasing the incidence of reintervention after PCI [2]. While the techniques and the devices were improved in the following years, the introduction of the coronary stent and its first-in-man implantation in 1986 by Jacques Puel, dramatically improved early and late results of percutaneous coronary intervention (PCI), yet introducing a novel clinical issue: stent thrombosis. This complication occurred in up to 10% of cases at that time, and while a treatment with warfarin alone or warfarin plus aspirin was common after PCI and stent implantation, the rate of stent thrombosis remained high. Only in 1998 two randomized trials demonstrated that dual antiplatelet therapy (DAPT), constituted by the combination of ASA and a platelet P2Y12 inhibitor, was more effective than warfarin and aspirin therapy in reducing the risk of stent thrombosis [3,4]. These studies have established DAPT the as the gold standard therapy after angioplasty and stent implantation [5–7]. At the same time, similar antithrombotic practices were implemented for other percutaneous cardiovascular interventions such as atrial septal defect [8,9] or patent foramen ovale (PFO) closure [5,10], and more recently transcatheter aortic valve implantation (TAVI) [11] and transcatheter mitral valve repair (TMVR), in which the evidence coming from the coronary intervention field has been extrapolated to structural heart interventions. The aim of the current review is to summarize the evidence that established the current standards and recommendation for DAPT type and duration after coronary intervention, comment on the current standards for personalized treatment decision-making, and discuss the most recent advances in terms of treatment combination of antiplatelet and direct acting oral anticoagulants (DOAC) for the secondary prevention of high ischemic risk patients and patients with concomitant PCI and non-valvular atrial fibrillation. Finally, we touch upon the current evidence, recommendations and future perspectives for antithrombotic therapy in patients undergoing structural heart interventions.

2. Type of Antithrombotic Treatment after PCI

2.1. Evidence for Clopidogrel

While ticlopidine was the first P2Y12 inhibitor to be associated with ASA for DAPT, its worse safety profile made it obsolete after the introduction of clopidogrel. In 2000, the CLASSIC study was the first comparative trial in which clopidogrel in association with ASA was compared with ticlopidine in association with ASA after PCI [12]. In this study, which randomized 1020 patients to the combination of clopidogrel and ASA vs. ticlopidine and ASA, clopidogrel provided better safety and tolerability (i.e., less allergy, skin or gastrointestinal disorders and neutropenia) with a similar bleeding and efficacy profile. The CURE trial compared clopidogrel vs. placebo in addition to ASA in patients who presented with acute coronary syndromes without ST-segment elevation undergoing invasive or non-invasive management. The first primary outcome—a composite of death from cardiovascular causes, nonfatal myocardial infarction, or stroke—was significantly reduced in the clopidogrel group by 20% as compared to placebo (relative risk (RR) 0.80; 95% CI 0.72–0.90; $p < 0.001$) [13]. The evidence provided by the landmark CURE trial established DAPT with clopidogrel as the standard of care after acute coronary syndrome (ACS) and after coronary stent implantation. However, its high inter-individual variability in platelet inhibition and a sizable proportion of non-responders patient [14] highlighted the need for more potent and consistent platelet inhibition that would be introduced with novel generation P2Y12 inhibitors.

2.2. Evidence for Prasugrel

Similar to clopidogrel, prasugrel is a prodrug which requires conversion to an active metabolite to ultimately irreversibly bind to the P2Y12 receptor and achieve antiplatelet effect (Figure 1). different from clopidogrel, prasugrel has a more rapid and greater antiplatelet effect [15,16]. These drugs have been tested head-to-head in TRITON TIMI 38 trial. In this study, 13,608 patients with moderate to high-risk ACS and a scheduled invasive strategy were randomized to receive either prasugrel or clopidogrel. The primary efficacy endpoint of death from cardiovascular causes, nonfatal myocardial infarction, or nonfatal stroke occurred in 12.1% of patients receiving clopidogrel and 9.9% of patients receiving prasugrel (HR 0.81; 95% confidence interval (CI)), 0.73–0.90; $p < 0.001$). There was also a significant reduction of myocardial infarction (9.7% for clopidogrel vs. 7.4% for prasugrel; $p < 0.001$), urgent target-vessel revascularization (3.7% vs. 2.5%; $p < 0.001$), and stent thrombosis (2.4% vs. 1.1%; $p < 0.001$) related to the use of Prasugrel. However, the higher efficacy of prasugrel was counterbalanced by an increased risk of major bleeding, including fatal bleeding. Patients with previous stroke or transient ischemic attack were harmed by prasugrel use (hazard ratio, 1.54; 95% CI, 1.02–2.32; $p = 0.04$), while patients with 75 years of age or older and patients weighing less than 60 kg had had no benefit from prasugrel compared to ticagrelor [17]. TRITON TIMI 38 did not include patients with ACS undergoing medical-management. This population was specifically evaluated in the TRILOGY ACS trial. In TRILOGY ACS, patients were randomly allocated to prasugrel or clopidogrel and managed exclusively with medical therapy without revascularization. Prasugrel ultimately failed to show superiority for the primary study outcome compared to Clopidogrel in ACS patient treated medically without revascularization [18].

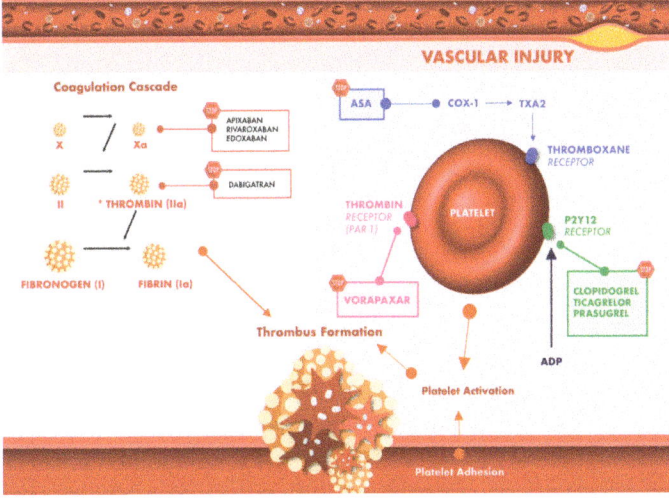

Figure 1. Antiplatelet and anticoagulant treatment strategies for secondary prevention of ischemic events.

Finally, the recent SASSICAIA trial (NCT02548611) explored the impact of prasugrel in patients undergoing elective PCI. In this study, patients with stable CAD and undergoing PCI were randomized to a loading dose with prasugrel or clopidogrel at the time of PCI. All patients after PCI were treated with clopidogrel alone and the primary outcome of all-cause death, any myocardial infarction, definite/probable stent thrombosis, stroke, or urgent vessel revascularization at 30 days was evaluated. Ultimately, there was no difference for the primary endpoint in the two study arms; hence, SASSICAIA trial failed to demonstrate that a prasugrel loading dose in elective patients reduces ischemic events as compared to an initial loading dose of clopidogrel.

2.3. Evidence for Ticagrelor

Ticagrelor is a P2Y12 inhibitor which binds reversibly the platelet receptor with a shorter plasma half-life. This has a more rapid onset and more pronounced platelet inhibition compared to clopidogrel (Figure 1) [19]. In the PLATO trial, 18,624 patients with acute coronary syndrome were randomized to Ticagrelor or Clopidogrel. In this study ticagrelor significantly reduced the rate of death from vascular causes, myocardial infarction, or stroke (9.8% vs. 11.7%; HR 0.84; 95% CI, 0.77–0.92; $p < 0.001$), but also increased non-coronary artery by-pass graft (CABG) related major bleeding [20]. In the ST Elevation Myocardial Infarction to Open the Coronary Artery (ATLANTIC) [21] study, 1862 patients with STEMI were randomized to pre-hospital administration of the loading dose of ticagrelor administered directly in the ambulance vs. in-hospital administration in the catheterization laboratory [21]. The two co-primary endpoints explored in the study (>70% resolution of ST-segment elevation before PCI and proportion of TIMI flow grade 3 at initial angiography) did not differ significantly between the two groups. The rates of definite stent thrombosis were lower in the pre-hospital administration group than in the in-hospital group (0% vs. 0.8%, $p = 0.008$ in the first 24 h; 0.2% vs. 1.2%, $p = 0.02$ at 30 days). No difference for major bleeding was observed with the two strategies.

2.4. Evidence for the Direct Comparison of Prasugrel and Ticagrelor

Despite having different pharmacological characteristics, prasugrel and ticagrelor demonstrated a similar efficacy profile in terms of platelet inhibition and percentage of patients with high on-treatment platelet reactivity [22]. On a clinical standpoint, while the two P2Y12 inhibitors proved superiority compared to clopidogrel in the two registration studies [17,20], a direct comparison between the two drugs has been provided only recently [23]. In the PRAGUE-18 study, 1230 patients with acute myocardial infarction (MI) treated with primary PCI were randomized to prasugrel or ticagrelor. The intended treatment duration was 12 months [24]. At one-year follow-up (although the study was ended prematurely for futility), the combined endpoint of cardiovascular death, MI, or stroke occurred in 6.6% of prasugrel and in 5.7% of ticagrelor patients (HR: 1.167; 95% CI: 0.742–1.835; $p = 0.503$). No significant differences for all bleeding (10.9% vs. 11.1%; $p = 0.999$) and TIMI major bleeding (0.9% vs. 0.7%; $p = 0.754$) were observed [24]. Rafique et al. explored the direct comparison of two P2Y12 inibhitors in the setting of primary PCI executing a network metanalysis of 37 studies: at one-year follow-up, prasugrel compared to ticagrelor was associated with a lower rate of MACE (OR: 0.77, 95% CI: 0.61–0.97), death for all causes (OR: 0.63, 95% CI: 0.46–0.87), but not CV death, MI or ST, with a similar rate of major bleeding [25]. While prior studies and meta-analysis have been inconclusive in unraveling possible differences in clinical outcomes between the two treatments, ISAR-REACT 5 was the first trial properly designed and sized to evaluate the direct comparison of ticagrelor vs. prasugrel [26]. In this multicenter, investigator-initiated, open-label trial 4018 patients with ACS undergoing invasive management were randomly assigned to either ticagrelor or prasugrel at the standard loading and maintenance doses. Importantly, according to guideline recommendations, patients randomized to the prasugrel arm were loaded only after angiography and to be assigned to a reduced maintenance dose if body weight was <60 kg or age >75 years. The primary endpoint of the study was a composite of death, myocardial infarction, or stroke at one year. The major secondary endpoint was bleeding according to BARC 3, 4 or 5 definition. At 12-month follow-up, the primary endpoint occurred 9.3% in the ticagrelor group and in 6.9% in the prasugrel group (HR, 1.36; 95% confidence interval (CI), 1.09–1.70; $p = 0.006$). The individual elements of the primary endpoint were all numerically in favor of prasugrel (death, 4.5% vs. 3.7%; MI, 4.8% vs. 3.0%; stroke, 1.1% vs. 1.0%). Stent thrombosis was similar between the two treatments. Surprisingly, no difference in terms of bleeding was observed among the two treatment arms, with a rate of BARC 3, 4 or 5 of 5.4% in the ticagrelor arm and 4.8% the prasugrel arm (HR 1.12; 95% CI, 0.83–1.51; $p = 0.46$) [26].

3. Duration of DAPT after PCI and Major Determinants for Treatment Selection

Randomized Trials

Numerous studies have tried in recent years to clarify which temporal window could be ideal after PCI or ACS (Table 1), and in general two major strategies have been presented relative to what was considered the standard of care for DAPT duration of 12 months [27]. A short DAPT encompasses a strategy of less than 12 months of treatment, and a long DAPT extends its duration beyond 12 months. With respect to a strategy of shortening DAPT duration, the first randomized study testing this assumption was the Efficacy of Xience/Promus Versus Cypher to Reduce Late Loss After Stenting (EXCELLENT). In this study, 1443 patients treated with drug-eluting stent (DES) implantation and randomized to 6 vs. 12 months DAPT, were evaluated to test the non-inferiority of the short DAPT strategy compared to the standard of care for the primary endpoint of cardiac death, myocardial infraction (MI), or ischemia-driven target vessel revascularization. Ultimately, six-month DAPT demonstrated non-inferior compared to the standard of care. In addition, TIMI major and minor bleeding were numerically higher in the 12-month group, but this difference was not statistically significant (HR 0.40; 95% CI: 0.13–1.27; $p = 0,12$) [28]. A similar hypothesis of non-inferiority of 6 vs. 12 months DAPT was also tested and observed in The Second Generation Drug-Eluting Stent Implantation Followed by Six-Versus Twelve-Month Dual Antiplatelet Therapy (SECURITY) [29] and in the Intracoronary Stenting and Antithrombotic Regimen: Safety and Efficacy of Six-month Dual Antiplatelet Therapy After Drug-Eluting Stenting (ISAR-SAFE) [30]. A different design was implemented in the Impact of Intravascular Ultrasound Guidance on Outcomes of XIENCE PRIME Stents in Long Lesions study [31]. In this case a factorial design was implemented and the first randomization was based on the routinely use of intravascular ultrasound PCI guidance, while the second randomization was for DAPT duration (6 vs. 12 months). At 12-month follow-up the composite of Cardiac death, MI, stroke, and TIMI major bleeding was similar between patients treated with 6- or 12-month DAPT (2.2% vs. 2.1%; $p = 0.85$). Interestingly, in the subgroup analysis for the primary endpoint patients treated with intravascular ultrasound guided stent implantation benefitted more from a shorter DAPT treatment as compared to those treated with angiographic guidance alone. In the specific setting of ACS, two randomized trials tested the feasibility of a shorter DAPT duration of six months as compared to the standard of care 12 months strategy: the SMART-DATE trial randomized 2712 patients to a DAPT for 6 or 12 months. At 18 months, the primary endpoint, a composite of all-cause death, MI, or stroke was recorded equally in the two study arms (4.7% vs. 4.2%) meeting the pre-specified non-inferiority hypothesis. However, a significant excess of MI was recorded in the short DAPT cohort [32]. A more specific setting was explored in the DAPT-STEMI trial where 870 patients with STEMI treated with primary PCI and second-generation DES that after six months of treatment with DAPT were randomized to another 12 months of DAPT therapy or to stop P2Y12 inhibitor and continue with aspirin only. The primary study endpoint was a composite of death, MI, revascularization, stroke, and major bleeding at 24 months after primary PCI. Short DAPT was found to be non-inferior as compared to the standard 12-month treatment duration (short DAPT 4.8% vs. long DAPT 6.6%; $p = 0.004$). However, these results should be interpreted with caution as the study enrolled a small sample size, and the event rate recorded was low compared to other studies in the literature [33]. The short DAPT therapy in high ischemic risk patient was the goal of the REDUCE trial (NCT02118870), which selected a population with a higher baseline ischemic risk to explore the non-inferiority of 3 vs. 12 months of DAPT in patients with ACS treated with PCI. The 1496 patients included in the study have been treated at index procedure exclusively with a bioabsorbable polymer DES. The primary endpoint was a composite of all cause death, MI, stent thrombosis, stroke, target vessel revascularization, or bleeding, with a wide, 5%, non-inferiority margin. The study reached non-inferiority with an event rate of 8.2% in the short DAPT arm and 8.4% in the long DAPT arm ($p < 0.001$). However, among secondary ischemic endpoints, stent thrombosis (1.2% vs. 0.4%; $p = 0.08$) and all-cause mortality (1.9% vs. 0.8%; $p = 0.07$) were numerically higher in the short DAPT arm, a trend which was consistent with that observed in the SMART-DATE trial [32]. Different temporal strategies have been considered in the design of the studies ITALIC [34] and NIPPON [35], respectively, 6 vs. 24 months of DAPT and 6 vs. 18 months of DAPT. These trials reached non-inferiority, but, again, the results from these studies should be interpreted with caution due to the study early termination and the wide non-inferiority margin selected.

Table 1. Randomized controlled trials of dual antiplatelet therapy duration in patients treated with percutaneous coronary intervention.

	Year	N	Study Design	Population Type	Type of Stent	Type of P2Y12 Inhibitor	DAPT Duration	Primary Endpoint	Event Rates (Short vs. Long)	Duration of Follow-Up
CREDO	2002	2116	Superiority of 12 mo DAPT *	ACS 67%	BMS 76.3% POBA 23.7%	Clopidogrel 100%	1 vs. 12	Death MI or stroke	11.5% vs. 8.5%	12 mo
PRODIGY	2012	1970	Superiority of 24 mo DAPT	ACS 75%	BMS 25% 1st gen DES 25% 2nd gen DES 50%	Clopidogrel 100%	6 vs. 24	All-cause death, MI, CVA	10% vs. 10.1%	24 mo
ARTIC INTERRUPTION	2012	1259	Superiority of 12 mo DAPT	ACS 34%	1st gen DES 41% 2nd gen DES 63%	Clopidogrel 91% Prasugrel 9%	12 vs. 18–24	All-cause death, MI, ST, stroke, TVR	4% vs. 4%.	17 mo
EXCELLENT	2012	1443	Non-inferiority of 6 mo DAPT	ACS 51%	1st gen DES 25% 2nd gen DES 75%	Clopidogrel 100%	6 vs. 12	Cardiac death, MI, TVR	4.8% vs. 4.3%	12 mo
RESET	2012	2117	Non-inferiority of 3 mo DAPT	ACS 59%	1st gen DES 21% 2nd gen DES 85%	Clopidogrel 100%	3 vs. 12	Cardiac death, MI, ST, TVR, major bleeding	4.7% vs. 4.7%	12 mo
OPTIMIZE	2013	3119	Non-inferiority of 3 mo DAPT	ACS 35%	2nd gen DES 100%	Clopidogrel 100%	3 vs. 12	All-cause death, MI, stroke, major bleeding	6% vs. 5.8%	12 mo
DES-LATE	2014	5045	Superiority of 24 mo DAPT	ACS 61%	1st gen DES 64% 2nd gen DES 30%	Clopidogrel 100%	12 vs. 36	Cardiac death, MI, stroke	2.4% vs. 2.6%	24 mo
DAPT	2014	9961	Superiority of 30 mo DAPT	ACS 43%	1st gen DES 38% 2nd gen DES 60%	Clopidogrel 65.3% Prasugrel 34.7%	12 vs. 30	Death, MI, stroke, ST.	7.3% vs. 4.7%	33 mo
SECURITY	2014	1399	Non-inferiority of 6 mo DAPT	28% ACS	2nd gen DES 100%	Clopidogrel 98.7% Prasugrel 0.2% Ticagrelor 0.4%	6 vs. 12	Cardiac death, MI, ST, or stroke	4.5% vs. 3.7%	12 mo
ISAR SAFE	2015	4000	Non-inferiority of 6 mo DAPT	ACS 40%	1st gen DES 10% 2nd gen DES 89%	Clopidogrel 100%	6 vs. 12	Death, MI, ST, stroke, major bleeding	1.5% vs. 1.6%	15 mo
ITALIC	2015	1822	Non-inferiority of 6 mo DAPT	ACS 24%	2nd gen DES 100%	Clopidogrel 98.6% Prasugrel 1.7% Ticagrelor 0.05%	6 vs. 24	Death, MI, TVR, stroke, major bleeding	1.6% vs. 1.5%	24 mo
I LOVE IT 2	2016	1829	Non-inferiority of 6 mo DAPT	ACS 64%	2nd gen DES 100%	Clopidogrel 100%	6 vs. 12	Cardiac death, target vessel MI	7.5% vs. 6.3%	18 mo
OPTIDUAL	2016	1385	Superiority of 48 mo DAPT	ACS 36%	1st gen DES 34% 2nd gen DES 59%	Clopidogrel 100%	12 vs. 48	Death, MI, stroke, ISTH major bleeding	7.5% vs. 5.8%	33 mo after randomization

Table 1. Cont.

	Year	N	Study Design	Population Type	Type of Stent	Type of P2Y12 Inhibitor	DAPT Duration	Primary Endpoint	Event Rates (Short vs. Long)	Duration of Follow-Up
IVUS XPL	2016	1400	Comparability of 6 vs. 12 mo DAPT	ACS 49%	2nd gen DES 100%	Clopidogrel 100%	6 vs. 12	Cardiac death, MI, stroke, or major bleeding	2.2% vs. 2.1%	12 mo
NIPPON	2016	3307	Non-inferiority of 6 mo DAPT	ACS 33%	2nd gen DES 100%	Clopidogrel 97.5% Prasugrel 0.1% Ticlopidine 2.3%	6 vs. 18	Death, MI, CVA, major bleeding	2.1% vs. 1.5%	18 mo
REDUCE	2017	1496	Non-inferiority of 3 mo DAPT	ACS 100%	2nd gen DES 100%	Clopidogrel 40.8% Prasugrel 10.4% Ticagrelor 48.9%	3 vs. 12	All-cause death, MI, ST, stroke, TVR, or bleeding	8.3% vs. 8.5%	12 mo
DAPT-STEMI	2017	861	Non-inferiority of 6 mo DAPT	ACS (STEMI) 100%	2nd gen DES 100%	Clopidogrel 42.0% Prasugrel 29.5% Ticagrelor 28.5%	6 vs. 12	All-cause mortality, MI, revascularization, stroke, and TIMI major bleeding	4.8% vs. 6.6%	24 mo
OPTIMA-C	2018	1368	Non-inferiority of 6 vs. 12 mo DAPT	ACS 50%	2nd gen DES 100%	Clopidogrel 100%	6 vs. 12	Cardiac death, TVR MI, Ischemia-driven TVR	1.2% vs. 0.6%	12 mo
SMART-DATE	2018	2712	Non-inferiority of 6 mo DAPT	ACS 100%	2nd gen DES 100%	Clopidogrel 80.7% Prasugrel/ Ticagrelor 19.3%	6 vs. 12	All-cause mortality, MI, stroke	4.7% vs. 4.2%	18 mo
GLOBAL LEADERS	2018	15,968	Superiority of 1 mo DAPT followed by 23 mo ticagrelor monotherapy vs. 12 mo DAPT followed by 12 mo ASA	ACS 47%	2nd gen DES 100%	Ticagrelor 46.8% Clopidogrel 53.2%	1 vs. 12	All-cause mortality non-fatal Q-wave MI	3.8% vs. 4.3%	24 mo
STOP DAPT 2	2019	3045	Non-inferiority of 1 month of DAPT followed by clopidogrel monotherapy compared with 12 mo DAPT	ACS 38.2%	2nd gen DES 100%	Clopidogrel 100%	1 vs. 12	CV death, MI, ischemic or hemorrhagic stroke, definite ST, or major or minor bleeding	2.4% vs. 3.7%	12 mo
SMART CHOICE	2019	2993	Non-inferiority of 3 mo of DAPT followed by P2Y12 inhibitor monotherapy compared with 12 mo DAPT	ACS 58.2%	2nd gen DES 100%	Clopidogrel 77.2% Prasugrel or Ticagrelor 22.8%	3 vs. 12	Death, MI or stroke	2.9% vs. 2.5%	12 mo

* The 12-month DAPT arm was associated to 300 mg clopidogrel loading dose before PCI, whereas the one-month DAPT arm was associated to placebo loading dose before PCI; ACS, acute coronary syndrome; BMS, bare metal stent; CV, cardiovascular; CVA, cerebrovascular accident; DAPT, dual antiplatelet therapy; DES, drug eluting stent; ISTH, International Society of Thrombosis and Hemostasis; MI, myocardial infarction; MO, months; POBA, plain old balloon angioplasty; ST, stent thrombosis; TIMI, The Thrombosysis in Myocardial Infarction; TVR, target vessel revascularization.

The rationale for a long DAPT strategy derives from the residual thrombotic risk during secondary prevention, which remains high despite potent P2Y12 inhibition [36]. Maintaining on a longer term a more potent and consistent platelet inhibition with DAPT should reduce the rate of ischemic complication due to plaque progression and rupture, yet may increase the risk of bleeding complications that have an equal negative impact on mortality [37,38]. The Dual-Antiplatelet Treatment Beyond one Year After Drug-Eluting Stent Implantation (ARCTIC INTERRUPTION) trial [39], an extended follow-up of the ARCTIC study, tested the superiority of ≥18 months DAPT vs. 12 months after stent implantation after an elective PCI. The primary efficacy endpoint occurred in 4% of patients in both study arms, while a significant excess of bleeding was detected in the prolonged DAPT arm. The PROlonging Dual antIplatelet treatment after Grading stent-induced intimal hYperplasia study (PRODIGY) trial [40], randomly allocated patients to a long DAPT strategy for 24 months vs. a short DAPT for six months showing no difference between the two strategies with respect to the study primary efficacy endpoint of death, MI, stroke, whereas an excess of actionable BARC 2, 3 or 5 bleeding was noted among patients allocated to the 24 month DAPT arm. The Dual Antiplatelet Therapy (DAPT) study was the first study with the adequate power to detect a difference for more rare ischemic events including stent thrombosis [41]. The study was funded by the American Food and Drug Administration and randomized 9961 patients who tolerated an uneventful course of DAPT of 12 months after stenting to two treatment strategies: interrupting DAPT at 12 months or continuing treatment up to 30 months. Extended DAPT resulted in a 1% absolute reduction in very late stent thrombosis and a 1.6% absolute reduction of major adverse cardiovascular and cerebrovascular events (MACCE). A total reduction of 2% of MI was also noted and this was ascribed in half of the cases to a different vessel from the one treated on a first place. Despite the sound reduction of ischemic events with a prolonged DAPT, this strategy was also burdened by a significant excess of major bleeding, with a doubtful or even negative impact on all cause mortality [41,42]. A landmark trial that further supported the potential extension of DAPT to the long term is the Prevention of Cardiovascular Events in Patients with Prior Heart Attack Using Ticagrelor Compared to Placebo on a Background of Aspirin–Thrombolysis in Myocardial Infarction 54 (PEGASUS-TIMI 54) study. PEGASUS investigated the potential benefit of extended DAPT therapy in patients with a prior myocardial infarction implementing two different Ticagrelor doses (90 mg twice daily and 60 mg twice a daily) on top of aspirin compared to placebo plus aspirin. The primary outcome was cardiovascular death, MI, or stroke, which occurred in 7.8% of the ticagrelor 90 mg bid group (hazard ratio (HR) vs. placebo 0.85, $p = 0.008$), 7.8% of the ticagrelor 60 mg bid group (HR vs. placebo 0.84, $p = 0.004$), and 9.0% of the placebo group. Ticagrelor was also associated with a significant increase in TIMI major bleeding, but no increase in intracranial hemorrhage [43]. Similar results were also observed, in a different population in THEMIS-PCI trial. This study evaluated the impact of DAPT with ticagrelor plus aspirin in patients with stable ischemic heart disease, type 2 diabetes, and prior PCI, compared to aspirin alone. At a median follow-up of 39.9 months, ticagrelor on top of aspirin was associated to a reduction of the primary efficacy outcome of cardiovascular death, MI, or stroke, which occurred in 7.3% of the ticagrelor/aspirin group and in 8.6% of the placebo/aspirin group ($p = 0.013$). The higher treatment efficacy was counterbalanced by an excess of bleeding, in fact the primary safety outcome of the study, TIMI major bleeding, occurred in 2.0% of the ticagrelor/aspirin group compared to 1.1% of the placebo/aspirin group ($p < 0.0001$). No difference in intracranial hemorrhage was observed. When the exploratory composite outcome of so-called "net irreversible harm"—a composite of all-cause death, MI, stroke, fatal bleeding, or intracranial hemorrhage—was explored, this occurred in 9.3% of the ticagrelor/aspirin group and in 11.0% of the placebo/aspirin group ($p = 0.005$) [44].

While DAPT type and duration selection is clearly associated with a trade-off between ischemia and bleeding [36,45], the optimal strategy, maximizing efficacy and safety should be individualized based on the patients' characteristics [46–50]. The type of clinical presentation (i.e., SCAD, unstable angina, non-STEMI, or STEMI) at the time of PCI is a major determinant of a patient's mortality risk, and may profoundly impact the probability of ischemic recurrences [51–53]. In the DAPT trial, 30.7%

presented with an acute coronary syndrome at the time of PCI. Long DAPT compared with standard DAPT regimen significantly reduced definite or probable stent thrombosis in patients both with MI (0.5 vs. 1.9%; $p = 0.001$) and without MI (0.4 vs. 1.1%; $p = 0.001$), yet the magnitude of the reduction of MACCE from longer DAPT was bigger among patients with MI (3.9 vs. 6.8%; $p = 0.001$) than among those without MI (4.4 vs. 5.3%; $p = 0.08$) at the time of presentation ($P_{int} = 0.03$) [41,54]. The ischemic risk after PCI is also associated to several anatomical or procedural characteristic [55]. The concept of PCI complexity is quantifiable using previously validated and guideline-endorsed criteria: PCI with ≥3 stents implanted and 3 ≥ lesions and/or coronary vessels treated; and/or bifurcation with 2 stents implanted, total stent length >60 mm, and/or treatment of a chronic total occlusion [56]. In these patients, long-term DAPT (≥12 month) compared with a short period of DAPT (three or six months), significantly reduced the risk of cardiac ischemic events with a greater effect in patients undergoing PCI with more complex features. On the other hand, the risk of bleeding, estimated through risk scores, is also a potent driver for treatment selection [57–60]. The PRECISE-DAPT score based on five-items (age, creatinine clearance, hemoglobin, white blood cell count, and prior spontaneous bleeding) showed potential to guide DAPT duration decision-making: individuals deemed at high bleeding risk (PRECISE-DAPT score ≥ 25), prolonged DAPT was associated with no ischemic benefit but a significant bleeding hazard, whereas, on the other side, among patients not deemed at high bleeding risk (PRECISE-DAPT score < 25) a long DAPT treatment was associated with a significant reduction in the composite ischemic endpoint of MI, definite stent thrombosis, stroke, and target vessel revascularization without a significant increase in bleeding events [58]. It is interesting to note that according to a recent retrospective study, patients who underwent complex PCI would benefit long-term DAPT only if not at high risk of bleeding at baseline (PRECISE DAPT < 25) [61,62]. Ultimately, international guidelines agree on the fact that coronary stent type is no more a driver mandating different DAPT duration, and preferential BMS use for anatomical [63] or clinical [64–67] reasons mandating shorter DAPT duration are no longer recommended [48].

4. From DAPT to Single Antiplatelet Therapy (SAPT), Evidence for Aspirin Withdrawal and Monotherapy with P2Y12 Inhibitor

Several clinical studies have been designed to test efficacy and safety of a strategy of early withdrawal of aspirin after PCI (Figure 2). In the One-Month Dual Antiplatelet Therapy Followed by Clopidogrel Monotherapy vs. Standard 12-Month Dual Antiplatelet Therapy With Clopidogrel After Drug-Eluting Stent Implantation (STOPDAPT-2) study, 3045 patients undergoing PCI (62% SCAD) were randomized to one month of DAPT followed by clopidogrel monotherapy for five years versus 12 months of DAPT followed by Aspirin monotherapy for five years. After the first year of follow-up, the primary endpoint of cardiovascular death, myocardial infarction (MI), definite stent thrombosis, stroke, or TIMI major/minor bleeding occurred in 2.4% of the one-month DAPT group and in 3.7% of the 12-month DAPT group (HR 0.64; 95% CI 0.42–0.98), reaching both non-inferiority and superiority of the experimental treatment compared to the 12 month DAPT arm (p non-inferiority < 0.001; p superiority = 0.04). This result was mostly driven by a significant 74% reduction of TIMI major or minor bleeding among patients treated with shorter DAPT (HR 0.26 95% CI 0.11–0.64; $p = 0.002$) [68]. However, since this study was exclusively conducted in an Asian population and with specific procedural standards (e.g., imaging guided PCI was carried out in >97% of patients) the external validity of these results may be limited.

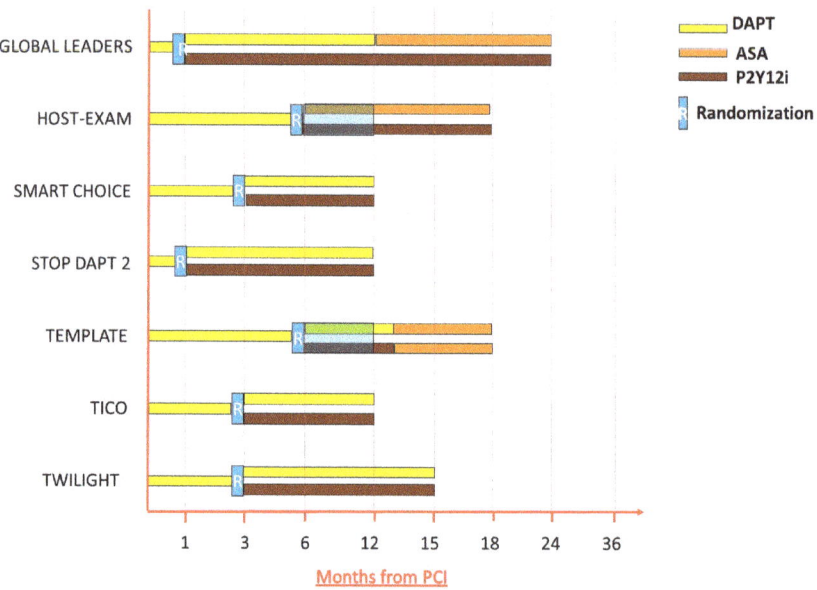

Figure 2. Design of clinical trials exploring aspirin withdrawal after percutaneous coronary intervention.

Similarly, the Comparison Between P2Y12 Antagonist Monotherapy and Dual Antiplatelet Therapy After DES (SMART-CHOICE) study compared a short treatment arm of three months of DAPT followed by P2Y12 inhibitor monotherapy with the standard 12-month duration of DAPT. The primary study hypothesis was the non-inferiority of the experimental treatment as compared to the standard treatment for the primary ischemic endpoint. In total, 2993 patients undergoing PCI (58% with ACS at presentation) were ultimately included. At 12-month follow-up, the primary outcome of all-cause death, MI, or stroke occurred in 2.9% of patients in the three-month DAPT arm and in 2.5% in the 12-month DAPT arm, meeting the pre-specified non-inferiority margin (p for non-inferiority = 0.007; p for superiority = 0.46). Actionable bleeding events accounted according to bleeding academic research consortium (BARC) Type 2, 3 or 5 criteria were significantly less in the short DAPT arm, mostly due to a reduction of minor bleeding [32].

The GLOBAL LEADER trial included 15,968 patients who underwent PCI for stable or unstable coronary disease that were randomized to DAPT of aspirin plus ticagrelor for one month, followed by ticagrelor monotherapy for 23 months versus DAPT for 12 months (aspirin/clopidogrel for stable coronary disease or aspirin/ticagrelor for unstable coronary disease), followed by aspirin monotherapy for 12 months [69]. The primary outcome was a composite of all-cause death or nonfatal myocardial infarction). The primary study hypothesis was to demonstrate the superiority of the experimental treatment for the composite ischemic endpoint at 24-month follow-up. Ultimately, at 24-month follow-up, there was an equipoise for the two treatment strategies for the primary study endpoint (p = 0.073). Importantly, adherence to the assigned treatment was as low as 78% at 24 months in the experimental arm, which may have reduced the pre-specified statistical power of the study [69,70].

Finally, the most recent TWILIGHT trial tested the impact of aspirin withdrawal at three months after PCI in 7119 high-risk patients who were randomized at three months after PCI to ticagrelor monotherapy for additional nine months or continuing standard DAPT with aspirin and ticagrelor. The trial specifically included patients that were deemed both at high ischemic and bleeding risk. At 12 months after PCI, the primary safety endpoint, a composite of BARC 2, 3 or 5 bleeding was reduced by 44% in the ticagrelor monotherapy arm (4.0% vs. 7.1%; HR 0.56; 95% CI 0.45–0.68; $p < 0.001$). No significant differences in MACE were observed in the two study arms, consistently to what observed in other studies of aspirin withdrawal.

Taken together, all the studies exploring aspirin withdrawal presented to date, show a consistent reduction of bleeding events by removing aspirin at different timepoints after PCI, with no apparent trade-off in ischemic events. However, some consideration regarding these studies should be highlighted. First, the STOP-DAPT 2 trial and SMART-CHOICE were exclusively conducted in an Asian population with very high usage of intravascular imaging for optimizing stent implantation, potentially limiting external validity of these findings to other centers with different practice. Second, the timing to randomization and effective aspirin withdrawal was of one month in three trials and three months in another. In addition, the baseline ischemic risk of the populations explored was different among trials; hence, it is not clear which is the optimal timing for safe aspirin withdrawal. In addition, whether potent P2Y12 inhibition should be preferred over a treatment with clopidogrel, in which high prevalence of drug non-responders may pose concerns for aspirin withdrawal should be clarified. In light of the recent results of the ISAR-REACT 5 trial, whether monotherapy with ticagrelor or with prasugrel should be preferred has not yet been studied.

5. Combination of Oral Anticoagulants and Antiplatelet Therapy in Patients at Higher Ischemic Risk or with Non-Valvular Atrial Fibrillation

5.1. Direct-Acting Oral Anticoagulants (DOAC) in Association to Antiplatelet Therapy in Patients at High Ischemic Risk

Despite the great progress in reducing the rate of events in patients at high ischemic risk, there is still a significant residual thrombotic risk in patients with coronary artery disease and prior vascular events, which is as high as 10% at 12 months after the occurrence of an ACS. [71] Novel pharmacological strategies focused on the long-term association of antiplatelet and anticoagulant drugs to further reduce the ischemic burden have been tested (Table 2). The Anti-Xa Therapy to Lower Cardiovascular Events in Addition to Standard Therapy in Subjects with Acute Coronary Syndrome–Thrombolysis in Myocardial Infarction 51 (ATLAS ACS 2-TIMI 51) study was based on this assumption and was the first testing the hypothesis that additional factor Xa inhibition on top of standard DAPT could further reduce the residual ischemic risk of patients after an acute coronary syndrome. The ATLAS ACS 2-TIMI 51 included a total of 15,526 patients with a recent ACS to receive twice-daily doses of either 2.5 mg or 5 mg of Rivaroxaban or placebo on top of standard DAPT with Aspirin and Clopidogrel. The primary efficacy end point was a composite of death from cardiovascular causes, myocardial infarction, or stroke, while the safety outcome was TIMI major bleeding not related to coronary-artery bypass grafting (CABG). After a mean treatment of 13 months, rivaroxaban significantly reduced the primary end point, as compared with placebo (HR in the rivaroxaban group, 0.84; 95% confidence interval, 0.74–0.96; $p = 0.008$), with a significant improvement observed for both the twice-daily 2.5-mg dose (9.1% vs. 10.7%, $p = 0.02$) and the twice-daily 5-mg dose (8.8% vs. 10.7%, $p = 0.03$). As compared with placebo, Rivaroxaban increased the rates of major bleeding not related to coronary-artery bypass grafting (2.1% vs. 0.6%, $p < 0.001$) and also of intracranial hemorrhage (0.6% vs. 0.2%, $p = 0.009$), yet not increasing fatal bleeding (0.3% vs. 0.2%, $p = 0.66$) [72]. Despite the promising results showed in the ATLAS ACS 2-TIMI 51, Rivaroxaban 2.5 mg was not widely introduced in practice with this indication mostly for the safety concerns due to the higher bleeding risk and most importantly to the introduction of the more potent P2Y12 inhibitors prasugrel and ticagrelor which are now preferred over clopidogrel in patients with ACS.

Table 2. Randomized controlled trials evaluating the effect of commercially available direct oral anticoagulants in patients with coronary artery disease.

	Randomization	N	Study Type	Recent ACS%	Age	Type of Antiplatelet Therapy Associated	F.U	Study Hypothesis	Primary Efficacy Endpoint	Primary Safety Endpoint	Conclusion
RE-DEEM	Dabigatran 50 mg bid 75 mg bid 110 mg bid 150 mg bid vs. Placebo	1861	Double Blind Phase 2	100%	61.8	Aspirin + Clopidogrel	6 month	Explore the rate of bleeding with dose escalating Dabigatran triple therapy	Reduction in D-dimer levels	Major or clinically relevant minor bleeding (ISTH, TIMI e GUSTO)	Dose-dependent increase in bleeding events with Dabigatran on top of antiplatelet therapy
ATLAS ACS-TIMI 46	Rivaroxaban 5 mg od (or 2.5 mg bid) or 20 mg od (or 10 mg bid) vs. Placebo	3491	Double Blind Phase 2	100%	58	Aspirin Alone or Aspirin + Thyenopiridine	6 month	Explore the rate of bleeding with dose escalating Rivaroxaban triple/dual therapy	Death, myocardial infarction, stroke, or severe recurrent ischemia requiring revascularization	TIMI major, TIMI minor, or requiring medical attention	Dose-dependent increase in bleeding events with Rivaroxaban on top of antiplatelet therapy
ATLAS ACS 2-TIMI 51	Rivaroxaban 2.5 mg bid or 5 mg bid vs. Placebo	15526	Double Blind Phase 3	100%	61.7	Aspirin + Thienopyridine	13 month	Rivaroxaban superior to placebo for the study primary efficacy endpoint	Death from cardiovascular causes, myocardial infarction, or stroke	Major non-CABG related bleeding (TIMI)	Rivaroxaban significantly reduced the primary efficacy endpoint
GEMINI ACS 1	Rivaroxaban 2.5 mg bid vs. Aspirin	3037	Double Blind Phase 2	100%	62.3	clopidogrel/ticagrelor	13 month	Estimate the bleeding risk of rivaroxaban compared with aspirin on top of standard P2Y12 inhibitor therapy	Cardiovascular death, myocardial infarction, stroke, or definite stent thrombosis	Non-CABG clinically signicant bleeding (TIMI)	Similar bleeding rate between rivaroxaban and aspirin on top of P2Y12i.
COMPASS	Rivaroxaban 2.5 mg bid + Aspirin Rivaroxaban 5 mg bid vs. Aspirin	27395	Double Blind Phase 3	0%	68	N.A.	23 month	Rivaroxaban superior to aspirin for the study primary efficacy endpoint	Cardiovascular death, myocardial infarction and stroke	Major or minor bleeding (ISTH)	Rivaroxaban 2.5 mg bid + aspirin significantly reduced the primary efficacy endpoint compared to aspirin alone
COMMANDER HF	Rivaroxaban 2.5 mg bid vs. Placebo	5022	Double Blind Phase 3	0%	66.4	N.A.	21 month	Rivaroxaban superior to placebo for the study primary efficacy endpoint	Death from any cause, myocardial infarction, or stroke	Fatal bleeding or bleeding into a critical space with a potential for permanent disability	No difference for the primary efficacy endpoint neither for the safety endpoint between rivaroxaban and placebo.

Table 2. Cont.

	Randomization	N	Study Type	Recent ACS%	Age	Type of Antiplatelet Therapy Associated	F.U	Study Hypothesis	Primary Efficacy Endpoint	Primary Safety Endpoint	Conclusion
APPRAISE	Apixaban 2.5 mg bid or 10 mg od 10 mg bid 20 mg od vs. Placebo	1715	Double Blind Phase 2	100%	60.8	Aspirin + Clopidogrel	6 month	Explore the rate of bleeding with dose escalating Apixaban triple/dual therapy	Cardiovascular death, myocardial infarction, severe recurrent ischemia, or ischemic stroke	Major or clinically relevant nonmajor bleeding (ISTH)	Dose-dependent increase in bleeding events with Apixaban on top of antiplatelet therapy
APPRAISE J	Apixaban 2.5 mg bid or 5 mg bid vs. Placebo	150	Double Blind Phase 2	100%	64.6	Aspirin + Clopidogrel	6 month	Explore the rate of bleeding with dose escalating Apixaban triple/dual therapy in a Japanese population	Deaths, nonfatal myocardial infarction, unstable angina and stroke	Major or clinically relevant nonmajor bleeding (ISTH)	Dose-dependent increase in bleeding events with Apixaban on top of antiplatelet therapy
APPRAISE II	Apixaban 5 mg bid vs. Placebo	7392	Double Blind Phase 3	100%	67	Apirin + Clopidogrel	8 month	Apixaban superior to placebo for the study primary endpoint	Cardiovascular death, myocardial infarction, or ischemic stroke	Major bleeding (TIMI)	Apixaban increased the number of major bleeding without a reduction in ischemic events
AFIRE	Rivaroxaban 15 mg or 10 mg vs. Rivaroxaban + Antiplatelet therapy	2236	Open Label Phase 4	0%	74	Aspirin or Clopidogrel	24 month	Rivaroxaban monotherapy non-inferior to the combination therapy for ischemia and superior for bleeding vs. Rivaroxaban + antiplatelet therapy	All-cause mortality, myocardial infarction, stroke, unstable angina requiring revascularization, or systemic embolism	Major bleeding (ISTH criteria)	Rivaroxaban monotherapy was non-inferior to the combination therapy for efficacy and superior for safety in patients with atrial fibrillation and stable coronary artery disease

Notes: ACS, acute coronary syndrome; bid, bis in die; CABG, coronary artery bypass grafting; F.U., follow up; GUSTO, Global Utilization Of Streptokinase And Tpa For Occluded Arteries; ISTH, International Society of Thrombosis and Hemostasis; MO, months; N.A., not available; od, once daily; TIMI, The Thrombolysis in Myocardial Infarction.

The APPRAISE-2 study tested the effect of Apixaban, at a dose of 5 mg twice daily in addition to standard antiplatelet therapy as compared with placebo in patients with a recent acute coronary syndrome and with high ischemic risk. The study was terminated prematurely after inclusion of 7392 patients because of an increase in clinically important bleeds, including fatal bleeds. The impact of apixaban on ischemic events could not be evaluated, because only 68% of the expected number of participants required to reach the pre-specified sample size was enrolled [73].

In the most recent Cardiovascular Outcomes for People Using Anticoagulation Strategies [74] trial, the role of factor Xa inhibition with Rvaroxaban was tested among chronic and stabilized patients with coronary artery disease (CAD) and in peripheral arterial disease (PAD) [74]. In this double-blind trial, the investigator randomly assigned 27,395 patients with stable atherosclerotic vascular disease to receive Rivaroxaban (2.5 mg twice daily) plus Aspirin (100 mg once daily), Rivaroxaban alone (5 mg twice daily), or Aspirin alone (100 mg once daily). The primary outcome was a composite of cardiovascular death, stroke, or myocardial infarction. The safety outcome was a modification of the International Society on Thrombosis and Haemostasis (ISTH) criteria for major bleeding and included fatal bleeding, symptomatic bleeding into a critical organ, bleeding into a surgical site requiring reoperation, and bleeding that led to hospitalization. With respect to the study primary endpoint, a treatment with rivaroxaban-plus-aspirin was associated to a significant 24% reduction of events as compared to aspirin-alone (379 patients vs. 496 patients; HR, 0.76; 95% CI, 0.66–0.86; $p < 0.001$), yet major bleeding were also more common in the rivaroxaban-plus-aspirin group (288 patients vs. 170 patients; HR, 1.70; 95% CI, 1.40–2.05; $p < 0.001$), mainly driven by nonfatal and non-intracranial bleedings. Rivaroxaban alone was not associated with lower rates of the primary endpoint compared with aspirin alone, but led to an excess of major bleeding events.

5.2. DOAC and Antiplatelet Therapy in Patients with Non-Valvular Atrial Fibrillation (AF) Undergoing PCI

The association of anticoagulant and antiplatelet therapies is needed in the case of the concomitant presence of atrial fibrillation and percutaneous coronary intervention or recent acute coronary syndrome. Multiple studies demonstrated on one side that anticoagulant is inferior to antiplatelet therapy after stenting, and on the other side that antiplatelet therapy is inferior to anticoagulant therapy for the prevention of thromboembolic events in patients with atrial fibrillation [75]. However, the prolonged association of these two treatments expose patients to a hazard of serious bleeding, which is 3–4-fold higher than the two treatments taken singularly [76]. Hence, multiple studies focused on the reduction of duration or intensity of the antithrombotic therapy in this setting (Table 3 and Figure 3). The What is the Optimal antiplatElet and anticoagulant therapy in patients with OAC and coronary StenTing [77] WOEST trial randomized 573 patients with an indication to long-term oral anticoagulation (of whom 69% of patients had AF) and who underwent PCI to a dual therapy of oral anticoagulants vitamin k antagonists plus clopidogrel or to a triple therapy of OAC plus Clopidogrel and Aspirin. Treatment was continued for one month after bare metal stent (BMS) placement and for one year after DES placement (65% of patients). The primary endpoint was the occurrence of any bleeding episode at one-year follow-up. Dual as compared to triple therapy was associated with a substantial reduction of all bleeding events at one year (19.4 vs. 44.4%; HR 0.36, 95% CI 0.26–0.50; $p < 0.001$) and also to a reduction of the combined secondary endpoint of death, myocardial infarction, stroke, target-vessel revascularization, and stent thrombosis (11.1 vs. 17.6%; HR 0.56, 95% CI 0.35–0.91; $p = 0.025$) [77]. While the study was not powered to detect differences among rare ischemic events, a significant reduction of all-cause death was observed among patients treated with a dual therapy strategy. Nevertheless, this result should be taken with caution due to the open-label design of the study. More recently, multiple studies evaluated both the impact of aspirin withdrawal among patients with indication to triple therapy and the concomitant effect of DOAC vs. the traditional treatment with Vitamin k antagonists. The PIONEER AF-PCI was the first to study this scenario and randomized 2124 patients with non-valvular AF who had undergone PCI with stenting to receive, in a 1:1:1 ratio, low-dose rivaroxaban (15 mg o.d.) plus a P2Y12 inhibitor (and no ASA), very-low-dose rivaroxaban (2.5 mg b.i.d.) plus DAPT, or standard therapy with a dose-adjusted VKA plus DAPT. The primary study endpoint consisted of clinically relevant bleeding according to the TIMI definition. At 12 months, the rate of the primary endpoint was lower in the two groups receiving rivaroxaban than in the group receiving standard therapy (16.8% for rivaroxaban 15 mg + P2Y12i, 18.0% for rivaroxaban 2.5 mg + DAPT, and 26.7% for VKA + DAPT). The lowest rate of bleeding was observed among patients treated with rivaroxaban 15 mg + P2Y12 inhibitor, and this strategy was associated with a 41% reduction of bleeding as compared to triple therapy (HR 0.59, 95% CI 0.47–0.76; $p < 0.001$) [78]. Rates of ischemic events were similar in the three groups. While the lowest dosage of rivaroxaban is not approved for thromboembolic protection in AF, rivaroxaban 15 mg may be preferred over the 20 mg od dosage in patients recently treated with PCI and treated with concomitant antiplatelet therapy as endorsed by international guidelines [7].

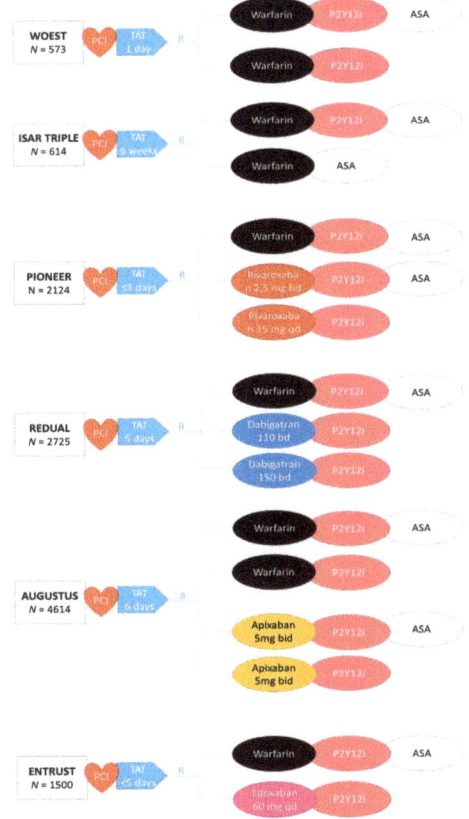

Figure 3. Design of clinical trials exploring the combination of oral anticoagulants and antiplatelet agents in patients with non-valvular atrial fibrillation undergoing percutaneous coronary intervention.

Table 3. Randomized controlled trials evaluating antithrombotic therapy type and duration in patients with non-valvular atrial fibrillation undergoing percutaneous coronary intervention.

	N	Randomization	P2Y12i Type	OAC Type	ACS	Age *	CHAD2Ds2 VASc	HAS BLEED	F.U.	Primary Endpoint	Results
WOEST	573	W-DT vs. W-TT	C (100%)	W	ACS 27%	70	1.5	N.A.	12 mo	Any bleeding (TIMI, GUSTO, BARC)	W-DT 19.4% vs. W-TT 44.4% HR 0.36 (95% CI 0.26–0.50) $p < 0.0001$
ISAR TRIPLE	614	W-TT 6 wk vs. W-TT 6 mo	C (100%)	W	ACS 32%	73	3.9	N.A.	9 mo	Death, MI, ST, stroke or major bleeding (TIMI)	6wkTT 9.8% vs. 6moTT 8.8% HR 1.14 (95% CI 0.68–1.9) $p = 0.63$
PIONEER AF PCI	2124	R-DT vs. W-TT vs. R-TT	C (94.3%)/ T (4.2%)/ p (1.3%)	W rivaroxaban 2.5 mg bid rivaroxaban 15 mg od	ACS 51.6%	70	n.a.	N.A.	12 mo	Major or minor bleeding (TIMI) or bleeding requiring medical attention	R-DT 16.8% vs. W-TT 26.7% HR 0.59 (CI 0.47–0.76) $p < 0.001$
RE-DUAL PCI	2725	D-DT110 or D-DT150 vs. W-TT	C (86%) T (12%)	W Dabigatran 110 mg bid Dabigatran 150 mg bid	ACS 50.5%	70	3.6	2.7	14 mo	Major or clinically relevant nonmajor bleeding event (ISTH)	D-DT110 15.4% vs. W-TT 26.9% HR 0.52 (95% CI 0.42–0.63) $p < 0.001$ D-DT150 20.2% vs. W-TT 25.7% HR 0.72 (95% CI 0.58–0.88) $p = 0.002$
AUGUSTUS	4614	Factorial A vs. W DT vs. TT	C (92.6%) T (6.2%) p (1.1%)	W Apixaban 5 mg bid **	ACS 37.3%	70.7	4	2.9	12 mo	Major or clinically relevant nonmajor bleeding (ISTH)	A 10.5% vs. W 14.7% HR 0.69 (95% CI 0.58–0.81) $p < 0.001$ DT 9% vs. TT 16.1% HR 1.89 (95% CI 1.59–2.24) $p < 0.001$
ENTRUST AF-PCI	1506	E-DT vs. W-TT	C (92%) T (8%) p (2%)	W Edoxaban 60 mg ***	ACS 52%	69	4	3	12 mo	Major or clinically relevant non-major bleeding (ISTH)	E-DT 17% vs. W-TT 20% HR 0.83 (0.65–1.05) p non-inferiority = 0.001 p superiority = 0.12

* Mean or median age in each trial is presented. ** 2.5 mg bid if dose reduction needed. *** 30 mg if dose reduction needed. N.A, Not Aviable; A, Apixaban; ACS, acute coronary syndrome; BARC, Bleeding Academic Research Consortium; bid, bis in die; C, clopidogrel; CI, confidence interval; D, Dabigatran; DT, dual therapy; E, Edoxaban; GUSTO, Global Utilization of Streptokinase and Tpa for Occluded arteries; HR, hazard ratio; ISTH, International Society of Thrombosis and Hemostasis; MI, myocardial infarction; mo, months; N.A., not available; OAC, oral anticoagulant; od, once daily; p, prasugrel; R, rivaroxaban; ST, stent thrombosis; T, ticagrelor; TIMI, The Thrombolysis in Myocardial Infarction; TT, triple therapy; W, warfarin; WK, weeks.

Similarly, the Randomized Evaluation of Dual Antithrombotic Therapy with Dabigatran versus Triple Therapy with Warfarin in Patients with Nonvalvular Atrial Fibrillation Undergoing Percutaneous Coronary Interventio trial [79], randomized 2725 patients with AF who had undergone PCI to triple therapy with warfarin plus a P2Y12 inhibitor (clopidogrel or ticagrelor) and aspirin, or to dual therapy with dabigatran (110 mg or 150 mg twice daily) plus a P2Y12 inhibitor (clopidogrel or ticagrelor, at the discretion of the treating physician) and no aspirin (110-mg and 150-mg dual-therapy groups). Different from the PIONEER AF-PCI trial, the RE-DUAL PCI trial randomized patients to both the approved doses of dabigatran for thromboembolic protection in AF. In addition, the triple therapy duration in this study was much shorter than observed in the previous WOEST and PIONEER AF-PCI, in which a significant proportion of triple therapy patients continued treatment up to 12 months. The primary end point was a composite of major or clinically relevant nonmajor bleeding according to the ISTH definition. The RE-DUAL PCI trial was designed to test both the non-inferiority and the superiority of the experimental treatment (i.e., dual therapy with DOAC) for the primary bleeding endpoint and also its non-inferiority with respect to the incidence of a composite of thromboembolic events and coronary ischemic events (myocardial infarction, stroke, or systemic embolism, death, or unplanned revascularization). After a mean follow-up of 14 months, the primary endpoint occurred in 15.4% of patients in the dual-therapy group with dabigatran 110-mg as compared with 26.9% in the triple-therapy group (HR, 0.52; 95% CI, 0.42–0.63; $p < 0.001$ for both non-inferiority and superiority) and in 20.2% of patients in the dual-therapy group with dabigatran 150-mg as compared to 25.7% in the triple-therapy group (HR, 0.72; 95% CI, 0.58–0.88; $p < 0.001$ for non-inferiority). Non-inferiority for the composite ischemic endpoint was also confirmed with both doses of dabigatran.

On the same line as in the previous two trials, the antithrombotic Therapy after Acute Coronary Syndrome or PCI in Atrial Fibrillation (AUGUSTUS) study evaluated the impact of a treatment with apixaban as compared to VKA in patients undergoing stenting or with a recent ACS. Different from the previous three studies, this used a two-by-two factorial design, i.e. not only the type of oral anticoagulant but also aspirin treatment was randomized. AUGUSTUS is thus the first trial to test both the concept of OAC type and dual vs. triple therapy separately. In total, 4614 patients were randomly allocated to apixaban 5 mg bid or VKA, and to aspirin or placebo, on top of a P2Y12 inhibitor (mostly clopidogrel) after a mean of seven days after the PCI/ACS occurrence. At six-month follow-up, the primary outcome of major or clinically relevant nonmajor bleeding was reported in 10.5% of the patients receiving apixaban, as compared with 14.7% of those receiving a vitamin k antagonist (HR, 0.69; 95% CI, 0.58–0.81; $p < 0.001$ for both non-inferiority and superiority) reaching both the prespecified non-inferiority and superiority of the experimental treatment. With respect to the second randomization, the primary endpoint occurred in 16.1% of those assigned to aspirin, as compared to 9.0% with placebo (HR, 1.89; 95% CI, 1.59–2.24; $p < 0.001$). A lower incidence of death or hospitalization was observed in patients treated with apixaban compared to vitamin k antagonists (23.5% vs. 27.4%; hazard ratio, 0.83; 95% CI, 0.74–0.93; $p = 0.002$). With respect to the secondary endpoint exploring ischemic events, this was similar among patients treated with apixaban or VKA and also for patients randomized to aspirin or placebo. Ischemic stroke was significantly reduced by 50% among patients in the apixaban arm. Despite the fact that this study was not powered to evaluate differences among study arms for the rare ischemic endpoints, a trend towards an excess of myocardial infarction and definite or probable stent thrombosis was observed among patients randomized to placebo (dual therapy) as compared to those assigned to aspirin (triple therapy) [80].

Finally, the recent Edoxaban Treatment Versus Vitamin K Antagonist in Patients With Atrial Fibrillation Undergoing Percutaneous Coronary Intervention (ENTRUST-AF-PCI) evaluated the safety and efficacy of edoxaban plus single antiplatelet therapy vs. VKA plus DAPT in subjects with atrial fibrillation following PCI with stent placement. Participants were randomly assigned (1:1) from four hours to five days after PCI to edoxaban (60 mg once daily) plus a P2Y12 inhibitor (mostly clopidogrel) for 12 months or a VKA in combination with a P2Y12 inhibitor and aspirin (100 mg once daily, for 1–12 months). The edoxaban dose was reduced to 30 mg per day if one or more factors were present (creatinine clearance 15–50 mL/min, bodyweight ≤60 kg, or concomitant use of specified potent p-glycoprotein inhibitors). The primary endpoint was a composite of major or clinically relevant non-major (CRNM) bleeding within 12 months. In the intention-to-treat analysis, major or CRNM bleeding events occurred in 128 (17%) patients randomized to Edoxaban and 152 (20%) patients to the VKA regimen; the relative risk reduction of 17% for the safety endpoint was enough to demonstrate the non-inferiority of the experimental treatment, but did not reach superiority (95% CI 0.65–1.05; $p = 0.0010$ for non-inferiority, $p = 0.12$ for superiority). In a post-hoc landmark analysis in which events occurring during the first two weeks after randomization were censored, experimental treatment with Edoxaban was associated to a significant 32% reduction of bleeding compared to triple therapy with VKA. No difference for ischemic events was observed, yet the study was not powered to detect differences for ischemic endpoints [81]. As already reported, none of these RCTs taken singularly was powered for ischemic endpoints, hence meta-analysis could provide important insights on this matter. However, the meta-analysis currently available in the literature drafted different conclusions. A first study-level network meta-analysis of four RCT and 10,026 patients, not including the more recent data from the ENTRUST trial, showed that dual therapy with both VKA or DOAC was associated to lower TIMI major or minor bleeding compared to triple therapy with VKA, and a similar risk of MACE, MI and ST [82]. On the contrary, a more recent patient-level meta-analysis including the recent results of the ENTRUST trial, showed a trend (although not significant) towards higher risk for stent thrombosis with dual therapy. Reconciling these inconsistencies will be a priority of future research to inform international practice guidelines. Ideally, more robust data may come from patient-level meta-analysis, which could also provide important insights on the subgroups that most benefit from each treatment.

Leveraging on the new evidence in the field, in particular the REDUAL-PCI and PIONEER-AF-PCI, a recent North American consensus statement on the management of antithrombotic therapy in patients with atrial fibrillation undergoing percutaneous coronary intervention [83] suggests a double-therapy approach as the default strategy for most patients. Instead, in selected patients at high ischemic/thrombotic and low bleeding risks, extending low-dose aspirin therapy (triple therapy) up to one month after PCI appear reasonable. In addition, in this setting, clopidogrel remains the P2Y12I of choice.

Finally, whether antiplatelet therapy should be stopped 12 months after PCI, leaving patients on treatment with OAC alone was a matter of debate. The recent Atrial Fibrillation and Ischemic Events with Rivaroxaban in Patients with Stable Coronary Artery Disease (AFIRE) trial compared rivaroxaban monotherapy compared with rivaroxaban/antiplatelet therapy after 12 months from PCI or CABG and up to 24 months in patients with atrial fibrillation and stable coronary artery disease. The study was prematurely interrupted for an excess of mortality in the combination therapy group treated with rivaroxaban plus antiplatelet therapy. The primary efficacy outcome of all-cause mortality, myocardial infarction, stroke, unstable angina requiring revascularization, or systemic embolism, occurred in 4.1%/patient-year in the rivaroxaban monotherapy group compared with 5.8%/patient-year in the rivaroxaban/antiplatelet therapy group (p for non-inferiority <0.0001). As expected, ISTH major bleeding occurred in 1.6%/patient-year in the rivaroxaban monotherapy group and in 2.8%/patient-year in the rivaroxaban/antiplatelet therapy group ($p = 0.01$).

6. Current Evidence for the Type and Duration of Antithrombotic Therapy in Percutaneous Structural Heart Interventions

6.1. Transcatheter Aortic Valve Implantation (TAVI)

Transcatheter Aortic Valve Implantation (TAVI) has been established as the method of choice for the treatment of severe aortic stenosis in patients with increased surgical risk [84,85]. Due to the vibrant activity in clinical trials, which is extending the indications of this treatment to different and lower risk clinical indications, TAVI could become the treatment of choice for most patients with aortic valve disease [86]. Secondary prevention with antithrombotic therapies after TAVI is primarily meant to reduce the risk of thrombosis of the valve components and prevent subsequent systemic thrombus embolization. While most of the events occurs during the first 48 h after valve implantation and are likely related to acute embolization of fibro-calcific valve material after valve implantation or catheter manipulation potentially damaging aortic wall, later ischemic events may be linked to thrombosis of the prosthesis surface or to unrecognized/new-onset of atrial fibrillation [87].

Current guidelines, mostly based on expert consensus extrapolated from the coronary stent experience, suggest as standard treatment strategy DAPT with aspirin and clopidogrel for 3–6 months after valve implantation, followed by a lifelong treatment with ASA. However, in patients with low hemorrhagic risk, a therapy with vitamin k antagonists in the first months after the procedure is also considered reasonable [84]. This latter indication is extrapolated from the experience with surgically-implanted valves, in which a short-term anticoagulation after bioprothetic valve implantation is common [84]. Despite the paucity of high-quality evidence in the field, several studies are evaluating possible antithrombotic treatment strategies after TAVI (Figure 4).

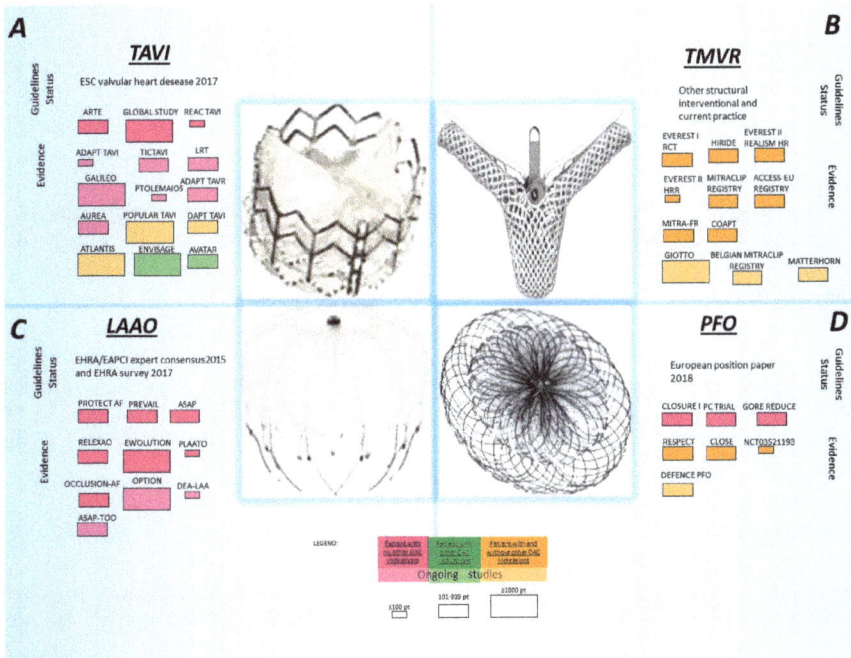

Figure 4. Clinical studies testing antithrombotic strategies for secondary prevention of percutaneous structural heart interventions. TAVI: transcatheter aortic valve implantation; TMVR: transcatheter mitral valve repair; LAAO: left atrial appendage occlusion; PFO: patent foramen ovale.

In the randomized Aspirin Versus Aspirin + Clopidogrel Following Transcatheter Aortic Valve Implantation Trial, 222 TAVI patients undergoing a balloon-expandable device implantation were randomized to DAPT (i.e., aspirin plus clopidogrel) or to aspirin alone. The primary endpoint of death, MI, stroke or transient ischemic attack, or major or life-threatening bleeding was similar between the two treatment groups but trended higher among patients assigned to DAPT (15.3% vs. 7.2%, $p = 0.065$) mostly due to an excess of major or life-threatening bleeding among patients treated with DAPT (10.8% vs. 3.6%, $p = 0.038$) [88]. Sherwood et al. tried to describe contemporary practice patterns of antiplatelet therapy and their relationship to outcomes post-TAVI trough a retrospective analysis of the NCDR STS/ACC TVT Registry. This analysis of 16,694 patients undergoing transfemoral TAVI reported that 81.1% patients were discharged on DAPT and 18.9% were discharged on SAPT. There was no difference in the main baseline characteristics among those assigned to DAPT or SAPT, whereas those assigned to DAPT had more CAD (64.6% vs. 52.3%; $p < 0.01$) and PAD (25.2% vs. 22.3%; $p < 0.01$). No difference in mortality (HR 0.92; 95% CI 0.81, 1.05) stroke (HR 1.04; CI 0.83, 1.31) or MI (HR 1.00; CI 0.72, 1.39) at one year was observed between DAPT and SAPT, but a significantly higher risk for major bleeding (HR 1.48; CI 1.10, 1.99) was observed with DAPT [89]. Current TAVI population carries an exaggerated bleeding risk, hence more potent platelet inhibition has to be justified by other concomitant indications rather that procedural alone. Whether the type and not only the number of the antiplatelet drugs implemented may have an impact in patients with TAVI is under investigation in the TICTAVI study (NCT02817789), which will evaluate the impact of ticagrelor monotherapy for 30 days after valve implantation vs. DAPT with clopidogrel and the soluble salt of aspirin lysine Acetylsalicylate.

Apart from antiplatelet therapy, various regimens of anticoagulant therapy are currently under investigation for secondary prevention after TAVI in patients without further indication to OAC. Based on the fact that valve thrombosis may be associated to a low shear stress thrombosis and that the current TAVI population has a high risk of new onset AF which was registered in up to 50% after valve implantation [90], use of OACs in this population may appear sound. The Global Study compares a rivAroxaban-based Antithrombotic Strategy with an antipLatelet-based Strategy After Transcatheter aortIc vaLve rEplacement to Optimise Clinical Outcomes (GALILEO) trial (NCT02556203) compared rivaroxaban 10 mg combined with aspirin for three months followed by rivaroxaban 10 mg monotherapy versus DAPT for three months followed by aspirin monotherapy in patients without an established indication for OAC [91]. The trial has been prematurely terminated due to an excess of death or thromboembolic events (11.4% vs. 8.8%), bleeding (4.2% vs. 2.4%) and all-cause death (6.8% vs. 3.3%) in patients allocated to rivaroxaban. Similarly, the ongoing DAPT versus OAC for a Short Time to Prevent Cerebral Embolism After TAVI (AUREA) trial (NCT01642134) will compare VKA with DAPT in patients without further indication to OAC. The primary study endpoint is the detection of new areas of cerebral infarction by MRI three months after TAVI. Further ongoing studies are evaluating the safety and efficacy of DOACs in patients undergoing TAVI. The ATLANTIS (Anti-Thrombotic Strategy After Trans-Aortic Valve Implantation for Aortic Stenosis trial) (NCT02664649) is testing the safety and efficacy of apixaban 5 mg bid compared to VKA in patients with an established indication for OAC, and apixaban 5 mg bid compared to DAPT/SAPT in patients without an indication for OAC. Similarly, the ENVISAGE AF trial (NCT02943785) is testing Edoxaban 30 and 60 mg vs. VKA in patients with AF and an indication for OAC.

Apart from secondary prevention of thromboembolic events, the evidence of clinically-evident valve thrombosis after biologic valve implantation has been described and require specific treatment to reduce the risk of embolization or prosthesis dysfunction. Prosthetic valve thrombosis is characterized by thrombus formation on the leaflets and metallic frames, with subsequent valve dysfunction with or without thromboembolism. Latib et al. reported in 4266 patients undergoing TAVI a total of 26 cases of PV thrombosis (0.61%) at a median timing from implantation of 181 days (interquartile range: 45–313 days) [92]. The most common clinical findings in these cases were presentation with progressive dyspnea, signs of heart failure or systemic embolization. Valve thrombosis could also be an incidental finding at the time of echocardiographic follow-up, detected by an increase transprosthetic gradient [93]. Valve thrombosis after TAVI could be acute (up to one day), subacute (ten days to one month), or late (more than one month) and its risk appears higher in the first three months post-implantation. Although the mechanisms are not completely clear, risk factors such as systemic pro-thrombotic state, valve malposition, prosthesis size, and the presence of low/high velocity flows after implantation [94] have been suggested as potential risk factors for this phenomenon. In addition, subclinical valve thrombosis has also been describing using novel imaging techniques but its clinical implications are still unclear. Makkar et al. showed that in patients with stroke after valvular implantation there was a reduction in the mobility of leafleats identifiable by CT scan as a hypo-attenuation on the valve leaflets after administration of contrast medium. In all cases, the reduction of leaflet motion was not related to an alteration of the valvular hemodynamics but seems to be related with an in increased risk of TIA/stroke (in the analysis of pooled RESOLVE and SAVORY cohorts). A treatment with OAC resolved leaflet hypomobility in all the patients treated, while other antithrombotic regimens did not prove effective [95]. Several observational studies showed a lower risk of valve thrombosis in patients on OAC treatment [96,97]. Latib et al. showed that, of 26 patients with valve thrombosis, 23 (88%) were treated with medical therapy, such as oral vitamin k antagonists with/without bridging heparin (unfractionated heparin or low-molecular–weight heparin). Anticoagulation was effective and resulted in significant decrease of the trans-prothesic aortic valve gradient or disappearance of the thrombotic mass in all patients [92]. The upcoming Comparison of a Rivaroxaban-based Strategy With an Antiplatelet-based Strategy Following Successful TAVR for the Prevention of Leaflet Thickening and Reduced Leaflet Motion as Evaluated by Four-dimensional, Volume-rendered Computed Tomography (GALILEO-4D) (NCT02833948) will also evaluate if anticoagulation compared to the usual double platelet inhibitor therapy after TAVRI may have an impact in reducing the risk of leaflet thrombosis, and its results are expected soon.

6.2. Evidence for MitraClip, Transcatheter Mitral Valve Interventions

Transcatheter mitral valve repair is indicated in moderate-to-severe or severe mitral insufficiency in patients with high surgical risk [98]. The MitraClip is currently the only system approved by the FDA and is based on the concept of "edge to edge" surgical repair to reduce valve insufficiency [99]. The procedure involves the passage of large bore catheter from the venous system, through atrial septal puncture in the left atrium, which may expose patients to peri-procedural and post-procedural ischemic events [100]. An incidence of 0.9% of ischemic stroke was documented on 30-day follow-up in the EVEREST RCT trial [98], 2.6% in the EVEREST-HRR and 2.4% in the EVEREST-REALISM registries [101] (Figure 4). Currently, neither international guidelines nor manufacturers provide precise recommendations for the type and duration of the antithrombotic therapy after the procedure and no specific studies have been yet carried out in this field. The current most commonly adopted antithrombotic treatments derive from the protocol recommendations of the first pivotal trials of the device. This generally consist of one month of DAPT with aspirin and clopidogrel followed by aspirin alone for 6–12 months. Transcatheter mitral valve replacement is flourishing and it is still at its inception. Multiple devices have been tested in first-in-man studies and the approach to antithrombotic therapy is still anecdotic and should be individualized based on the specific device used. Given the slow blood flow on the atrial side of the prosthesis together with the high rate of AF in these patients, the risk of device thrombosis is potentially high and merits consideration at the time of antithrombotic treatment selection.

6.3. Percutaneous Patent Foramen Ovale (PFO) Occlusion

Patent foramen ovale (PFO) and atrial septal defects [8] represent the most prevalent cardiac anomaly in the general population [102,103]. The presence of PFOs may predispose to paradoxical right-to-left atrium embolism, of which the most dreadful consequence is cryptogenic stroke, representing a major cause of embolic stroke in younger patients. Several devices have been developed in the last 20 years to physically occlude the PFO and prevent right-to-left shunt embolism [104,105] and systemic embolization. While these devices are effective for the scope, several procedural and long-term complications exist, including atrial rupture, pericardial tamponade, septal perforation, and acute/late thrombus formation of the device [106]. Thrombus formation can be a consequence of the incorrect measurement of the device [107,108]. More typically thrombosis could be triggered by the metal structure of the device, owing to endothelialization defects within the first four weeks [109]. However experimental studies in vivo have shown that the endothelialization process can last up to three months [110], or even up to five years post implantation [111] in some reports. Independent predictors of thrombotic formation are atrial fibrillation and presence of septal aneurysm [109]. Antithrombotic therapy is therefore crucial after device implantation, but the strategies remain controversial, and no randomized studies have been published to assess the optimal antithrombotic strategy in this scenario

(Figure 4). In many centers, the antithrombotic strategy of choice is DAPT with ASA plus clopidogrel for 6–8 weeks followed by ASA alone for an additional 4–8 months. DAPT for 1–6 months followed by single antiplatelet therapy for at least five years is recommended in a recent consensus document endorsed by the EAPCI [112]. In contrast, the latest American Academy of Neurology guidelines recommended lifelong antithrombotic therapy after PFO closure [113]. In the REDUCE trial, 664 patients with previous cryptogenic stroke were randomized in a 2:1 ratio to undergo PFO closure with the Gore Occluder. Antiplatelet therapy consisted of ASA alone (59%), clopidogrel alone (25.9%) or a combination of aspirin and P2Y12 inhibitor (i.e., clopidogrel or dypiridamole, <10%) and was similar in the two study groups. Follow-up was continued during a median of 3.2 years after the procedure, and in this period antiplatelet was maintained. The risk of recurrent stroke was significantly lower with PFO closure plus antiplatelet therapy than with antiplatelet therapy alone (1.4% vs. 5.4%, $p = 0.002$) [114]. Device thrombosis was reported in two patients in the closure group. In the CLOSE trial, 663 patients with a recent stroke attributed to PFO were assigned in a 1:1:1 ratio to PFO closure (11 different devices were used) plus long-term antiplatelet therapy, oral anticoagulation alone or antiplatelet therapy alone. The PFO closure group received DAPT for three months, followed by SAPT for a median follow-up of 5.5 years. Among patients assigned to oral anticoagulation, 93% received VKA and 7% DOACs. In the antiplatelet therapy group, 87% received ASA alone, 10% Clopidogrel alone and 3% ASA plus dipyridamole throughout the study period. At 12-month echocardiography evaluation, 93% of patients who underwent closure had no or minimal residual shunt. The rate of recurrent stroke at five years was significantly lower with PFO closure plus long-term antiplatelet therapy than with antiplatelet therapy alone (0% vs. 4.9%, $p < 0.001$) [115]. Within the comparison of antiplatelet therapy or anticoagulant therapy, recurrent stroke at five years was observed in 3.8% of patients assigned to antiplatelet therapy vs. 1.5% of patients assigned to oral anticoagulant therapy, however statistical significance was not analyzed because the study was not powered to compare outcomes in these groups, hence any conclusion regarding the indirect comparison of PFO closure and anticoagulant therapy cannot be extrapolated from this study. One device thrombosis was reported, and no significant differences in terms of major bleeding were recorded. In the RESPECT trial, 980 patients with previous cryptogenic ischemic stroke were randomly assigned to undergo PFO closure (Amplatz PFO occluder) or receive medical therapy for a median follow-up of 5.9 years. Patient undergoing PFO closure received ASA plus clopidogrel daily for one month, followed by ASA alone for five months. In the medical-therapy group, four regimens were allowed: ASA alone, clopidogrel alone, warfarin with a goal INR of 2–3, and ASA plus dipyridamole. After a median follow-up of 5.9 years, closure of PFO was associated with a lower rate of recurrent ischemic stroke than medical therapy (3.6% vs. 5.8%, $p = 0.007$). There were two cases of device thrombosis treated successfully with intravenous heparin. Wintzer-Wehekind et al. in a retrospective analysis 453 patient after PFO closure reported a low but clinically relevant risk of bleeding, which exceeded the risk of ischemic events in their cohort. As expected, all major bleeding events occurred in patients receiving antiplatelet therapy, and only one fifth of the patients stopped the antithrombotic therapy within one year after PFO closure. Antiplatelet therapy discontinuation was not associated with any increase in ischemic events. The authors concluded that, in patients without any other risk factors, shorter-term (≤1 year) antiplatelet treatment after PFO closure is a safer option [116].

6.4. Left Atrial Appendage Occlusion (LAAO)

Imaging studies have shown that 90% of thrombotic formations detected in patients with non-valvular atrial fibrillation are located in the left atrial appendage [117,118]. For this reason, percutaneous LAA occlusion (LAAO) has become an alternative to anticoagulation for patients that are ineligible or contraindicated to the medical treatment [119].

The first case of LAA surgical occlusion was reported in 1949 [120], while the first device for percutaneous exclusion was the PLAATO [121]. This was followed by introduction of the Watchman device (Boston Scientific) in 2002 and the Amplatzer cardiac plug in 2008, which are currently the most used devices in clinical practice. Watchman remains the only device studied in properly sized randomized trials, such as PROTECT AF [122] and the PREVAIL [123].

The device-oriented need for antithrombotic therapy after percutaneous LAAO has been tackled differently in various randomized studies and is meant to reduce the risk of device thrombosis, which is associated with an increased risk of stroke (Figure 4). Device thrombosis was observed in 4.2% of patients in the PROTECT AF trial with a stroke rate attributable to this event of 0.6%. Device thrombosis in other recent registries ranged from 1.3% to 7.2% [124]. While most of the data currently available are obtained from the Watchman device, there is currently a similar approach to antithrombotic therapy irrespective of the type and size of device implanted. Complete device endothelization has been observed after 90 days in animal models, but this time may be protracted in humans, and interindividual variability may be significant, adding uncertainty regarding the optimal type and duration of the antithrombotic therapy after LAAO. In the PROTECT AF trial, which included patients with AF without concomitant high bleeding risk, VKA with a target INR of 2–3 was implemented for 45 days after LAAO and was followed by DAPT for six months and then lifelong aspirin monotherapy. The same approach was used in the PREVAIL trial [123]. A different approach has been used in registries including high bleeding risk patients. The ASAP study included patients with an absolute contraindication to oral anticoagulation, and in this setting the protocol mandated six months of DAPT followed by lifelong aspirin [122]. Much more variability have been observed in recent real-world registries, which reflect the extreme heterogeneity of this patient population often requiring a personalized approach. In the EWOLUTION registry for example, antithrombotic regimens after LAAO were as follows: warfarin in 16%, DOAC in 11%, DAPT in 60%, SAPT in 7%, and no therapy in 6% [125]. In a survey by European Heart Rhythm association, showed that DAPT for six weeks to six months followed by aspirin monotherapy was the most common regimen, while 41% of centers would prescribe no therapy after LAAO and less than 10% would follow the antithrombotic regimen advocated by the PROTECT AF protocol [126].

While a randomized comparison on the efficacy of different antithrombotic strategies is lacking, a recent propensity matched analysis of 1527 patients from various trials and registries implementing the WATCHMAN device compared OAC vs. antiplatelet therapy after LAAO. The OAC arm included patients treated with OAC for 45 days after device implantation followed by six months of single or dual antiplatelet therapy. The antiplatelet therapy arm included patients managed with antiplatelet therapy alone, either dual or single, for various durations. While the rate of hard endpoints, including bleeding and thromboembolic events, was similar between the two treatment groups, a significant excess of device thrombosis was observed in the group among managed with antiplatelet therapy alone (OAC 1.4% vs. APT 3.1%; $p = 0.018$). While this comparison was not randomized and there was a high heterogeneity of treatment types and duration among the two study arms (e.g., APT included both DAPT and SAPT for various duration), this study stressed the importance of specific antithrombotic treatment after LAAO. In a retrospective series of 487 patients undergoing WATCHMAN or ACP/Amulet implantation, 208 received SAPT therapy only or no antithrombotic therapy after LAAO. In this series device thrombosis was as high as 7.2%, and in multivariable analysis DAPT or OAC therapy were protective for device thrombosis compared to SAPT or no therapy, raising concerns on the safety of such treatment strategy after LAAO [124].

While awaiting future randomized clinical trials which are urgently needed to shed light on the optimal antithrombotic treatment strategy after LAAO, the European Heart Rhythm Association/European Association of Percutaneous Cardiovascular Interventions (EHRA/EAPCI) expert consensus statement recommends treatment with OAC for at least six weeks followed by DAPT for six months and a single antiplatelet drug thereafter in patients without contraindications for OAC. Instead, patients ineligible to OAC should be managed with DAPT for 1–6 month followed by aspirin monotherapy indefinitely [125]. In addition, evidence coming from real-world registries, supported the safety of treatment with DOAC post-LAAC, and updates in international LAAC device labeling now admits three-month DAPT or direct OAC therapy post-LAAC, if the standard regimen with 45 days of warfarin followed by DAPT up to six months is not an option.

Importantly, since the risk of device thrombosis varies based on both patients' characteristics and device placement, personalization of the treatment type and duration taking into consideration these variables together with the baseline bleeding risk should always be a priority. The most recognized predictors of stroke and device thrombosis are left ventricular ejection fraction <40%, female sex, smoking, higher CHA2DS2-VASc score, spontaneous echocardiographic contrast, pre-existing LAA thrombus, and LAA peak emptying velocity [127–129]. Other mechanical factors such as deep implantation of the device forming a neoappendage or failure of disc apposition and significant residual device leak (>5 mm) are other factors of additional thromboembolic risk.

7. Conclusions

Antithrombotic agents are among the most prescribed treatments in cardiology, and their implementation for secondary prevention of spontaneous vascular or device-related thrombotic complications after percutaneous cardiovascular interventions has been extensively explored. While dual antiplatelet therapy after PCI and stenting has been studied in the last two decades, the search for the optimal antithrombotic therapy after structural interventions is still in its infancy. Intensification or prolongation of the antithrombotic strategy is generally associated with a superior efficacy for ischemic events prevention but also to an excess of bleeding, which should be avoided. Patient-centered data informing decision-making and treatment personalization represent the main objective of future research, in order to optimize the balance between ischemic and bleeding complications.

Author Contributions: A.C.: Conceived the review, drafted and critically revised the text. P.M.: Conceived the review, drafted and critically revised the text. G.L.: Conceived the review, G.M.-G.: Conceived the review, drafted and critically revised the text Critically revised the text. V.G.-R.: Critically revised the text. A.P.: Critically revised the text. F.D.: Conceived the review, drafted and critically revised the text G.G.: Conceived the review, drafted and critically revised the text. F.C.: Conceived the review, drafted and critically revised the text. S.C.: Critically revised the text. F.S.: Critically revised the text. S.G.: critically revised the text.

Funding: This research received no external funding.

Conflicts of Interest: The authors declare no conflict of interest.

Abbreviations

ACS	Acute coronary syndrome
AF	Atrial fibrillation
ASA	Aspirin
BARC	Bleeding Academic Research Consortium
BMS	Bare metal stent
CABG	Coronary artery bypass graft surgery
CAD	Coronary artery disease
CI	Confidence interval
DAPT	Dual antiplatelet therapy
DAT	Dual antithrombotic therapy
DES	Drug eluting stent
DOAC	Direct Oral anticoagulant
HR	Hazard ratio
ISTH	International Society on Thrombosis and Haemostasis
LAA	Left atrial appendage
LAAO	Left atrial appendage occlusion
MACCE	Major Adverse Cardiovascular and Cerebrovascular Events
MI	Myocardial infraction
NSTEMI	Non ST-segment Elevated Myocardial Infarction
OAC	Oral anticoagulant

P2Y12i	Receptor P2Y12 inhibitor
PAD	Peripheral arterial disease
PCI	Percutaneous coronary intervention
PFO	Patent foramen ovale
PTCA	Percutaneous transluminal coronary angioplasty
PV	Prosthetic Valve
RCT	Randomized controlled trial
SAPT	Single antiplatelet therapy
TAT	Triple antithrombotic therapy
TAVI	Transcatheter aortic valve implantation
TVMR	Transcatheter mitral valve repair
VKA	Vitamin k antagonist

References

1. Gruntzig, A.R.; Senning, A.; Siegenthaler, W.E. Nonoperative dilatation of coronary-artery stenosis: Percutaneous transluminal coronary angioplasty. *N. Engl. J. Med.* **1979**, *301*, 61–68. [CrossRef] [PubMed]
2. Thornton, M.A.; Gruentzig, A.R.; Hollman, J.; King, S.B., 3rd; Douglas, J.S. Coumadin and aspirin in prevention of recurrence after transluminal coronary angioplasty: A randomized study. *Circulation* **1984**, *69*, 721–727. [CrossRef] [PubMed]
3. Schömig, A.; Neumann, F.-J.; Kastrati, A.; Schühlen, H.; Blasini, R.; Hadamitzky, M.; Walter, H.; Zitzmann-Roth, E.-M.; Richardt, G.; Alt, E.; et al. A Randomized comparison of antiplatelet and anticoagulant therapy after the placement of coronary-artery stents. *N. Engl. J. Med.* **1996**, *334*, 1084–1089. [CrossRef] [PubMed]
4. Leon, M.B.; Baim, D.S.; Popma, J.J.; Gordon, P.C.; Cutlip, D.E.; Ho, K.K.L.; Giambartolomei, A.; Diver, D.J.; Lasorda, D.M.; Williams, D.O.; et al. A clinical trial comparing three antithrombotic-drug regimens after coronary-artery stenting. *N. Engl. J. Med.* **1998**, *339*, 1665–1671. [CrossRef] [PubMed]
5. Valgimigli, M.; Costa, F.; Byrne, R.; Haude, M.; Baumbach, A.; Windecker, S. Dual antiplatelet therapy duration after coronary stenting in clinical practice: Results of an EAPCI survey. *EuroIntervention* **2015**, *11*, 68–74. [CrossRef] [PubMed]
6. Collet, J.P.; Roffi, M.; Byrne, R.A.; Costa, F.; Valgimigli, M.; Task Force for the Management of Dual Antiplatelet Therapy in Coronary Artery Disease of the European Society of Cardiology (ESC); ESC Scientific Document Group. Case-based implementation of the 2017 ESC focused update on dual antiplatelet therapy in coronary artery disease. *Eur. Heart J.* **2018**, *39*, e1–e33. [CrossRef] [PubMed]
7. Valgimigli, M.; Bueno, H.; Byrne, R.A.; Collet, J.P.; Costa, F.; Jeppsson, A.; Juni, P.; Kastrati, A.; Kolh, P.; Mauri, L.; et al. 2017 ESC focused update on dual antiplatelet therapy in coronary artery disease developed in collaboration with EACTS: The task force for dual antiplatelet therapy in coronary artery disease of the European Society of Cardiology (ESC) and of the European Association for Cardio-Thoracic Surgery (EACTS). *Eur. Heart J.* **2017**, *53*, 34–78. [CrossRef]
8. Task Force, M.; Montalescot, G.; Sechtem, U.; Achenbach, S.; Andreotti, F.; Arden, C.; Budaj, A.; Bugiardini, R.; Crea, F.; Cuisset, T.; et al. 2013 ESC guidelines on the management of stable coronary artery disease: The task force on the management of stable coronary artery disease of the European Society of Cardiology. *Eur. Heart J.* **2013**, *34*, 2949–3003. [CrossRef]
9. King, T.D.; Thompson, S.L.; Steiner, C.; Mills, N.L. Secundum atrial septal defect: Nonoperative closure during cardiac catheterization. *JAMA* **1976**, *235*, 2506–2509. [CrossRef]
10. Bridges, N.D.; Hellenbrand, W.; Latson, L.; Filiano, J.; Newburger, J.W.; Lock, J.E. Transcatheter closure of patent foramen ovale after presumed paradoxical embolism. *Circulation* **1992**, *86*, 1902–1908. [CrossRef]
11. Cribier, A.; Eltchaninoff, H.; Bash, A.; Borenstein, N.; Tron, C.; Bauer, F.; Derumeaux, G.; Anselme, F.; Laborde, F.o.; Leon, M.B. Percutaneous transcatheter implantation of an aortic valve prosthesis for calcific aortic stenosis. *Circulation* **2002**, *106*, 3006–3008. [CrossRef] [PubMed]

12. Bertrand, M.E.; Rupprecht, H.-J.R.; Urban, P.; Gershlick, A.H.; CLASSICS Investigators. Double-blind study of the safety of Clopidogrel with and without a loading dose in combination with aspirin compared with Ticlopidine in combination with aspirin after coronary stenting. *Circulation* **2000**, *102*, 624–629. [CrossRef] [PubMed]
13. Yusuf, S.; Zhao, F.; Mehta, S.R.; Chrolavicius, S.; Tognoni, G.; Fox, K.K. Effects of clopidogrel in addition to aspirin in patients with acute coronary syndromes without ST-segment elevation. *N. Engl. J. Med.* **2001**, *345*, 494–502. [CrossRef]
14. Serebruany, V.L.; Steinhubl, S.R.; Berger, P.B.; Malinin, A.I.; Bhatt, D.L.; Topol, E.J. Variability in platelet responsiveness to clopidogrel among 544 individuals. *J. Am. Coll. Cardiol.* **2005**, *45*, 246–251. [CrossRef] [PubMed]
15. Brandt, J.T.; Payne, C.D.; Wiviott, S.D.; Weerakkody, G.; Farid, N.A.; Small, D.S.; Jakubowski, J.A.; Naganuma, H.; Winters, K.J. A comparison of prasugrel and clopidogrel loading doses on platelet function: Magnitude of platelet inhibition is related to active metabolite formation. *Am. Heart J.* **2007**, *153*, 66.e9–66.e16. [CrossRef] [PubMed]
16. Jernberg, T.; Payne, C.D.; Winters, K.J.; Darstein, C.; Brandt, J.T.; Jakubowski, J.A.; Naganuma, H.; Siegbahn, A.; Wallentin, L. Prasugrel achieves greater inhibition of platelet aggregation and a lower rate of non-responders compared with clopidogrel in aspirin-treated patients with stable coronary artery disease. *Eur. Heart J.* **2006**, *27*, 1166–1173. [CrossRef]
17. Wiviott, S.D.; Braunwald, E.; McCabe, C.H.; Montalescot, G.; Ruzyllo, W.; Gottlieb, S.; Neumann, F.-J.; Ardissino, D.; De Servi, S.; Murphy, S.A.; et al. Prasugrel versus clopidogrel in patients with acute coronary syndromes. *N. Engl. J. Med.* **2007**, *357*, 2001–2015. [CrossRef]
18. Roe, M.T.; Armstrong, P.W.; Fox, K.A.A.; White, H.D.; Prabhakaran, D.; Goodman, S.G.; Cornel, J.H.; Bhatt, D.L.; Clemmensen, P.; Martinez, F.; et al. Prasugrel versus clopidogrel for acute coronary syndromes without revascularization. *N. Engl. J. Med.* **2012**, *367*, 1297–1309. [CrossRef]
19. Husted, S.; Emanuelsson, H.; Heptinstall, S.; Sandset, P.M.; Wickens, M.; Peters, G. Pharmacodynamics, pharmacokinetics, and safety of the oral reversible P2Y12 antagonist AZD6140 with aspirin in patients with atherosclerosis: A double-blind comparison to clopidogrel with aspirin. *Eur. Heart J.* **2006**, *27*, 1038–1047. [CrossRef]
20. Wallentin, L.; Becker, R.C.; Budaj, A.; Cannon, C.P.; Emanuelsson, H.; Held, C.; Horrow, J.; Husted, S.; James, S.; Katus, H.; et al. Ticagrelor versus clopidogrel in patients with acute coronary syndromes. *N. Engl. J. Med.* **2009**, *361*, 1045–1057. [CrossRef]
21. Montalescot, G.; van't Hof, A.W.; Lapostolle, F.; Silvain, J.; Lassen, J.F.; Bolognese, L.; Cantor, W.J.; Cequier, A.; Chettibi, M.; Goodman, S.G.; et al. Prehospital ticagrelor in ST-segment elevation myocardial infarction. *N. Engl. J. Med.* **2014**, *371*, 1016–1027. [CrossRef] [PubMed]
22. Rollini, F.; Franchi, F.; Cho, J.R.; DeGroat, C.; Bhatti, M.; Muniz-Lozano, A.; Singh, K.; Ferrante, E.; Wilson, R.E.; Dunn, E.C.; et al. A head-to-head pharmacodynamic comparison of prasugrel vs. ticagrelor after switching from clopidogrel in patients with coronary artery disease: Results of a prospective randomized study. *Eur. Heart J.* **2016**, *37*, 2722–2730. [CrossRef]
23. Marquis-Gravel, G.; Costa, F.; Boivin-Proulx, L.A. "Ticagrelor or Prasugrel, Doctor?" The basis for decision in clinical practice. *Can. J. Cardiol.* **2019**, *35*, 1283–1285. [CrossRef] [PubMed]
24. Motovska, Z.; Hlinomaz, O.; Kala, P.; Hromadka, M.; Knot, J.; Varvarovsky, I.; Dusek, J.; Jarkovsky, J.; Miklik, R.; Rokyta, R.; et al. 1-Year outcomes of patients undergoing primary angioplasty for myocardial infarction treated with Prasugrel versus Ticagrelor. *J. Am. Coll. Cardiol.* **2018**, *71*, 371–381. [CrossRef] [PubMed]
25. Rafique, A.M.; Nayyar, P.; Wang, T.Y.; Mehran, R.; Baber, U.; Berger, P.B.; Tobis, J.; Currier, J.; Dave, R.H.; Henry, T.D. Optimal P2Y12 inhibitor in patients with ST-segment elevation myocardial infarction undergoing primary percutaneous coronary intervention: A network meta-analysis. *JACC Cardiovasc. Interv.* **2016**, *9*, 1036–1046. [CrossRef] [PubMed]
26. Schüpke, S.; Neumann, F.-J.; Menichelli, M.; Mayer, K.; Bernlochner, I.; Wöhrle, J.; Richardt, G.; Liebetrau, C.; Witzenbichler, B.; Antoniucci, D.; et al. Ticagrelor or Prasugrel in patients with acute coronary syndromes. *N. Engl. J. Med.* **2019**, *381*, 1524–1534. [CrossRef] [PubMed]
27. Costa, F.; Windecker, S.; Valgimigli, M. Dual antiplatelet therapy duration: Reconciling the inconsistencies. *Drugs* **2017**, *77*, 1733–1754. [CrossRef] [PubMed]

28. Gwon, H.-C.; Hahn, J.-Y.; Park, K.W.; Song, Y.B.; Chae, I.-H.; Lim, D.-S.; Han, K.-R.; Choi, J.-H.; Choi, S.-H.; Kang, H.-J.; et al. Six-month versus 12-month dual antiplatelet therapy after implantation of drug-eluting stents. *Circulation* **2012**, *125*, 505–513. [CrossRef]
29. Colombo, A.; Chieffo, A.; Frasheri, A.; Garbo, R.; Masotti-Centol, M.; Salvatella, N.; Oteo Dominguez, J.F.; Steffanon, L.; Tarantini, G.; Presbitero, P.; et al. Second-generation drug-eluting stent implantation followed by 6- versus 12-month dual antiplatelet therapy: The SECURITY randomized clinical trial. *J. Am. Coll. Cardiol.* **2014**, *64*, 2086–2097. [CrossRef]
30. Schulz-Schüpke, S.; Byrne, R.A.; Ten Berg, J.M.; Neumann, F.J.; Han, Y.; Adriaenssens, T.; Tölg, R.; Seyfarth, M.; Maeng, M.; Zrenner, B.; et al. ISAR-SAFE: A randomized, double-blind, placebo-controlled trial of 6 vs. 12 months of clopidogrel therapy after drug-eluting stenting. *Eur. Heart J.* **2015**, *36*, 1252–1263. [CrossRef]
31. Hong, S.J.; Shin, D.H.; Kim, J.S.; Kim, B.K.; Ko, Y.G.; Choi, D.; Her, A.Y.; Kim, Y.H.; Jang, Y.; Hong, M.K.; et al. 6-month versus 12-month dual-antiplatelet therapy following long everolimus-eluting stent implantation: The IVUS-XPL randomized clinical trial. *JACC Cardiovasc. Interv.* **2016**, *9*, 1438–1446. [CrossRef] [PubMed]
32. Hahn, J.-Y.; Song, Y.B.; Oh, J.-H.; Chun, W.J.; Park, Y.H.; Jang, W.J.; Im, E.-S.; Jeong, J.-O.; Cho, B.R.; Oh, S.K.; et al. Effect of P2Y12 inhibitor monotherapy vs dual antiplatelet therapy on cardiovascular events in patients undergoing percutaneous coronary intervention: The SMART-CHOICE randomized clinical trial. *JAMA* **2019**, *321*, 2428–2437. [CrossRef] [PubMed]
33. Kedhi, E.; Fabris, E.; van der Ent, M.; Buszman, P.; von Birgelen, C.; Roolvink, V.; Zurakowski, A.; Schotborgh, C.E.; Hoorntje, J.C.A.; Eek, C.H.; et al. Six months versus 12 months dual antiplatelet therapy after drug-eluting stent implantation in ST-elevation myocardial infarction (DAPT-STEMI): Randomised, multicentre, non-inferiority trial. *BMJ* **2018**, *363*, k3793. [CrossRef] [PubMed]
34. Gilard, M.; Barragan, P.; Noryani, A.A.L.; Noor, H.A.; Majwal, T.; Hovasse, T.; Castellant, P.; Schneeberger, M.; Maillard, L.; Bressolette, E.; et al. 6- versus 24-month dual antiplatelet therapy after implantation of drug-eluting stents in patients nonresistant to Aspirin: The randomized, multicenter ITALIC trial. *J. Am. Coll. Cardiol.* **2015**, *65*, 777–786. [CrossRef] [PubMed]
35. Nakamura, M.; Iijima, R.; Ako, J.; Shinke, T.; Okada, H.; Ito, Y.; Ando, K.; Anzai, H.; Tanaka, H.; Ueda, Y.; et al. Dual antiplatelet therapy for 6 versus 18 months after biodegradable polymer drug-eluting stent implantation. *JACC Cardiovasc. Interv.* **2017**, *10*, 1189–1198. [CrossRef] [PubMed]
36. Udell, J.A.; Bonaca, M.P.; Collet, J.P.; Lincoff, A.M.; Kereiakes, D.J.; Costa, F.; Lee, C.W.; Mauri, L.; Valgimigli, M.; Park, S.J.; et al. Long-term dual antiplatelet therapy for secondary prevention of cardiovascular events in the subgroup of patients with previous myocardial infarction: A collaborative meta-analysis of randomized trials. *Eur. Heart J.* **2016**, *37*, 390–399. [CrossRef]
37. Valgimigli, M.; Costa, F.; Lokhnygina, Y.; Clare, R.M.; Wallentin, L.; Moliterno, D.J.; Armstrong, P.W.; White, H.D.; Held, C.; Aylward, P.E.; et al. Trade-off of myocardial infarction vs. bleeding types on mortality after acute coronary syndrome: Lessons from the Thrombin Receptor Antagonist for Clinical Event Reduction in Acute Coronary Syndrome (TRACER) randomized trial. *Eur. Heart J.* **2017**, *38*, 804–810. [CrossRef]
38. Costa, F.; Valgimigli, M. The optimal duration of dual antiplatelet therapy after coronary stent implantation: To go too far is as bad as to fall short. *Cardiovasc. Diagn. Ther.* **2018**, *8*, 630–646. [CrossRef]
39. Albaladejo, P.; Charbonneau, H.; Samama, C.M.; Collet, J.P.; Marret, E.; Piriou, V.; Genty, C.; Bosson, J.L. Bleeding complications in patients with coronary stents during non-cardiac surgery. *Thromb. Res.* **2014**, *134*, 268–272. [CrossRef]
40. Valgimigli, M.; Campo, G.; Monti, M.; Vranckx, P.; Percoco, G.; Tumscitz, C.; Castriota, F.; Colombo, F.; Tebaldi, M.; Fucà, G.; et al. Short- versus long-term duration of dual-antiplatelet therapy after coronary stenting. *Circulation* **2012**, *125*, 2015–2026. [CrossRef]
41. Mauri, L.; Kereiakes, D.J.; Yeh, R.W.; Driscoll-Shempp, P.; Cutlip, D.E.; Steg, P.G.; Normand, S.-L.T.; Braunwald, E.; Wiviott, S.D.; Cohen, D.J.; et al. Twelve or 30 months of dual antiplatelet therapy after drug-eluting stents. *N. Engl. J. Med.* **2014**, *371*, 2155–2166. [CrossRef] [PubMed]
42. Costa, F.; Adamo, M.; Ariotti, S.; Navarese, E.P.; Biondi-Zoccai, G.; Valgimigli, M. Impact of greater than 12-month dual antiplatelet therapy duration on mortality: Drug-specific or a class-effect? A meta-analysis. *Int. J. Cardiol.* **2015**, *201*, 179–181. [CrossRef] [PubMed]
43. Bonaca, M.P.; Bhatt, D.L.; Cohen, M.; Steg, P.G.; Storey, R.F.; Jensen, E.C.; Magnani, G.; Bansilal, S.; Fish, M.P.; Im, K.; et al. Long-term use of Ticagrelor in patients with prior myocardial infarction. *N. Engl. J. Med.* **2015**, *372*, 1791–1800. [CrossRef] [PubMed]

44. Bhatt, D.L.; Steg, P.G.; Mehta, S.R.; Leiter, L.A.; Simon, T.; Fox, K.; Held, C.; Andersson, M.; Himmelmann, A.; Ridderstråle, W.; et al. Ticagrelor in patients with diabetes and stable coronary artery disease with a history of previous percutaneous coronary intervention (THEMIS-PCI): A phase 3, placebo-controlled, randomised trial. *Lancet* **2019**, *394*, 1169–1180. [CrossRef]
45. Navarese, E.P.; Andreotti, F.; Schulze, V.; Kolodziejczak, M.; Buffon, A.; Brouwer, M.; Costa, F.; Kowalewski, M.; Parati, G.; Lip, G.Y.; et al. Optimal duration of dual antiplatelet therapy after percutaneous coronary intervention with drug eluting stents: Meta-analysis of randomised controlled trials. *BMJ* **2015**, *350*, h1618. [CrossRef]
46. Valgimigli, M.; Ariotti, S.; Costa, F. Duration of dual antiplatelet therapy after drug-eluting stent implantation: Will we ever reach a consensus? *Eur. Heart J.* **2015**, *36*, 1219–1222. [CrossRef]
47. Adamo, M.; Costa, F.; Vranckx, P.; Leonardi, S.; Navarese, E.P.; Garcia-Garcia, H.M.; Valgimigli, M. Does smoking habit affect the randomized comparison of 6 versus 24-month dual antiplatelet therapy duration? Insights from the PRODIGY trial. *Int. J. Cardiol.* **2015**, *190*, 242–245. [CrossRef]
48. Valgimigli, M.; Bueno, H.; Byrne, R.A.; Collet, J.P.; Costa, F.; Jeppsson, A.; Juni, P.; Kastrati, A.; Kolh, P.; Mauri, L.; et al. 2017 ESC focused update on dual antiplatelet therapy in coronary artery disease developed in collaboration with EACTS. *Eur. J. Cardiothorac. Surg.* **2018**, *53*, 34–78. [CrossRef]
49. Gargiulo, G.; Ariotti, S.; Santucci, A.; Piccolo, R.; Baldo, A.; Franzone, A.; Magnani, G.; Marino, M.; Esposito, G.; Windecker, S.; et al. Impact of sex on 2-year clinical outcomes in patients treated with 6-month or 24-month dual-antiplatelet therapy duration: A pre-specified analysis from the PRODIGY trial. *JACC Cardiovasc. Interv.* **2016**, *9*, 1780–1789. [CrossRef]
50. Gargiulo, G.; Costa, F.; Ariotti, S.; Biscaglia, S.; Campo, G.; Esposito, G.; Leonardi, S.; Vranckx, P.; Windecker, S.; Valgimigli, M. Impact of proton pump inhibitors on clinical outcomes in patients treated with a 6- or 24-month dual-antiplatelet therapy duration: Insights from the PROlonging Dual-antiplatelet treatment after Grading stent-induced Intimal hyperplasia studY trial. *Am. Heart J.* **2016**, *174*, 95–102. [CrossRef]
51. McAllister, K.S.L.; Ludman, P.F.; Hulme, W.; de Belder, M.A.; Stables, R.; Chowdhary, S.; Mamas, M.A.; Sperrin, M.; Buchan, I.E. A contemporary risk model for predicting 30-day mortality following percutaneous coronary intervention in England and Wales. *Int. J. Cardiol.* **2016**, *210*, 125–132. [CrossRef] [PubMed]
52. Costa, F.; Vranckx, P.; Leonardi, S.; Moscarella, E.; Ando, G.; Calabro, P.; Oreto, G.; Zijlstra, F.; Valgimigli, M. Impact of clinical presentation on ischaemic and bleeding outcomes in patients receiving 6- or 24-month duration of dual-antiplatelet therapy after stent implantation: A pre-specified analysis from the PRODIGY (Prolonging Dual-Antiplatelet Treatment After Grading Stent-Induced Intimal Hyperplasia) trial. *Eur. Heart J.* **2015**, *36*, 1242–1251. [CrossRef] [PubMed]
53. Crimi, G.; Leonardi, S.; Costa, F.; Ariotti, S.; Tebaldi, M.; Biscaglia, S.; Valgimigli, M. Incidence, prognostic impact, and optimal definition of contrast-induced acute kidney injury in consecutive patients with stable or unstable coronary artery disease undergoing percutaneous coronary intervention. insights from the all-comer PRODIGY trial. *Catheter. Cardiovasc. Interv.* **2015**, *86*, E19–E27. [CrossRef] [PubMed]
54. Costa, F.; Valgimigli, M. Impact of clinical presentation on dual antiplatelet therapy duration: Let's re-evaluate our priorities. *J. Am. Coll. Cardiol.* **2015**, *66*, 1203–1204. [CrossRef]
55. Costa, F.; Adamo, M.; Ariotti, S.; Ferrante, G.; Navarese, E.P.; Leonardi, S.; Garcia-Garcia, H.; Vranckx, P.; Valgimigli, M. Left main or proximal left anterior descending coronary artery disease location identifies high-risk patients deriving potentially greater benefit from prolonged dual antiplatelet therapy duration. *EuroIntervention* **2016**, *11*, e1222–e1230. [CrossRef]
56. Giustino, G.; Chieffo, A.; Palmerini, T.; Valgimigli, M.; Feres, F.; Abizaid, A.; Costa, R.A.; Hong, M.-K.; Kim, B.-K.; Jang, Y.; et al. Efficacy and safety of dual antiplatelet therapy after complex PCI. *J. Am. Coll. Cardiol.* **2016**, *68*, 1851–1864. [CrossRef]
57. Costa, F.; Tijssen, J.G.; Ariotti, S.; Giatti, S.; Moscarella, E.; Guastaroba, P.; De Palma, R.; Ando, G.; Oreto, G.; Zijlstra, F.; et al. Incremental value of the CRUSADE, ACUITY, and HAS-BLED risk scores for the prediction of hemorrhagic events after coronary stent implantation in patients undergoing long or short duration of dual antiplatelet therapy. *J. Am. Heart Assoc.* **2015**, *4*, e002524. [CrossRef]
58. Costa, F.; van Klaveren, D.; James, S.; Heg, D.; Räber, L.; Feres, F.; Pilgrim, T.; Hong, M.-K.; Kim, H.-S.; Colombo, A.; et al. Derivation and validation of the predicting bleeding complications in patients undergoing stent implantation and subsequent dual antiplatelet therapy (PRECISE-DAPT) score: A pooled analysis of individual-patient datasets from clinical trials. *Lancet* **2017**, *389*, 1025–1034. [CrossRef]

59. Yeh, R.W.; Secemsky, E.A.; Kereiakes, D.J.; Normand, S.L.; Gershlick, A.H.; Cohen, D.J.; Spertus, J.A.; Steg, P.G.; Cutlip, D.E.; Rinaldi, M.J.; et al. Development and validation of a prediction rule for benefit and harm of dual antiplatelet therapy beyond 1 year after percutaneous coronary intervention. *JAMA* **2016**, *315*, 1735–1749. [CrossRef]
60. Ando, G.; Costa, F. Bleeding risk stratification in acute coronary syndromes. Is it still valid in the era of the radial approach? *Postepy Kardiol. Interwencyjnej* **2015**, *11*, 170–173. [CrossRef]
61. Costa, F.; Van Klaveren, D.; Feres, F.; James, S.; Räber, L.; Pilgrim, T.; Hong, M.-K.; Kim, H.-S.; Colombo, A.; Steg, P.G.; et al. Dual antiplatelet therapy duration based on ischemic and bleeding risks after coronary stenting. *J. Am. Coll. Cardiol.* **2019**, *73*, 741–754. [CrossRef] [PubMed]
62. Giustino, G.; Costa, F. Characterization of the individual patient risk after percutaneous coronary intervention: At the crossroads of bleeding and thrombosis. *JACC Cardiovasc. Interv.* **2019**, *12*, 831–834. [CrossRef] [PubMed]
63. Costa, F.; Brugaletta, S.; Pernigotti, A.; Flores-Ulmanzor, E.; Ortega-Paz, L.; Cequier, A.; Iniguez, A.; Serra, A.; Jimenez-Quevedo, P.; Mainar, V.; et al. Does large vessel size justify use of bare-metal stents in primary percutaneous coronary intervention? *Circ. Cardiovasc. Interv.* **2019**, *12*, e007705. [CrossRef] [PubMed]
64. Ariotti, S.; Adamo, M.; Costa, F.; Patialiakas, A.; Briguori, C.; Thury, A.; Colangelo, S.; Campo, G.; Tebaldi, M.; Ungi, I.; et al. Is bare-metal stent implantation still justifiable in high bleeding risk patients undergoing percutaneous coronary intervention?: A pre-specified analysis from the ZEUS trial. *JACC Cardiovasc. Interv.* **2016**, *9*, 426–436. [CrossRef]
65. Ariotti, S.; Costa, F.; Valgimigli, M. Coronary stent selection and optimal course of dual antiplatelet therapy in patients at high bleeding or thrombotic risk: Navigating between limited evidence and clinical concerns. *Curr. Opin. Cardiol.* **2015**, *30*, 325–332. [CrossRef]
66. Crimi, G.; Leonardi, S.; Costa, F.; Adamo, M.; Ariotti, S.; Valgimigli, M. Role of stent type and of duration of dual antiplatelet therapy in patients with chronic kidney disease undergoing percutaneous coronary interventions. Is bare metal stent implantation still a justifiable choice? A post-hoc analysis of the all comer PRODIGY trial. *Int. J. Cardiol.* **2016**, *212*, 110–117. [CrossRef]
67. Varenne, O.; Cook, S.; Sideris, G.; Kedev, S.; Cuisset, T.; Carrié, D.; Hovasse, T.; Garot, P.; Mahmoud, R.E.; Spaulding, C.; et al. Drug-eluting stents in elderly patients with coronary artery disease (SENIOR): A randomised single-blind trial. *Lancet* **2018**, *391*, 41–50. [CrossRef]
68. Watanabe, H.; Domei, T.; Morimoto, T.; Natsuaki, M.; Shiomi, H.; Toyota, T.; Ohya, M.; Suwa, S.; Takagi, K.; Nanasato, M.; et al. Effect of 1-month dual antiplatelet therapy followed by Clopidogrel vs 12-month dual antiplatelet therapy on cardiovascular and bleeding events in patients receiving PCI: The STOPDAPT-2 randomized clinical trial. *JAMA* **2019**, *321*, 2414–2427. [CrossRef]
69. Vranckx, P.; Valgimigli, M.; Jüni, P.; Hamm, C.; Steg, P.G.; Heg, D.; van Es, G.A.; McFadden, E.P.; Onuma, Y.; van Meijeren, C.; et al. Ticagrelor plus aspirin for 1 month, followed by ticagrelor monotherapy for 23 months vs aspirin plus clopidogrel or ticagrelor for 12 months, followed by aspirin monotherapy for 12 months after implantation of a drug-eluting stent: A multicentre, open-label, randomised superiority trial. *Lancet* **2018**, *392*, 940–949. [CrossRef]
70. Valgimigli, M.; Garcia-Garcia, H.M.; Vrijens, B.; Vranckx, P.; McFadden, E.P.; Costa, F.; Pieper, K.; Vock, D.M.; Zhang, M.; Van Es, G.A.; et al. Standardized classification and framework for reporting, interpreting, and analysing medication non-adherence in cardiovascular clinical trials: A consensus report from the Non-adherence Academic Research Consortium (NARC). *Eur. Heart J.* **2019**, *40*, 2070–2085. [CrossRef]
71. Costa, F.; Brugaletta, S. Antithrombotic therapy in acute coronary syndrome: Striking a happy medium. *Rev. Esp. Cardiol. (Engl. Ed.)* **2018**, *71*, 782–786. [CrossRef]
72. Mega, J.L.; Braunwald, E.; Wiviott, S.D.; Bassand, J.P.; Bhatt, D.L.; Bode, C.; Burton, P.; Cohen, M.; Cook-Bruns, N.; Fox, K.A.; et al. Rivaroxaban in patients with a recent acute coronary syndrome. *N. Engl. J. Med.* **2012**, *366*, 9–19. [CrossRef] [PubMed]
73. Alexander, J.H.; Lopes, R.D.; James, S.; Kilaru, R.; He, Y.; Mohan, P.; Bhatt, D.L.; Goodman, S.; Verheugt, F.W.; Flather, M.; et al. Apixaban with antiplatelet therapy after acute coronary syndrome. *N. Engl. J. Med.* **2011**, *365*, 699–708. [CrossRef] [PubMed]
74. Eikelboom, J.W.; Connolly, S.J.; Bosch, J.; Dagenais, G.R.; Hart, R.G.; Shestakovska, O.; Diaz, R.; Alings, M.; Lonn, E.M.; Anand, S.S.; et al. Rivaroxaban with or without Aspirin in stable cardiovascular disease. *N. Engl. J. Med.* **2017**, *377*, 1319–1330. [CrossRef] [PubMed]

75. Connolly, S.J.; Group, T.A.W. Clopidogrel plus aspirin versus oral anticoagulation for atrial fibrillation in the Atrial fibrillation Clopidogrel Trial with Irbesartan for prevention of Vascular Events (ACTIVE W): A randomised controlled trial. *Lancet* **2006**, *367*, 1903–1942.
76. Sorensen, R.; Hansen, M.L.; Abildstrom, S.Z.; Hvelplund, A.; Andersson, C.; Jorgensen, C.; Madsen, J.K.; Hansen, P.R.; Kober, L.; Torp-Pedersen, C.; et al. Risk of bleeding in patients with acute myocardial infarction treated with different combinations of aspirin, clopidogrel, and vitamin K antagonists in Denmark: A retrospective analysis of nationwide registry data. *Lancet* **2009**, *374*, 1967–1974. [CrossRef]
77. Dewilde, W.J.; Oirbans, T.; Verheugt, F.W.; Kelder, J.C.; De Smet, B.J.; Herrman, J.P.; Adriaenssens, T.; Vrolix, M.; Heestermans, A.A.; Vis, M.M.; et al. Use of clopidogrel with or without aspirin in patients taking oral anticoagulant therapy and undergoing percutaneous coronary intervention: An open-label, randomised, controlled trial. *Lancet* **2013**, *381*, 1107–1115. [CrossRef]
78. Gibson, C.M.; Mehran, R.; Bode, C.; Halperin, J.; Verheugt, F.W.; Wildgoose, P.; Birmingham, M.; Ianus, J.; Burton, P.; van Eickels, M.; et al. Prevention of bleeding in patients with atrial fibrillation undergoing PCI. *N. Engl. J. Med.* **2016**, *375*, 2423–2434. [CrossRef]
79. Cannon, C.P.; Bhatt, D.L.; Oldgren, J.; Lip, G.Y.H.; Ellis, S.G.; Kimura, T.; Maeng, M.; Merkely, B.; Zeymer, U.; Gropper, S.; et al. Dual antithrombotic therapy with Dabigatran after PCI in atrial fibrillation. *N. Engl. J. Med.* **2017**, *377*, 1513–1524. [CrossRef]
80. Lopes, R.D.; Heizer, G.; Aronson, R.; Vora, A.N.; Massaro, T.; Mehran, R.; Goodman, S.G.; Windecker, S.; Darius, H.; Li, J.; et al. Antithrombotic therapy after acute coronary syndrome or PCI in atrial fibrillation. *N. Engl. J. Med.* **2019**, 10.1056/NEJMoa1817083. [CrossRef]
81. Vranckx, P.; Valgimigli, M.; Eckardt, L.; Tijssen, J.; Lewalter, T.; Gargiulo, G.; Batushkin, V.; Campo, G.; Lysak, Z.; Vakaliuk, I.; et al. Edoxaban-based versus vitamin K antagonist-based antithrombotic regimen after successful coronary stenting in patients with atrial fibrillation (ENTRUST-AF PCI): A randomised, open-label, phase 3b trial. *Lancet* **2019**, *394*, 1335–1343. [CrossRef]
82. Lopes, R.D.; Hong, H.; Harskamp, R.E.; Bhatt, D.L.; Mehran, R.; Cannon, C.P.; Granger, C.B.; Verheugt, F.W.A.; Li, J.; Berg, J.M.T.; et al. Safety and efficacy of antithrombotic strategies in patients with atrial fibrillation undergoing percutaneous coronary intervention: A network meta-analysis of randomized controlled trials. *JAMA Cardiol.* **2019**, *4*, 747–755. [CrossRef] [PubMed]
83. Angiolillo, D.J.; Goodman, S.G.; Bhatt, D.L.; Eikelboom, J.W.; Price, M.J.; Moliterno, D.J.; Cannon, C.P.; Tanguay, J.-F.; Granger, C.B.; Mauri, L.; et al. Antithrombotic therapy in patients with atrial fibrillation treated with oral anticoagulation undergoing percutaneous coronary intervention. *Circulation* **2018**, *138*, 527–536. [CrossRef] [PubMed]
84. Nishimura, R.A.; Otto, C.M.; Bonow, R.O.; Carabello, B.A.; John, P.; Erwin, I.; Fleisher, L.A.; Jneid, H.; Mack, M.J.; McLeod, C.J.; et al. 2017 AHA/ACC focused update of the 2014 AHA/ACC guideline for the management of patients with valvular heart disease: A report of the American College of Cardiology/American Heart Association task force on clinical practice guidelines. *Circulation* **2017**, *70*, 252–289. [CrossRef] [PubMed]
85. Baumgartner, H.; Falk, V.; Bax, J.J.; De Bonis, M.; Hamm, C.; Holm, P.J.; Iung, B.; Lancellotti, P.; Lansac, E.; Rodriguez Muñoz, D.; et al. 2017 ESC/EACTS guidelines for the management of valvular heart disease. *Eur. Heart J.* **2017**, *38*, 2739–2791. [CrossRef] [PubMed]
86. Mack, M.J.; Leon, M.B.; Thourani, V.H.; Makkar, R.; Kodali, S.K.; Russo, M.; Kapadia, S.R.; Malaisrie, S.C.; Cohen, D.J.; Pibarot, P.; et al. Transcatheter aortic-valve replacement with a balloon-expandable valve in low-risk patients. *N. Engl. J. Med.* **2019**, *380*, 1695–1705. [CrossRef] [PubMed]
87. Amat-Santos, I.J.; Rodés-Cabau, J.; Urena, M.; DeLarochellière, R.; Doyle, D.; Bagur, R.; Villeneuve, J.; Côté, M.; Nombela-Franco, L.; Philippon, F.; et al. Incidence, predictive factors, and prognostic value of new-onset atrial fibrillation following transcatheter aortic valve implantation. *J. Am. Coll. Cardiol.* **2012**, *59*, 178–188. [CrossRef]
88. Rodés-Cabau, J.; Masson, J.-B.; Welsh, R.C.; Garcia del Blanco, B.; Pelletier, M.; Webb, J.G.; Al-Qoofi, F.; Généreux, P.; Maluenda, G.; Thoenes, M.; et al. Aspirin versus Aspirin plus Clopidogrel as antithrombotic treatment following transcatheter aortic valve replacement with a balloon-expandable valve: The ARTE (Aspirin versus Aspirin + Clopidogrel following transcatheter aortic valve implantation) randomized clinical trial. *JACC Cardiovasc. Interv.* **2017**, *10*, 1357–1365. [CrossRef]

89. Sherwood, M.W.; Vemulapalli, S.; Harrison, J.K.; Dai, D.; Vora, A.N.; Mack, M.J.; Holmes, D.R.; Rumsfeld, J.S.; Cohen, D.J.; Thourani, V.H.; et al. Variation in post-TAVR antiplatelet therapy utilization and associated outcomes: Insights from the STS/ACC TVT registry. *Am. Heart J.* **2018**, *204*, 9–16. [CrossRef]
90. Kalra, R.; Patel, N.; Doshi, R.; Arora, G.; Arora, P. Evaluation of the incidence of new-onset atrial fibrillation after aortic valve replacement. *JAMA Intern. Med.* **2019**, *179*, 1122–1130. [CrossRef]
91. Windecker, S.; Tijssen, J.; Giustino, G.; Guimarães, A.H.C.; Mehran, R.; Valgimigli, M.; Vranckx, P.; Welsh, R.C.; Baber, U.; van Es, G.-A.; et al. Trial design: Rivaroxaban for the prevention of major cardiovascular events after transcatheter aortic valve replacement: Rationale and design of the GALILEO study. *Am. Heart J.* **2017**, *184*, 81–87. [CrossRef] [PubMed]
92. Latib, A.; Naganuma, T.; Abdel-Wahab, M.; Danenberg, H.; Cota, L.; Barbanti, M.; Baumgartner, H.; Finkelstein, A.; Legrand, V.; de Lezo, J.S.; et al. Treatment and clinical outcomes of transcatheter heart valve thrombosis. *Circ. Cardiovasc. Interv.* **2015**, *8*, e001779. [CrossRef] [PubMed]
93. Dangas, G.D.; Weitz, J.I.; Giustino, G.; Makkar, R.; Mehran, R. Prosthetic heart valve thrombosis. *J. Am. Coll. Cardiol.* **2016**, *68*, 2670–2689. [CrossRef] [PubMed]
94. Puri, R.; Auffret, V.; Rodés-Cabau, J. Bioprosthetic valve thrombosis. *J. Am. Coll. Cardiol.* **2017**, *69*, 2193–2211. [CrossRef]
95. Makkar, R.R.; Fontana, G.; Jilaihawi, H.; Chakravarty, T.; Kofoed, K.F.; De Backer, O.; Asch, F.M.; Ruiz, C.E.; Olsen, N.T.; Trento, A.; et al. Possible subclinical leaflet thrombosis in bioprosthetic aortic valves. *N. Engl. J. Med.* **2015**, *373*, 2015–2024. [CrossRef]
96. Holy, E.W.; Kebernik, J.; Allali, A.; El-Mawardy, M.; Richardt, G.; Abdel-Wahab, M. Comparison of dual antiplatelet therapy versus oral anticoagulation following transcatheter aortic valve replacement: A retrospective single-center registry analysis. *Cardiol. J.* **2017**, *24*, 649–659. [CrossRef]
97. Jose, J.; Sulimov, D.S.; El-Mawardy, M.; Sato, T.; Allali, A.; Holy, E.W.; Becker, B.; Landt, M.; Kebernik, J.; Schwarz, B.; et al. Clinical bioprosthetic heart valve thrombosis after transcatheter aortic valve replacement: Incidence, characteristics, and treatment outcomes. *JACC Cardiovasc. Interv.* **2017**, *10*, 686–697. [CrossRef]
98. Feldman, T.; Foster, E.; Glower, D.D.; Kar, S.; Rinaldi, M.J.; Fail, P.S.; Smalling, R.W.; Siegel, R.; Rose, G.A.; Engeron, E.; et al. Percutaneous repair or surgery for mitral regurgitation. *N. Engl. J. Med.* **2011**, *364*, 1395–1406. [CrossRef]
99. Maisano, F.; La Canna, G.; Colombo, A.; Alfieri, O. The evolution from surgery to percutaneous mitral valve interventions: The role of the edge-to-edge technique. *J. Am. Coll. Cardiol.* **2011**, *58*, 2174–2182. [CrossRef]
100. Glower, D.D.; Kar, S.; Trento, A.; Lim, D.S.; Bajwa, T.; Quesada, R.; Whitlow, P.L.; Rinaldi, M.J.; Grayburn, P.; Mack, M.J.; et al. Percutaneous mitral valve repair for mitral regurgitation in high-risk patients: Results of the EVEREST II study. *J. Am. Coll. Cardiol.* **2014**, *64*, 172–181. [CrossRef]
101. Lim, D.S.; Reynolds, M.R.; Feldman, T.; Kar, S.; Herrmann, H.C.; Wang, A.; Whitlow, P.L.; Gray, W.A.; Grayburn, P.; Mack, M.J.; et al. Improved functional status and quality of life in prohibitive surgical risk patients with degenerative mitral regurgitation after transcatheter mitral valve repair. *J. Am. Coll. Cardiol.* **2014**, *64*, 182–192. [CrossRef] [PubMed]
102. Harper, R.W.; Mottram, P.M.; McGaw, D.J. Closure of secundum atrial septal defects with the amplatzer septal occluder device: Techniques and problems. *Catheter. Cardiovasc. Interv.* **2002**, *57*, 508–524. [CrossRef]
103. Windecker, S.; Wahl, A.; Chatterjee, T.; Garachemani, A.; Eberli, F.R.; Seiler, C.; Meier, B. Percutaneous closure of patent foramen ovale in patients with paradoxical embolism. *Circulation* **2000**, *101*, 893–898. [CrossRef] [PubMed]
104. Clergeau, M.-R.; Hamon, M.L.; Morello, R.M.; Saloux, E.; Viader, F.; Hamon, M. Silent cerebral infarcts in patients with pulmonary embolism and a patent foramen ovale. *Stroke* **2009**, *40*, 3758–3762. [CrossRef] [PubMed]
105. Pell, A.C.H.; Hughes, D.; Keating, J.; Christie, J.; Busuttil, A.; Sutherland, G.R. Fulminating fat embolism syndrome caused by paradoxical embolism through a patent foramen ovale. *N. Engl. J. Med.* **1993**, *329*, 926–929. [CrossRef] [PubMed]
106. Braun, M.; Gliech, V.; Boscheri, A.; Schoen, S.; Gahn, G.; Reichmann, H.; Haass, M.; Schraeder, R.; Strasser, R.H. Transcatheter closure of patent foramen ovale (PFO) in patients with paradoxical embolism. Periprocedural safety and mid-term follow-up results of three different device occluder systems. *Eur. Heart J.* **2004**, *25*, 424–430. [CrossRef]

107. Brandt, R.R.; Neumann, T.; Neuzner, J.; Rau, M.; Faude, I.; Hamm, C.W. Transcatheter closure of atrial septal defect and patent foramen ovale in adult patients using the Amplatzer occlusion device: No evidence for thrombus deposition with antiplatelet agents. *J. Am. Soc. Echocardiogr.* **2002**, *15*, 1094–1098. [CrossRef]
108. Rickers, C.; Hamm, C.; Stern, H.; Hofmann, T.; Franzen, O.; Schräder, R.; Sievert, H.; Schranz, D.; Michel-Behnke, I.; Vogt, J.; et al. Percutaneous closure of secundum atrial septal defect with a new self centring device ("angel wings"). *Heart* **1998**, *80*, 517–521. [CrossRef]
109. Krumsdorf, U.; Ostermayer, S.; Billinger, K.; Trepels, T.; Zadan, E.; Horvath, K.; Sievert, H. Incidence and clinical course of thrombus formation on atrial septal defect and patent foramen ovale closure devices in 1,000 consecutive patients. *J. Am. Coll. Cardiol.* **2004**, *43*, 302–309. [CrossRef]
110. Kuhn, M.A.; Latson, L.A.; Cheatham, J.P.; McManus, B.; Anderson, J.M.; Kilzer, K.L.; Furst, J. Biological response to Bard Clamshell Septal Occluders in the canine heart. *Circulation* **1996**, *93*, 1459–1463. [CrossRef]
111. Davies, A.; Ekmejian, A.; Collins, N.; Bhagwandeen, R. Multidisciplinary assessment in optimising results of percutaneous patent foramen ovale closure. *Heart Lung Circ.* **2017**, *26*, 246–250. [CrossRef] [PubMed]
112. Pristipino, C.; Sievert, H.; D'Ascenzo, F.; Louis Mas, J.; Meier, B.; Scacciatella, P.; Hildick-Smith, D.; Gaita, F.; Toni, D.; Kyrle, P.; et al. European position paper on the management of patients with patent foramen ovale. General approach and left circulation thromboembolism. *Eur. Heart J.* **2019**, *40*, 3182–3195. [CrossRef]
113. Messé, S.R.; Gronseth, G.; Kent, D.M.; Kizer, J.R.; Homma, S.; Rosterman, L.; Kasner, S.E. Practice advisory: Recurrent stroke with patent foramen ovale (update of practice parameter): Report of the guideline development, dissemination, and implementation subcommittee of the American Academy of Neurology. *Neurology* **2016**, *87*, 815–821. [CrossRef] [PubMed]
114. Søndergaard, L.; Kasner, S.E.; Rhodes, J.F.; Andersen, G.; Iversen, H.K.; Nielsen-Kudsk, J.E.; Settergren, M.; Sjöstrand, C.; Roine, R.O.; Hildick-Smith, D.; et al. Patent foramen ovale closure or antiplatelet therapy for cryptogenic stroke. *N. Engl. J. Med.* **2017**, *377*, 1033–1042. [CrossRef] [PubMed]
115. Mas, J.-L.; Derumeaux, G.; Guillon, B.; Massardier, E.; Hosseini, H.; Mechtouff, L.; Arquizan, C.; Béjot, Y.; Vuillier, F.; Detante, O.; et al. Patent foramen ovale closure or anticoagulation vs. antiplatelets after stroke. *N. Engl. J. Med.* **2017**, *377*, 1011–1021. [CrossRef] [PubMed]
116. Wintzer-Wehekind, J.; Alperi, A.; Houde, C.; Côté, J.-M.; de Freitas Campos Guimaraes, L.; Côté, M.; Rodés-Cabau, J. Impact of discontinuation of antithrombotic therapy following closure of patent foramen ovale in patients with cryptogenic embolism. *Am. J. Cardiol.* **2019**, *123*, 1538–1545. [CrossRef] [PubMed]
117. Lincoff, A.M.; Mehran, R.; Povsic, T.J.; Zelenkofske, S.L.; Huang, Z.; Armstrong, P.W.; Steg, P.G.; Bode, C.; Cohen, M.G.; Buller, C.; et al. Effect of the REG1 anticoagulation system versus bivalirudin on outcomes after percutaneous coronary intervention (REGULATE-PCI): A randomised clinical trial. *Lancet* **2016**, *387*, 349–356. [CrossRef]
118. Blackshear, J.L.; Odell, J.A. Appendage obliteration to reduce stroke in cardiac surgical patients with atrial fibrillation. *Ann. Thorac. Surg.* **1996**, *61*, 755–759. [CrossRef]
119. Stoddard, M.F.; Dawkins, P.R.; Prince, C.R.; Ammash, N.M. Left atrial appendage thrombus is not uncommon in patients with acute atrial fibrillation and a recent embolic event: A transesophageal echocardiographic study. *J. Am. Coll. Cardiol.* **1995**, *25*, 452–459. [CrossRef]
120. Madden, J.L. Resection of the left auricular appendix: A prophylaxis for recurrent arterial emboli. *JAMA* **1949**, *140*, 769–772. [CrossRef]
121. Ostermayer, S.H.; Reisman, M.; Kramer, P.H.; Matthews, R.V.; Gray, W.A.; Block, P.C.; Omran, H.; Bartorelli, A.L.; Della Bella, P.; Di Mario, C.; et al. Percutaneous Left Atrial Appendage Transcatheter Occlusion (PLAATO System) to prevent stroke in high-risk patients with non-rheumatic atrial fibrillation: Results from the international multi-center feasibility trials. *J. Am. Coll. Cardiol.* **2005**, *46*, 9–14. [CrossRef]
122. Reddy, V.Y.; Möbius-Winkler, S.; Miller, M.A.; Neuzil, P.; Schuler, G.; Wiebe, J.; Sick, P.; Sievert, H. Left atrial appendage closure with the watchman device in patients with a contraindication for oral anticoagulation: The ASAP study (ASA plavix feasibility study with watchman left atrial appendage closure technology). *J. Am. Coll. Cardiol.* **2013**, *61*, 2551–2556. [CrossRef] [PubMed]
123. Holmes, D.R.; Kar, S.; Price, M.J.; Whisenant, B.; Sievert, H.; Doshi, S.K.; Huber, K.; Reddy, V.Y. Prospective randomized evaluation of the watchman left atrial appendage closure device in patients with atrial fibrillation versus long-term warfarin therapy: The PREVAIL trial. *J. Am. Coll. Cardiol.* **2014**, *64*, 177–179. [CrossRef] [PubMed]

124. Fauchier, L.; Cinaud, A.; Brigadeau, F.; Lepillier, A.; Pierre, B.; Abbey, S.; Fatemi, M.; Franceschi, F.; Guedeney, P.; Jacon, P.; et al. Device-related thrombosis after percutaneous left atrial appendage occlusion for atrial fibrillation. *J. Am. Coll. Cardiol.* **2018**, *71*, 1528–1536. [CrossRef] [PubMed]
125. Boersma, L.V.; Ince, H.; Kische, S.; Pokushalov, E.; Schmitz, T.; Schmidt, B.; Gori, T.; Meincke, F.; Protopopov, A.V.; Betts, T.; et al. Efficacy and safety of left atrial appendage closure with WATCHMAN in patients with or without contraindication to oral anticoagulation: 1-year follow-up outcome data of the EWOLUTION trial. *Heart Rhythm* **2017**, *14*, 1302–1308. [CrossRef]
126. Tilz, R.R.; Potpara, T.; Chen, J.; Dobreanu, D.; Larsen, T.B.; Haugaa, K.H.; Dagres, N. Left atrial appendage occluder implantation in Europe: Indications and anticoagulation post-implantation. Results of the European Heart Rhythm Association survey. *Europace* **2017**, *19*, 1737–1742. [CrossRef] [PubMed]
127. Saw, J.; Tzikas, A.; Shakir, S.; Gafoor, S.; Omran, H.; Nielsen-Kudsk, J.E.; Kefer, J.; Aminian, A.; Berti, S.; Santoro, G.; et al. Incidence and clinical impact of device-associated thrombus and peri-device leak following left atrial appendage closure with the amplatzer cardiac plug. *JACC Cardiovasc. Interv.* **2017**, *10*, 391–399. [CrossRef]
128. Plicht, B.; Konorza, T.F.M.; Kahlert, P.; Al-Rashid, F.; Kaelsch, H.; Jánosi, R.A.; Buck, T.; Bachmann, H.S.; Siffert, W.; Heusch, G.; et al. Risk factors for thrombus formation on the amplatzer cardiac plug after left atrial appendage occlusion. *JACC Cardiovasc. Interv.* **2013**, *6*, 606–613. [CrossRef]
129. Sedaghat, A.; Schrickel, J.-W.; Andrié, R.; Schueler, R.; Nickenig, G.; Hammerstingl, C. Thrombus formation after left atrial appendage occlusion with the amplatzer amulet device. *JACC Clin. Electrophysiol.* **2017**, *3*, 71–75. [CrossRef]

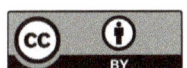 © 2019 by the authors. Licensee MDPI, Basel, Switzerland. This article is an open access article distributed under the terms and conditions of the Creative Commons Attribution (CC BY) license (http://creativecommons.org/licenses/by/4.0/).

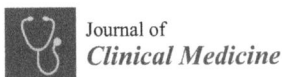

Review

Radial Artery Access for Percutaneous Cardiovascular Interventions: Contemporary Insights and Novel Approaches

Renato Francesco Maria Scalise [1], Armando Mariano Salito [1], Alberto Polimeni [2], Victoria Garcia-Ruiz [3], Vittorio Virga [1], Pierpaolo Frigione [1], Giuseppe Andò [1], Carlo Tumscitz [4] and Francesco Costa [1,*]

1. Department of Clinical and Experimental Medicine, Policlinic "G. Martino", University of Messina, 98100 Messina, Italy; rfm.scalise@gmail.com (R.F.M.S.); armandosalito@gmail.com (A.M.S.); vittorio.virga@yahoo.it (V.V.); pfrigione@homail.com (P.F.); gando@unime.it (G.A.)
2. Division of Cardiology, Department of Medical and Surgical Sciences, Magna Graecia University, 88100 Catanzaro, Italy; polimeni@unicz.it
3. UGC del Corazón, Servicio de Cardiología, Hospital Clínico Universitario Virgen de la Victoria, 29010 Málaga, Spain; mavigaru@gmail.com
4. Department of Cardiology, Azienda Ospedaliero Universitaria di Ferrara, Via Aldo Moro, 8, Cona, 30010 Ferrara, Italy; Tumscitz@gmail.com
* Correspondence: dottfrancescocosta@gmail.com; Tel.: +39-090-221-23-41; Fax: +39-090-221-23-81

Received: 13 September 2019; Accepted: 12 October 2019; Published: 18 October 2019

Abstract: Since its introduction, the transradial access for percutaneous cardiovascular procedures has been associated with several advantages as compared to transfemoral approach, and has become the default for coronary angiography and intervention. In the last 30 years, a robust amount of evidence on the transradial approach has been mounted, promoting its diffusion worldwide. This article provides a comprehensive review of radial artery access for percutaneous cardiovascular interventions, including the evidence from clinical trials of transradial vs. transfemoral approach, technical considerations, access-site complications and limitations, alternative forearm accesses (e.g., ulnar and distal radial artery), and ultimately the use of the radial approach for structural interventions.

Keywords: radial; ulnar; distal radial; snuffbox; percutaneous coronary intervention; aortic valvuloplasty

1. Introduction

The radial artery has progressively become during the last decade the standard access site for percutaneous coronary diagnostic and interventional procedures. The first report of transradial access (TRA) for cardiovascular diagnostics dates to 1947, when Radner performed an aortography via radial artery employing a cut-down technique [1]. Afterwards, in 1989, Campeau published the first case series of 100 transradial coronary angiographies performed through the radial access, emphasizing the safety and the fast mobilization of patients with this approach [2]. Hereafter, in 1993, Kiemeneij described three cases of transradial coronary stenting [3]. On the basis of this pioneering work, TRA gradually diffused supported by a growing body of evidence. As compared to the transfemoral approach (TFA), the radial artery has a more superficial location that allows an easier localization and compression resulting in a lower rate of hemorrhagic complications. Furthermore, the absence of damageable structures reduces the risk of complications due to the puncture itself, while the vascular reserve provided by ulnar artery limits distal ischemic injury of the hand. In addition, the radial access improves patient comfort and accelerates mobilization. On the contrary, radial interventions may result tricky in case of tortuous anatomies of the subclavian axis and results in a more difficult coronary cannulation and catheter manipulation. This results in a significant learning curve for operators that trained with femoral approach as a standard access site. While radial access provides undoubted advantages in most of coronary interventional cases, femoral access remains the preferred route for complex high-risk coronary interventions or when bulky devices are necessary (e.g., mechanical circulatory support, structural procedures etc.). The purpose of this review is to provide a comprehensive overview of the evidence, technical considerations, and future perspectives of the radial artery and other forearm arterial approaches for cardiovascular interventions.

2. Evidence Supporting Transradial Artery Access

A solid body of evidence have mounted in the last 10 years regarding the advantages provided by the radial approach for coronary interventions (Table 1). The Mortality benefit Of Reduced Transfusion after percutaneous coronary intervention via the Arm or Leg (MORTAL) registry [4], a large retrospective study including 30,900 patients treated with percutaneous coronary intervention (PCI), showed for the first time a reduced need for blood transfusion and 1-year mortality with TRA as compared to TFA. These preliminary findings were confirmed by other observational studies. The lack of randomized evidence confronting radial vs. femoral approach was filled by the RadIal Vs. femorAL access for coronary intervention (RIVAL) trial [5], the first randomized comparison between TRA and TFA for PCI in patients with acute coronary syndromes. The RIVAL trial enrolled 7021 patients, which were randomly assigned to TRA ($N = 3507$) or TFA ($N = 3514$) at the time of vascular access. The primary endpoint, a composite of death, myocardial infarction, stroke, or non-coronary artery bypass graft (CABG)-related major bleeding at 30 days, was similar in both groups (3.7% in TRA vs. 4.0% in TFA; HR 0.92, 95% CI 0.72–1.17; $P = 0.50$). No difference for ischemic endpoints was observed between the two treatment arms, neither a difference in terms of the primary safety endpoint of non-CABG major bleeding. Post-hoc analysis including an alternative definition of bleeding showed a significant reduction of major bleeding with TRA. Major vascular complications were more common in the TFA group (1.4% vs. 3.7%; $P < 0.0001$), whereas the need for access-site crossover (i.e., transition between the randomly assigned access to an alternative access) was more common in the TRA group (7.6% vs. 2.0%; $P < 0.0001$). The subgroups analysis of the primary endpoint revealed a significant interaction favoring TRA over TFA in highest tertile volume radial centers (HR: 0.49, 95% CI: 0.28–0.87; $P = 0.015$) and in patients presenting with ST-segment elevated myocardial infarction (STEMI) (HR: 0,60, 95% CI: 0.38–0.94; $P = 0.026$). In particular, in patients with STEMI approached via TRA a lower rate of the composite of death, MI and stroke (P int = 0.011), and death for all causes (P int = 0.001) was also observed, in line with the hypothesis that a more intensive antithrombotic regimen implemented in STEMI patients could unveil the benefit of the radial access.

The overall neutral findings of the RIVAL trial contrasted with the previous evidence from observational studies. A possible explanation for this inconsistency could be found in a deeper evaluation of this study. A subsequent analysis of the RIVAL trial showed that all the access-site major bleeding reported in the radial arm were due to intra-aortic balloon pump use and radial-to-femoral crossover, which were assigned to the radial cohort in keeping with the intention-to-treat analysis. After relocating these events in the femoral group in the as-treated analysis, a significant relationship between femoral approach and access-site major bleeding was found also for the study safety endpoint (0 vs. 18 events) [5]. Finally, the RIVAL trial may have been underpowered to observe differences in non–CABG-related major bleeding, hence reducing its ability to find superiority for the radial approach on the primary endpoint [5].

In line with the STEMI subgroup analysis of the RIVAL trial, the Radial versus Femoral Randomized Investigation in ST-Elevation Acute Coronary Syndrome (RIFLE-STEACS) trial, tested the superiority of TRA vs. TFA in patients presenting with STEMI [6]. This study enrolled 1001 patients undergoing primary or rescue PCI. The primary endpoint of the study was a composite of death, myocardial infarction, target lesion revascularization, stroke or non–CABG-related major bleeding defined by Bleeding Academic Research Consortium (BARC) at 30-days. TRA was ultimately associated with a significant reduction of the primary endpoint (13.6% in TRA vs. 21% in TFA; $P = 0.003$), reduced non–CABG-related major bleeding (7.8% in TRA vs. 12.2% in TFA; $P = 0.026$) and overall mortality (5.2% in TRA vs. 9.2% in TFA; $P = 0.02$). These impressive results should be closely analyzed to understand major differences with the RIVAL study. All operators in the RIFLE-STEACS were experienced and highly skilled performing more than 200 PCI per year with the radial approach. Furthermore, the mortality and the bleeding event-rate observed in the RIFLE-STEACS population was higher compared to previous studies, likely owing to the inclusion of a higher risk population with extensive use of GPIIb/IIIa inhibitors. Moreover, a subsequent analysis using the more stringent Thrombosis in Myocardial Infarction (TIMI) bleeding definition revealed no difference in access-site bleeding among the two treatment arms [6].

Table 1. Clinical studies for Radial vs. Femoral approach in percutaneous coronary intervention.

Trial, Year	N. of Patients	STEMI%	NSTE-ACS%	All-Cause Mortality%	MACE%	Access-Site Bleeding%	Major Bleeding%
RIVAL, 2011							
Radial	3507	27	73	1.3	3.2	1.4	0.7
Femoral	3514	29	71	1.5	3.2	3.7	0.9
RIFLE-STEACS, 2012							
Radial	500	100	-	5.2	7.2	2.6	1.8
Femoral	501	100		9.2	11.4	6.8	2.8
STEMI-RADIAL, 2014							
Radial	348	100	-	2.3	3.4	0.6	1.4
Femoral	359	100		3.1	4.2	5.3	7.2
MATRIX, 2015							
Radial	4197	48	52	1.6	8.8	0.4	1.5
Femoral	207	48	52	2.2	10.2	1	2.3
SAFARI-STEMI, 2019							
Radial	1136	100	-	1.5	4	-	1.1
Femoral	1156	100		1.3	3.4		1.3

STEMI: ST-Elevation myocardial infraction. NSTE-ACS: non-ST-Elevation acute coronary syndrome. MACE: major adverse cardiovascular events.

Subsequently, the STEMI-RADIAL trial, a multicenter randomized study, compared TRA and TFA in patients undergoing primary PCI performed by high-volume operators experienced in both access sites. The study enrolled 707 patients with STEMI who were randomized to TRA ($N = 348$) or TFA ($N = 359$) before the primary PCI [7]. The primary endpoint, a composite of major bleeding and vascular access-site complications at 30 days, was significantly lower in the radial cohort (1.4% vs. 7.2%; $P < 0.0001$). Likewise, the net adverse clinical events (NACE) rate, a composite of death, myocardial infarction, stroke, major bleeding and vascular complications was lower in the radial cohort (4.6% vs. 11%; $P = 0.0028$). The mortality at 30 days was similar in both group (2.3% in the TRA group vs. 3.1% in TFA group; $P = 0.64$).

A paramount contribution in the field was given by the Minimizing Adverse Hemorrhagic Events by TRansradial Access Site and Systemic Implementation of angioX (MATRIX) program [8,9]. This large multicenter study was designed to assess if TRA or bivalirudin, compared with TFA or unfractionated heparin, decrease the 30-day incidence of ischemic or and/or bleeding events in patients with acute coronary syndrome undergoing early invasive management. The MATRIX access [10], the first trial from this program, was a multicenter superiority trial comparing TRA versus TFA. The study population was composed of 8404 patients with acute coronary syndrome, with or without ST-segment elevation myocardial infarction, undergoing coronary angiography and PCI which were randomized to TRA ($N = 4197$) or TFA ($N = 4207$). The two co-primary endpoints were Major Adverse Cardiovascular Events (MACE) at 30 days and NACE at 30 days using the BARC major bleeding definition. Results showed a similar MACE rate in both groups (8.8% in TRA group vs. 10.3% in TFA group; RR: 0.85, 95% CI: 0.74–0.99; $P = 0.0307$, non-significant α of 0.025) whereas NACE rate was lower in patients of TRA group (9.8% vs. 11.7%, RR: 0.83, 95% CI: 0.73–0.96; $P = 0.092$). The benefit in radial access was mainly due to a significant reduction of non-CABG-related major bleeding (1.6% in TRA group vs. 2.3%, RR: 0.67, 95% CI: 0.49–0.92; $P = 0.013$) and all-cause mortality (1.6% in TRA group vs. 2.2% in TFA group, RR: 0.72, 95% CI: 0.53–0.99; $P = 0.045$). Results remained consistent also at a longer-term follow-up of one year [11].

A meta-analysis of the these four multicenter randomized trials (RIVAL, RIFLE-STEACS, STEMI-RADIAL, and MATRIX access) including a total of 17,133 patients (8552 in TRA group and 8581 in TFA group) demonstrated that TRA reduced mortality (RR: 0.73, 95% CI: 0.59–0.90; $P = 0.003$), major adverse cardiovascular events (RR: 0.86, 95% CI: 0.75–0.98; $P = 0.025$) and major bleeding (RR: 0.57, 95% CI: 0.37–0.88, $P = 0.011$) with no effect on myocardial infarction or stroke. Yet, a minimal procedural time delay (standardized mean difference of 0.11 min; 95% CI: 0.04–0.18 min; $P = 0.002$) and a higher rate of access-site crossover (6.3% vs. 1.7% $P = 0.001$) was associated with TRA [12]. These results remained consistent in a second subanalysis including also observational studies [13].

Recently, the SAFARI-STEMI trial, presented at the American College of Cardiology in 2019 [14] compared TRA and TFA in 4884 patients undergoing primary PCI for STEMI. At interim analysis, due to lower than expected rate of the primary outcome, the study was terminated for futility. Finally, just 2292 patients were enrolled a randomized to TRA ($N = 1136$) or TFA ($N = 1156$). Results showed no difference in 30-day all-cause mortality (1.8% in TRA group vs. 1.6% in TFA group; $P = 0.83$), reinfarction (1.8% in TRA group vs. 1.6% in TFA group; $P = 0.83$), stroke (1.0% in TRA group vs. 0.4% in TFA group; $P = 0.12$) and a composite endpoint including death, reinfarction and stroke (4.0% in TRA group vs. 3.4% in TFA group; $P = 0.45$). Unexpectedly, the bleeding rate was comparable between the two groups independently from bleeding definition used (1.1% in TRA group vs. 1.3% in TFA group; $P = 0.74$).

3. Technical Factors and Access-Site Complications

The radial artery originates, together with the ulnar artery, from the brachial artery bifurcation at the proximal border of the antecubital fossa (Figure 1).

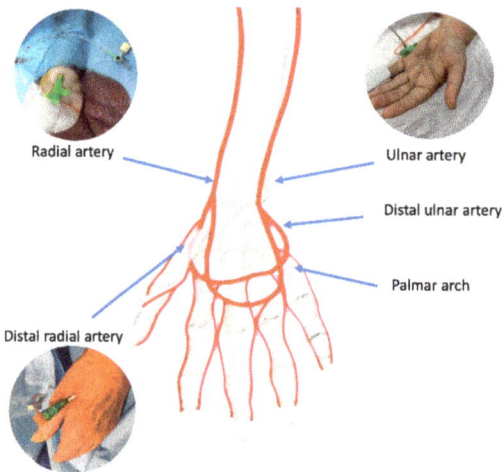

Figure 1. Arterial anatomy of the wrist/hand and potential vascular accesses.

The radial artery can be divided in three segments: the proximal segment laying in the forearm, the middle segment running in the back of the wrist, and the distal segment transitioning from the wrist to the dorsal side in the hand through the anatomical snuffbox. An intricate anastomotic network formed by the deep palmar arch, deriving mainly from the radial artery, and the superficial palmar arch deriving mainly by the ulnar artery provides the hand a dual blood supply. As observed in post-mortem studies [15] this anastomotic circle can present highly variable patterns. Sometimes, a superficial palmar branch can stem from the radial artery in the forearm and it can converge in the distal ulnar artery segment, completing the superficial palmar arch; in the same way, a deep palmar branch can stem from distal ulnar artery and it can converge in the distal radial artery completing the deep palmar arch. Theoretically, the patency of palmar connection between radial and ulnar artery is essential to prevent hand ischemic complications if the radial or the ulnar artery occludes. Several non-invasive tests have been proposed to evaluate the palmar arch circulation: the Allen test, the modified Allen test, and the Barbeau test. In the modified Allen test, the patient first has to lift the hand and clench the fist, then the operator compresses both radial and ulnar artery to block the flow and finally the patients opens the fingers, the operator removes ulnar artery compression and counts the time necessary to recolor the hand. The test is normal if blushing appears within 5 s, it is intermediate if blushing appears between 6 and 10 s, it is abnormal if blushing takes more than 10 s to appear. Similarly, the Barbeau test is performed in a similar manner as the modified Allen test but implements the evaluation of the plethysmographic waveform and pulse oximetry evaluation of the hand [16]. Recently, the laser Doppler scan, a novel promising non-invasive diagnostic technique, has been described [17]. It uses a low-power laser beam and generates color maps of blood perfusion. This test allows quick and easy diagnosis of radial artery occlusion after catheterization in an operator-independent manner [18].

Nevertheless, the effectiveness of these non-invasive tests is debatable and did not appear essential to prevent hand ischemia.

The Predictive Value of Allen's Test Result in Elective Patients Undergoing Coronary Catheterization Through Radial Approach (RADAR) study [19] evaluated prospectively the safety and feasibility of TRA approach in relation to the Allen test. The study enrolled 203 patients undergoing elective or urgent coronary catheterization which were divided based on Allen test results in three groups: normal ($N = 83$), intermediate ($N = 60$) and abnormal ($N = 60$). Every patient was subjected to serial assessments of thumb capillary lactate (the primary endpoint), thumb plethysmography, ulnar frame count, handgrip strength tests, and discomfort ratings. No statistically significant difference emerged among the 3 study groups for lactate (mean: 1.85 ± 0.93 mmol/L in normal group, 1.85 ± 0.66 mmol/L in intermediate group, and 1.97 ± 0.71 mmol/L in abnormal group; $P = 0.59$), handgrip strength test results, and discomfort ratings after the procedure or at other time points during the study. In patients with abnormal or intermediate results, plethysmography revealed ulnopalmar collateralization improvements while the ulnar frame count was reduced, indicating augmented ulnar flow after TRA.

The ACRA anatomy study (Assessment of Disability After Coronary Procedures Using Radial Access) [20] evaluated the clinical relevance of the palmar arch incompleteness and the correlation to commonly used patency tests. This study enrolled 234 patients undergoing TRA cardiac catheterization. Patients were valued angiographically to define the hand vascular anatomy and with modified Allen test and Barbeau test before TRA. Furthermore, a functional evaluation of the hand was assessed at baseline and 2-year follow-up by the QuickDASH, a shortened version of the 30-item DASH (Disabilities of the Arm, Shoulder and Hand) questionnaire. Results showed that incompleteness of the superficial palmar arch was present in 46% of patients, meanwhile the deep palmar arch was complete in all patients. Modified Allen test and Barbeau test results were associated with incompleteness of the superficial palmar arch ($P = 0.001$ and $P = 0.001$). The modified Allen test sensitivity and sensibility for superficial palmar arch incompleteness were 33% and 86% respectively with a cut-off of >10 s and 59% and 60% respectively with a cut-off of >5 s. The Barbeau test sensitivity and specificity were 7% and 98% respectively for type D and a 21% and 93% respectively for types C and D combined. The upper-extremity dysfunction had no correlation with superficial palmar arch incompleteness ($P = 0.77$). These results suggested that while the incompleteness of the superficial palm arch is common, a complete deep palmar arch guarantees the blood supply to distal districts, and the preprocedural patency tests do no add benefit to prevent ischemic complications of the hand.

The ACRA-perfusion [21], a prespecified sub-study of the ACRA anatomy study, focused on how transradial approach may impair digital perfusion. Sequential laser Doppler perfusion imaging was used to evaluate digital perfusion in 100 patients undergoing elective transradial cardiac catheterization in comparison with contralateral hand. The primary outcome was thumb perfusion at baseline, during radial access, at TR band application and at discharge. The vascular anatomy was assessed with angiography and the upper-extremity function was measured by QuickDASH questionnaire at baseline and follow-up. Results showed a reduced tissue perfusion during radial access and during TR band application both in the homolateral thumb (−32% and −32%, respectively) than in contralateral thumb (−34% and −21%, respectively). No perfusion difference emerged during TRA between the homolateral and the contralateral thumb (arbitrary flux units: 217; IQR, 112–364 vs. 209; IQR, 99–369; $P = 0.59$). There was no association between reduced thumb perfusion and superficial palmar arch incompleteness (complete superficial palmar arch 56% vs. incomplete superficial palmar arch 71%; $P = 0.13$). Digital perfusion at discharge remained below baseline levels but showed an improving trend (homolateral −11% and contralateral −14%). Reduced digital perfusion during TRA was not associated with hand dysfunction at 18 months.

The radial approach procedure begins with the administration of local anesthetic to limit the patient's discomfort, usually a modest dose (1–2 mL) is used to not distort the normal anatomy. The radial artery cannulation is commonly obtained close to the styloid process with two different techniques: the Seldinger and the modified Seldinger technique [22]. The Seldinger technique employs a catheter-over-needle system which is used first to pass the anterior wall and subsequently, when blood fills the needle, the posterior wall; the needle is then removed and the catheter is slowly draw back until a pulsatile blood flow is obtained; finally a 0.021-inch guidewire is advanced, the catheter is removed, and the introducer over the wire is placed. The modified Seldinger technique employs a micro-puncture needle entering arterial lumen, as soon the blood flows through the needle a 0.018 inch or 0.021 inch guidewire is advanced into the vessel, the needle is removed, and an introducer over the wire is placed. A randomized evaluation of these two techniques was performed in 412 patients undergoing TRA catheterization [23]. 210 patients were approached with the Seldinger technique and 212 with the modified Seldinger technique. Results showed a statistically significant advantage for the Seldinger technique regarding time to gain radial artery access (mean time in seconds 78.3 ± 37.7 vs. 134.2 ± 87.5; $P < 0.001$) and total procedure time (mean time in minutes 17.1 ± 6.4 vs. 19.3 ± 7.1; $P < 0.01$), while no difference emerged in post-procedural hematoma (0.5% vs. 1.5%, $P > 0.2$), and radial artery occlusion at 24 h (8% vs. 7.9%; $P > 0.5$) or at 30 days (4.3% vs. 3.9%; $P > 0.5$). A meta-analysis comparing all available studies on the use of 5-Fr versus 6-Fr system in coronary procedures through the TRA showed a significant lower contrast medium administration (MD = −22.20 (−36.43 to −7.9), $P < 0.01$) and bleedings (OR = 0.58 (0.38–0.90), $P = 0.02$) of 5-Fr system, without compromising procedural success (OR = 0.95 (0.53–1.69), $P = 0.86$) or procedure length (OR = 0.55 (−2.58 to 3.69), $P = 0.73$), compared to the 6-Fr system [24].

Introducer sheaths of different sizes are available on the market and many operators usually prefer longer sheaths (23 cm) as compared to short sheaths (13 cm) due to a supposed spasm reduction and easier catheter manipulation. A randomized controlled trial investigated the impact of length and hydrophilic coating of the introducer sheath on radial artery spasm, radial artery occlusion, and local vascular complications in patients undergoing elective transradial coronary procedures [25]. This study enrolled 790 patients, which were randomly assigned to long (23-cm) or short (13-cm) and hydrophilic-coated or uncoated introducer sheaths. Results showed a reduction of radial artery spasm (19.0% vs. 39.9%, OR: 2.87; 95% CI: 2.07 to 3.97; $P = 0.001$) and patient reported discomfort (15.1% vs. 28.5%, OR: 2.27; 95% CI: 1.59 to 3.23; $P = 0.001$) in patients receiving a hydrophilic-coated sheath while no difference emerged between long and short sheaths.

The R-RADAR study [26] (The Rotterdam Radial Access Research Ultrasound-Based Radial Artery Evaluation for Diagnostic and Therapeutic Coronary Procedures) investigated structural changes of the radial artery wall after catheterization to define predictors of radial pulsation loss, occlusion, local pain, or functional impairment of the upper extremity. This prospective, single-center study enrolled 90 patients undergoing TRA coronary angiography or intervention, which were scanned with a high-resolution 40-MHz ultrasound (US) before cannulation, at 3 h and 30 days after procedure. All patients presented acute injuries, predominantly dissection and intramural hematoma, but these were not associated with loss of radial pulsation, occlusion, local pain, or functional impairment at 30 days. An intimal thickening and total wall thickness increase was observed at 3 h after puncture and persisted at 30 days, while a modest luminal inner caliber reduction was observed at the puncture site. Radial occlusion and pulsation loss rate at 30 days were 3.9% and 9.2% respectively. Smaller radial artery lumen at baseline was associated with an increased risk of radial pulsation loss at 30 days (OR 1.23; $P = 0.049$). The number of radial puncture attempts was associated with 30-day pulsation loss (OR, 2.64; $P = 0.027$), artery occlusion (OR, 3.49; $P = 0.022$), and symptoms (OR 2.24; $P = 0.05$).

The utility of US for guiding TRA was evaluated in the RAUST study (Radial Artery access with Ultrasound Trial) [27]. This prospective multicenter trial enrolled 698 patients undergoing transradial cardiac catheterization that were randomized to needle insertion with palpation ($N = 351$) or real-time US guidance ($N = 347$). The primary endpoints were the first-pass success rate, the total number of attempts needed for access, and the time to access. US guidance was related to a number attempts reduction mean: 1.65 ± 1.2 vs. 3.05 ± 3.4; $P < 0.0001$; median: 1 (IQR: 1 to 2) vs. 2 (1 to 3); $P < 0.0001$ and to a first-pass success rate improvement (64.8% vs. 3.9%; $P < 0.0001$) with a consensual time to access reduction (mean: 88 ± 78 s vs. 108 ± 112 s; $P = 0.006$; median: 64 (IQR: 45 to 94) vs. 74 (IQR: 49 to 120); $P = 0.01$). Crossover from palpation to US guidance was necessary in 10 patients with subsequent successful sheath insertion rate of 80%. US guidance also reduced the difficult access rate procedures (2.4% vs. 18.6% for ≥5 attempts; $P < 0.001$; 3.7% vs. 6.8% for ≥5 min; $P = 0.07$).

The right-sided controls position in the catheterization laboratory predisposes to a right radial approach (RRA) that both operator and the patients generally prefer [28]. Despite this, the left arterial access (LRA) offers a direct entrance to the left subclavian artery with a better support for guides or catheters and ease left internal mammary artery cannulation. Furthermore, the LRA has been associated with a reduced procedural duration and a higher rate of procedural success mainly due to the low prevalence of left subclavian artery tortuosity. Controversial data emerged comparing right and LRA about radiation exposure duration.

The Transradial approach left vs. right and procedural times during percutaneous coronary procedures (TALENT) [29] study evaluated the safety and efficacy of LRA compared with RRA for coronary procedures focusing on fluoroscopy time for coronary angiography and PCI (primary endpoints). Patients age and operator experience were also analyzed. This dual-center study enrolled 1540 patients which were randomized to RRA ($N = 770$) or LRA ($N = 770$); 1467 patients underwent coronary angiography (diagnostic group: 732 with LRA approach and 735 with RRA) and 688 patients underwent percutaneous coronary procedures (PCI group: 344 each group). Fluoroscopy time (median: 149 s, IQR 95–270 s), as well as Dose Area Product (DAP) (median: 10.7 Gy cm^2, IQR 6–20.5 Gy cm^2), were significantly lower with LRA in the diagnostic group when compared with RRA (median: 168 s, IQR 110–277 s; $P = 0.0025$ and 12.1 Gy cm^2, IQR 7–23.8 Gy cm^2; $P = 0.004$, respectively). No significant differences emerged in the PCI group in fluoroscopy time (median: 614 s, IQR 367–1087 s for LRA vs. 695 s for RRA, IQR 415–1235 s; $P = 0.087$) and DAP (median: 53.7 Gy cm^2, IQR 29–101 Gy cm^2 for LRA vs. 63.1 Gy cm^2 for RRA, IQR 31–119 Gy cm^2; $P = 0.17$). Subgroup analyses revealed that the differences between left and RRA were linked to patients age (≥70 years old) and to operator experience.

The REVEREE (Randomized Evaluation of Vascular Entry Site and Radiation Exposure) trial [30] evaluated radiation exposure during cardiac catheterization comparing TFA with LRA and RRA. This study enrolled 1493 patients undergoing cardiac catheterization that were randomized in a 1:1:1 fashion. The primary endpoint was air kerma, the secondary endpoints included DAP, fluoroscopy time, operator dose per procedure, number of cineangiograms, and number of catheters. Results showed no significant differences among the three group concerning the primary endpoint (medians: TFA: 421 mGy, IQR 337–574 mGy; LRA: 454 mGy IQR: 331–643 mGy; RRA 483 mGy, IQR: 382–592 mGy; $P = 0.146$), and DAP (medians: TFA: 25.5 Gy cm^2 IQR: 19.6–34.5 Gy cm^2; LRA: 26.6 Gy cm^2 IQR: 19.5–37.5 Gy cm^2; RRA 27.7 Gy cm^2, IQR: 21.9–34.4 Gy cm^2; $P = 0.40$), or fluoroscopy time (medians: TFA 1.3 min IQR: 1.0–1.7 min; LRA: 1.3 min, IQR: 1.0–1.7 min, and RRA: 1.32 min, IQR: 1.0–1.7 min; $P = 0.19$). Conversely operator exposure was significantly higher in the LRA group (3 mrem, IQR: 2–5 mrem) compared with TFA (2 mrem, IQR: 2–4 mrem; $P = 0.001$) and TRA (3 mrem, QR: 2 to 5 mrem; $P = 0.0001$).

The RAD-MATRIX [31], a sub-study of the MATRIX [10] investigated if TRA access procedures compared to TFA increases the radiation exposure risk of operator or patient. A total of 18 expert operators, performing 777 procedures in 767 patients were recruited and randomized to TRA or TFA. Each operator was equipped with lithium fluoride thermoluminescent dosimeter to measure radiation exposure on the thorax (primary endpoint), on the wrist and on the head (secondary endpoints). Results showed an equivalent dose at the thorax significantly higher with TRA (77 µSv, IQR: 39.9 µSv to 112 µSv) than TFA access (41 µSv, IQR: 23.4 mSv to 58.5 µSv; $P = 0.019$) which was still significant after normalization of operator radiation dose by fluoroscopy time or DAP. Otherwise, there was no difference in radiation dose at wrist or head among the two cohort. Similar thorax operator dose was observed for RRA (84 µSv) and LRA (52 µSv; $P = 0.15$). Operator effective dose was significantly higher with RRA than LRA (2.6 vs. 1.6 µSv; $P = 0.016$). A subsequent analysis [32] was performed to appraise the determinants of operator radiation overexposure with RRA. Operator radiation exposure was investigated in relation to the right arm position and the upper leaded glass size. Results showed a greater-than-10-fold difference in radiation at thorax level among the 14 operators who agreed to participate (from 21.5 to 267 µSv and from 0.35 to 3.5 µSv/Gy*cm^2 after DAP normalization). Thorax dose was higher among operators who positioned the instrumented right arm far from the body (110.4 µSv, interquartile range 71.5–146.5 µSv), when compared to those that placed the instrumented right arm adjacent to the right leg (46.1 µSv, 31.3–56.8 µSv; $P = 0.02$) and the difference persisted after normalization by DAP ($P = 0.028$). In the same way, smaller full glass shield was associated with a higher radiation exposure when compared to a larger composite shield (147.5 and 60 µSv, respectively, $P = 0.016$).

Apart from the evident impact on vascular complications and access-site bleeding, the implementation of the radial access showed several additional clinical benefits [33,34]. In the AKI-MATRIX [35] study, the radial vs. femoral access impact on post-procedural acute kidney injury was explored. Renal function evaluation regarded 8210 patients, 4109 in the TRA cohort and 4101 in the TFA cohort. The primary endpoint was acute kidney injury defined as an absolute (>0.5 mg/dl) or a relative (>25%) increase in serum creatinine. Results showed an overall lower acute kidney injury rate with TRA compared to TFA (15.4% vs. 17.4%, OR 0.87; 95% CI: 0.77 to 0.98; $P = 0.0181$). In particular, a >25% relative serum creatinine increase regarded the 15.4% of the TRA cohort patients and the 17.3% of the TFA cohort patients (OR: 0.87; 95% CI: 0.77 to 0.98; $P = 0.0195$), while a >0.5 mg/dl absolute serum creatinine increase occurred in the 4.3% of patients in the TRA cohort and in the 5.4% of patients in the TFA cohort (OR: 0.77; 95% CI: 0.63 to 0.95; $P = 0.0131$). By applying the Kidney Disease Improving Global Outcomes criteria, acute kidney disease rate was 3-fold less prevalent with TRA access (OR: 0.85; 95% CI: 0.70 to 1.03; $P = 0.090$), with stage 3 acute kidney injury in the 0.68% of patients in the TRA cohort and in the 1.12% of patients in the TFA cohort ($P = 0.0367$). Post-intervention dialysis was needed in the 0.15% of patients in the TRA cohort and in the 0.34% of patients in the TFA cohort ($P = 0.0814$).

A subsequent analysis evaluated how radial and femoral access relate to bleeding, acute kidney injury and all-cause mortality to clarify the correlation between these different types of events [36]. A multistate and competing risk models highlighted large relative risk reductions in mortality for TRA compared with TFA access for the transition from acute kidney injury to death (HR 0.55, 95% CI

0.31–0.97) and for the pathway from PCI to acute kidney injury to death (HR 0.49, 95% CI 0.26–0.92). On the contrary, there was little evidence for a difference between TRA and TFA groups for the transition from bleeding to death (HR 1.05, 95% CI 0.42–2.64) and the pathway from PCI to bleeding to death (HR 0.84, 95% CI 0.28–2.49). These results suggest that radial approach benefit on mortality is mainly driven by acute kidney injury prevention while bleeding role in this association was minor [33,36].

4. The Distal Radial Approach

The distal radial artery (Figure 2) approach was first introduced by anesthesiologists for perioperative patient monitoring [37] at the anatomical snuffbox or at the dorsum of the hand. This access is obtained where the vessel runs superficially, at the intersection of the thumb and first finger over the bony structures of the snuffbox or at the dorsum of the hand, distal to the tendon of the extensor pollicis longus muscle. The technique described by Kiemeneij [38] and Davies and Gilchrist [39] starts with a subcutaneous injection of 1–5 cc of local anesthetic, then the artery is punctured with a 21-gauge open needle, directed to point of highest pulsation, from lateral to medial with a 30–45° angle. When the blood flows through the needle a flexible, soft, J-shaped 0.21 metallic wire is inserted and the needle is removed. A small skin incision before introducer placement is sometimes necessary because the skin is thicker and harder than at the forearm [40]. A through-and-through technique should be avoided, especially if the artery is approached at the snuffbox, for the high risk of puncturing the periosteum of the scaphoid or trapezium bones, which can be painful [38]. Hemostasis is obtained compressing the artery against the base of the 1st or 2nd metacarpal bone and an elastic bandage might be necessary [39]. Theorized advantages of distal radial approach are a decreased risk of radial artery occlusion at the forearm, lower bleeding risk, lower vascular access-site complication rate [41] and an improved operator and patient comfort, especially when approaching left radial artery [40]. Ongoing randomized controlled trials are evaluating the feasibility and safety of distal radial approach compared to radial approach in various settings, including patients with STEMI [42].

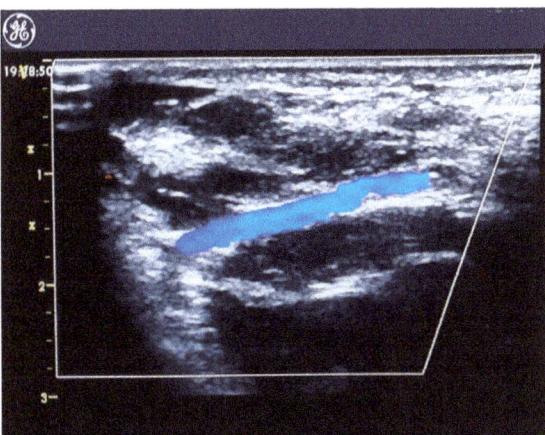

Figure 2. Echocolordoppler image of the distal radial artery.

5. Radial Artery Approach Limitations

Radial artery occlusion (RAO) after radial artery interventions remains an important issue after TRA. Despite this did not show a significant impact of hand ischemia, RAO may prevent future use of the radial artery for interventional purposes, for using the radial artery as an arterial conduit for CABG or in the need for fistula for dialysis.

For this reason, several studies evaluated strategies to reduce the risk of RAO and optimize radial puncture.

The PROPHET (Prevention of radial artery occlusion-patent hemostasis evaluation trial) study [43] enrolled 436 consecutive patients undergoing cardiac catheterization which were randomized to conventional compression or compression maintaining radial artery patency using plethysmography. Results showed that implementation of patent hemostasis is highly effective in reducing RAO (59% decrease at 24 h and 75% decrease at 30 days; $P < 0.05$).

The PROPHET-II study [44] investigated whether ipsilateral ulnar compression increases radial artery flow and could impact the incidence of RAO. This trial enrolled 3000 patients undergoing diagnostic cardiac catheterization, which were randomized to standard patent hemostasis or prophylactic ipsilateral ulnar compression in addition to patent hemostasis. Plethysmography was used to evaluate radial artery patency resulting in a lower RAO occurrence at 30 day in patients with patent hemostasis and prophylactic ulnar compression (0.9% vs. 3.0%; $P = 0.0001$).

The effect of duration of hemostatic compression on RAO was evaluated in a retrospective study [45] that involved 400 consecutive patients undergoing transradial PCI. Half of patients received hemostatic compression for 6 h after the procedure, and the other group for 2 h. Shorter duration of hemostatic compression was associated with a lower incidence of early RAO (5.5% vs.12%; $P = 0.025$) and chronic RAO (3.5% vs. 8.5%; $P = 0.035$) without differences in bleeding complications although maintaining radial patency during hemostatic compression, eliminates the adverse effect of duration of compression.

Use of anticoagulants, administered directly into the radial artery or intravenously, during the procedure has been demonstrated to reduce the incidence of RAO [46,47], particularly a dose-dependent effect of unfractionated heparin [48,49].

The artery spasm may determine friction between the artery wall and devices used during TRA and this endothelial stress can contribute to RAO development. For this reason, the use of vasodilators has been proposed. Nitroglycerin administered into radial artery before sheath removal was associated with RAO incidence reduction [50], as well as and the use of verapamil or verapamil in combination with nitroglycerin is effective in preventing radial artery spasm [51].

On top of the added risk of long-term RAO, the radial artery has some intrinsic anatomical limitations that impedes its use in specific types of intervention. The smaller caliber of the artery, which is 2.5–3.5 times smaller than the common femoral artery, restrict its use in case of larger devices. For this reason, the femoral artery remain the default access in procedures where bulky device are needed such as transcatheter aortic valve implantation (TAVI) [52], mechanical circulatory support including intra-aortic balloon pump (IABP), Impella (Abiomed, Danvers, Massachusetts), or veno-arterial extracorporeal membrane oxygenation (ECMO) [53]. Furthermore, femoral approach is still the preferred access site for some complex procedures, particularly angioplasty of coronary chronic total occlusion [54,55].

6. The Ulnar Artery Approach

The ulnar artery represents an alternative access for percutaneous procedures, and it is increasingly being used when radial access is not available (Table 2) [56–62]. The ulnar artery stems at the inferior margin of the antecubital fossa as a large branch of the brachial artery. It passes in the forearm on the ulnar bone side deep to the flexor muscles and it reaches the hand through the Guyon canal. As compared to the radial artery, the ulnar artery has a lower incidence of anatomical variations, loops, and tortuosity; furthermore, the ulnar artery has a modest concentration of adrenergic receptors that limit the arterial spasm [60]. Conversely the deeper position of the vessel and the absence of a bony structure to compress against expose to a higher rate of access-site complication and impose a heavier compression [58]. The access technique for the ulnar artery is similar to the radial, and both the Seldinger technique and the modified Seldinger technique can be used. The ulnar nerve passes lateral to the ulnar artery, so it is recommended to start the puncture on the medial side of the ulnar artery to avoid pain and spasm.

Table 2. Clinical studies of transradial vs. transulnar approach.

First Author, Year	N. of Patients (TUA/TRA)	STEMI% (TUA/TRA)	NSTEMI% (TUA/TRA)	Successful Vascular Access% (TUA/TRA)	Crossover to Other Approach% (TUA/TRA)	Arterial Access Time (min) (TUA/TRA)	PCI% (TUA/TRA)	Bleeding or Hematoma% (TUA/TRA)	Occlusion% (TUA/TRA)	MACE% (TUA/TRA)
Aptecar, 2006	216/215	17.5/16.7	22.5/27.6	93.1/95.5	6.9/4.2	NR	43.5/44.2	6.8/8.1	5.7/4.7	2.1/4.2
Li, 2010	118/122	4.2/4.9	77.1/73	98.3/100	1.7/0	NR	65/69.2	5.9/5.7	1.7/4.9	0/0
Hahalis, 2013	462/440	14.1/13.2	37.4/38.4	67.7/99.1	32.3/5.9	NR	36.4/32.7	3.2/0.5	10.4/4.3	2.8/3.4
Geng, 2014	271/264	14.4/13.6	72.7/70.4	91.5/95.1	8.5/4.2	NR	62.4/52.3	13.2/7.9	1.9/5.8	9.4/8.7
Liu, 2014	317/319	19.6/20.4	75.9/77.4	92.7/95.9	1.6/1.9	6.3 ± 1.3/5.9 ± 1.2	100/100	4.1/9.4	6.3/4.7	1.9/2.5
Gokhroo, 2016	1270/1262	48.3/45.2	27.6/30.6	95.6/96.2	4.4/3.8	5.6 ± 2.1/5.9 ± 1.7	NR	6.2/6.7	6.1/6.6	2.9/3.2
Bi, 2017	220/225	NR	NR	90.9/92.9	9.1/7.1	NR	66.8/62.2	28.6/11.5	2.7/9.3	NR

STEMI: ST-Elevation myocardial infarction. NSTEMI: non-ST-Elevation myocardial infarction. MACE: major adverse cardiovascular events.

The PCVI-CUBA [63], a single-center randomized study, compared efficacy and safety of the transulnar access (TUA) and the TRA in patients undergoing coronary angiography and PCI. This study enrolled 431 patients who were randomized to TUA ($N = 216$) or TRA ($N = 215$). Results showed no difference among the two groups for successful vascular access (93.1% in the TUA group vs. 95.5% in the TRA group; $P = 0.84$), procedural success (95.2% in the TUA group vs. 96.2% in the TRA group; $P = 0.82$), arterial occlusion (5.7% in the TUA group vs. 4.7% in the TRA group, $P = 0.76$) and major bleeding (5.5% in the TUA group vs. 8.1 in the TRA group, $P = 0.47$). Procedural time (mean 14 ± 8.2 min vs. 12.7 ± 6.7 min $P = 0.06$), fluoroscopy time (mean 5.6 ± 5.1 min vs. 5.2 ± 4.2 min, $P = 0.35$) and X-ray DAP (mean 7559 ± 4865 mGy/cm^2 vs. 7195 ± 4850 mGy/cm^2 $P = 0.43$) were similar between the two group. Freedom from MACE at 30 days was comparable between the two groups (97.8% for ulnar group and 95.8% for radial group, $P = 0.41$).

Another single-center, randomized study [64] evaluated the safety and efficacy of the TUA versus the TRA for coronary angiography and PCI. This study randomized 240 patients undergoing coronary angiography, followed or not by intervention. Results showed a comparable artery stenosis rate between the two groups at 1 day (11.0% in TUA group vs. 12.3% in the TRA group; $P = 0.758$) and at 30 days (5.1% in the ulnar group vs. 6.6% in the radial group; $P = 0.627$). Arterial occlusion rate was similar in the two cohort at 1 day (5.1% in the TUA group vs. 1.7% in the TRA group, $P = 0.627$) and at 30 days (6.6% in the TUA group vs. 4.9% in the TRA group; $P = 0.164$). Minor bleeding was similar between the two groups (5.9% in the TUA group vs. 5.7% in the TRA group; $P = 0.949$).

In contrast to these single-center studies, the AURA of ARTEMIS trial [62] failed to demonstrate the non-inferiority of a default TUA compared to TRA. This prospective randomized multicenter study enrolled 902 patients undergoing diagnostic coronary angiography and PCI who were randomized to TRA ($N = 440$) or TUA ($N = 462$). The primary endpoint was a composite of crossover to another arterial access, MACE, and major vascular complications of the arm at 60 days. The trial was early stopped because the first interim analysis showed the inferiority of the TUA for primary outcome (42.2% vs. 18.0%; $P < 0.0001$). After adjustment for operator clustering, the difference in the primary endpoint became inconclusive (24.30%; 99.99% CI, −7.98% to 56.58%; $P = 0.03$ at $\alpha = 0.0001$). Moreover, the crossover rate, which driven most of the difference for the primary endpoint, was higher in the TUA group, with a difference of 26.34% (95% CI, 21.53%–31.27%; $P < 0.001$).

A subsequent single-center randomized study [59] including 535 consecutive patients evaluated safety and feasibility of TUA for coronary catheterization. The primary endpoints were the success of artery cannulation and the access-site-related complications at day 30 (hematoma, artery stenosis, artery occlusion, arteriovenous fistula, pseudoaneurysm, and nerve injury). Results showed a comparable successful puncture rate between the two cohort (91.5% in the TUA group vs. 95.1% in TRA group; $P > 0.05$). Hematoma occurrence was similar in between the two groups (7.7% in the TUA group vs. 4.2% in the TRA group; $P = 0.100$). Ulnar nerve injury occurred in one patient in the TUA group. Asymptomatic arterial occlusion rate was similar in the two group (1.1% in the TUA group vs. 3.0% in TRA group; $P = 0.137$). Freedom from MACE rate was also similar between the two group (90.6% in the TUA vs. 91.3% in the TRA group; $P = 0.985$).

A randomized single-center, trial [65] compared the clinical outcomes of 445 patients undergoing coronary artery intervention with TUA ($N = 220$) and TRA ($N = 225$). At 1-year follow-up, the primary outcome, arterial occlusion of a forearm artery, was lower in the TUA group (2.7% vs. 9.3%; $P = 0.007$). The occlusion rate of approached vessel was lower in TUA group (OR 3.85, P 0.006). A higher of incidence of hematomas (13.2% vs. 5.8%, $P = 0.01$) and symptoms of discomfort (15.5% vs. 5.8%, $P = 0.002$) emerged in the TUA group.

Finally, the AJmer ULnar ARtery Working Group Study (AJULAR) study [56], a single-center, randomized study, tested the non-inferiority on TUA as compared to TRA when performed by an experienced operator (at least 150 TRA/year and 50 TUA performed). This study enrolled 2532 patients undergoing cardiac catheterization who were randomized to TUA ($N = 1270$) or TRA ($N = 1262$). The primary endpoint was a composite of MACE during hospital stay, crossover to another arterial access, major vascular events during hospital stay (large hematoma with hemoglobin drop of ≥3 g%) or vessel occlusion rate. Secondary endpoints were each component of the primary endpoint, failed attempts (≥3 attempts prior to successful cannulation), procedural and fluoroscopy times, contrast volume used, and vasospasm. Results showed a similar occurrence of primary endpoint (14.6% in TUA group vs. 14.4% in TRA group; RR: 1.01; 95% CI: 0.83–1.2; $P = 0.92$ at $\alpha = 0.05$). The secondary endpoints were all comparable among the two groups, except large hematoma, for which non-inferiority could not be proved. Twelve patients in the TUA group suffered transient paresthesia.

A meta-analysis [66] of six randomized controlled of TUA vs. TRA has been presented, including 5299 patients undergoing percutaneous coronary procedure. Results showed a comparable incidence of MACE between the two access sites (RR 0.90; 95% CI 0.66–1.23) but an excess of vascular complications in the TUA group (RR 3.58; CI 2.67–4.79, $P < 0.00001$). No difference for arterial access time, fluoroscopy time, and contrast load was observed.

7. Radial Access for Non-Coronary Cardiovascular Interventions

The exponential growth of the technique expanded TRA use also to endovascular peripheral artery disease interventions and some selected structural heart disease interventions [66–68] TRA has been reported as primary access-site for alcohol septal ablation [69] paravalvular leak closure [70], ventricular septal defect closure [71], or balloon aortic valvuloplasty (BAV) [72]. Also, more extensively, TRA has been used as secondary access for transcatheter aortic valve replacement (TAVR), patent ductus arteriosus closure, and endovascular repair of abdominal or thoracic aneurysm [68].

In the domain of structural heart interventions, BAV can be a useful tool in patients with severe aortic stenosis who require urgent non-cardiac surgery or safely bridge to either to Surgical Aortic Valve Replacement (SAVR) or TAVR [72]. In addition, population's mean age in western countries is increasing and it is increasingly important to avoid futile TAVR procedures. Still, there is no clear evidence on which patients should be preliminarily excluded from aortic valve intervention because of excessive risk or clinical futility. In this setting BAV as bridge to TAVR, might serve as a stratification method in uncertain TAVR recipients.

Yet, considering the higher rate of comorbidities in this frail population, the rate of vascular complications and the relative attributable mortality remain high [73].

For this reason, using alternative vascular approaches, which may reduce the risk of such complications is attractive. Mini-invasive radial BAV reduces the rate of vascular complications with feasibility and efficacy comparable with standard femoral approach [74].

Implementation of large-bore access sites from the femoral artery and increasing sheath-artery diameter ratio invariably increases the rate of vascular complications [75]. Moreover, during transfemoral TAVR, CT studies of the ilio-femoral arteries confirmed the need for a <1:1 lumen to sheath ratio to avoid risk of vascular damage and serious adverse events [72].

Yet, owing to specific histologic characteristics of the radial artery wall, the 1:1 safety rule could be less important in this scenario. The radial artery wall is thicker than that of other arteries [76] and the prevalent muscular tunica has unique elastic features resulting more compliant than the other arterial vessels, in which progressive elastic fiber degeneration often increases stiffness in older patients [77].

These features, together with the more superficial position and the easier compression, could explain the lower incidence of vascular complications during radial BAV.

The first step to perform radial BAV is obtaining two radial accesses with standard technique, or ulnar access in case radial access would be unavailable. In case only one radial access is possible a mono-lateral approach could be performed, even if two different arterial accesses provide opportunity to switch quickly to the contralateral access, check the hemodynamic efficacy of rapid pacing and the possibility to inject contrast.

After obtaining vascular accesses, the aortic valve should be crossed with conventional 0.035" guidewire. Then a pigtail catheter is advanced in the left ventricle and basal peak-to-peak and mean gradients are measured. In this phase, vascular tortuosity of the epi-aortic branches could hinge on catheter control. In this case, switching from one radial access to the contralateral could be useful. After placing a stiff 0.035″ guidewire in the left ventricle carefully avoiding mitral chordae along the path, the 6 French sheath should be exchanged with an 8 or 9 French femoral sheath (depending on the compatibility of the aortic balloon's manufacturer used). A very short sheath is preferable (5.5 cm) but longer sheaths can be equally used if they are advanced no more than 5–6 cm inside the artery (Figure 3a–b).

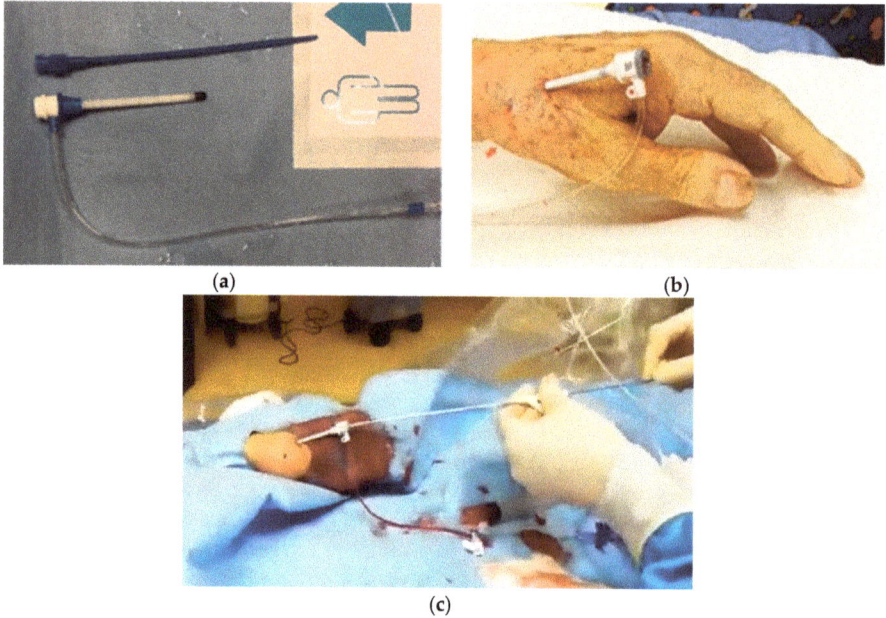

Figure 3. Vascular access for radial balloon aortic valvuloplasty. (**a**) Brite Tip 5.5 cm pediatric 8 French sheath (CORDIS, Ireland). (**b**) regular 11 cm 8F sheath, 5 cm out of the distal radial artery. (**c**) Vascular access for radial balloon aortic valvuloplasty: "Push and pull" maneuver for balloon retrieval.

When the sheath is in place, advancement of the aortic valvuloplasty balloon is usually very easy. When the balloon is across the aortic valve the two electric alligator-connectors should be connected to the distal end of the stiff guidewire placed inside the left ventricle and to a needle placed on the patient's skin and connected to a temporary pacemaker [78]. Alternatively, a transvenous temporary pacemaker stimulating in the right ventricle could be placed through the standard routes. One rapid 160–200 bpm burst should be attempted before the balloon is advanced through the valve to test pacing efficacy. Once the balloon is advanced through the aortic valve and rapid pacing is started the balloon is inflated making sure to maintain position inside the valve. When several inflations have been performed (usually 2–3), the balloon should be exchanged with a pigtail catheter to measure the final pressure gradient.

The balloon could be then retrieved: this is usually easy until it reaches the radial artery. Ideally, two operators should coordinate a "push and pull" maneuverer to minimize the friction of the balloon on the arterial wall in this phase (Figure 3c) and perform a gentle retrieval through the sheath. At this stage of the procedure the patient may complain of acute but transient pain in the forearm region.

It is advisable to perform a careful hemostasis of the radial artery to minimize the risk of occlusion. Good results have been described with patent hemostasis.

According to the experience gained with the radial BAV pilot study and the subsequent ongoing multicenter SOFTLY2 Register, mini-invasive radial BAV is feasible in most patients, regardless of the body weight. Nevertheless, there are some contraindications to the procedure that, even if uncommon, they should to be highlighted: first, the presence of a very small artery with a high take-off of the artery above the elbow or a diffusely diseased radial artery, which is often discovered after several failed attempt to advance diagnostic catheters over the elbow. In addition, severe loops or accessory radial artery anatomy, could increase the risk of arterial rupture. Finally, the evidence of Monkeberg's disease of the forearm arteries (extended calcifications) should discourage any procedure's attempt.

8. Conclusions

TRA is now established as the standard of care access for percutaneous coronary diagnostic and intervention. While TRA already demonstrated a sizable benefit in terms of hard endpoints compared to TFA, a continuously growing body of evidence is focused on surpassing current TRA limitations and expanding alternative vascular accesses, as TUA or distal radial artery for cardiovascular interventions. The recent implementation of TRA as primary or secondary access site for peripheral and structural interventions might provide some of the advantages already observed in the coronary domain also in these new techniques. Nevertheless, owing to the intrinsic anatomical limitations of the TRA preventing large-bore device use, mastering best practices for femoral access remain a priority for future generations of interventional cardiologists.

Author Contributions: R.F.M.S.: Conceived the review, drafted and critically revised the text. A.M.S.: Conceived the review, drafted and critically revised the text. A.P.: Critically revised the text. V.G.-R.: Critically revised the text. V.V.: Critically revised the text. P.F.: Critically revised the text. G.A.: Critically revised the text. C.T.: Conceived the review, drafted and critically revised the text. F.C.: Conceived the review, drafted and critically revised the text.

Funding: This research received no external funding.

Conflicts of Interest: The authors declare no conflict of interest.

References

1. Radner, S. Thoracal Aortography by Catheterization from the Radial Artery: Preliminary Report of a New Technique. *Acta Radiol.* **1948**, *29*, 178–180. [CrossRef] [PubMed]
2. Campeau, L. Percutaneous radial artery approach for coronary angiography. *Catheter. Cardiovasc. Diagn.* **1989**, *16*, 3–7. [CrossRef]
3. Kiemeneij, F.; Jan Laarman, G. Percutaneous transradial artery approach for coronary stent implantation. *Catheter. Cardiovasc. Diagn.* **1993**, *30*, 173–178. [CrossRef]
4. Chase, A.J.; Fretz, E.B.; Warburton, W.P.; Klinke, W.P.; Carere, R.G.; Pi, D.; Berry, B.; Hilton, J.D. Association of the arterial access site at angioplasty with transfusion and mortality: The M.O.R.T.A.L study (Mortality benefit Of Reduced Transfusion after percutaneous coronary intervention via the Arm or Leg). *Heart* **2008**, *94*, 1019–1025. [CrossRef] [PubMed]
5. Cantor, W.J.; Mehta, S.R.; Yuan, F.; Džavík, V.; Worthley, M.; Niemelä, K.; Valentin, V.; Fung, A.; Cheema, A.N.; Widimsky, P.; et al. Radial versus femoral access for elderly patients with acute coronary syndrome undergoing coronary angiography and intervention: Insights from the RIVAL trial. *Am. Heart J.* **2015**, *170*, 880–886. [CrossRef] [PubMed]
6. Romagnoli, E.; Biondi-Zoccai, G.; Sciahbasi, A.; Politi, L.; Rigattieri, S.; Pendenza, G.; Summaria, F.; Patrizi, R.; Borghi, A.; Di Russo, C.; et al. Radial Versus Femoral Randomized Investigation in ST-Segment Elevation Acute Coronary Syndrome. *J. Am. Coll. Cardiol.* **2012**, *60*, 2481–2489. [CrossRef] [PubMed]
7. Bernat, I.; Horak, D.; Stasek, J.; Mates, M.; Pesek, J.; Ostadal, P.; Hrabos, V.; Dusek, J.; Koza, J.; Sembera, Z.; et al. ST-Segment Elevation Myocardial Infarction Treated by Radial or Femoral Approach in a Multicenter Randomized Clinical Trial. *J. Am. Coll. Cardiol.* **2014**, *63*, 964–972. [CrossRef]
8. Valgimigli, M. Design and rationale for the Minimizing Adverse haemorrhagic events by TRansradial access site and systemic Implementation of angioX program. *Am. Heart J.* **2014**, *168*, 838–845.e6. [CrossRef]

9. On Behalf of the Matrix Investigators; Valgimigli, M.; Calabrò, P.; Cortese, B.; Frigoli, E.; Garducci, S.; Rubartelli, P.; Andò, G.; Santarelli, A.; Galli, M.; et al. Scientific Foundation and Possible Implications for Practice of the Minimizing Adverse Haemorrhagic Events by Transradial Access Site and Systemic Implementation of AngioX (MATRIX) Trial. *J. Cardiovasc. Trans. Res.* **2014**, *7*, 101–111. [CrossRef]
10. Valgimigli, M.; Gagnor, A.; Calabró, P.; Frigoli, E.; Leonardi, S.; Zaro, T.; Rubartelli, P.; Briguori, C.; Andò, G.; Repetto, A.; et al. Radial versus femoral access in patients with acute coronary syndromes undergoing invasive management: A randomised multicentre trial. *Lancet* **2015**, *385*, 2465–2476. [CrossRef]
11. Valgimigli, M.; Frigoli, E.; Leonardi, S.; Vranckx, P.; Rothenbühler, M.; Tebaldi, M.; Varbella, F.; Calabrò, P.; Garducci, S.; Rubartelli, P.; et al. Radial versus femoral access and bivalirudin versus unfractionated heparin in invasively managed patients with acute coronary syndrome (MATRIX): Final 1-year results of a multicentre, randomised controlled trial. *Lancet* **2018**, *392*, 835–848. [CrossRef]
12. Andò, G.; Capodanno, D. Radial Versus Femoral Access in Invasively Managed Patients with Acute Coronary Syndrome: A Systematic Review and Meta-analysis. *Ann. Intern. Med.* **2015**, *163*, 932. [CrossRef] [PubMed]
13. Andò, G.; Capodanno, D. Radial Access Reduces Mortality in Patients with Acute Coronary Syndromes. *JACC Cardiovasc. Interv.* **2016**, *9*, 660–670. [CrossRef] [PubMed]
14. Le May, M.R.; Wells, G.; So, D.Y. The safety and efficacy of femoral access vs. radial access in STEMI. In Proceedings of the ACC 2019, New Orleans, LA, USA, 18 March 2019.
15. Brzezinski, M.; Luisetti, T.; London, M.J. Radial Artery Cannulation: A Comprehensive Review of Recent Anatomic and Physiologic Investigations. *Anesth. Analg.* **2009**, *109*, 1763–1781. [CrossRef]
16. Barbeau, G.R.; Arsenault, F.; Dugas, L.; Simard, S.; Larivière, M.M. Evaluation of the ulnopalmar arterial arches with pulse oximetry and plethysmography: Comparison with the Allen's test in 1010 patients. *Am. Heart J.* **2004**, *147*, 489–493. [CrossRef]
17. De Rosa, S.; Passafaro, F.; Polimeni, A.; Sorrentino, S.; Indolfi, C. A novel quick and easy test for radial artery occlusion with the laser Doppler scan. *JACC Cardiovasc. Interv.* **2014**, *7*, e89–e90. [CrossRef]
18. Indolfi, C.; Passafaro, F.; Sorrentino, S.; Spaccarotella, C.; Mongiardo, A.; Torella, D.; Polimeni, A.; Sabatino, J.; Curcio, A.; De Rosa, S. Hand Laser Perfusion Imaging to Assess Radial Artery Patency: A Pilot Study. *J. Clin. Med.* **2018**, *7*, 319. [CrossRef]
19. Valgimigli, M.; Campo, G.; Penzo, C.; Tebaldi, M.; Biscaglia, S.; Ferrari, R. Transradial Coronary Catheterization and Intervention Across the Whole Spectrum of Allen Test Results. *J. Am. Coll. Cardiol.* **2014**, *63*, 1833–1841. [CrossRef]
20. Van Leeuwen, M.A.H.; Hollander, M.R.; van der Heijden, D.J.; van de Ven, P.M.; Opmeer, K.H.M.; Taverne, Y.J.H.J.; Ritt, M.J.P.F.; Kiemeneij, F.; van Mieghem, N.M.; van Royen, N. The ACRA Anatomy Study (Assessment of Disability After Coronary Procedures Using Radial Access): A Comprehensive Anatomic and Functional Assessment of the Vasculature of the Hand and Relation to Outcome After Transradial Catheterization. *Circ. Cardiovasc. Interv.* **2017**, *10*. [CrossRef]
21. van Leeuwen, M.A.H.; van der Heijden, D.J.; Hollander, M.R.; Mulder, M.J.; van de Ven, P.M.; Ritt, M.J.P.F.; Kiemeneij, F.; van Mieghem, N.M.; van Royen, N. ACRA Perfusion Study: The Impact of Transradial Intervention on Digital Hand Perfusion. *Circ. Cardiovasc. Interv.* **2019**, *12*. [CrossRef]
22. Rao, S.V.; Stone, G.W. Arterial access and arteriotomy site closure devices. *Nat. Rev. Cardiol.* **2016**, *13*, 641–650. [CrossRef] [PubMed]
23. Pancholy, S.B.; Sanghvi, K.A.; Patel, T.M. Radial artery access technique evaluation trial: Randomized comparison of seldinger versus modified seldinger technique for arterial access for transradial catheterization. *Catheter. Cardiovasc. Interv.* **2012**, *80*, 288–291. [CrossRef]
24. Polimeni, A.; Passafaro, F.; De Rosa, S.; Sorrentino, S.; Torella, D.; Spaccarotella, C.; Mongiardo, A.; Indolfi, C. Clinical and Procedural Outcomes of 5-French versus 6-French Sheaths in Transradial Coronary Interventions. *Medicine* **2015**, *94*, e2170. [CrossRef] [PubMed]
25. Rathore, S.; Stables, R.H.; Pauriah, M.; Hakeem, A.; Mills, J.D.; Palmer, N.D.; Perry, R.A.; Morris, J.L. Impact of Length and Hydrophilic Coating of the Introducer Sheath on Radial Artery Spasm During Transradial Coronary Intervention. *JACC Cardiovasc. Interv.* **2010**, *3*, 475–483. [CrossRef]
26. Costa, F.; van Leeuwen, M.A.H.; Daemen, J.; Diletti, R.; Kauer, F.; van Geuns, R.-J.; Ligthart, J.; Witberg, K.; Zijlstra, F.; Valgimigli, M.; et al. The Rotterdam Radial Access Research: Ultrasound-Based Radial Artery Evaluation for Diagnostic and Therapeutic Coronary Procedures. *Circ. Cardiovasc. Interv.* **2016**, *9*. [CrossRef] [PubMed]

27. Seto, A.H.; Roberts, J.S.; Abu-Fadel, M.S.; Czak, S.J.; Latif, F.; Jain, S.P.; Raza, J.A.; Mangla, A.; Panagopoulos, G.; Patel, P.M.; et al. Real-Time Ultrasound Guidance Facilitates Transradial Access. *JACC Cardiovasc. Interv.* **2015**, *8*, 283–291. [CrossRef] [PubMed]
28. Bertrand, O.F.; Rao, S.V.; Pancholy, S.; Jolly, S.S.; Rodés-Cabau, J.; Larose, É.; Costerousse, O.; Hamon, M.; Mann, T. Transradial Approach for Coronary Angiography and Interventions. *JACC Cardiovasc. Interv.* **2010**, *3*, 1022–1031. [CrossRef]
29. Sciahbasi, A.; Romagnoli, E.; Burzotta, F.; Trani, C.; Sarandrea, A.; Summaria, F.; Pendenza, G.; Tommasino, A.; Patrizi, R.; Mazzari, M.; et al. Transradial approach (left vs. right) and procedural times during percutaneous coronary procedures: TALENT study. *Am. Heart J.* **2011**, *161*, 172–179. [CrossRef]
30. Pancholy, S.B.; Joshi, P.; Shah, S.; Rao, S.V.; Bertrand, O.F.; Patel, T.M. Effect of Vascular Access Site Choice on Radiation Exposure During Coronary Angiography. *JACC Cardiovasc. Interv.* **2015**, *8*, 1189–1196. [CrossRef]
31. Sciahbasi, A.; Frigoli, E.; Sarandrea, A.; Rothenbühler, M.; Calabrò, P.; Lupi, A.; Tomassini, F.; Cortese, B.; Rigattieri, S.; Cerrato, E.; et al. Radiation Exposure and Vascular Access in Acute Coronary Syndromes. *J. Am. Coll. Cardiol.* **2017**, *69*, 2530–2537. [CrossRef]
32. Sciahbasi, A.; Frigoli, E.; Sarandrea, A.; Calabrò, P.; Rubartelli, P.; Cortese, B.; Tomassini, F.; Zavalloni, D.; Tebaldi, M.; Calabria, P.; et al. Determinants of radiation dose during right transradial access: Insights from the RAD-MATRIX study. *Am. Heart J.* **2018**, *196*, 113–118. [CrossRef] [PubMed]
33. Andò, G.; Costa, F.; Boretti, I.; Trio, O.; Valgimigli, M. Benefit of radial approach in reducing the incidence of acute kidney injury after percutaneous coronary intervention: A meta-analysis of 22,108 patients. *Int. J. Cardiol.* **2015**, *179*, 309–311. [CrossRef] [PubMed]
34. Andò, G.; Costa, F.; Trio, O.; Oreto, G.; Valgimigli, M. Impact of vascular access on acute kidney injury after percutaneous coronary intervention. *Cardiovasc. Revasc. Med.* **2016**, *17*, 333–338. [CrossRef] [PubMed]
35. Andò, G.; Cortese, B.; Russo, F.; Rothenbühler, M.; Frigoli, E.; Gargiulo, G.; Briguori, C.; Vranckx, P.; Leonardi, S.; Guiducci, V.; et al. Acute Kidney Injury After Radial or Femoral Access for Invasive Acute Coronary Syndrome Management. *J. Am. Coll. Cardiol.* **2017**, *69*, 2592–2603. [CrossRef]
36. Rothenbühler, M.; Valgimigli, M.; Odutayo, A.; Frigoli, E.; Leonardi, S.; Vranckx, P.; Turturo, M.; Moretti, L.; Amico, F.; Uguccioni, L.; et al. Association of acute kidney injury and bleeding events with mortality after radial or femoral access in patients with acute coronary syndrome undergoing invasive management: Secondary analysis of a randomized clinical trial. *Eur. Heart J.* **2019**, *40*, 1226–1232. [CrossRef]
37. Amato, J.J.; Solod, E.; Cleveland, R.J. A "second" radial artery for monitoring the perioperative pediatric cardiac patient. *J. Pediatr. Surg.* **1977**, *12*, 715–717. [CrossRef]
38. Kiemeneij, F. Left distal transradial access in the anatomical snuffbox for coronary angiography (ldTRA) and interventions (ldTRI). *EuroIntervention* **2017**, *13*, 851–857. [CrossRef]
39. Davies, R.E.; Gilchrist, I.C. Back hand approach to radial access: The snuff box approach. *Cardiovasc. Revasc. Med.* **2018**, *19*, 324–326. [CrossRef]
40. Babunashvili, A.; Dundua, D. Recanalization and reuse of early occluded radial artery within 6 days after previous transradial diagnostic procedure. *Catheter. Cardiovasc. Interv.* **2011**, *77*, 530–536. [CrossRef]
41. Indolfi, C.; Passafaro, F.; Mongiardo, A.; Spaccarotella, C.; Torella, D.; Sorrentino, S.; Polimeni, A.; Emanuele, V.; Curcio, A.; De Rosa, S. Delayed sudden radial artery rupture after left transradial coronary catheterization: A case report. *Medicine* **2015**, *94*, e634. [CrossRef]
42. Lee, S.H. Wonju Severance Christian Hospital, Wonju, Gangwon-do, Korea, Comparison of Success Rate Between Distal Radial Approach and Radial Approach in STEMI. Available online: https://clinicaltrials.gov/ct2/show/NCT03611725 (accessed on 20 September 2019).
43. Pancholy, S.; Coppola, J.; Patel, T.; Roke-Thomas, M. Prevention of radial artery occlusion-Patent hemostasis evaluation trial (PROPHET study): A randomized comparison of traditional versus patency documented hemostasis after transradial catheterization: Prevention of Radial Artery Occlusion. *Catheter. Cardiovasc. Interv.* **2008**, *72*, 335–340. [CrossRef] [PubMed]
44. Pancholy, S.B.; Bernat, I.; Bertrand, O.F.; Patel, T.M. Prevention of Radial Artery Occlusion After Transradial Catheterization: The PROPHET-II Randomized Trial. *JACC Cardiovasc. Interv.* **2016**, *9*, 1992–1999. [CrossRef] [PubMed]
45. Pancholy, S.B.; Patel, T.M. Effect of duration of hemostatic compression on radial artery occlusion after transradial access. *Catheter. Cardiovasc. Interv.* **2012**, *79*, 78–81. [CrossRef] [PubMed]

46. Rao, S.V.; Bernat, I.; Bertrand, O.F. Remaining challenges and opportunities for improvement in percutaneous transradial coronary procedures. *Eur. Heart J.* **2012**, *33*, 2521–2526. [CrossRef]
47. Wagener, J.F.; Rao, S.V. Radial artery occlusion after transradial approach to cardiac catheterization. *Curr. Atheroscler. Rep.* **2015**, *17*, 489. [CrossRef]
48. Pancholy, S.B. Strategies to prevent radial artery occlusion after transradial PCI. *Curr. Cardiol. Rep.* **2014**, *16*, 505. [CrossRef]
49. Spaulding, C.; Lefèvre, T.; Funck, F.; Thébault, B.; Chauveau, M.; Ben Hamda, K.; Chalet, Y.; Monségu, H.; Tsocanakis, O.; Py, A.; et al. Left radial approach for coronary angiography: Results of a prospective study. *Catheter. Cardiovasc. Diagn.* **1996**, *39*, 365–370. [CrossRef]
50. Dharma, S.; Kedev, S.; Patel, T.; Kiemeneij, F.; Gilchrist, I.C. A novel approach to reduce radial artery occlusion after transradial catheterization: Postprocedural/prehemostasis intra-arterial nitroglycerin. *Catheter. Cardiovasc. Interv.* **2015**, *85*, 818–825. [CrossRef]
51. Kwok, C.S.; Rashid, M.; Fraser, D.; Nolan, J.; Mamas, M. Intra-arterial vasodilators to prevent radial artery spasm: A systematic review and pooled analysis of clinical studies. *Cardiovasc. Revasc. Med.* **2015**, *16*, 484–490. [CrossRef]
52. Webb, J.G.; Wood, D.A. Current status of transcatheter aortic valve replacement. *J. Am. Coll. Cardiol.* **2012**, *60*, 483–492. [CrossRef]
53. Werdan, K.; Gielen, S.; Ebelt, H.; Hochman, J.S. Mechanical circulatory support in cardiogenic shock. *Eur. Heart J.* **2014**, *35*, 156–167. [CrossRef] [PubMed]
54. Alaswad, K.; Menon, R.V.; Christopoulos, G.; Lombardi, W.L.; Karmpaliotis, D.; Grantham, J.A.; Marso, S.P.; Wyman, M.R.; Pokala, N.R.; Patel, S.M.; et al. Transradial approach for coronary chronic total occlusion interventions: Insights from a contemporary multicenter registry. *Catheter. Cardiovasc. Interv.* **2015**, *85*, 1123–1129. [CrossRef] [PubMed]
55. Tanaka, Y.; Moriyama, N.; Ochiai, T.; Takada, T.; Tobita, K.; Shishido, K.; Sugitatsu, K.; Yamanaka, F.; Mizuno, S.; Murakami, M.; et al. Transradial Coronary Interventions for Complex Chronic Total Occlusions. *JACC Cardiovasc. Interv.* **2017**, *10*, 235–243. [CrossRef] [PubMed]
56. Gokhroo, R.; Kishor, K.; Ranwa, B.; Bisht, D.; Gupta, S.; Padmanabhan, D.; Avinash, A. Ulnar Artery Interventions Non-Inferior to Radial Approach: AJmer Ulnar ARtery (AJULAR) Intervention Working Group Study Results. *J Invasive Cardiol.* **2016**, *28*, 1–8. [PubMed]
57. Liu, J.; Fu, X.-H.; Xue, L.; Wu, W.-L.; Gu, X.-S.; Li, S.-Q. A comparative study of transulnar and transradial artery access for percutaneous coronary intervention in patients with acute coronary syndrome. *J. Interv. Cardiol.* **2014**, *27*, 525–530. [CrossRef]
58. Kedev, S.; Zafirovska, B.; Dharma, S.; Petkoska, D. Safety and feasibility of transulnar catheterization when ipsilateral radial access is not available. *Catheter. Cardiovasc. Interv.* **2014**, *83*, E51–E60. [CrossRef]
59. Geng, W.; Fu, X.; Gu, X.; Jiang, Y.; Fan, W.; Wang, Y.; Li, W.; Xing, K.; Liu, C. Safety and feasibility of transulnar versus transradial artery approach for coronary catheterization in non-selective patients. *Chin. Med. J.* **2014**, *127*, 1222–1228.
60. Deshmukh, A.R.; Kaushik, M.; Aboeata, A.; Abuzetun, J.; Burns, T.L.; Nubel, C.A.; White, M.D.; Lanspa, T.J.; Hunter, C.B.; Mooss, A.N.; et al. Efficacy and safety of transulnar coronary angiography and interventions—A single center experience. *Catheter. Cardiovasc. Interv.* **2014**, *83*, E26–E31. [CrossRef]
61. Kwan, T.W.; Ratcliffe, J.A.; Chaudhry, M.; Huang, Y.; Wong, S.; Zhou, X.; Pancholy, S.; Patel, T. Transulnar catheterization in patients with ipsilateral radial artery occlusion. *Catheter. Cardiovasc. Interv.* **2013**, *82*, E849–E855. [CrossRef]
62. Hahalis, G.; Tsigkas, G.; Xanthopoulou, I.; Deftereos, S.; Ziakas, A.; Raisakis, K.; Pappas, C.; Sourgounis, A.; Grapsas, N.; Davlouros, P.; et al. Transulnar compared with transradial artery approach as a default strategy for coronary procedures: A randomized trial. The Transulnar or Transradial Instead of Coronary Transfemoral Angiographies Study (the AURA of ARTEMIS Study). *Circ. Cardiovasc. Interv.* **2013**, *6*, 252–261. [CrossRef]
63. Aptecar, E.; Pernes, J.-M.; Chabane-Chaouch, M.; Bussy, N.; Catarino, G.; Shahmir, A.; Bougrini, K.; Dupouy, P. Transulnar versus transradial artery approach for coronary angioplasty: The PCVI-CUBA study. *Catheter. Cardiovasc. Interv.* **2006**, *67*, 711–720. [CrossRef] [PubMed]

64. Li, Y.-Z.; Zhou, Y.-J.; Zhao, Y.-X.; Guo, Y.-H.; Liu, Y.-Y.; Shi, D.-M.; Wang, Z.-J.; Jia, D.-A.; Yang, S.-W.; Nie, B.; et al. Safety and efficacy of transulnar approach for coronary angiography and intervention. *Chin. Med. J.* **2010**, *123*, 1774–1779. [PubMed]
65. Bi, X.; Wang, Q.; Liu, D.; Gan, Q.; Liu, L. Is the Complication Rate of Ulnar and Radial Approaches for Coronary Artery Intervention the Same? *Angiology* **2017**, *68*, 919–925. [CrossRef] [PubMed]
66. Fernandez, R.; Zaky, F.; Ekmejian, A.; Curtis, E.; Lee, A. Safety and efficacy of ulnar artery approach for percutaneous cardiac catheterization: Systematic review and meta-analysis. *Catheter. Cardiovasc. Interv.* **2018**, *91*, 1273–1280. [CrossRef] [PubMed]
67. Sanghvi, K.; Kurian, D.; Coppola, J. Transradial intervention of iliac and superficial femoral artery disease is feasible. *J. Interv. Cardiol.* **2008**, *21*, 385–387. [CrossRef] [PubMed]
68. Allende, R.; Ribeiro, H.B.; Puri, R.; Urena, M.; Abdul-Jawad, O.; del Trigo, M.; Veiga, G.; del Rosario Ortas, M.; Paradis, J.-M.; De Larochellière, R.; et al. The transradial approach during transcatheter structural heart disease interventions: A review. *Eur. J. Clin. Investig.* **2015**, *45*, 215–225. [CrossRef]
69. Sawaya, F.J.; Louvard, Y.; Spaziano, M.; Morice, M.-C.; Hage, F.; El-Khoury, C.; Roy, A.; Garot, P.; Hovasse, T.; Benamer, H.; et al. Short and long-term outcomes of alcohol septal ablation with the trans-radial versus the trans-femoral approach: A single center-experience. *Int. J. Cardiol.* **2016**, *220*, 7–13. [CrossRef]
70. Osken, A.; Aydin, E.; Akdemir, R.; Gunduz, H. Percutaneous Closure of an Aortic Prosthetic Paravalvular Leak with Device in a Patient Presenting with Heart Failure. *Heart Views* **2015**, *16*, 56–58. [CrossRef]
71. Sanghvi, K.; Selvaraj, N.; Luft, U. Percutaneous closure of a perimembranous ventricular septal defect through arm approach (radial artery and basilic vein). *J. Interv. Cardiol.* **2014**, *27*, 199–203. [CrossRef]
72. Saia, F.; Marrozzini, C.; Moretti, C.; Ciuca, C.; Taglieri, N.; Bordoni, B.; Dall'ara, G.; Alessi, L.; Lanzillotti, V.; Bacchi-Reggiani, M.L.; et al. The role of percutaneous balloon aortic valvuloplasty as a bridge for transcatheter aortic valve implantation. *EuroIntervention* **2011**, *7*, 723–729. [CrossRef]
73. Kumar, A.; Paniagua, D.; Hira, R.S.; Alam, M.; Denktas, A.E.; Jneid, H. Balloon Aortic Valvuloplasty in the Transcatheter Aortic Valve Replacement Era. *J. Invasive Cardiol.* **2016**, *28*, 341–348. [PubMed]
74. Tumscitz, C.; Campo, G.; Tebaldi, M.; Gallo, F.; Pirani, L.; Biscaglia, S. Safety and Feasibility of Transradial Mini-Invasive Balloon Aortic Valvuloplasty: A Pilot Study. *JACC Cardiovasc. Interv.* **2017**, *10*, 1375–1377. [CrossRef] [PubMed]
75. Kadakia, M.B.; Herrmann, H.C.; Desai, N.D.; Fox, Z.; Ogbara, J.; Anwaruddin, S.; Jagasia, D.; Bavaria, J.E.; Szeto, W.Y.; Vallabhajosyula, P.; et al. Factors associated with vascular complications in patients undergoing balloon-expandable transfemoral transcatheter aortic valve replacement via open versus percutaneous approaches. *Circ. Cardiovasc. Interv.* **2014**, *7*, 570–576. [CrossRef] [PubMed]
76. van Son, J.A.; Smedts, F.; Vincent, J.G.; van Lier, H.J.; Kubat, K. Comparative anatomic studies of various arterial conduits for myocardial revascularization. *J. Thorac. Cardiovasc. Surg.* **1990**, *99*, 703–707.
77. Gkaliagkousi, E.; Douma, S. The pathogenesis of arterial stiffness and its prognostic value in essential hypertension and cardiovascular diseases. *Hippokratia* **2009**, *13*, 70–75.
78. Faurie, B.; Abdellaoui, M.; Wautot, F.; Staat, P.; Champagnac, D.; Wintzer-Wehekind, J.; Vanzetto, G.; Bertrand, B.; Monségu, J. Rapid pacing using the left ventricular guidewire: Reviving an old technique to simplify BAV and TAVI procedures. *Catheter. Cardiovasc. Interv.* **2016**, *88*, 988–993. [CrossRef]

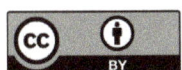

© 2019 by the authors. Licensee MDPI, Basel, Switzerland. This article is an open access article distributed under the terms and conditions of the Creative Commons Attribution (CC BY) license (http://creativecommons.org/licenses/by/4.0/).

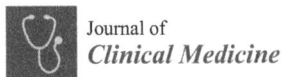

Review

Right Heart Catheterization—Background, Physiological Basics, and Clinical Implications

Grzegorz M. Kubiak [1], Agnieszka Ciarka [2], Monika Biniecka [3] and Piotr Ceranowicz [4],*

[1] Department of Cardiac, Vascular and Endovascular Surgery and Transplantology, Silesian Centre for Heart Diseases, Medical University of Silesia, 41-800 Zabrze, Poland
[2] Department of Cardiovascular Diseases, University Hospitals Leuven, University of Leuven, Herestraat 49, Leuven 3000, Belgium
[3] KardioMed Silesia, M. Curie-Skłodowskiej 10C, 41-800 Zabrze, Poland
[4] Department of Physiology, Faculty of Medicine, Jagiellonian University Medical College, 31-008 Kraków, Poland
* Correspondence: piotr.ceranowicz@uj.edu.pl

Received: 5 July 2019; Accepted: 25 August 2019; Published: 28 August 2019

Abstract: The idea of right heart catheterization (RHC) grew in the milieu of modern thinking about the cardiovascular system, influenced by the experiments of William Harvey, which were inspired by the treatises of Greek philosophers like Aristotle and Gallen, who made significant contributions to the subject. RHC was first discovered in the eighteenth century by William Hale and was subsequently systematically improved by outstanding experiments in the field of physiology, led by Cournand and Dickinson Richards, which finally resulted in the implementation of pulmonary artery catheters (PAC) into clinical practice by Jeremy Swan and William Ganz in the early 1970s. Despite its premature euphoric reception, some further analysis seemed not to share the early enthusiasm as far as the safety and effectiveness issues were concerned. Nonetheless, RHC kept its significant role in the diagnosis, prognostic evaluation, and decision-making of pulmonary hypertension and heart failure patients. Its role in the treatment of end-stage heart failure seems not to be fully understood, although it is promising. PAC-guided optimization of the treatment of patients with ventricular assist devices and its beneficial introduction into clinical practice remains a challenge for the near future.

Keywords: right heart catheterization; pulmonary hypertension; heart failure; diagnosis; prognostic evaluation; clinical implications

1. Introduction

1.1. Aim of the Review

To elucidate the state of the art of right heart catheterization, focusing on the background of the initial experiments and its physiological meaning, which leads to its implementation in clinical practice. To indicate potential directions for future research.

1.2. From Greek Philosophy into Modern Understanding

Right heart catheterization (RHC) has emerged as an invasive procedure with a potent role among the current armory of clinical diagnostic tools, including computed tomography (CT), magnetic resonance imaging (MRI), and genetical immunoassays sampling [1,2]. The birth of this technique is strictly associated with the genial English physiologist and physician William Harvey (1578–1657), who actually proposed a theoretical model of the functioning of an animal circulatory system, which he unveiled in the work entitled Exercitatio Anatomica de Motu Cordis et Sanguinis in Animalibus and published in 1628 in Frankfurt [3].

The work, containing 17 chapters within 72 pages, irretrievably changed the modern understanding of the blood circulation. It is important to keep in mind that Galen was the first person to make extraordinary contributions to the concepts of physiology and medicine that turned out to be widely accepted paradigms. He believed that the circulatory system consisted of two separated parts: venous, originating from the liver, and arterial, originating from the heart. The idea of two separate, unidirectional systems of distribution rather than a unified system of circulation remained unchallenged for many centuries. Harvey, although heavily influenced by his potent predecessor, unwillingly found himself in the position of a revolutionary antagonizer. Harvey's way of thinking and analyzing different phenomena was heavily influenced by another ancient Greek philosopher, Aristotle [4,5]. The Aristotelian way of thinking would be to engage not only rigorous mathematical calculations but also analogies to the natural phenomena covered by physics, biology, and other empirical sciences.

"De motu cordis" was released in Europe during the Thirty Years' War, described as one of the most destructive and violent periods in human history. This era was characterized by different political, religious, and cultural movements (the Reformation, Counter-reformation, and forming of the Anglican Church). During these times of overwhelming crime, plagues, and the rising wave of inquisition, the signs of independent thinking, especially when based on evidence and experiments, were unwanted and considered dangerous [6,7].

1.3. Pioneers of Right Heart Catheterization

As time passed, further attempts to experimentally evaluate the circulatory system were made. In 1711, Stephen Hale reported the measurement of cardiac output (CO) with the use of brass pipes introduced into equine veins and arteries [8–11]. The technical aspects of these examinations were further improved by Claude Bernard, who challenged the pulmonary combustion model of circulation, claiming that the blood temperature varies significantly between the systemic and pulmonary circulatory system [12]. Since his previous attempts to encounter surgical techniques in the temperature measurement appeared to be inaccurate, Bernard developed the technique of exposing the jugular vein and carotid artery of a horse in order to perform the measurements above. Bernard proved the technical feasibility of those examinations, which were continued by another two French physiologists, Baptiste Chauveau and Étienne Marey [13–15]. The collaboration of these has been linked to the virtual beginning of intracardiac pressure recordings.

The innovative dual-lumen catheter device was designed to simultaneously assess the intracardiac pressures of the left ventricle and the aorta, as well as the atrium and the right ventricle. These experiments discovered the so far unreported phenomena of ventricular pressure curves, isometric phase of ventricular contraction, interventricular synchrony, and the chronology of valve closing. It is worth noting that Marey was also renowned as a pioneer of electrocardiography, with significant contributions in the field made by the discovery of the refractory period in 1875 and the first recording of electrocardiogram with the use of capillary electrometer in 1876 [16].

Remarkably, it was nearly three decades before Willem Einthoven reported his invention, which was about to revolutionize the modern diagnosis and treatment of cardiovascular disorders. In his late years, Marey, being somehow possessed by the idea of a general visualization of the motion of different species present in the environment, turned his professional activity towards chronophotography, which he documented in books entitled *Le mouvement* and *Le vol des oiseaux* [17].

1.4. Nobel Prize for the Famous Three

German scientists Fritz Bleichroeder, Ernst Unger, and W. Loeb continued the pathway of right heart catheterization in animals, and performed self-experiments in that field; however, these were scarcely documented [18]. A breakthrough came when a recently graduated doctor Werner Forssmann performed the first in-vivo catheterization of his own heart, which took place in Eberswalde in 1929 [19–24]. This experiment was an act of bravery which took the human cardiac catheterization from theory into practice in a short period of time. Forssmann's attitude towards the National Socialist

German Workers' Party (NSDAP) arose from the phase of an early euphoria into the late deception and was basically indifferent from the typical attitude of his fellow countrymen [25].

The denazification process, to which he had been submitted in the late 1940s, did not alter his recognition in the area of right catheterization, for which he was awarded the Nobel Prize in 1956, along with Doctors André Cournand and Dickinson Richards. Remarkably, Doctors Cournand and Richards, during their work at the Department of Physiology of the Bellevue Hospital in New York, made an extraordinary contribution to the refinement of the antecedents techniques; they were the first to report a reliable measurement of CO using the Fick principle [26].

1.5. Jeremy Swan and William Ganz—Catheterization in Clinical Practice

Moreover, they understood the phenomenon of oxygen debt in the setting of "clinical shock", which they managed to treat successfully with the implementation of a human serum albumin [27]. These observations set the stage for future scientific research in the field of different kinds of shock, their risk stratification and management [28,29]. Interestingly, Cournand positively verified the usefulness of a ballistocardiogram and its correlation with the results of invasive measurement of CO performed using the Fick principle [30]. Having proven that the catheter might be uneventfully left in the right heart cavities for a prolonged period, exceeding twenty-four hours, some further improvements were made, which eventually evolved into the discovery of the pulmonary capillary/artery wedge pressure (PCWP/PAWP).

Its monitoring, first demonstrated by Hellems and co-workers, was a fairly safe technique of estimating left atrial pressure in the absence of mitral regurgitation [31]. Remarkably, another innovation was associated with the introduction of a balloon at the end of the tip, whose presence facilitated migration with the blood flow [32,33]. Another improvement was associated with the utilization of the thermodilution method to precisely assess CO. Needless to say, it added important information that, along with the modifications above, appears safe and reliable [34,35]. To see the milestones of RHC, please refer to Figure 1.

1.6. Technique of the Measurement and Basic Definitions

The preferred access point is the internal jugular vein. Its patency and anatomical conditions are reassured during an ultrasound examination, which is believed to reduce access site complications [36–39]. The currently used Seldinger technique is based on the principle of a guiding wire that enters into the vessel lumen. After an anatomical evaluation of a correct position, a special, dedicated sheath with a valve is inserted into the lumen, enabling easy access into the internal jugular vein and the subsequent structures [40–43]. A Swan-Ganz (S-G) catheter, basically not different from the prototype used by its inventors in 1970, is inserted via the internal jugular vein into the right atrium, ventricle, and pulmonary arteries. In some cases, RHC might be technically demanding, particularly in individuals with severely dilated right ventricle (RV) due to pulmonary hypertension, severe tricuspid regurgitation (TR), or other obstacles located in the right heart, like pacemaker leads or artificial valves. In these cases, the use of fluoroscopic guidance or even the angioplasty wire in order to acquire an adequate PAWP may be beneficial. An unreliable PAWP value may be verified by a direct left ventricular end-diastolic pressure (LVEDP) measurement via the arterial access [44]. Several potential pitfalls may occur during RHC. It should be underlined that PAWP is vulnerable to errors in parameter of key importance in the diagnosis of pulmonary hypertension (PH). It might be either over- or, more often, under-wedged, which may lead to a misdiagnosis and, consequently, inappropriate treatment [45]. Since the PAWP is heavily dependent on respiration, it is a subject of debate whether it should be measured at the end-expiration or averaged during spontaneous breathing [44,45]. It applies mainly to the patients with respiratory disorders, in whom there is an intrathoracic pressure swing influencing the intracardiac conditions [45].

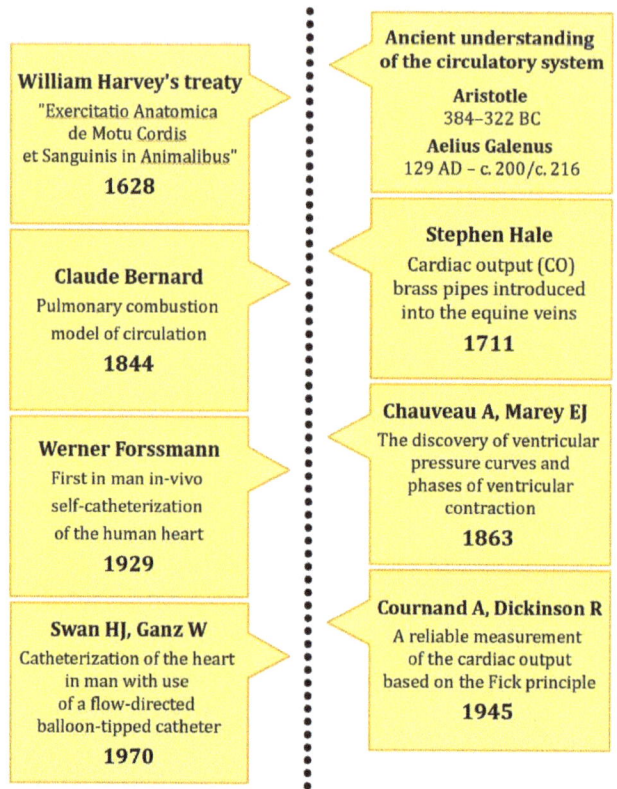

Figure 1. The milestones of right heart catheterization (RHC).

2. Physiological Aspects of Right Heart Catheterization

The European Society of Cardiology (ESC) and the European Respiratory Society (ERS) recommend performing the zeroing of the transducer at the mid-thoracic line (with the reference point defined by the crossing of the frontal plane at the mid-thoracic level, the transverse plane at the level of the fourth anterior intercostal space, and the midsagittal plane in a supine patient halfway between the anterior sternum and the bed surface [1,46]). It is important to emphasize the role of an adequate calibration of the pressure transducer; however, the theoretical and experimental background of right ventricle elasticity, along with the associations concerning volumes in different clinical states and different species, falls beyond the scope of the current review [47–56]. For research purposes, it is recommended to perform a single-beat estimation of the right ventricular end-systolic pressure–volume relationship [57–59]. To see the typical pressure curves and values assessed during RHC within the physiological states please refer to Figure 2.

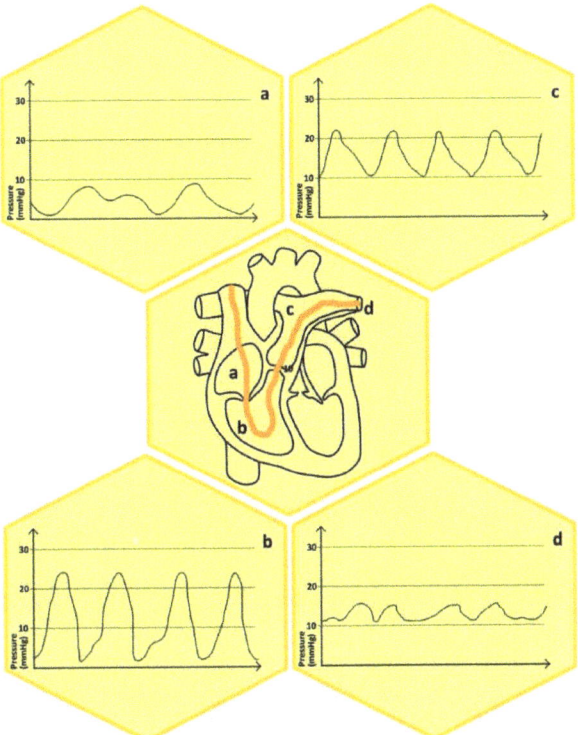

Figure 2. Typical pressure curves and values assessed during RHC within the physiological states. (**a**) right atrium, (**b**) right ventricle, (**c**) pulmonary artery, (**d**) tip of the catheter in a small artery.

After zeroing, the measurements of the right atrium, right ventricle, pulmonary artery, and capillary wedge pressure are performed. The currently accepted and recommended measurement of cardiac output is the thermodilution method, in which a constant amount of saline (usually 10 cL) is injected into the bloodstream—the difference in the temperature is analyzed by the thermistor and recorded. It is important to collect at least three to five results of CO in order to acquire reliable values, especially given that it affects the decision-making process in the real-life clinical setting (eligibility for heart transplantation, mechanical circulatory support–mono/bi–ventricular assist device). It is noteworthy that inaccurately measured, reduced CO will result in raised pulmonary vascular resistance (PVR), according to the equation (PAPm (PAPm—pulmonary artery pressure mean)—PAWP/CO = PVR). In clinical practice, the assessment of the CO by the use of thermodilution is preferred to the evaluation by the Fick method. The latter, in which the cardiac output is calculated as the quotient of oxygen uptake (O2) and the difference of the arterial and mixed venous oxygen content, is advised in the case of tricuspid regurgitation. The main limitation of the Fick method is caused by the fact that the bedside measurement of oxygen uptake is technically demanding. To see the basic definitions and range of normal values please refer to Table 1.

Table 1. Basic definitions and the range of normal values.

Parameter	Abbreviation	Normal Value	Definitions/Comments
Heart rate	HR	60–100 bpm	number of beats per minute
Stroke volume	SV	60–100 mL/beat	the amount of blood pumped by each ventricle of the heart during contraction
Cardiac output	CO	4.0–8.0 L/min	volume of blood being pumped within the minute
Body surface area	BSA	1.6–1.9 m^2	the measured or calculated surface area of a human body
Cardiac index	CI	2.5–4.0 L/min/m^2	CO/BSA
Central Venous Pressure	CVP	2–6 mmHg	superior vena cava pressure—might be used to estimate preload and right atrial pressure
Right atrial pressure	RAP	2–6 mmHg	usually RAP~CVP
Pulmonary artery pressure (systolic/diastolic/mean) (s/d/m)	PAPs/d/m	15–30/8–15/9–18 mmHg	assessed by a Swan-Ganz catheter placed in either RPA or LPA
Pulmonary artery wedge pressure	PAWP	6–12 mmHg	the inflated balloon of the catheter tip passively transmits the pressure of LA
Transpulmonary gradient	TPG	≤12 mm Hg	PAPm—PAWPm
Pulmonary vascular resistance	PVR	<3.125 WU	PAPm—PAWPm/CO
Diastolic pulmonary gradient	DPG	<7 mmHg	PAPd—PAWPm
Systemic vascular resistance	SVR	10–15 WU	SBPm—RAPm/CO

Table legend: SBPm–systemic blood pressure mean, WU–Wood Units.

3. Clinical Practice Implications

3.1. Safety of Right Heart Catheterization—The Evaluation of Clinical Outcomes

Since there existed a vital need to monitor the severely ill patients' pulmonary artery, catheterization has been widely introduced into clinical practice, including pediatrics, cardiac surgery, invasive treatments in different kinds of clinical settings, including a wide variety of shock states originating from the circulatory and/or septic background [60–68]. The use of this technology, mainly without appropriate guidance or experience, resulted in few complications, reported thereafter in the form of case reports [69–75].

These complications had different natures—from relatively mild dissections in the puncture site to serious ones with systemic clinical implications, like tricuspid valve chord rupture or pulmonary hemorrhages. Apparently, the learning curve and equipment imperfections could have been blamed to some extent; however, re-evaluation of this clinical modality of invasive cardiovascular system assessment, according to the evidence-based medicine, rapidly generated interest in the community of intensive care practitioners and physicians [76–82].

The Study to Understand Prognoses and Preferences for Outcomes and Risks of Treatments (SUPPORT) lead by Connors and co-investigators was the first prospective cohort study designed to address the issue of pulmonary artery catheter (PAC) effectiveness and costs [76]. PAC (formerly called the Swan-Ganz catheter) did not have any favorable effect, moreover it significantly raised the cost of treatment. This work has been succeeded by others, like Wheeler et al., who evaluated one thousand patients with acute lung injuries and stated that PAC did not have a positive influence on the course of the management process in comparison to the central venous catheter and should, therefore, not be used in this clinical condition [77]. Harvey and co-workers did not report any benefit from the PAC-guided treatment in severely ill patients enrolled within the "PAC-man" trial in the United Kingdom [78]. Ramsey et al. [82] retrospectively analyzed the outcomes of PAC use in non-emergent coronary artery bypass graft surgery and stated that not only did PAC not have any beneficial effect in reducing complications, but it was also associated with a two-fold increase in mortality, extended the length of hospital stay, and significantly raised the costs [82]. It referred predominantly to the low volume centers in which the PAC-derived data were apparently inadequately interpreted. These studies gradually changed the clinical practice in the USA, resulting in a decrease in PAC use in response, which was reported by Wiener and Ikuta [83,84].

3.2. The Position of Right Heart Catheterization in the Diagnostic and Management Algorithm of Heart Failure

RHC is currently often used to monitor patients and guide the therapy to optimize filling pressures and volume overloads. Some centers use it excessively in almost all patients, highlighting the point that this technique is basically less prone to subjective inter-observer variability. The Evaluation Study of Congestive Heart Failure and Pulmonary Artery Catheterization Effectiveness (ESCAPE) (85) investigators assessed the results of using RHC in 433 patients enrolled randomly in either an interventional or conservative arm. Remarkably, RHC was used intentionally to optimize pharmacological treatment, not only for those that did not prove any benefit; additionally, it was associated with a higher risk of adverse events, predominantly PAC infection [85]. Sionis [86] and co-workers analyzed the data of cardiogenic shock (CS) patients included in the CardShock registry. Eighty-two of them (37.4%) diagnosed with PAC received goal-oriented therapy consisting of mechanical ventilation, renal replacement therapy, and mechanical assist devices more often as compared to the routinely assessed group of patients ($p < 0.01$). Nevertheless, PAC use was not associated with any survival benefit within a 30-day observation period, even after propensity score-matching analysis. Doshi et al. [87] compared the trends in the utilization of PAC between 2005 and 2014 in a total of over six million of patients with heart failure (HF) with reduced or preserved ejection fraction (HFrEF/HFpEF respectively). They found that the PAC utilization per 1000 hospitalizations significantly declined from 2005 to 2010 in both HFrEF and HFpEF. On the contrary, from 2010 to 2014, the use of PAC per 1000 hospitalizations increased in both HFrEF and HFpEF. The temporary decline in risk-adjusted mortality during the study period for HFrEF and HFpEF is mostly associated with the improvements in HF therapies. Hernandez [88] and co-authors retrospectively analyzed the trends in PAC utilization between 2004 and 2014 in a total of 9,431,944 patients admitted with the primary diagnosis of HF ($n = 8,516,528$), or who developed CS ($n = 915,416$) during the index hospitalization. They observed a decline in the use of PAC in patients with HF, from 8 PAC used per 1000 admissions in 2004 to 6 PAC used per 1000 admissions in 2007. Additionally, there has been a constant rise in PAC use to 12 PAC per 1000 admissions in 2014 ($p < 0.001$). Interestingly, there has been a gradual decline in the use of PAC in patients with CS, from 123 PAC used per 1000 admissions in 2004 to 78 PAC per 1000 admissions in 2014 ($p < 0.001$). Moreover, patients with PAC had increased hospital costs, length of stay, and mechanical circulatory support use. In patients with HF, PAC use was associated with a higher mortality. In those with CS, PAC was associated with a lower mortality and lower in-hospital cardiac arrest; the paradox was also present after propensity score-matching.

Nevertheless, it should be addressed that PAC-guided therapy improved filling pressures and reduced the rates of atrium/brain natriuretic peptides (ANP/BNP) and patients' quality of life expressed by trade-off protocol. Moreover, its use did not have any impact on overall mortality and, last but not least, its implementation was not assessed in a triage of patients with cardiogenic shock or eligible for ventricular assist device (VAD)/orthotopic heart transplantation (OHT). On the other hand, Tehrani et al. proposed a different, team-based therapy for CS on the base of RHC data. This approach enabled a significant reduction in mortality from 47% in 2016 to 76.6% in 2018 ($p < 0.01$) [89]. Ma et al. re-evaluated publicly accessible data on the previously mentioned ESCAPE trial to discriminate the potential prognostic role of the invasively derived parameters [90]. Their post-hoc analysis revealed that a group of patients characterized by a single hemodynamic target, defined as PCWP + RAP ≥ 30 mmHg (congestion index), was associated with poor prognosis and increased relative risk (RR) of death (RR 5.76), death-or-transplantation (DT) (RR 4.92), and death-or-rehospitalization (DR) (RR 1.80) at six months follow-up. Moreover, this group had 45.3% mortality, 54.7% DT, and 84.9% DR at six months, contrasting with the cohort of PCWP + RAP < 30 mmHg, which had 8.7% mortality, 13.0% DT, and 58.7% DR at six months. These observations suggest that the PAC-guided treatment of filling pressures and volume overload in the specific groups of most demanding patients with end-stage heart failure or after VADs implantations needs to be assessed in randomized controlled trials [91–95], especially given that the progress in the management of HF through the last decade, including pharmacology and technical possibilities, has been promising [96]. To see the recapitulative table with the major studies and findings, please refer to Table 2, depicted below.

3.3. Position of the RHC in the Diagnostic Algorithm of Pulmonary Hypertension

RHC is currently considered a gold standard in the assessment of PH, which by definition is associated with the elevation of PAPm above 25 mmHg at rest [1,2,97]. Clinical investigation, electrocardiogram, chest radiograph, and echocardiography are the first-line examinations in this entity; however, RHC is obligatory not only to establish the definite diagnosis but also to differentiate between the subtypes of PH and prognosticate response to treatment and survival rate. Guidelines, along with the World Health Organization, classify PH into five groups of etiologic entities characterized by different hemodynamic profiles.

Pre-capillary PH is characterized by PAPm ≥ 25 mmHg, and PAWP ≤ 15 mmHg may occur in clinical groups 1, 3–5, where groups 2 and 5 in special conditions consist of different forms of post-capillary PH, which is characterized by PAPm ≥ 25 mmHg and PAWP > 15 mmHg. It can be further divided into isolated postcapillary PH with DPG (diastolic pressure gradient) < 7 mmHg and/or PVR ≤ 3 Wood Units (WU), or a combined form of either pre–and post-capillary component with DPG ≥ 7 mmHg and/or PVR > 3 WU. It needs to be underlined that the role of DPG in the diagnosis of PH has decreased recently, since it is challenging to prove its influence on a patient's prognosis [98,99]. The physiological characteristics of pulmonary hypertension presented from the clinical point of view are depicted in Figure 3.

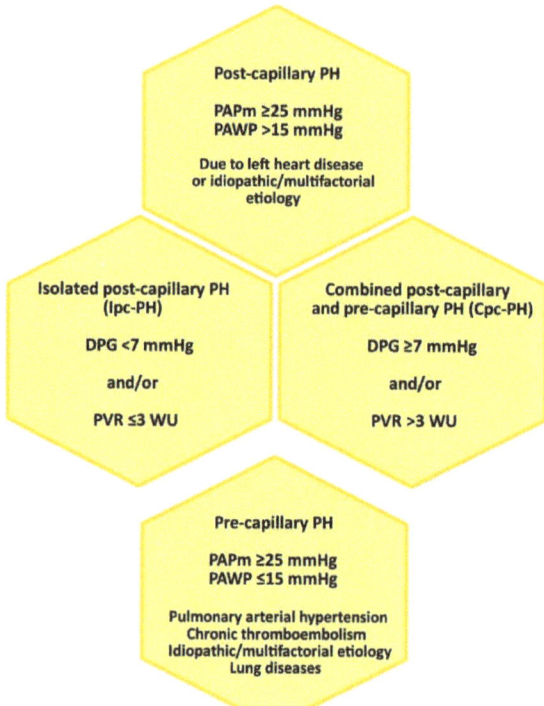

Figure 3. The clinical characteristics of pulmonary hypertension on the base of current guidelines. PH—pulmonary hypertension, PAPm—pulmonary artery pressure mean, PAWP—pulmonary artery wedge pressure, DPG—diastolic pressure gradient, PVR—pulmonary vascular resistance.

Table 2. Summary of the most important studies describing the role pulmonary artery catheters.

Author, Reference Number, and the Year of Publication	Number of Patients and the Time of Observation	Primary Condition Diagnosed/Treated	Results and Main Findings
Connors [76], 1996 "SUPPORT"	5735 pts, 180 days	Severe illness. RHC group versus no RHC group: Acute respiratory failure: 589 (27%) versus 1200 (34%) Multiorgan system failure: 1235 (57%) versus 1245 (35%) Congestive heart failure: 209 (10%) versus 247 (7%) Other: 151 (7%) versus 859 (24%)	1. Patients with RHC had an increased 30-day mortality (odds ratio, 1.24; 95% confidence interval, 1.03–1.49); 2. The mean cost (25th, 50th, 75th percentiles) per hospital stay was $49 300 ($17,000, $30,500, $56,600) with RHC and $35,700 ($11,300, $20,600, $39,200) without RHC; 3. Mean length of stay in the ICU was 14.8 (5, 9, 17) days with RHC and 13.0 (4, 7, 14) days without RHC; 4. Conclusions: After adjustment for treatment selection bias, RHC was associated with increased mortality and increased utilization of resources.
Wheeler [77], 2006	1000 pts, 60 days	Acute lung injury (ALI)	5. Patients randomized into PAC versus CVC guided therapy; 6. The rates of death during the first 60 days before discharge home were similar in the PAC and CVC groups (27.4% and 26.3%, respectively; $p = 0.69$); 7. Complications were uncommon and were reported at similar rates in each group: 0.08 ± 0.01 per catheter inserted in the PAC group and 0.06 ± 0.01 per catheter inserted in the CVC group ($p = 0.35$); 8. Conclusions: The routine use of PAC in the ALI group of pts is discouraged.
Harvey [78], 2005 "PAC-Man"	1014 pts, 90 days	Acute respiratory failure (13%), Multiorgan dysfunction (65–66%), Decompensated heart failure (11%), Other (10–11%)	9. No difference in hospital mortality between patients managed with or without a PAC (68% (346 of 506) versus 66% (333 of 507), $p = 0.39$); 10. No clear evidence of benefit or harm by managing critically ill patients with a PAC; 11. Nearly 10% of pts in the PAC arm suffered from the complications (none of these were fatal).
Ramsey [82], 2004	13,907 pts, 7–8 days	Aortocoronary bypass for heart revascularization—any type	12. The relative risk of in-hospital mortality was 2.10 for the PAC group compared with the patients who did not receive a PAC (95% confidence interval (CI), 1.40 to 3.14; $p < 0.001$); 13. The mortality risk was significantly higher in hospitals with the lowest third of PAC use (odds ratio, 3.35; 95% CI, 1.74 to 6.47; $p < 0.001$); 14. Not significantly increased in the highest two thirds of users (odds ratio, 1.62; 95% CI, 0.99 to 2.66; $p = 0.09$); 15. Days spent in critical care were similar, although total length of hospital stay was 0.26 days longer in the PAC group ($p < 0.001$); 16. Hospital costs were $1402 higher in the PAC group.
Binanay [85], 2005 "ESCAPE"	433 pts, 180 days	Severe symptomatic heart failure despite recommended therapies	17. The use of the PAC did not significantly affect the primary end point of days alive and out of the hospital during the first six months (133 days versus 135 days; hazard ratio (HR), 1.00 (95% confidence interval (CI), 0.82–1.21); $p = 0.99$); 18. Mortality (43 patients (10%) versus 38 patients (9%); odds ratio (OR), 1.26 (95% CI, 0.78–2.03); $p = 0.35$), or the number of days hospitalized (8.7 versus 8.3; HR, 1.04 (95% CI, 0.86–1.27); $p = 0.67$); 19. In-hospital adverse events were more common among patients in the PAC group (47 (21.9%) versus 25 (11.5%); $p = 0.04$); 20. There were no deaths related to PAC use; 21. No difference for in-hospital plus 30-day mortality (10 (4.7%) versus 11 (5.0%); OR, 0.97 (95% CI, 0.38–2.22); $p = 0.97$);

Table 2. *Cont.*

Author, Reference Number, and the Year of Publication	Number of Patients and the Time of Observation	Primary Condition Diagnosed/Treated	Results and Main Findings
Sionis [86], 2019 "CardShock"	219 pts, 82 (37.4%) received PAC, 30 days	Patients with cardiogenic shock included in the CardShock Study	22. Cardiogenic shock patients who managed with a PAC received more frequent treatment with inotropes and vasopressors, mechanical ventilation, renal replacement therapy, and mechanical assist devices ($p < 0.01$); 23. Overall 30-day mortality was 36.5%. Pulmonary artery catheter use did not affect mortality even after propensity score matching analysis (hazard ratio = 1.17 (0.59–2.32), $p = 0.66$).
Doshi [87], 2018	6,645,363 pts, in hospital stay between 3–17 days	HFrEF—3,225,529 hospitalizations HFpEF—3,419,834 hospitalizations	24. Per 1000 hospitalizations, the use of PAC declined from 2005 to 2010 in both HFrEF (12.9 to 7.9, $p < 0.001$) and HFpEF (12.9 to 5.5, $p < 0.001$); 25. From 2010 to 2014, the use of PAC per 1000 hospitalizations increased in both HFrEF (7.9 to 9.7, $p < 0.001$) and HFpEF (5.5 to 6.7, $p < 0.001$); 26. The temporal decline in risk-adjusted mortality during the study period for HFrEF (odds ratio, 3.93 in 2005–2006 to 2.7 in 2013–2014, $p < 0.001$) and HFpEF (odd ratio, 2.72 in 2005–2006 to 2.62 in 2013–2014, $p < 0.001$); 27. The length of stay and cost were significantly higher with PAC use in both HFrEF and HFpEF.
Hernandez [85], 2019	9,431,944 pts, in hospital stay between 2–20 days	HF ($n = 8,516,528$) index manifestation CS ($n = 915,416$) developed during the index hospitalization	28. Overall, patients with PAC had increased hospital costs, length of stay, and mechanical circulatory support use; 29. In patients with HF, PAC use was associated with higher mortality (9.9% versus 3.3% OR 3.96 $p < 0.001$); 30. In those with CS, PAC was associated with lower mortality (35.1% versus 39.2% OR 0.91 $p < 0.001$); 31. And lower in-hospital cardiac arrest (14.9% versus 18.3% OR 0.77 $p < 0.001$); 32. This paradox persisted after propensity score matching.
Tehrani [88], 2019	204 consecutive pts, 30-day survival	CS	33. Compared with a 30-day survival of 47% in 2016, the 30-day survival in 2017 and 2018 increased to 57.9% and 76.6%, respectively ($p < 0.01$); 34. Independent predictors of 30-day mortality were age ≥ 71 years, diabetes mellitus, dialysis, ≥36 h of vasopressor use at time of diagnosis, lactate levels ≥ 3.0 mg/dL, CPO < 0.6 W, and PAPi < 1.0 at 24 h after diagnosis and the implementation of therapies; 35. Either 1 or 2 points were assigned to each variable, and a three-category risk score was determined: 0 to 1 (low), 2 to 4 (moderate), and ≥5 (high); 36. Conclusions: A standardized team-based approach may improve CS outcomes; 37. A score incorporating demographic, laboratory, and hemodynamic data may be used to quantify risk and guide clinical decision-making for all phenotypes of CS.

Table legend: PAC—pulmonary artery catheter, CVC—central venous catheter, ALI—Acute Lung Injury, HR—Hazard ratio, OR—Odds ratio, CI—confidence interval, HFrEF/HFpEF—heart failure with reduced/preserved ejection fraction, CS—cardiogenic shock, CPO—cardiac power output, PAPi—pulmonary arterial pulsatility index.

The performance of vasorecactivity testing is recommended in the arterial form of PH, where it contributes significantly to the choice of the treatment regimen [100]. The encouraged vasoreactive agent is nitric oxide (NO), with a dose of 10–20 ppm, and the test is interpreted as reactive, whether the reduction in mean PAP is 10 mmHg or higher. However, the absolute value should be 40 mmHg or less [1,99]. Patients presenting significant reductions in pulmonary pressures in vasoreactivity testing during RHC may benefit from calcium channel blockers therapy, although the absolute number of these cases is quite restricted [101,102].

Some experienced heart centers use the vasoreactivity testing in heart failure scenario associated with type 2 PH as a part of the integral stratification prior to OHT. Paradoxically, increased PVR above 2.5 WU was associated with unfavorable prognosis only if it was associated with a decrease in systolic blood pressure below 85 mmHg during vasoreactive testing with sodium nitroprusside [103,104]. These data, although not standardized, sustain the theoretical assumptions that reversibility testing has the prognostic competence to discriminate the patients prone to developing acute right ventricle failure after OHT.

4. Conclusions

RHC, although present in experimental physiology and medicine since the beginning of the seventeenth century, still has safety concerns. These, however, are predominantly related to its depersonalized, randomly assigned utilization, regardless of its risk-to-benefit ratio to the patients. RHC is indispensable in PH diagnosis settlement, treatment monitoring, and decision-making. Moreover, it is imperative prior to OHT to stratify the risk of early post-operative RV failure, which might be useful in the end-stage heart failure group of patients (including VADs) in the optimization of pharmacotherapy.

Funding: The work was partly financed from Jagiellonian University Medical College.

Conflicts of Interest: The authors declare no conflict of interest.

References

1. Galiè, N.; Humbert, M.; Vachiery, J.-L.; Gibbs, S.; Lang, I.; Torbicki, A.; Simonneau, G.; Peacock, A.; Vonk Noordegraaf, A.; Beghetti, M.; et al. 2015 ESC/ERS Guidelines for the Diagnosis and Treatment of Pulmonary Hypertension. *Rev. Esp. Cardiol. Engl. Ed.* **2016**, *69*, 177. [PubMed]
2. Task Force for Diagnosis and Treatment of Pulmonary Hypertension of European Society of Cardiology (ESC); European Respiratory Society (ERS); International Society of Heart and Lung Transplantation (ISHLT); Galiè, N.; Hoeper, M.M.; Humbert, M.; Torbicki, A.; Vachiery, J.-L.; Barbera, J.A.; Beghetti, M.; et al. Guidelines for the Diagnosis and Treatment of Pulmonary Hypertension. *Eur. Respir. J.* **2009**, *34*, 1219–1263.
3. Pasipoularides, A. Greek Underpinnings to His Methodology in Unraveling De Motu Cordis and What Harvey Has to Teach Us Still Today. *Int. J. Cardiol.* **2013**, *168*, 3173–3182. [CrossRef] [PubMed]
4. Lo Presti, R. The Theory of the Circulation of Blood and (Different) Paths of Aristotelianism. Girolamo Franzosi's De Motu Cordis et Sanguinis in Animalibus pro Aristotele et Galeno Adversus Anatomicos Neotericos Libri Duo: Teleology versus Mechanism? *Gesnerus* **2014**, *71*, 271–289. [PubMed]
5. Pasipoularides, A. Historical Perspective: Harvey's Epoch-Making Discovery of the Circulation, Its Historical Antecedents, and Some Initial Consequences on Medical Practice. *J. Appl. Physiol.* **2013**, *114*, 1493–1503. [CrossRef] [PubMed]
6. Outram, Q. The Socio-Economic Relations of Warfare and the Military Mortality Crises of the Thirty Years' War. *Med. Hist.* **2001**, *45*, 151–184. [CrossRef] [PubMed]
7. Bruning, H. Life at German universities at the time of the Thirty Years War. *Med. Monatsschr.* **1954**, *8*, 830–832.
8. Hoff, H.E.; Geddes, L.A.; McCrady, J.D. The Contributions of the Horse to Knowledge of the Heart and Circulation. 1. Stephen Hales and the Measurement of Blood Pressure. *Conn. Med.* **1965**, *29*, 795–800.
9. Geddes, L.A.; Hoff, H.E.; Mccrady, J.D. Some aspects of the cardiovascular physiology of the horse. *Cardiovasc. Res. Cent. Bull.* **1965**, *4*, 80–95.

10. Geddes, L.A.; McCrady, J.D.; Hoff, H.E. The Contribution of the Horse to Knowledge of the Heart and Circulation. II. Cardiac Catheterization and Ventricular Dynamics. *Conn. Med.* **1965**, *29*, 864–876.
11. Braun, R. Voyaging in the Vein: Medical Experimentation with Heart Catheters in the Twentieth Century. *Nuncius* **2011**, *26*, 132–158. [CrossRef] [PubMed]
12. Cournand, A. Historical Details of Claude Bernard's Invention of a Technique for Measuring the Temperature and the Pressure of the Blood within the Cavities of the Heart. *Trans. N. Y. Acad. Sci.* **1980**, *39*, 1–14. [CrossRef] [PubMed]
13. Bourassa, M.G. The History of Cardiac Catheterization. *Can. J. Cardiol.* **2005**, *21*, 1011–1014. [PubMed]
14. Sette, P.; Dorizzi, R.M.; Azzini, A.M. Vascular Access: An Historical Perspective from Sir William Harvey to the 1956 Nobel Prize to André F. Cournand, Werner Forssmann, and Dickinson W. Richards. *J. Vasc. Access.* **2012**, *13*, 137–144. [CrossRef] [PubMed]
15. Fye, W.B. Jean-Baptiste Auguste Chauveau. *Clin. Cardiol.* **2003**, *26*, 351–353. [CrossRef] [PubMed]
16. Barold, S.S. Willem Einthoven and the Birth of Clinical Electrocardiography a Hundred Years Ago. *Card. Electrophysiol. Rev.* **2003**, *7*, 99–104. [CrossRef] [PubMed]
17. Silverman, M.E. Etienne-Jules Marey: 19th Century Cardiovascular Physiologist and Inventor of Cinematography. *Clin. Cardiol.* **1996**, *19*, 339–341. [CrossRef] [PubMed]
18. Cournand, A. Cardiac Catheterization; Development of the Technique, Its Contributions to Experimental Medicine, and Its Initial Applications in Man. *Acta Med. Scand. Suppl.* **1975**, *579*, 3–32. [PubMed]
19. Forssmann, W. Die Sondierung des rechten Herzens [Probing of the right heart]. *Klin. Wochenschr.* **1929**, *8*, 2085–2087. [CrossRef]
20. Forssmann, W. Ueber Kontrastdarstellung der Hohlen des lebenden rechten Herzens und der Lungenschlagader [On contrast demonstration of the chambers of the living right heart and the pulmonary artery]. *Münchener Med. Wochenschr.* **1931**, *78*, 489–492.
21. Meyer, J.A. Werner Forssmann and Catheterization of the Heart, 1929. *Ann. Thorac. Surg.* **1990**, *49*, 497–499. [CrossRef]
22. Hansson, N.; Packy, L.-M.; Halling, T.; Groß, D.; Fangerau, H. From Nobody to Nobel laureate? The case of Werner Forßmann. *Urologe A* **2015**, *54*, 412–419. [CrossRef] [PubMed]
23. Hollmann, W. Werner Forssmann, Eberswalde, the 1956 Nobel Prize for Medicine. *Eur. J. Med. Res.* **2006**, *11*, 409–412. [PubMed]
24. Forssmann-Falck, R. Werner Forssmann: A Pioneer of Cardiology. *Am. J. Cardiol.* **1997**, *79*, 651–660. [CrossRef]
25. Packy, L.-M.; Krischel, M.; Gross, D. Werner Forssmann—A Nobel Prize Winner and His Political Attitude before and after 1945. *Urol. Int.* **2016**, *96*, 379–385. [CrossRef] [PubMed]
26. Cournand, A.; Riley, R.L.; Breed, E.S.; Baldwin, E.D.; Richards, D.W.; Lester, M.S.; Jones, M. Measurement of cardiac output in man using the technique of catheterization of the right auricle or ventricle. *J. Clin. Investig.* **1945**, *24*, 106–116. [CrossRef]
27. Cournand, A.; Noble, R.P.; Breed, E.S.; Lauson, H.D.; Baldwin, E.d.F.; Pinchot, G.B.; Richards, D.W. Chemical, clinical, and immunological studies on the products of human plasma fractionation. viii. clinical use of concentrated human serum albumin in shock, and comparison with whole blood and with rapid saline infusion. *J. Clin. Investig.* **1944**, *23*, 491–505. [CrossRef]
28. Kubiak, G.M.; Tomasik, A.R.; Bartus, K.; Olszanecki, R.; Ceranowicz, P. Lactate in Cardiogenic Shock—Current Understanding and Clinical Implications. *J. Physiol. Pharmacol.* **2018**, *69*, 15–21.
29. Kubiak, G.M.; Jacheć, W.; Wojciechowska, C.; Traczewska, M.; Kolaszko, A.; Kubiak, L.; Jojko, J.; Nowalany-Kozielska, E. Handheld Capillary Blood Lactate Analyzer as an Accessible and Cost-Effective Prognostic Tool for the Assessment of Death and Heart Failure Occurrence during Long-Term Follow-Up. *Dis. Markers* **2016**, *2016*, 5965782. [CrossRef]
30. Cournand, A.; Ranges, H.A.; Riley, R.L. Comparison of results of the normal ballistocardiogram and a direct fick method in measuring the cardiac output in man. *J. Clin. Investig.* **1942**, *21*, 287–294. [CrossRef]
31. Hellems, H.K.; Haynes, F.W.; Dexter, L. Pulmonary Capillary Pressure in Man. *J. Appl. Physiol.* **1949**, *2*, 24–29. [PubMed]
32. Swan, H.J.; Ganz, W.; Forrester, J.; Marcus, H.; Diamond, G.; Chonette, D. Catheterization of the Heart in Man with Use of a Flow-Directed Balloon-Tipped Catheter. *N. Engl. J. Med.* **1970**, *283*, 447–451. [CrossRef] [PubMed]

33. Lategola, M.; Rahn, H. A Self-Guiding Catheter for Cardiac and Pulmonary Arterial Catheterization and Occlusion. *Proc. Soc. Exp. Biol. Med.* **1953**, *84*, 667–668. [CrossRef] [PubMed]
34. Ganz, W.; Donoso, R.; Marcus, H.S.; Forrester, J.S.; Swan, H.J. A New Technique for Measurement of Cardiac Output by Thermodilution in Man. *Am. J. Cardiol.* **1971**, *27*, 392–396. [CrossRef]
35. Ganz, W.; Tamura, K.; Marcus, H.S.; Donoso, R.; Yoshida, S.; Swan, H.J. Measurement of Coronary Sinus Blood Flow by Continuous Thermodilution in Man. *Circulation* **1971**, *44*, 181–195. [CrossRef] [PubMed]
36. Saugel, B.; Scheeren, T.W.L.; Teboul, J.-L. Ultrasound-Guided Central Venous Catheter Placement: A Structured Review and Recommendations for Clinical Practice. *Crit. Care* **2017**, *21*, 225. [CrossRef] [PubMed]
37. Brass, P.; Hellmich, M.; Kolodziej, L.; Schick, G.; Smith, A.F. Ultrasound Guidance versus Anatomical Landmarks for Internal Jugular Vein Catheterization. *Cochrane Database Syst. Rev.* **2015**, *1*, CD006962. [CrossRef]
38. Brass, P.; Hellmich, M.; Kolodziej, L.; Schick, G.; Smith, A.F. Ultrasound Guidance versus Anatomical Landmarks for Subclavian or Femoral Vein Catheterization. *Cochrane Database Syst. Rev.* **2015**, *1*, CD011447. [CrossRef]
39. Parienti, J.-J.; Mongardon, N.; Mégarbane, B.; Mira, J.-P.; Kalfon, P.; Gros, A.; Marqué, S.; Thuong, M.; Pottier, V.; Ramakers, M.; et al. Intravascular Complications of Central Venous Catheterization by Insertion Site. *N. Engl. J. Med.* **2015**, *373*, 1220–1229. [CrossRef]
40. Ge, X.; Cavallazzi, R.; Li, C.; Pan, S.M.; Wang, Y.W.; Wang, F.-L. Central Venous Access Sites for the Prevention of Venous Thrombosis, Stenosis and Infection. *Cochrane Database Syst. Rev.* **2012**, *3*, CD004084. [CrossRef]
41. Hsu, C.C.-T.; Kwan, G.N.C.; Evans-Barns, H.; Rophael, J.A.; van Driel, M.L. Venous Cutdown versus the Seldinger Technique for Placement of Totally Implantable Venous Access Ports. *Cochrane Database Syst. Rev.* **2016**, *8*, CD008942. [CrossRef] [PubMed]
42. Muralidhar, K. Left Internal versus Right Internal Jugular Vein Access to Central Venous Circulation Using the Seldinger Technique. *J. Cardiothorac. Vasc. Anesth.* **1995**, *9*, 115–116. [CrossRef]
43. Meyer, P.; Cronier, P.; Rousseau, H.; Vicaut, E.; Choukroun, G.; Chergui, K.; Chevrel, G.; Maury, E. Difficult Peripheral Venous Access: Clinical Evaluation of a Catheter Inserted with the Seldinger Method under Ultrasound Guidance. *J. Crit. Care* **2014**, *29*, 823–827. [CrossRef] [PubMed]
44. D'Alto, M.; Dimopoulos, K.; Coghlan, J.G.; Kovacs, G.; Rosenkranz, S.; Naeije, R. Right Heart Catheterization for the Diagnosis of Pulmonary Hypertension: Controversies and Practical Issues. *Heart Fail. Clin.* **2018**, *14*, 467–477. [CrossRef] [PubMed]
45. Rosenkranz, S.; Preston, I.R. Right heart catheterisation: Best practice and pitfalls in pulmonary hypertension. *Eur. Respir. Rev.* **2015**, *24*, 642–652. [CrossRef] [PubMed]
46. Kovacs, G.; Avian, A.; Pienn, M.; Naeije, R.; Olschewski, H. Reading Pulmonary Vascular Pressure Tracings. How to Handle the Problems of Zero Leveling and Respiratory Swings. *Am. J. Respir. Crit. Care Med.* **2014**, *190*, 252–257. [CrossRef] [PubMed]
47. Taquini, A.C.; Fermoso, J.D.; Aramendia, P. Behaviour of the right ventricle following acute constriction of the pulmonary artery. *Circ. Res.* **1960**, *8*, 315–318. [CrossRef] [PubMed]
48. Suga, H.; Sagawa, K.; Shoukas, A.A. Load independence of the instantaneous pressure-volume ratio of the canine left ventricle and effects of epinephrine and heart rate on the ratio. *Circ. Res.* **1973**, *32*, 314–322. [CrossRef] [PubMed]
49. Brown, K.A.; Ditchey, R.F. Human right ventricular end-systolic pressure-volume relation defined by maximal elastance. *Circulation* **1988**, *78*, 81–91. [CrossRef]
50. Lambermont, B.; Ghuysen, A.; Kolh, P.; Tchana-Sato, V.; Segers, P.; Gérard, P.; Morimont, P.; Magis, D.; Dogné, J.M.; Masereel, B.; et al. Effects of endotoxic shock on right ventricular systolic function and mechanical efficiency. *Cardiovasc. Res.* **2003**, *59*, 412–418. [CrossRef]
51. Kuehne, T.; Yilmaz, S.; Steendijk, P.; Moore, P.; Groenink, M.; Saaed, M.; Weber, O.; Higgins, C.B.; Ewert, P.; Fleck, E.; et al. Magnetic resonance imaging analysis of right ventricular pressure-volume loops: In vivo validation and clinical application in patients with pulmonary hypertension. *Circulation* **2004**, *110*, 2010–2016. [CrossRef] [PubMed]
52. Dell'Italia, L.J.; Walsh, R.A. Application of a time-varying elastance model to right ventricular performance in man. *Cardiovasc. Res.* **1988**, *22*, 864–874. [CrossRef] [PubMed]

53. Tedford, R.J.; Mudd, J.O.; Girgis, R.E.; Mathai, S.C.; Zaiman, A.L.; Housten-Harris, T.; Boyce, D.; Kelemen, B.W.; Bacher, A.C.; Shah, A.A.; et al. Right ventricular dysfunction in systemic sclerosis associated pulmonary arterial hypertension. *Circ. Heart Fail.* **2013**, *6*, 953–963. [CrossRef] [PubMed]
54. Rondelet, B.; Dewachter, C.; Kerbaul, F.; Kang, X.; Fesler, P.; Brimioulle, S.; Naeije, R.; Dewachter, L. Prolonged overcirculation-induced pulmonary arterial hypertension as a cause of right ventricular failure. *Eur. Heart J.* **2012**, *33*, 1017–1026. [CrossRef] [PubMed]
55. Faber, M.J.; Dalinghaus, M.; Lankhuizen, I.M.; Steendijk, P.; Hop, W.C.; Schoemaker, R.G.; Duncker, D.J.; Lamers, J.M.; Helbing, W.A. Right and left ventricular function after chronic pulmonary artery banding in rats assessed with biventricular pressure-volume loops. *Am. J. Physiol. Heart Circ. Physiol.* **2006**, *291*, H1580–H1586. [CrossRef] [PubMed]
56. Rex, S.; Missant, C.; Segers, P.; Rossaint, R.; Wouters, P.F. Epoprostenol treatment of acute pulmonary hypertension is associated with a paradoxical decrease in right ventricular contractility. *Intensive Care Med.* **2008**, *34*, 179–189. [CrossRef] [PubMed]
57. Brimioulle, S.; Wauthy, P.; Ewalenko, P.; Rondelet, B.; Vermeulen, F.; Kerbaul, F.; Naeije, R. Single-Beat Estimation of Right Ventricular End-Systolic Pressure-Volume Relationship. *Am. J. Physiol. Heart Circ. Physiol.* **2003**, *284*, H1625–H1630. [CrossRef]
58. Sunagawa, K.; Yamada, A.; Senda, Y.; Kikuchi, Y.; Nakamura, M.; Shibahara, T.; Nose, Y. Estimation of the Hydromotive Source Pressure from Ejecting Beats of the Left Ventricle. *IEEE Trans. Biomed. Eng.* **1980**, *27*, 299–305. [CrossRef]
59. Trip, P.; Kind, T.; van de Veerdonk, M.C.; Marcus, J.T.; de Man, F.S.; Westerhof, N.; Vonk-Noordegraaf, A. Accurate Assessment of Load-Independent Right Ventricular Systolic Function in Patients with Pulmonary Hypertension. *J. Heart Lung Transplant.* **2013**, *32*, 50–55. [CrossRef]
60. Katz, R.W.; Pollack, M.M.; Weibley, R.E. Pulmonary artery catheterization in pediatric intensive care. *Adv. Pediatr.* **1983**, *30*, 169–190.
61. Monnet, X.; Richard, C.; Teboul, J.L. The pulmonary artery catheter in critically ill patients. Does it change outcome? *Minerva Anestesiol.* **2004**, *70*, 219–224. [PubMed]
62. Aikawa, N.; Martyn, J.A.; Burke, J.F. Pulmonary artery catheterization and thermodilution cardiac output determination in the management of critically burned patients. *Am. J. Surg.* **1978**, *135*, 811–817. [CrossRef]
63. Moser, K.M.; Spragg, R.G. Use of the balloon-tipped pulmonary artery catheter in pulmonary disease. *Ann. Intern. Med.* **1983**, *98*, 53–58. [CrossRef] [PubMed]
64. Gilbertson, A.A. Pulmonary artery catheterization and wedge pressure measurement in the general intensive therapy unit. *Br. J. Anaesth.* **1974**, *46*, 97–104. [CrossRef] [PubMed]
65. Risk, S.C.; Brandon, D.; D'Ambra, M.N.; Koski, E.G.; Hoffman, W.J.; Philbin, D.M. Indications for the use of pacing pulmonary artery catheters in cardiac surgery. *J. Cardiothorac. Vasc. Anesth.* **1992**, *6*, 275–279. [CrossRef]
66. McGee, W.T.; Mailloux, P.; Jodka, P.; Thomas, J. The pulmonary artery catheter in critical care. *Semin. Dial.* **2006**, *19*, 480–491. [CrossRef]
67. Mora, C.T.; Seltzer, J.L.; McNulty, S.E. Evaluation of a new design pulmonary artery catheter for intraoperative ventricular pacing. *J. Cardiothorac. Anesth.* **1988**, *2*, 303–308. [CrossRef]
68. Zaidan, J.R.; Freniere, S. Use of a pacing pulmonary artery catheter during cardiac surgery. *Ann. Thorac Surg.* **1983**, *35*, 633–636. [CrossRef]
69. McNabb, T.G.; Green, L.H.; Parker, F.L. A Potentially Serious Complication with Swan-Ganz Catheter Placement by the Percutaneous Internal Jugular Route. *Br. J. Anaesth.* **1975**, *47*, 895–897. [CrossRef]
70. Colvin, M.P.; Savege, T.M.; Lewis, C.T. Pulmonary Damage from a Swan-Ganz Catheter. *Br. J. Anaesth.* **1975**, *47*, 1107–1110.
71. Katz, S.A.; Cohen, E.L. Urologic Complication Associated with Swan-Ganz Catheter. *Urology* **1975**, *6*, 716–718. [CrossRef]
72. Sink, J.D.; Comer, P.B.; James, P.M.; Loveland, S.R. Evaluation of Catheter Placement in the Treatment of Venous Air Embolism. *Ann. Surg.* **1976**, *183*, 58–61. [CrossRef] [PubMed]
73. Smith, W.R.; Glauser, F.L.; Jemison, P. Ruptured Chordae of the Tricuspid Valve. The Consequence of Flow-Directed Swan-Ganz Catheterization. *Chest* **1976**, *70*, 790–792. [CrossRef] [PubMed]
74. Rubin, S.A.; Puckett, R.P. Pulmonary Artery—Bronchial Fistula: A New Complication of Swan-Ganz Catheterization. *Chest* **1979**, *75*, 515–516. [CrossRef] [PubMed]

75. Connors, J.P.; Sandza, J.G.; Shaw, R.C.; Wolff, G.A.; Lombardo, J.A. Lobar Pulmonary Hemorrhage. An Unusual Complication of Swan-Ganz Catheterization. *Arch. Surg.* **1980**, *115*, 883–885. [CrossRef] [PubMed]
76. Connors, A.F.; Speroff, T.; Dawson, N.V.; Thomas, C.; Harrell, F.E., Jr.; Wagner, D.; Desbiens, N.; Goldman, L.; Wu, A.W.; Califf, R.M.; et al. The Effectiveness of Right Heart Catheterization in the Initial Care of Critically Ill Patients. *JAMA* **1996**, *276*, 889–897. [CrossRef]
77. National Heart, Lung, and Blood Institute Acute Respiratory Distress Syndrome (ARDS) Clinical Trials Network; Wheeler, A.P.; Bernard, G.R.; Thompson, B.T.; Schoenfeld, D.; Wiedemann, H.P.; deBoisblanc, B.; Connors, A.F., Jr.; Hite, R.D.; Harabin, A.L. Pulmonary-artery versus central venous catheter to guide treatment of acute lung injury. *N. Engl. J. Med.* **2006**, *354*, 2213–2224.
78. Harvey, S.; Harrison, D.A.; Singer, M.; Ashcroft, J.; Jones, C.M.; Elbourne, D.; Brampton, W.; Williams, D.; Young, D.; Rowan, K.; et al. Assessment of the clinical effectiveness of pulmonary artery catheters in management of patients in intensive care (PAC-Man): A randomised controlled trial. *Lancet* **2005**, *366*, 472–477. [CrossRef]
79. Cohen, M.G.; Kelly, R.V.; Kong, D.F.; Menon, V.; Shah, M.; Ferreira, J.; Pieper, K.S.; Criger, D.; Poggio, R.; Ohman, E.M.; et al. Pulmonary artery catheterization in acute coronary syndromes: Insights from the GUSTO IIb and GUSTO III trials. *Am. J. Med.* **2005**, *118*, 482–488. [CrossRef]
80. Richard, C.; Warszawski, J.; Anguel, N.; Deye, N.; Combes, A.; Barnoud, D.; Boulain, T.; Lefort, Y.; Fartoukh, M.; Baud, F.; et al. Early use of the pulmonary artery catheter and outcomes in patients with shock and acute respiratory distress syndrome: A randomized controlled trial. *JAMA* **2003**, *290*, 2713–2720. [CrossRef]
81. Rhodes, A.; Cusack, R.J.; Newman, P.J.; Grounds, R.M.; Bennett, E.D. A randomised, controlled trial of the pulmonary artery catheter in critically ill patients. *Intensive Care Med.* **2002**, *28*, 256–264. [CrossRef] [PubMed]
82. Ramsey, S.D.; Saint, S.; Sullivan, S.D.; Dey, L.; Kelley, K.; Bowdle, A. Clinical and economic effects of pulmonary artery catheterization in nonemergent coronary artery bypass graft surgery. *J. Cardiothorac. Vasc. Anesth.* **2000**, *14*, 113–118. [CrossRef]
83. Wiener, R.S.; Welch, H.G. Trends in the use of the pulmonary artery catheter in the United States, 1993–2004. *JAMA* **2007**, *298*, 423–429. [CrossRef] [PubMed]
84. Ikuta, K.; Wang, Y.; Robinson, A.; Ahmad, T.; Krumholz, H.M.; Desai, N.R. National Trends in Use and Outcomes of Pulmonary Artery Catheters Among Medicare Beneficiaries, 1999–2013. *JAMA Cardiol.* **2017**, *2*, 908–913. [CrossRef] [PubMed]
85. Binanay, C.; Califf, R.M.; Hasselblad, V.; O'Connor, C.M.; Shah, M.R.; Sopko, G.; Stevenson, L.W.; Francis, G.S.; Leier, C.V.; Miller, L.W.; et al. Evaluation Study of Congestive Heart Failure and Pulmonary Artery Catheterization Effectiveness: The ESCAPE Trial. *JAMA* **2005**, *294*, 1625–1633.
86. Sionis, A.; Rivas-Lasarte, M.; Mebazaa, A.; Tarvasmäki, T.; Sans-Roselló, J.; Tolppanen, H.; Varpula, M.; Jurkko, R.; Banaszewski, M.; Silva-Cardoso, J.; et al. Current Use and Impact on 30-Day Mortality of Pulmonary Artery Catheter in Cardiogenic Shock Patients: Results From the CardShock Study. *J. Intensive Care Med.* **2019**. [CrossRef]
87. Doshi, R.; Patel, H.; Shah, P. Pulmonary artery catheterization use and mortality in hospitalizations with HFrEF and HFpEF: A nationally representative trend analysis from 2005 to 2014. *Int. J. Cardiol.* **2018**, *269*, 289–291. [CrossRef]
88. Hernandez, G.A.; Lemor, A.; Blumer, V.; Rueda, C.A.; Zalawadiya, S.; Stevenson, L.W.; Lindenfeld, J. Trends in Utilization and Outcomes of Pulmonary Artery Catheterization in Heart Failure with and Without Cardiogenic Shock. *J. Card. Fail.* **2019**, *25*, 364–371. [CrossRef]
89. Tehrani, B.N.; Truesdell, A.G.; Sherwood, M.W.; Desai, S.; Tran, H.A.; Epps, K.C.; Singh, R.; Psotka, M.; Shah, P.; Cooper, L.B.; et al. Standardized Team-Based Care for Cardiogenic Shock. *J. Am. Coll. Cardiol.* **2019**, *73*, 1659–1669. [CrossRef]
90. Ma, T.S.; Paniagua, D.; Denktas, A.E.; Jneid, H.; Kar, B.; Chan, W.; Bozkurt, B. Usefulness of the Sum of Pulmonary Capillary Wedge Pressure and Right Atrial Pressure as a Congestion Index That Prognosticates Heart Failure Survival (from the Evaluation Study of Congestive Heart Failure and Pulmonary Artery Catheterization Effectiveness Trial). *Am. J. Cardiol.* **2016**, *118*, 854–859.

91. Uriel, N.; Sayer, G.; Addetia, K.; Fedson, S.; Kim, G.H.; Rodgers, D.; Kruse, E.; Collins, K.; Adatya, S.; Sarswat, N. Hemodynamic Ramp Tests in Patients with Left Ventricular Assist Devices. *JACC Heart Fail.* **2016**, *4*, 208–217. [CrossRef] [PubMed]
92. Estep, J.D.; Vivo, R.P.; Krim, S.R.; Cordero-Reyes, A.M.; Elias, B.; Loebe, M.; Bruckner, B.A.; Bhimaraj, A.; Trachtenberg, B.H.; Ashrith, G. Echocardiographic Evaluation of Hemodynamics in Patients with Systolic Heart Failure Supported by a Continuous-Flow LVAD. *J. Am. Coll. Cardiol.* **2014**, *64*, 1231–1241. [CrossRef] [PubMed]
93. Uriel, N.; Levin, A.P.; Sayer, G.T.; Mody, K.P.; Thomas, S.S.; Adatya, S.; Yuzefpolskaya, M.; Garan, A.R.; Breskin, A.; Takayama, H. Left Ventricular Decompression During Speed Optimization Ramps in Patients Supported by Continuous-Flow Left Ventricular Assist Devices: Device-Specific Performance Characteristics and Impact on Diagnostic Algorithms. *J. Card. Fail.* **2015**, *21*, 785–791. [CrossRef] [PubMed]
94. Dean, D.A.; Jia, C.X.; Cabreriza, S.E.; D'Alessandro, D.A.; Dickstein, M.L.; Sardo, M.J.; Chalik, N.; Spotnitz, H.M. Validation study of a new transit time ultrasonic flow probe for continuous great vessel measurements. *ASAIO J.* **1996**, *42*, M671–M676. [CrossRef] [PubMed]
95. Salerno, C.T.; Sundareswaran, K.S.; Schleeter, T.P.; Moanie, S.L.; Farrar, D.J.; Walsh, M.N. Early elevations in pump power with the HeartMate II left ventricular assist device do not predict late adverse events. *J. Heart Lung. Transplant.* **2014**, *33*, 809–815. [CrossRef] [PubMed]
96. Allen, L.A.; Rogers, J.G.; Warnica, J.W.; Disalvo, T.G.; Tasissa, G.; Binanay, C.; O'Connor, C.M.; Califf, R.M.; Leier, C.V.; Shah, M.R.; et al. High Mortality without ESCAPE: The Registry of Heart Failure Patients Receiving Pulmonary Artery Catheters without Randomization. *J. Card. Fail.* **2008**, *14*, 661–669. [CrossRef] [PubMed]
97. Hoeper, M.M.; Bogaard, H.J.; Condliffe, R.; Frantz, R.; Khanna, D.; Kurzyna, M.; Langleben, D.; Manes, A.; Satoh, T.; Torres, F.; et al. Definitions and Diagnosis of Pulmonary Hypertension. *J. Am. Coll. Cardiol.* **2013**, *62* (Suppl. 25), D42–D50. [CrossRef] [PubMed]
98. Kovacs, G.; Dumitrescu, D.; Barner, A.; Greiner, S.; Grünig, E.; Hager, A.; Köhler, T.; Kozlik-Feldmann, R.; Kruck, I.; Lammers, A.E.; et al. Definition, clinical classification and initial diagnosis of pulmonary hypertension: Updated recommendations from the Cologne Consensus Conference 2018. *Int. J. Cardiol.* **2018**, *272*, S11–S19. [CrossRef] [PubMed]
99. Dragu, R.; Hardak, E.; Ohanyan, A.; Adir, Y.; Aronson, D. Prognostic value and diagnostic properties of the diastolic pulmonary pressure gradient in patients with pulmonary hypertension and left heart disease. *Int. J. Cardiol.* **2019**, *290*, 138–143. [CrossRef]
100. Rich, S.; Kaufmann, E.; Levy, P.S. The Effect of High Doses of Calcium-Channel Blockers on Survival in Primary Pulmonary Hypertension. *N. Engl. J. Med.* **1992**, *327*, 76–81. [CrossRef]
101. Sitbon, O.; Humbert, M.; Jaïs, X.; Ioos, V.; Hamid, A.M.; Provencher, S.; Garcia, G.; Parent, F.; Hervé, P.; Simonneau, G. Long-Term Response to Calcium Channel Blockers in Idiopathic Pulmonary Arterial Hypertension. *Circulation* **2005**, *111*, 3105–3111. [CrossRef] [PubMed]
102. Badesch, D.B.; Abman, S.H.; Ahearn, G.S.; Barst, R.J.; McCrory, D.C.; Simonneau, G.; McLaughlin, V.V.; American College of Chest Physicians. Medical Therapy for Pulmonary Arterial Hypertension: ACCP Evidence-Based Clinical Practice Guidelines. *Chest* **2004**, *126* (Suppl. 1), 35S–62S. [CrossRef] [PubMed]
103. Costard-Jäckle, A.; Fowler, M.B. Influence of Preoperative Pulmonary Artery Pressure on Mortality after Heart Transplantation: Testing of Potential Reversibility of Pulmonary Hypertension with Nitroprusside Is Useful in Defining a High Risk Group. *J. Am. Coll. Cardiol.* **1992**, *19*, 48–54. [CrossRef]
104. Zakliczynski, M.; Zebik, T.; Maruszewski, M.; Swierad, M.; Zembala, M. Usefulness of Pulmonary Hypertension Reversibility Test with Sodium Nitroprusside in Stratification of Early Death Risk after Orthotopic Heart Transplantation. *Transplant. Proc.* **2005**, *37*, 1346–1348. [CrossRef] [PubMed]

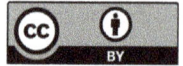

© 2019 by the authors. Licensee MDPI, Basel, Switzerland. This article is an open access article distributed under the terms and conditions of the Creative Commons Attribution (CC BY) license (http://creativecommons.org/licenses/by/4.0/).

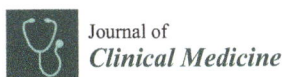

Review

Utilization of Percutaneous Mechanical Circulatory Support Devices in Cardiogenic Shock Complicating Acute Myocardial Infarction and High-Risk Percutaneous Coronary Interventions

Rabea Asleh and Jon R. Resar *

Division of Cardiology, Department of Medicine, Johns Hopkins University School of Medicine, Baltimore, MD 21205, USA
* Correspondence: jresar@jhmi.edu; Tel.: +1-(410)-614-1132

Received: 30 June 2019; Accepted: 8 August 2019; Published: 13 August 2019

Abstract: Given the tremendous progress in interventional cardiology over the last decade, a growing number of older patients, who have more comorbidities and more complex coronary artery disease, are being considered for technically challenging and high-risk percutaneous coronary interventions (PCI). The success of performing such complex PCI is increasingly dependent on the availability and improvement of mechanical circulatory support (MCS) devices, which aim to provide hemodynamic support and left ventricular (LV) unloading to enable safe and successful coronary revascularization. MCS as an adjunct to high-risk PCI may, therefore, be an important component for improvement in clinical outcomes. MCS devices in this setting can be used for two main clinical conditions: patients who present with cardiogenic shock complicating acute myocardial infarction (AMI) and those undergoing technically complex and high-risk PCI without having overt cardiogenic shock. The current article reviews the advancement in the use of various devices in both AMI complicated by cardiogenic shock and complex high-risk PCI, highlights the available hemodynamic and clinical data associated with the use of MCS devices, and presents suggestive management strategies focusing on appropriate patient selection and optimal timing and support to potentially increase the clinical benefit from utilizing these devices during PCI in this high-risk group of patients.

Keywords: mechanical circulatory support; percutaneous coronary intervention; cardiogenic shock; acute myocardial infarction; outcome; patient selection

1. Introduction

Recent advances in percutaneous coronary intervention (PCI) technologies, including mechanical circulatory support (MCS) devices, have facilitated treatment of high-risk patients with complex coronary artery disease (CAD) and low left ventricular (LV) systolic function as well as patients with acute myocardial infarction (AMI) complicated by cardiogenic shock. These high-risk patients would otherwise be poor candidates for coronary artery bypass grafting (CABG) due to high surgical morbidity and mortality risks, and the ability to provide adequate hemodynamic support using MCS devices would potentially enable safer PCI and improve outcomes as compared to unprotected PCI strategy, surgical revascularization, or medical therapy alone [1]. However, despite the preemptive improvement in hemodynamics with the use of MCS devices [2], randomized trials using intraaortic balloon pump (IABP) or Impella 2.5 devices have not demonstrated significant reduction in mortality during high-risk and complex PCI as compared to unprotected PCI [3,4]. A clinical benefit from the use of MCS in the setting of cardiogenic shock complicating AMI has also not yet been conclusively demonstrated [5,6]. Besides possible methodological flaws in these trials, other important factors might have contributed to the lack of benefit seen in these studies and should be taken into consideration, such as inadequate hemodynamic support, inappropriate patient selection, and deferred or inappropriate timing of device insertion during the course of cardiogenic shock and also in relation to PCI.

In light of the development of new generation MCS devices with greater hemodynamic support and lower device-associated complications combined with careful planning and optimal timing of device utilization, a growing body of data is suggestive of improvement in procedural success and clinical outcomes [7,8], and thus opens the door for future research in this field to examine the benefit of optimal MCS use in the setting of high risk PCI among a highly selective group of patients. Herein, we provide the most updated data available on MCS in two different situations involving high risk patients undergoing PCI: (1) high risk patients without cardiogenic shock undergoing complex PCI, and (2) patients with AMI complicated by cardiogenic shock.

2. High-Risk Percutaneous Coronary Interventions

Over the last few decades, there has been a tremendous progression in coronary interventional techniques that enables performance of PCI in complex coronary lesions (heavily calcified and type C) that would previously not have been amenable to intervention. This includes improved guide catheters and wires, mother-child guide catheters, low-profile balloons, coronary atherectomy devices, dedicated chronic total occlusion devices and algorithms, and superior stent designs that enhance deliverability to achieve complete multivessel revascularization including those involving chronic totally occluded coronary vessels. However, each aspect of PCI, beginning from guide catheter engagement and ending with balloon inflation and stent deployment, is associated with potential risk of vascular damage and impairment of myocardial perfusion. For instance, patients at advanced age, with increased comorbidities, and underlying left ventricular dysfunction, may pose a clinical challenge, as complex PCI among these patients may incur a substantial risk that overweighs any benefit achieved from revascularization [4]. On the other hand, utilization of PCI even in older adults with AMI and cardiogenic shock has been shown to be associated with substantial reduction in mortality in a recent contemporary analysis involving older adults ≥75 years of age [9]. Although clinical judgment is important, one should not, therefore, exclude patients from PCI solely based on advanced age in the absence of clear contraindications.

Among high-risk patients with active ischemia, the need and the type of revascularization should be discussed by Heart Team in an individual base. The recommendation with respect to the type of revascularization (PCI versus CABG) should be generally guided by important criteria including the predicted surgical mortality (based on the Society of Thoracic Surgeons (STS) score), the anatomical complexity of CAD (based on the SYNTAX (Synergy between Percutaneous Coronary Intervention with Taxus and Cardiac Surgery) score), and the anticipated completeness of revascularization. The risks of periprocedural complications should be weighed up against the anticipated improvement in quality of life and long-term freedom from death, MI, and repeat vascularization for electing whether conservative therapy, PCI, or CABG is the recommended strategy. According to the current ESC guidelines [10], when suitable coronary anatomy for both procedures and low predicted surgical mortality exist, patients with three-vessel disease and diabetes in particular achieve greater benefit from CABG than PCI regardless of the SYNTAX score, while in patients without diabetes CABG is favored over PCI only when SYNTAX score is intermediate or high (>22). In the presence of significant left main CAD, CABG is preferred for patients with SYNTAX score >22 irrespective of the diabetic state. However, in the presence of complex CAD anatomy (i.e., unprotected left main CAD or three-vessel disease) and high surgical mortality (i.e., previous cardiac surgery, severe comorbidities, and frailty) precluding CABG, high-risk PCI with MCS protection may be suggested as an alternative strategy for achieving complete revascularization safely in this high-risk group of patients. Although high-risk PCI has not been well defined, it can be generally categorized into three major groups based on patient characteristics, lesion characteristics, and clinical presentation [2,11] (Table 1). Patient characteristics include increased age, comorbidities (such as diabetes mellitus, chronic kidney disease, and chronic obstructive lung disease), reduced left ventricular systolic function, and prior myocardial infarction [12–14]. Lesion characteristics include anatomical and procedural variables that determine the complexity of PCI from the technical perspectives and the potential risk of complications. These include PCI of unprotected left main stenosis, bifurcation disease, heavily calcified lesions, saphenous vein grafts, and chronic total occlusions [15,16]. Finally, the clinical characteristics, among which acute coronary syndrome presentation and heart failure symptoms are important elements to take into consideration when assessing PCI risk [17]. An example of a high-risk PCI that can be facilitated by MCS is in an elderly patient with comorbidities who presents acutely with reduced LV systolic function and has a heavily calcified left main bifurcation or three-vessel coronary artery disease.

Table 1. High-Risk Percutaneous Coronary Intervention Characteristics.

Patient Characteristics
Increased age
Comorbidities (diabetes mellitus, chronic lung disease, prior myocardial infarction, peripheral arterial disease, frailty)
Severe LV systolic dysfunction (EF < 20–30%)
Severe renal function impairment (eGFR < 30 mL/min/1.73 m^2).
Lesion Characteristics
Severe three-vessel coronary artery disease
Unprotected left main stenosis
Bifurcation disease or ostial stenosis
High SYNTAX score or type C lesions
Chronic total occlusions
Saphenous vein graft disease
Heavily calcified lesions requiring coronary atherectomy
Clinical Presentation
Acute coronary syndrome
Heart failure symptoms (dyspnea, orthopnea, PND, exercise intolerance, peripheral edema)
Arrhythmias (atrial fibrillation with RVR, ventricular tachycardia)
Elevated LV end-diastolic pressure
Severe mitral regurgitation (or other valvular disease)

Abbreviations: EF, ejection fraction; eGFR, estimated glomerular filtration rate; LV, left ventricular; PND, paroxysmal nocturnal dyspnea; RVR, rapid ventricular response; SYNTAX, Synergy between Percutaneous Coronary Intervention with Taxus and Cardiac Surgery.

As high-risk PCI is associated with increased risk of myocardial ischemia and hemodynamic compromise that may lead to circulatory collapse, the purpose of MCS is to diminish myocardial oxygen consumption and provide adequate cardiac output and myocardial perfusion during the procedure. Use of appropriate MCS devices allows adequate time to safely perform complex PCI with optimal results in these high-risk patients who would not otherwise tolerate complete revascularization [18]. It is critical, therefore, that MCS device insertion in this setting is performed prior to PCI as this enables confident proceeding with revascularization without the risk of circulatory collapse that may subsequently require emergent bailout MCS implementation. Although several patient- and lesion-specific variables are well-recognized predictors of adverse outcomes after PCI, a risk score to assess the need for MCS during PCI has not yet been developed and warrants further research. Despite the lack of a risk calculator, most interventional cardiologists would now consider the use of MCS devices in patients with severely reduced LV systolic function and complex coronary artery disease involving a large territory (such as sole-remaining vessel, unprotected left main, or three-vessel disease) [11].

3. Cardiogenic Shock Complicating Acute Myocardial Infarction

Cardiogenic shock is defined as the combination of sustained systemic tissue hypoperfusion and decreased cardiac output despite adequate circulatory volume and LV filling pressure. Specific clinical and hemodynamic criteria that define cardiogenic shock include systolic blood pressure of <90 mmHg for >30 min, cardiac index <2.2 L/min/m^2 with hemodynamic support or <1.8 L/min/m^2 without support, pulmonary capillary wedge pressure (PCWP) >15 mmHg, and evidence of end-organ damage (such as urinary output <30 mL/h, high lactate levels, or cool extremities) [19,20]. Cardiogenic shock can develop because of various pathologies that affect the heart with AMI involved in the majority of cases. It occurs in 6–10% of patients with AMI and remains a leading cause of death with in-hospital mortality exceeding 50% despite the implementation of guideline-directed medical therapy and early myocardial reperfusion by primary PCI [21,22]. Consequently, patients with cardiogenic shock complicating MI represent a high-risk group of patients with compromised cardiac function and hemodynamics who are more susceptible to circulatory collapse during PCI [23]. Indeed, even though a substantial improvement in PCI techniques and pharmacology has occurred over time, this has not translated to further improvement in outcomes beyond what is achieved with prompt revascularization in the setting of cardiogenic shock [5,6]. Therefore, utilization of percutaneous MCS devices to augment cardiac output and decrease LV filling pressures by LV unloading may act as a successful adjunct to PCI as a bridge to myocardial recovery in these critically ill patients [24].

4. Hemodynamic Effects of Percutaneous Mechanical Circulatory Support Devices

The hemodynamic condition in steady state as well as in various cardiac abnormalities is illustrated by the pressure-volume loop, which provides fundamental information to the understanding of the underlying hemodynamic imbalance and the anticipated effect with the use of each type of the available MCS devices (Figure 1) [11,18]. Pressure-volume loops not only provides a platform for explaining ventricular mechanics, such as contractile and relaxation properties, stroke volume, and cardiac work, but provides a platform for understanding the determinants of myocardial oxygen consumption represented mainly by LV work [11,18,25,26]. Each one of these hemodynamic variables can be compromised based on the clinical presentation. In AMI, for example, patients may mainly present with decreased myocardial contractility and stroke volume in addition to increased myocardial oxygen demand and diminished coronary blood flow (Figure 1B). In cardiogenic shock, LV contractility and stroke volume are severely reduced, while LV end-diastolic volume (LVEDV) and pressure (LVEDP) as well as myocardial oxygen demand are considerably increased (Figure 1C). In the setting of mechanical support, the change in the volume-pressure loops is dependent on the type of the MCS device and the amount of support [18,27,28]. IABP provides modest hemodynamic support demonstrated by modest reduction in both LV systolic and diastolic pressures with afterload reduction and increase in stroke volume (Figure 1D). Percutaneous LV assist devices (including Impella and TandemHeart) result in remarkable reduction in LV systolic and diastolic pressures, LV volumes, and stroke volume resulting in significant decrease in LV work. Unlike the other forms of support, continuous pumping of blood directly from the LV by Impella is not dependent on blood ejection through the aortic valve and LV unloading can, therefore, be augmented by increasing the flow rate, thus resulting in further reduction in LV filling pressures and in myocardial oxygen demand (Figure 1E). Venoarterial extracorporeal membrane oxygenation (VA-ECMO) has the capacity to assume responsibility for the entire cardiac output providing biventricular support in combination with full gas exchange. Strictly on a hemodynamic basis and without an LV venting strategy, use of VA-ECMO results in increased LV systolic and diastolic pressures and reduced stroke volume, with a final flow-dependent increase in afterload and LVEDP (Figure 1F). Therefore, LV venting assisted by Impella or IABP may be ultimately required to mitigate LV loading and decrease left-sided filling pressures and myocardial oxygen demand, especially when the aortic valve remains persistently closed during ECMO support indicating a maximal LV loading condition.

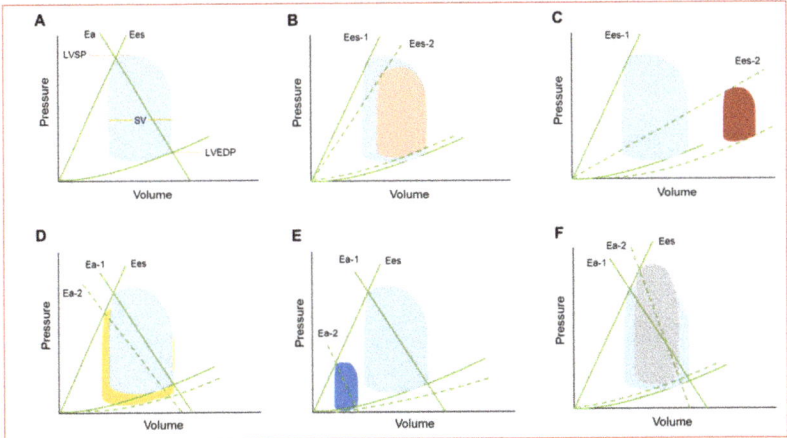

Figure 1. (**A**) Normal pressure-volume (PV) loop. Effective arterial elastance (Ea) is the slope of the line extending from the left ventricular (LV) end-diastolic pressure-volume point through the end-systolic pressure-volume point of the loop. Ea is determined by the total peripheral resistance and heart rate and gives an estimate of the LV afterload. End-systolic elastance (Ees) is the slope of the line extending from the volume-axis intercept V_0 through the end-systolic pressure-volume point of the loop and represents the ventricular contractility. The width of the PV loop represents stroke volume (SV), which can be extracted by calculating the difference between the end-diastolic and end-systolic volumes. (**B**) PV loop in the setting of acute myocardial infarction (AMI) showing decreased contractility (Ees) and SV in addition to increased LV end-diastolic pressure (LVEDP). (**C**) PV loop of patients with cardiogenic shock showing severe reduction in contractility (Ees) and SV in addition to markedly increased LVEDP and LV end-diastolic volume (LVEDV). (**D**) Illustration of PV loop change after intraaortic balloon (IABP) counterpulsation showing mildly reduced LVEDP and LV end systolic pressure (LVESP) resulting in modest afterload (Ea) reduction and increase in SV. (**E**) PV loop with percutaneous LV assist device support (Impella or TandemHeart) showing marked reduction in LVEDP, LVESP, and SV, with a net effect of substantial afterload, preload, and LV workload reduction. (**F**) LV loop with veno-arterial extracorporeal membrane oxygenation (VA-ECMO) without LV venting increases LVEDP and LVESP, while reduces stroke volume and an ultimate increase in afterload (Ea) and LV loading.

5. Available Percutaneous Mechanical Circulatory Support Devices

Several percutaneous MCS devices are currently available to assist interventional cardiologists during high-risk PCIs both for patients undergoing a complex PCI and for those requiring PCI in the setting of cardiogenic sock complicating AMI. Types of available percutaneous MCS devices and comparisons of their characteristics and hemodynamic impact are presented in Table 2 [29,30]. Generally, the goal of MCS devices is to improve cardiac power (defined as the product of mean arterial blood pressure and cardiac output), which has been demonstrated to be a strong predictor of outcomes in patients with cardiogenic shock [31,32]. Therefore, each device has its unique impact on cardiovascular hemodynamics, but an ideal MCS device should ultimately provide circulatory support to achieve adequate systemic tissue perfusion, by increasing mean arterial pressure, while concurrently decreasing myocardial oxygen demand, by reducing both LV volume (preload) and pressure (afterload).

Table 2. Comparison of Technical and Clinical Features of Contemporary Percutaneous Mechanical Circulatory Support Devices.

Features	IABP	Impella 2.5	Impella CP	iVAC 2L	TandemHeart	VA-ECMO
Inflow/outflow	Aorta	LV→aorta	LV→aorta	LV→aorta	LA→aorta	RA→aorta
Mechanism of action	Pneumatic	Axial flow	Axial flow	Pulsatile flow	Centrifugal flow	Centrifugal flow
Insertion approach	Pc (FA)	Pc (FA)	Pc (FA)	Pc (FA)	Pc (FA/FV)	Pc (FA/FV)
Sheath size	7–8 F	13 F	14 F	17 F	Venous: 21 F Arterial: 12–19 F	Venous: 17–21 F Arterial: 16–19 F
Flow (L/min)	0.3–0.5	Max 2.5	3.7–4.0	Max 2.8	Max 4.0	Max 7.0
Pump speed (RPM)	N/A	Max 51,000	Max 51,000	40 mL/beat	Max 7500	Max 5000
Duration of support	2–5 days	6 h–10 days	6 h–10 days	6 h–10 days	Up to 14 days	7–10 days
LV function dependency	+	–	–	–	–	–
Synchrony with the cardiac cycle	+	–	–	–	–	–
LV unloading	+	++	+++	+	+++	–
Afterload	↓	→	→	→	←	↑↑
MAP	↑	↑↑	↑↑	↑↑	↑↑	↑↑
Cardiac index	↑	↑↑	↑↑↑	↑↑↑	↑↑↑	↑↑↑
PCWP	↓	→	↓↓	→	↓↓	[↑]
LVEDP	↓	↓↓	↓↓	↓↓	↓↓↓	[↑]
Coronary perfusion	↑	↑	↑	↑	↓↔	[↑]
Myocardial oxygen demand	↓	↓↓	↓↓	↓↓	↓	[↑]
Anticoagulation	+	+	+	+	+	+
Implant complexity	+	++	++	++	++	++
Management complexity	+	++	++	++	+++	+++
Complications	Limb ischemia, bleeding	Hemolysis, limb ischemia, bleeding	Hemolysis, limb ischemia, bleeding	Hemolysis, limb ischemia, bleeding	Limb ischemia, bleeding, hemolysis	Bleeding, limb ischemia, hemolysis
Contraindications	Moderate-to-severe AR, severe PAD	Severe AS/AR, mechanical AoV, LV thrombus, CI to AC	Severe AS/AR, mechanical AoV, LV thrombus, CI to AC	Severe AS/AR, mechanical AoV, CI to AC	Moderate-to-severe AR, severe PAD, CI to AC, LA thrombus	Moderate-to-severe AR, severe PAD, CI to AC
CE-certification	+	+	+	+	+	+
FDA approval	+	+	+	–	+	+

Abbreviations: AC, anticoagulation; AoV, aortic valve; AR, aortic regurgitation; AS, aortic stenosis; CI, contraindication; FA, femoral artery; FDA, US Food and Drug Administration; FV, femoral vein; LV, left ventricle; LVEDP, left ventricular end-diastolic pressure; IABP, intraaortic balloon pump; MAP, mean arterial pressure; Max, maximum; PAD, peripheral arterial disease; Pc, percutaneous; PCWP, pulmonary capillary wedge pressure; PS, peripheral surgical; RA, right atrium; RPM, rotations per minute; VA-ECMO, venoarterial extracorporeal membrane oxygenation.

5.1. Intraaortic Balloon Bump

Since its introduction in the 1960s, IABP remains the most widely used device for temporary support in hemodynamically unstable patients due to its greater availability and ease of insertion as compared to other temporary devices [33]. It is typically inserted via femoral arterial access, though axillary or subclavian approaches are also feasible and have the advantage of enabling ambulation among stabilized patients. IABP support is driven by electrocardiogram (ECG)-guided balloon inflation with helium (due to its low viscosity that facilitates easy transfer in and out of the balloon in addition to its rapid absorption in blood in case of balloon rupture) at the onset of diastole and deflation at the onset of LV systole. This diastolic pressure augmentation results in increased coronary perfusion, decreased afterload, decreased cardiac work, and decreased myocardial oxygen demand. Despite these favorable effects, the increase in cardiac output is usually minimal and it may not, therefore, provide adequate support to improve end-organ perfusion in patients with severe cardiogenic shock. Moreover, optimal support is dependent on the underlying heart work and also on other factors, such as a stable electrical rhythm, optimal balloon position and sizing, and the timing of balloon inflation in diastole and deflation in systole [34].

The complications associated with IABP use are mainly vascular, including limb ischemia, vascular injury, and stroke [35]. Although it rarely occurs, trauma to the aorta or ostia of the visceral arteries can result in life-threatening complications, including acute renal failure, bowel ischemia, and atheroembolic events. Other complications include bleeding, infection, and thrombocytopenia. Anticoagulation therapy (usually with heparin) is generally recommended for patients supported with an IABP to prevent ischemic complications though no definitive evidence exists to support this approach and some centers do not use anticoagulation with 1:1 pumping, particularly in patients at high bleeding risk. IABP is contraindicated in patients with severe peripheral arterial or aortic disease and in those with moderate or severe aortic valve regurgitation. With the emergence of newer short term support strategies that provide greater hemodynamic support and ventricular unloading, the role of IABP support in the setting of cardiogenic shock or high risk PCI will continue to decline as experience grows with more promising short-term MCS therapies. According to the current European Society of Cardiology (ESC) guidelines, IABP is not indicated for patients with cardiogenic shock complicating AMI (Class III) [10], and a recent study has found that IABP is considered one of the medical reversals in clinical practice as this widespread therapeutic strategy bolstered by retrospective studies and previous guidelines was strongly challenged by subsequent large prospective and randomized studies showing no clinical benefit of its utilization in this clinical setting [36].

5.2. Impella Devices

The Impella pumps are continuous nonpulsatile microaxial flow devices that are deployed into the LV across the aortic valve and unload the LV by pumping blood from the LV cavity to the ascending aorta. The Impella 2.5 and CP pumps (Abiomed Inc, Danvers, MA, USA) can be placed percutaneously and provide maximal flow rates of 2.5 and 3.0–4.0 L/min, respectively, while the Impella 5.0 and Impella LD (Abiomed Inc, Danvers, MA, USA) devices are larger LV assist axial-flow pumps that require surgical cutdown and provide up to 5.0 L/min of cardiac output [14,37,38]. Similarly, the right-sided Impella RP is designed for right ventricular (RV) hemodynamic support by propelling blood from the inferior vena cava and right atrium (RA) to the pulmonary arteries and can also be deployed percutaneously. The percutaneous Impella devices for LV support are inserted most commonly through the femoral artery and then advanced in a retrograde fashion to the LV with a flexible pigtail loop that stabilizes the pump in the LV chamber and protects from LV perforation. Impella insertion requires large-bore arterial cannulation (13-F for Impella 2.5 and 14-F for Impella CP) and therefore, it is essential to ensure adequate femoral and iliac arterial diameters to enable device delivery via a femoral approach. Alternatively, though less commonly used, axillary or subclavian arterial accesses can be used to deliver these pumps percutaneously. For high-risk PCI, the device is usually removed at the end of the procedure. However, in patients with persistent cardiogenic shock despite revascularization, Impella should be retained for further hemodynamic support, a condition that may pose some challenges and thus requires careful assessment and management in the cardiac care unit. Optimal device functioning is crucial and largely depends on appropriate positioning in the LV cavity, as device migration can lead to low flow, ventricular arrhythmias, and hemolysis [39]. In such cases, bedside transthoracic echocardiography-guided device repositioning is usually successful without the need for fluoroscopy [11].

Unlike IABP, Impella (as other percutaneous ventricular assist devices) functions independently of the remaining LV function and does not require synchronization with the cardiac cycle. Therefore, Impella devices are more helpful than IABP in patients with severely depressed LV function who present with significant arrhythmias. Impella results in effective LV unloading thus resulting in decreased LV filling pressures (LVEDP) and myocardial oxygen consumption, while improving cardiac output, mean arterial pressure, and coronary perfusion [40]. All the hemodynamic parameters, including cardiac output, are more markedly improved with Impella use compared with an IABP. Additionally, the more powerful Impella CP and 5.0 devices provide greater hemodynamic support than Impella 2.5 and thereby are more beneficial in patients with profound cardiogenic shock requiring greater hemodynamic support [30].

Despite the improvement in hemodynamic parameters, device-related complications are not rare and can be clinically meaningful, thereby contradicting the potential hemodynamic benefits that can be achieved with the use of Impella devices in some cases. As with any mechanical support device, common complications associated with Impella include vascular trauma, limb ischemia, and bleeding requiring blood transfusion. Moreover, hemolysis is frequently encountered during Impella support due to mechanical erythrocyte shearing, but usually improves after repositioning the device. Based on the Impella EUROSHOCK Registry [39], utilization of Impella 2.5 in the setting of acute cardiogenic shock was found to be associated bleeding at the vascular access site requiring blood transfusion in 24% of cases and hemolysis requiring blood transfusion in 7.5% of cases after a mean Impella support duration of approximately 48 h. Impella may also worsen right-to-left shunting and hypoxemia among patients with a preexisting ventricular or atrial septal defect. As device technology continues to improve and the Impella-associated complications continue to decrease, the use of Impella devices has been steadily increasing over the last several years [41]. This is also owing to its relative ease of deployment and more efficient hemodynamic support compared with other MCS devices.

Impella should not be used in patients with a mechanical aortic valve or LV thrombus as well as in those with severe peripheral arterial disease or who cannot tolerate systemic anticoagulation therapy. Although severe aortic stenosis and regurgitation are considered relative contraindication, the use of Impella in this setting has been shown to be feasible and may be considered in selected high-risk patients with severe aortic stenosis and cardiogenic shock or those with severe LV dysfunction and CAD who require high-risk PCI and/or balloon aortic valvuloplasty as well as in selected patients who develop hemodynamic collapse during transcatheter aortic valve replacement (TAVR) [42].

5.3. TandemHeart

The TandemHeart (CardiacAssist) system is an extracorporeal, centrifugal, continuous flow pump, which is available on the market for left, right, and biventricular failure. For LV support, TandemHeart device is percutaneously inserted to pump blood extracorporeally from the left atrium through a transseptal cannula back into the femoral/iliac artery through an arterial cannula using a centrifugal pump that provides 3 to 5 L/min of continuous flow at 3000 to 7500 rpm, respectively [11,37]. The transseptal inflow cannula is a 21-F and contains a large end-hole and 14 side holes that enable effective blood aspiration from the left atrium while the arterial outflow cannula ranges in size between 15-F and 19-F according to the flow rate via the iliofemoral arterial system [43]. The pump is also FDA-approved and available in market for an oxygenator to be added to the circuit thereby allowing for blood oxygenation with simultaneous LV unloading. As with Impella support, anticoagulation (typically with unfractionated heparin) is required with a recommended activated clotting time (ACT) goal of about 250–300 s prior to device activation.

By propelling blood from the left atrium directly to the arterial system, TandemHeart results in a significantly reduced LV preload, filling pressures, and myocardial oxygen demand, while cardiac output and mean arterial pressures are improved. However, because LV output through the aortic valve competes with the retrograde flow from the device, LV afterload increases as the device support is augmented, which may ultimately result in aortic valve closure requiring LV venting [44,45].

Similar to other percutaneous MCS devices, TandemHeart use may infrequently cause limb ischemia and vascular injury [37]. Additionally, as transseptal puncture is needed to insert a large caliber venous cannula, expertise with this technique is crucial for TandemHeart application in clinical practice, which may limit its widespread use, particularly among inexperienced interventional cardiologists not regularly performing transseptal punctures in their practice. Although rare, unique complications related to the transseptal puncture required for MCS with TandemHeart may occur and include cardiac tamponade, hemolysis, and thrombus or air embolism. Finally, device migration with dislodgement of the left atrial cannula to the RA during patient transport or leg movement may cause significant right-to-left shunt, resulting in severe hypoxemia and hemodynamic collapse. Severe peripheral arterial disease, left atrial thrombus, and profound coagulopathy are considered contraindications for TandemHeart use. Moreover, limited experience exists regarding the use of this device among patients with moderate to severe aortic regurgitation or those with ventricular septal defect [46].

5.4. Venoarterial Extracorporeal Membrane Oxygenation (VA-ECMO)

Based on the Extracorporeal Life Support Organization (ELSO) registry data, the number of ECMO devices and the number of centers utilizing ECMO are markedly increasing [47,48]. VA-ECMO provides both circulatory and oxygenation support, and therefore it is ideally used in patients with biventricular failure who develop cardiogenic shock and impaired oxygenation requiring cardiopulmonary resuscitation at the time PCI is initiated [49]. This is unlike venovenous ECMO (VV-ECMO), which is reserved for patients with respiratory failure but without significant cardiac dysfunction. When percutaneously inserted, VA-ECMO bypasses both the right and left side of the heart by draining deoxygenated blood from a central vein or RA with an 18-F to 21-F venous cannula and pumping oxygenated blood, after passing via an extracorporeal membrane oxygenator, into the iliofemoral arterial circulation (14-F to 19-F arterial cannula). The VA-ECMO system provides cardiac flow between 3 and 7 L/min depending on cannula sizes and can potentially be maintained for several days to weeks among patients with persistent cardiogenic shock as a bridge to recovery, permanent LV assist device implantation, or heart transplantation. Due to the substantial hemodynamic support provided by VA-ECMO, the hemodynamic and metabolic derangement resulted from cardiogenic shock is generally corrected within hours of device activation. Unfractionated heparin is typically used during ECMO support but other anticoagulants, such as bivalirudin, particularly in patients with heparin-induced thrombocytopenia who are unable to receive heparin, have been increasingly used as alternatives. The extent of anticoagulation during ECMO support is largely dependent on the type of membrane oxygenator and ranges from 180–250 s [50].

VA-ECMO support results in a remarkable increase in cardiac output and mean arterial pressure. However, its use is limited by retrograde blood flow leading to LV afterload mismatch, inadequate LV decompression, and high myocardial oxygen demand. The concurrent use of IABP or Impella can add further support by direct unloading of the LV and reducing ventricular wall stress [51,52]. Recently, a novel electrocardiogram (ECG)-synchronized, pulsatile VA-ECMO system, labeled i-cor (Xenios AG), has been introduced. The i-cor system consists of an ECG-triggered diagonal pump, which has a feature of diastolic augmentation and a capacity of providing a support up to 8 L/min. The main difference of the i-cor pump is the ability to generate a physiological pulse and to manage rotational timing to synchronize the pulse with the cardiac cycle of the native heart in order to provide adequate and physiologic circulatory support. By decreasing extracorporeal blood flow during systole and increasing flow during diastole, i-cor assist device flow decreases afterload and LV end-diastolic pressure and improves LV function and coronary flow compared with standard continuous VA-ECMO flow [53–55]. The first-in-man study, involving 15 patients with cardiogenic shock (71% due to AMI), showed that the i-cor pump was safe and applicable in clinical practice and implicated a hemodynamic benefit [56]. A multicenter study designed to test the safety and feasibility of this innovative pulsatile cardiac-synchronous MCS system in a larger population (the "SynCor" trial) is still ongoing.

One of the recent advancements in the percutaneous extracorporeal life support (ECLS) technology is the development of the Lifebridge B2T "bridge to therapy" system (Zoll Medical GmbH, Köln, Germany), which is a miniaturized and portable heart-lung support system similar in design to standard ECMO systems with an ability to provide cardiovascular stabilization and sufficient end-organ perfusion immediately after circulatory arrest. The Lifebridge system enables rapid application within 5 min due to its automated set-up and portable design in addition to less cumbersome transportation of the patient than standard ECMO equipment due to its smaller size and suitcase configuration. Other technical features include a battery life of 2 h, an overall weight of 18 kg (39.6 lb.), and a maximal blood flow of 6 L/min. Real-world clinical data of the German Lifebridge Registry involving 444 patients from 60 tertiary cardiovascular centers has been recently published [57] showing that this transportable automated ECLS system was safely applicable for hemodynamic stabilization with acceptable complications. However, mortality rates remained extremely high in these critically ill patients with immediate survival rates of 36% and 16% at 30-days after device implementation, especially in those with high lactate levels on admission.

Adverse events related to VA-ECMO include bleeding (with excessive anticoagulation), thromboembolic events in the circuit or systemically (if anticoagulation is inadequate), cannula-induced vascular injuries, infection, stroke (ischemic or hemorrhagic), hemolysis, and limb ischemia [58]. To reduce the risk of limb ischemia, a second antegrade arterial sheath can be inserted into the superficial femoral artery and when fed by the main arterial cannula can provide secured antegrade perfusion to the limb. Contraindications to peripheral VA-ECMO include patients with severe chronic organ dysfunction (renal failure, cirrhosis, or emphysema), prolonged cardiopulmonary resuscitation without adequate tissue perfusion, severe peripheral arterial disease, and patients unable to receive anticoagulation [11].

5.5. Other Percutaneous Mechanical Support Devices

Percutaneous LV MCS pumps under investigation include the pulsatile iVAC 2L (PulseCath BV, Arnhem, The Netherlands), which has been recently evaluated prospectively in a pilot study of 14 patients undergoing high-risk PCI demonstrating 100% angiographic success [59]. The Aortix (Procyrion, Houston, TX, USA) and Reitan (Cardiobridge, Hechingen, Germany) devices are other investigational devices that are deployed in the descending aorta similar to the IABP.

Apart from LV support, RV failure refractory to medical therapy is increasingly becoming a clinical challenge, thereby prompting the development of devices to specifically provide RV support. Large inferior AMI may cause predominant RV failure with cardiogenic shock with or without severe LV dysfunction. When cardiogenic shock is persistent despite maximal medical therapy, the options for MCS in this setting include VA-ECMO, surgical implantation of RVAD or total artificial heart (TAH), and heart transplantation [60]. The recent development of Impella RP launched an evolving field of percutaneous mechanical therapies for refractory RV failure. Impella RP is an intracardiac microaxial pump designed predominantly for management of primary RV failure, particularly in the setting of AMI, and can be inserted through the femoral vein to eject blood from the inferior vena cava directly to the pulmonary artery. The safety and reliability of the RP Impella has been established in the prospective RECOVER RIGHT study for severe isolated RV dysfunction [61]. Like LV Impella devices, complications that may occur with RP Impella support include bleeding, thrombosis, hemolysis, or infection.

6. Clinical Benefit of Percutaneous MCS Devices for PCI

The most recent clinical practice guidelines regarding the use of percutaneous MCS for PCI and management of ACS recommend consideration of the use of these devices in the setting of high-risk PCI and AMI complicated by cardiogenic shock [11]. However, despite accumulating evidence of hemodynamic improvement using various MCS devices, a convincing clinical benefit based on randomized controlled trials has not yet been demonstrated among this population. Because this is an extremely high-risk group of patients, improving clinical outcomes can be challenging and further research is still necessary to examine the optimal device features, the timing of support, and the appropriate patient for achieving maximal clinical benefit from these devices during PCI. The salient findings of contemporary studies examining the effect of MCS devices on outcomes in cardiogenic shock complicating AMI and high-risk PCI are summarized in Tables 3 and 4, respectively.

6.1. Intraaortic Balloon Bump

In the setting of PCI with cardiogenic shock complicating AMI, a previous retrospective study has suggested a potential benefit with early IABP support placed prior to PCI showing decreased rates of in-hospital mortality and cardiac adverse events compared with IABP placed only following PCI [62]. In a meta-analysis by Sjauw et al. [63], no mortality benefit or improvement in LV ejection fraction were found with utilizing IABP among patients undergoing PCI for ST-elevation myocardial infarction (STEMI), while higher stroke and bleeding rates were observed in the IABP group. Furthermore, among patients with cardiogenic shock undergoing PCI, there was a 6% increase in 30-day mortality [63]. Not only were randomized studies analyzed but cohort studies were also included in this meta-analysis; therefore, it could be subject to selection bias as sicker patients with more profound cardiogenic shock were more likely to be supported with IABP. In the SHOCK trial [64], IABP was not been shown to reduce mortality or major adverse events in patients with cardiogenic shock or high-risk PCI except in patients with STEMI. Subsequently, the IABP-SHOCK II trial [5], a prospective randomized controlled trial designed to study the effect of IABP involving 600 patients with AMI and cardiogenic shock undergoing early revascularization, showed no improvement in survival with IABP at 30 days [5] and subsequently at 1 year [65] and 6 years [66] post AMI. Moreover, there were no significant differences in any of the secondary clinical and laboratory (including lactate and creatinine) endpoints, and there were no significant differences in subgroup analyses. Based on the current guidelines, IABP is largely recommended in patients with mechanical complications post AMI or during transport of unstable patients from PCI centers without to centers with on-site cardiac surgery [12,67].

Among patients undergoing PCI without evident cardiogenic shock, IABP use was tested in the CRISP-AMI (Counterpulsation to Reduce Infarct Size Pre-PCI Acute Myocardial Infarction) trial [68]; a 30-center randomized controlled trial involving 337 patients with anterior STEMI, which found that routine IABP placement immediately prior to PCI had no significant effect on the infarct size as assessed by magnetic resonance imaging 3 to 5 days post PCI or on survival rates after 6 months of follow-up. Similarly, in a nonrandomized study using the National Cardiovascular Data Registry database, IABP utilization in high-risk PCI was not associated with lower mortality, and wide regional variations in the use of IABP was noted among the different centers [69]. Finally, the BCIS-1 trial [3], a prospective randomized controlled trial involving 301 patients randomized to routine IABP versus provisional IABP support for high-risk PCI, found no significant differences in mortality between the two groups. However, a long-term follow-up of more than four years showed a 34% relative reduction in all-cause mortality risk with routine IABP in patients with severe ischemic cardiomyopathy undergoing high-risk PCI, which might be attributed to lower incidence of procedural hypotension with preplanned IABP insertion [70].

Given these conflicting results and the controversy surrounding its benefit, the use of IABP in the setting of STEMI complicated with cardiogenic shock is decreasing and its routine use has been recently downgraded to class III (harm) by the ESC [10] and to class IIa (should be considered) by the American Heart Association (AHA)/American College of Cardiology (ACC) [71] guidelines. Furthermore, due to the introduction of new devices, such as Impella, and the continuous advancement in MCS technology, which provides superior hemodynamic support and potentially more favorable outcomes, the future role of IABP in management of cardiogenic shock and ventricular unloading may continue to decline.

6.2. Impella Devices

There are currently limited available data to establish a significant clinical benefit of Impella use in patients with cardiogenic shock undergoing PCI. Impella devices provide greater hemodynamic support with a more pronounced cardiac output augmentation and LV unloading than IABP. In 2008, the ISAR-SHOCK (Impella LP 2.5 versus IABP in Cardiogenic SHOCK) trial [72] was the first randomized clinical study to assess the safety and efficacy of Impella 2.5 in the setting of AMI complicated by cardiogenic shock as compared to IABP. Twenty-five patients were randomized to the Impella 2.5 LP device or IABP, and the primary endpoint was a change in cardiac index after 30 min of support. All patients received PCI of the infarct-related artery and remained in shock. Patients supported with an Impella had greater increase in cardiac index and mean arterial blood pressure after 30 min of support. However, there was no difference in mortality or in the rates of bleeding or limb ischemia between the two groups [72]. Subsequently, the safety and efficacy of Impella 2.5 LP was examined in the EUROSHOCK multicenter registry [39] involving 120 patients with severe cardiogenic shock refractory to conventional therapy, among which cardiopulmonary resuscitation was performed in more than 40%, showing high overall in-hospital mortality rates reaching 64% without survival benefit in the group treated with an Impella. Similarly, the IMPRESS in Severe SHOCK (IMPella versus IABP Reduces mortality in STEMI patients treated with primary PCI in Severe cardiogenic SHOCK) trial [6] enrolled 48 mechanically ventilated patients with severe cardiogenic shock after AMI who were randomized 1:1 to Impella CP or IABP and followed for all-cause mortality at 30 days and 6 months post AMI. Importantly, 44 (92%) patients had cardiac arrest prior to randomization with interquartile time till return of spontaneous circulation ranging from 15 to 52 min and a considerable proportion of patients (46%) died due to anoxic brain damage. The overall mortality in the study was 50% and there were no significant differences between the two arms (50% versus 46% at 30 days and 50% versus 50% at 6 months in the IABP and Impella CP groups, respectively), thus reflecting a very high risk cohort presenting with late-stage cardiogenic shock [6,73]. The only study reporting a mortality benefit of Impella in the setting of cardiogenic shock complicating AMI was by Karatolios et al. [74], who conducted a retrospective, single-center study including 90 patients suffering from AMI and cardiogenic shock treated with Impella (n = 27) or medical treatment alone (n = 63). Patients in the Impella group were sicker, evidenced by higher lactate levels, longer low cardiac output duration, and lower LV ejection fraction than those treated medically. When 20 patients of each group were matched, patients supported with Impella had decreased rates of in-hospital (35% versus 80%; $p = 0.01$) and 6-month (40% versus 80%; $p = 0.02$) mortality [74]. More recently, using IABP-SHOCK II trial inclusion and exclusion criteria, a retrospective analysis of 237 patients with AMI and cardiogenic shock treated with Impella 2.5 (~30% of patients) or Impella CP (~70% of patients) were propensity matched to the same number of patients from the IABP-SHOCK II trial [75]. There was no significant difference in 30-day all-cause mortality. Moreover, severe or life-threatening bleedings as well as peripheral vascular complications occurred more often in the Impella group. Limiting the analysis to IABP-treated patients as the control group showed comparable results with no evidence of favorable outcomes with Impella use [75]. Finally, a meta-analysis including 588 patients from the main aforementioned studies, the use of MCS with Impella in the setting of AMI and cardiogenic shock was not associated with improved short-time survival but there were higher rates of complications when compared with IABP and medical treatment [76]. It is important to recognize, however, that the vast majority of patients included in these studies were in profound cardiogenic shock and after cardiac arrest. As the use of Impella in patients with less severe shock or pre-shock conditions was not the focus of these studies, its effect on outcomes cannot, therefore, be addressed based on the current data and further studies are still warranted in these settings.

The effectiveness and safety of Impella support for planned high-risk coronary interventions have been investigated in small studies showing encouraging results. In the AMC MAC1 study [77], 19 consecutive high-risk and poor surgical candidates with moderate-to-severe LV dysfunction (ejection fraction < 40%) underwent PCI of an unprotected left main or the last remaining vessel with Impella 2.5 support showing 100% procedural success and no important device-related adverse events, thereby demonstrating safety and feasibility of utilizing Impella devices for high-risk PCI. This has also been confirmed in the PROTECT I trial [78], a prospective and multicenter study, which showed that Impella 2.5 system is safe, easy to implant, and provides excellent hemodynamic support for a mean duration of 1.7 h (range: 0.4–2.5 h) during high-risk PCI. The real-world use of the Impella 2.5 in complex high-risk PCI showed an angiographic revascularization success of 99% in the overall cohort and in 90% of patients with multivessel revascularization. Survival rates were 91% and 81% at 6 months and 12 months, respectively, despite including inoperable patients with a high prevalence of LV dysfunction, New York Heart Association (NYHA) class III and IV heart failure, and chronic renal dysfunction [14].

The largest prospective randomized clinical study to examine the effect of hemodynamic support with Impella in patients undergoing high-risk PCI was the PROTECT II trial [4]. In this multi-center study, 452 patients with complex three-vessel disease or unprotected left main CAD and severely depressed LV function were assigned to IABP or Impella 2.5 during non-emergent high-risk PCI. The composite primary endpoint of 30-day incidence of 11 major adverse events was similar between the Impella and IABP groups (35.1% for Impella 2.5 versus 40.1% for IABP, $p = 0.227$ in the intention-to-treat population, and 34.3% versus 42.2%, $p = 0.092$ in the per-protocol population). Impella did provide greater hemodynamic support and at 90-day follow-up there was a trend towards a decreased incidence of adverse events with Impella in the intention-to-treat population (40.6% versus 49.3%, $p = 0.066$) and significantly decreased events in the per-protocol population (40.0% versus 51.0%, $p = 0.023$) [4]. A subsequent analysis of the outcomes using a prognostic ally important definition of AMI based on new Q-waves or >8× increase in creatinine kinase-MB, demonstrated that that Impella resulted in improved event-free survival after 90 days of follow-up, supporting a late benefit that could be attributed to more stable procedural hemodynamics that facilitate the performance of more complete revascularization and complex PCI procedures, such as rotational atherectomy and bifurcation coronary disease intervention, more safely [79]. A more recent consecutive real-world cohort of high-risk PCI patients, new generation MCS devices (including Impella CP, Heartmate PHP, and PulseCath iVAC2L) have demonstrated a significant reduction in the composite endpoint of serious peri-procedural adverse events, including cardiac arrest and 30-day mortality despite worse LV function and higher Synergy between Percutaneous Coronary Intervention with TAXUS and Cardiac Surgery (SYNTAX)-I score observed in patients protected with MCS [8]. Interestingly, patients under age of 75, with a SYNTAX-I score > 32, and with an LV ejection fraction < 30% derived most potential benefit from MCS utilization during PCI. These promising findings indicate that the more powerful LV support obtained using new generation MCS devices may be necessary for improving clinical outcomes, which has not been evidently seen using the IABP or Impella 2.5 devices.

6.3. TandemHeart

Small studies have shown a significant improvement in hemodynamics with TandemHeart use, but were underpowered to show improvement in survival. In an observational study by Kar et al. [43], TandemHeart placement in patients with severe cardiogenic shock refractory to conventional inotropic or IABP therapy was associated with improvement in cardiac index (increased from 0.5 to 3 L/min/m^2), PCWP (decreased from 31 to 17 mmHg), and mixed venous oxygen saturation (increased from 49 to 69%), as well as improvement in kidney function (urine output increased from 70 to 1200 mL/day and creatinine decreased from 1.5 to 1.2 mg/dL) and lactic acid level (decreased from 11 to 1.5 mg/dL). However, overall mortality (40.2% at 30 days and 45.3% at 6 months) and bleeding complications remained high [43]. In a small randomized study involving patients in cardiogenic shock after AMI, with intended PCI to the infarcted artery, who were assigned to either IABP (n = 20) or TandemHeart (n = 21), hemodynamic and metabolic parameters was more effectively reversed by TandemHeart than by IABP treatment. However, adverse events, such as severe bleeding and limb ischemia, were encountered more frequently after TandemHeart support, and 30-day mortality was similar [80]. Similarly, a small randomized trial of patients presenting within 24 h of the development of cardiogenic shock and assigned to IABP or TandemHeart showed superior hemodynamic parameters with TandemHeart, even in patients failing IABP, but no significant differences in in-hospital mortality or severe adverse events when compared with IABP alone [81].

Data on the use of TandemHeart in high-risk PCI is limited to observational studies. A study from the Mayo Clinic summarized data on 54 consecutive patients undergoing high-risk PCI using a TandemHeart device for support, demonstrating feasibility and safety of this device to allow performance of high-risk and complex intervention [82]. All patients were deemed high risk for surgery and underwent complex PCI, with a Society of Thoracic Surgery (STS) mortality risk score of 13%, a median SYNTAX score of 33, and the majority of patients underwent left main and multivessel PCI. Procedural success was achieved in 97% of cases, with hemodynamic improvement during the procedure, and 6-month survival was 87%. However, major vascular complications occurred in 13% of cases [82]. Additional small series of patients undergoing TandemHeart-assisted high-risk PCI have shown comparable results. A meta-analysis of usefulness of percutaneous MCS devices, including eight cohort studies with 205 patients supported by TandemHeart and 12 studies with 1346 patients supported with Impella 2.5 during high-risk PCI, found 30-day mortality rates of 8% and major bleeding rates of 3.6% with TandemHeart compared with 3.5% and 7.1% with Impella 2.5, respectively. Overall periprocedural outcomes were comparable between the two groups [83].

6.4. Venoarterial Extracorporeal Membrane Oxygenation (VA-ECMO)

While ECMO provides excellent cardiopulmonary support with a relative ease of implementation, its use in the setting of AMI and shock is limited by the need for specialized perfusion expertise and nursing as well as the possibility for increased LV stroke work and myocardial oxygen demand, which can precipitate further myocardial ischemia. Additionally, there is need for large bore cannulas and aggressive antithrombotic therapy which increase the risk of bleeding. A recent single-center study [84] reported a 67% survival to discharge rate among 18 consecutive patients who received femoral VA-ECMO in the cardiac catheterization lab for severe shock due to ACS. The average length of ECMO support was 3.2 days and 17 (94%) patients required at least one blood transfusion with higher bleeding rates observed among those treated with glycoprotein IIb/IIIa inhibitors [84]. In another small retrospective study [85], a total of 15 patients undergoing VA-ECMO placement for AMI with refractory cardiogenic shock were analyzed. One-third of patients presented with out-of-hospital resuscitation and 60% had IABP placed for LV venting. The survival rate after 30 days was 47% and vascular complications occurred in 53% of patients. There is a growing utilization of VA-ECMO in patients suffering from cardiac arrest requiring prolonged cardiopulmonary resuscitation (CPR) showing acceptable survival rate and outcome [86]. A meta-analysis including 1866 patients treated with VA-ECMO for cardiogenic shock or cardiac arrest showed an approximate overall survival of 30% and significant associated morbidity with the performance of this intervention [58]. These data suggest that use of VA-ECMO should be individualized based on risk-benefit analysis derived from vascular anatomy and comorbidities to maximize clinical benefit. Finally, LV unloading during VA-ECMO treatment for cardiogenic shock appears beneficial either with predominant use of IABP [51] or Impella [87] demonstrating significant improvement in survival with the two unloading tools.

7. Recommendations for MCS Use During PCI

A suggested algorithmic approach to MCS use during PCI for cardiogenic shock complicating AMI and high-risk PCI without cardiogenic shock is depicted in Figure 2. Interventional cardiologists are challenged with a growing number of patients in need of coronary revascularization but who are hemodynamically unstable or deemed poor surgical candidates and too high risk for PCI. The use of percutaneous MCS devices has been proven to be feasible and safe in clinical conditions previously considered for conservative therapy only. However, data on survival benefit as a result of utilizing these percutaneous devices is still lacking. It is not therefore surprising that there has been a modest adoption of these devices in the current practice, reflecting the equivocal results from the current evidence base in addition to the uncertainty as to which patients MCS will add a real benefit. Optimal timing of device insertion is also an important variable. In light of the currently available data, it is reasonable that utilization of MCS devices in clinical practice should be advocated in an individualized manner based on a detailed review of the risks and benefits rather than as a standard of care for every complex procedure. The recommendations on the use of a specific MCS device are based on the anticipated hemodynamic effects and risks as well as clinical outcome data. Based on the recent SCAI/ACC/HFSA/STS Clinical Expert Consensus Statement published in 2015 [11], percutaneous MCS may be considered in carefully selected patients with severe cardiogenic shock complicating AMI unresponsive to pharmacologic support as a bridge to recovery following PCI or definitive therapy. The evidence is stronger in the setting of mechanical complications post MI, such as ischemic mitral regurgitation when hemodynamic derangement is usually acute and more substantial and the benefit from these devices is more pronounced. There is an increasing indication for temporary MCS use during and after primary PCI for patients presenting with large AMI causing severe LV dysfunction, and RV mechanical support with Impella RP can be considered for RV infarction complicated by cardiogenic shock. Early insertion of MCS devices is essential to attenuate the sequelae that may result from persistent cardiac ischemia and systemic hypoperfusion. The type of MCS device is dependent on multiple factors including the amount of hemodynamic support needed and the ultimate goal of support as well as technical characteristics that should be taken into consideration, such as the ease or deployment, and availability of these devices. IABP is more often used due to the ease of insertion and availability although the benefit of its utility is questionable in patients with AMI and cardiogenic shock. Impella 2.5 or CP provide more powerful hemodynamic support and can be inserted as rapidly as an IABP in experienced centers and are thus considered more favorable devices in appropriate patients. Finally, TandemHeart, VA-ECMO, or Impella 5 (which requires surgical cutdown for delivery) should be reserved for patients who continue to deteriorate despite such support. In patients who present with biventricular or cardiopulmonary failure, VA-ECMO is recommended as the first choice. For isolated RV failure with cardiogenic shock, Impella RP is an available percutaneous MCS option that may be considered in such cases [28].

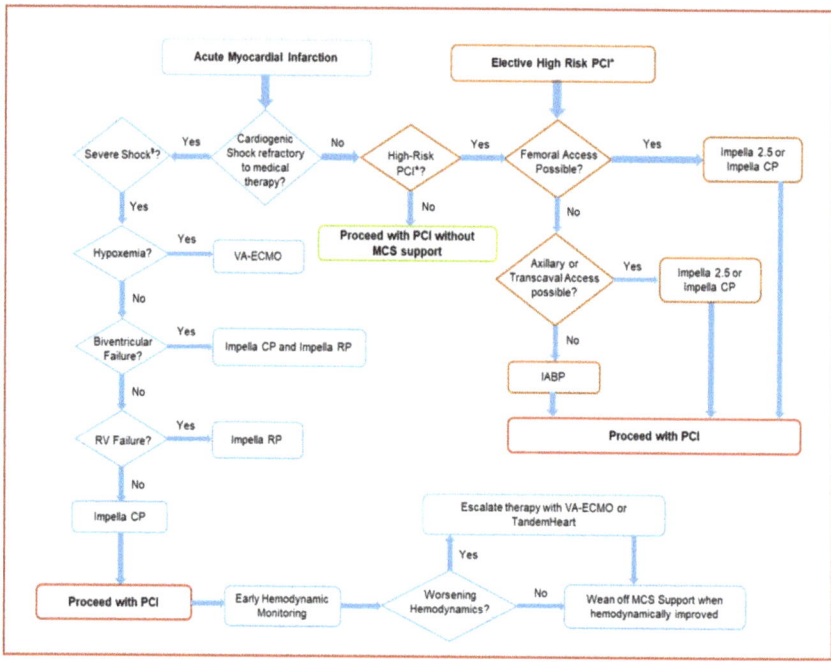

Figure 2. Suggested algorithmic approach for MCS in patients with cardiogenic shock complicating AMI and high-risk PCI. MCS, mechanical circulatory support; AMI, acute myocardial infarction; PCI, percutaneous coronary intervention. IABP, intraaortic balloon bump; VA-ECMO, venoarterial extracorporeal membrane oxygenation. * High-risk PCI is defined as presented in Table 1 and mainly include comorbidities, severe LV dysfunction (EF < 35%), and complex coronary artery disease involving a large territory, such as unprotected left main, sole-remaining vessel, or three-vessel disease. ‡ Severe cardiogenic shock is defined as markedly abnormal hemodynamic parameters (systolic blood pressure < 90 mmHg, heart rate > 120 beats per minute, cardiac index < 1.5 L/min/m^2, pulmonary capillary wedge pressure/left ventricular end-diastolic pressure > 30 mmHg), metabolic (lactate > 4 mg/dL), and clinical (confusion, cool extremities, on ≥2 vasopressors/inotropes) parameters.

For prophylactic percutaneous MCS use in the setting of high-risk PCI, great emphasis should be on identifying the patient's anatomic, hemodynamic, and procedural features that indicate adjunctive MCS support may be necessary and also determine the optimal device to utilize [2]. The current recommendation is to consider using MCS devices in patients with severe LV dysfunction (EF < 35%) or recent presentation with decompensated heart failure in the setting of complex coronary artery disease involving a large territory, such as unprotected left main, sole-remaining vessel, or three-vessel disease. Generally, patients with anticipated noncomplex PCI may be considered for IABP as the first-line MCS option with Impella as back up support, whereas those with anticipated technically challenging or prolonged procedure (rotational atherectomy or bifunctional stenting) may be considered for Impella, TandemHeart, or VA-ECMO depending on vascular anatomy, RV function, expertise, and availability [2,88]. The more severe the clinical and anatomic circumstances, the greater the potential benefit of MCS use [11]. MCS support should be initiated before the start of the PCI and in most cases can be removed immediately after the intervention. In cases with hemodynamic derangement after PCI, prolonged MCS support should be considered until hemodynamic improvement. Continuous hemodynamic monitoring with pulmonary arterial catheter in encouraged as early as possible to tailor therapy and help with determining the amount and duration of MCS support needed. Finally, the use of MCS devices in the emergent setting has been suggested to be cost-effective compared with surgical ECMO or ventricular assist device support [89], as well as in the elective setting when compared with IABP [90].

8. Future Directions

The majority of studies involving the new MCS devices for cardiogenic shock and high risk PCI have demonstrated superior hemodynamic improvement as compared to IABP but these studies were largely underpowered to find mortality benefit and therefore should be regarded as feasibility trials and a basis for larger clinical trials in the future. The DanGer Shock study [91] is an ongoing prospective randomized multicenter study with planned enrollment of 360 patients with AMI complicated by cardiogenic shock randomized 1:1 immediately after shock diagnosis to either Impella CP prior to PCI or current guideline-driven therapy. Patients with coma after out of hospital cardiac arrest are excluded. The primary endpoint is all-cause mortality at 180 days. The DanGer trial will be the first adequately powered randomized controlled trial to examine whether MCS with Impella CP improves survival among patients with cardiogenic shock complicating AMI and will therefore provide fundamental knowledge on the use of transvalvular LV unloading in this setting [91].

Despite the lack of current evidence, we believe that advanced MCS devices may improve clinical outcomes, including survival, in a selected group of patients and in specific circumstances. Future studies should largely focus on three major considerations when examining the clinical benefit of MCS. First, the optimal MCS device design and amount of support needed to achieve hemodynamic as well as metabolic improvement is unclear. For instance, in the IMPRESS in Severe Shock trial, one third of the patients died due to refractory cardiogenic shock and lactate levels remained high in many patients while being on Impella CP support, suggesting that the actual level of support was not sufficient [6,73]. Second, appropriate patient selection is a key factor that should be emphasized in future studies. Because utilization is currently determined based on subjective criteria, many patients may survive without MCS while others with irreversible anoxic brain injury from prolonged shock may not survive even with adequate hemodynamic support. Additionally, patients with shock and multiorgan dysfunction are at significantly higher risk of bleeding due to increased inflammation and coagulopathy which may progress to disseminated intravascular coagulation. Therefore, studies focusing on identifying patients are higher risk of device-associated complications among whom the harm of these complications may outweigh the benefit is clinically meaningful for mitigating device complications. For example, lactate has been shown to be an important biomarker for risk stratification in the setting of cardiogenic shock. Among patients undergoing extracorporeal cardiopulmonary resuscitation due to cardiac arrest, lactate clearance was the sole predictor of neurological outcome as assessed by the Glasgow Outcome Scale (GOS) [92] and in patients with refractory cardiogenic shock requiring VA-ECMO support, lactate levels and lactate clearance during ECMO therapy were predictive markers for 30-day mortality [93]. In patients with cardiac arrest, lactate levels prior to ECMO initiation was significantly associated with increased risk of all-cause mortality at 90 days. Interestingly, lactate was found to be more predictive of outcome than duration of cardiopulmonary resuscitation or absence of return of spontaneous circulation [94]. These findings suggest that early metabolic assessment by measuring plasma lactate levels may be an important prognostic marker for risk stratification when considering MCS in patients with cardiogenic shock. One study has shown that high body mass index (BMI) was an additional predictor of 30-day mortality in patients with AMI and cardiogenic shock supported by VA-ECMO [95]. However, the influence of BMI on outcomes among patients supported by other MCS devices is unclear.

Third, the timing of MCS device insertion in relation to primary PCI among patients with AMI and cardiogenic shock can be critical to achieve survival benefit and future studies should focus on determining the optimal timing of MCS, which remains elusive. Recent studies have shown in an animal model that mechanical support with LV unloading reduces infarct size and favorably mediates key biological pathways associated with inflammation and maladaptive cardiac remodeling when mechanical support is initiated prior to coronary reperfusion compared with early reperfusion without support [96–99]. In a prospective safety and feasibility first-in-human study known as the Door to Unloading With Impella CP System in Acute Myocardial Infarction to Reduce Infarct Size (DTU), LV unloading with the Impella CP with a 30-min delay prior to reperfusion in patient with STEMI is feasible with similar rates of adverse cardiovascular events and 30-day mean infarct size and without prohibitive safety signals [100]. These data suggest that LV unloading prior to PCI initiation in the setting of myocardial ischemia may be pivotal to achieve significant benefit from MCS devices but clinical evidence from randomized control trials is still awaiting. In support of this hypothesis, in the setting of AMI and cardiogenic shock, data from the catheter-based ventricular assist device registry have shown that early MCS implantation (either the Impella 2.5 or Impella CP) before PCI, prior to escalating doses of inotropes or vasopressors and within 75 min from shock onset, was independently associated with improved survival compared with later MCS support [24]. Similarly, data from a quality improvement registry including over 15,000 patients with AMI complicated by cardiogenic shock and supported with Impella have shown wide variation in outcomes across centers with higher survival rates seen when Impella was used as first support strategy, when invasive hemodynamic monitoring was used, and at higher institutional Impella implantation volume [101]. A meta-analysis of 3 available studies on the use of early Impella in patients with AMI and cardiogenic shock found that early initiation of Impella decreased in-hospital or 30-day mortality by 48% compared with late initiation of Impella [102].

Based on these promising retrospective data, and after the FDA's approval of Impella for cardiogenic shock complicating AMI, investigators have organized the construct of a multicenter national shock protocol now referred to as the "National Cardiogenic Shock Initiative" (NCSI) emphasizing invasive hemodynamic monitoring and rapid initiation of percutaneous MCS support. The analysis of the first 171 patients enrolled in NCSI was recently published [7] and included patients presenting with AMI and cardiogenic shock using the same inclusion and exclusion criteria from the "SHOCK" trial (with an additional exclusion criteria of IABP use prior to MCS). The majority of patients were supported with Impella CP (92%) prior to PCI (74%) with an average door to support of 85 min in STEMI cases. Moreover, right heart catheterization with hemodynamic monitoring was performed in 92% of cases. The use of a protocol-based approach showed improved survival compared with previously reported studies [7]. Despite the limitations of being an observational single arm study, these findings highlight the importance of early MCS prior to PCI for achieving the most benefit from MCS. Future studies are still warranted to confirm these promising findings. Finally, it is necessary to derive efficient risk scores for identifying patients at high risk of developing cardiogenic shock following AMI as this may aid in risk stratification and potential prophylactic utilization of MCS during PCI to mitigate subsequent hemodynamic derangement in this high-risk population [103].

Another field of future research is the percutaneous LV unloading strategy using Impella in combination with VA-ECMO (ECMELLA) to improve outcomes in patients with refractory cardiogenic shock [87,104]. In an all-comers retrospective study, percutaneous LV unloading with Impella on top of VA-ECMO showed improved outcomes, including higher 30-day survival, as compared to predicted outcomes by established risk scores [87]. In addition to the ECMELLA approach, previous studies have also suggested that a combination of VA-ECMO plus IABP is safe and associated with improved in-hospital survival in cardiogenic shock patients [105]. However, given the retrospective nature of these studies, prospective and randomized studies are still warranted to further investigate this therapeutic strategy.

Table 3. Main Clinical Studies of Percutaneous MCS devices in AMI with Cardiogenic Shock.

First Author/Study (Ref. #)	N	Study Type	Study Arms	Definition	Primary Endpoint	Salient Findings
IABP						
IABP-SHOCK-II [5,65,66]	600	RCT	IABP versus no IABP	AMI with cardiogenic shock (SBP < 90 mmHg for >30 min or need for vasoactive agents, pulmonary congestion, impaired organ perfusion)	30-day, 1-year, 6-year all-cause mortality	No difference in survival at 30 days [5], 1 year [65], and 6 years [66]. No differences recurrent MI, stroke, ischemic comp, severe bleeding, or sepsis.
TACTICs [106]	57	RCT	Fibrinolytic therapy with IABP versus without IABP	AMI with sustained hypotension and heart failure with signs of hypoperfusion	6-month all-cause Mortality	No survival benefit except for patients with Killip III/IV supported with IABP.
Waksman et al. [107]	45	Prospective, nonrandomized	Fibrinolytic therapy with IABP versus without IABP	AMI complicated by cardiogenic shock	In-hospital and 1-year all-cause mortality	In-hospital and 1-year survival improved with IABP after early revascularization with fibrinolytic therapy.
NRMI [108]	23,180	Observational	Fibrinolytic or PCI with IABP versus no IABP	AMI with cardiogenic shock at initial presentation or during hospitalization	In-hospital all-cause mortality	IABP was associated with decreased in-hospital mortality in patients received fibrinolysis but not PCI.
Hariss et al. [62]	48	Observational	IABP prior to PCI versus late IABP	AMI complicated by cardiogenic shock	In-hospital all-cause mortality	Early IABP was associated with decreased in-hospital mortality compared with late IABP.
Sjauw et al. [63]	1009 (RCTs) 10,529 (cohort studies)	Meta-analysis (7 RCTs, 9 cohort studies)	IABP versus no IABP	AMI complicated by cardiogenic shock	30-day all-cause mortality	No survival benefit or improvement in LV ejection fraction with IABP.

Table 3. Cont.

First Author/Study (Ref. #)	N	Study Type	Study Arms	Definition	Primary Endpoint	Salient Findings
Impella						
ISAR-SHOCK [72]	25	RCT	Impella 2.5 versus IABP	AMI complicated by cardiogenic shock	Change in the CI at 30 min post implantation	Superior hemodynamics with Impella. Mortality was similar between the two groups.
EUROSHOCK [39]	120	Observational	Impella 2.5	AMI complicated by cardiogenic shock	30-day all-cause mortality	30-day mortality was high at 64% despite improvement in hemodynamic and metabolic parameters with Impella.
IMPRESS in Severe Shock [6]	48	RCT	Impella CP versus IABP	AMI with severe shock (SBP < 90 mmHg or the need for vasoactive agents, and all required mechanical ventilation)	30-day all-cause mortality	Mortality occurred in 50% of patients with no significant survival benefit with Impella.
Karatolios et al. [74]	90	Observational	Impella versus medical therapy	AMI with post-cardiac arrest cardiogenic shock	In-hospital all-cause mortality	Impella group had better survival at discharge and after 6 months despite being a sicker group.
Schrage et al. [75]	237	Observational	Impella 2.5 (~30%), Impella CP (~70%) versus IABP (matched from IABP-SHOCK trial)	AMI with cardiogenic shock (SBP < 90 mmHg for >30 min or need for vasoactive agents, pulmonary congestion, impaired organ perfusion)	30-day all-cause mortality	Impella was not associated with lower 30-day mortality. Severe bleedings and peripheral vascular complications were more common with Impella use.
Wernly et al. [76]	588	Meta-analysis (4 studies)	Impella versus IABP or medical therapy alone	AMI with cardiogenic shock	30-day all-cause mortality	No improvement in short-term survival with Impella. Higher risk of major bleeding and peripheral ischemic events with Impella.

Table 3. Cont.

First Author/Study (Ref. #)	N	Study Type	Study Arms	Definition	Primary Endpoint	Salient Findings
Cheng et al. [109]	100	Meta-analysis (3 RCTs; 1 for Impella versus IABP and 2 for TandemHeart versus IABP))	Impella or TandemHeart versus IABP	AMI with cardiogenic shock	30-day all-cause mortality	No significant differences in 30-day mortality. Improved hemodynamics with Impella and TandemHeart. Higher rates of bleeding with TandemHeart and of hemolysis with Impella.
Alushi et al. [110]	116	Observational	Impella 2.5 (~30%), Impella CP (~70%) versus IABP	AMI with cardiogenic shock	30-day all-cause mortality	No significant differences in 30-day mortality. Impella significantly reduced the inotropic score, lactate levels, and improved LVEF compared with IABP. Higher rates of bleeding with Impella.
TandemHeart						
Kar et al. [43]	117	Observational	TandemHeart	Severe cardiogenic shock despite vasopressor and IABP support	30-day all-cause mortality	30-day mortality: 40%. Improvement in hemodynamics refractory to vasopressors and IABP.
Thiele et al. [80]	41	RCT	TandemHeart versus IABP	AMI with cardiogenic shock (CI < 2.1 L/min/m^2, lactate > 2)	Change in cardiac index	Hemodynamic and metabolic parameters were reversed more effectively by TandemHeart. 30-day mortality was similar. Bleeding and ischemic events were more common with TandemHeart.
Burkhoff et al. [81]	42	RCT	TandemHeart versus IABP	Severe cardiogenic shock (most had AMI and failed IABP)	30-day all-cause mortality	Similar mortality rates and adverse events at 30 days. Superior hemodynamics with TandemHeart.

Table 3. *Cont.*

First Author/Study (Ref. #)	N	Study Type	Study Arms	Definition	Primary Endpoint	Salient Findings
VA-ECMO						
Esper et al. [84]	18	Observational	VA-ECMO	Severe cardiogenic shock due to ACS	Survival to hospital discharge	Survival rates at discharge: 67%. High bleeding rates (94% required blood transfusion).
Negi et al. [85]	15	Observational	VA-ECMO	AMI with severe cardiogenic shock (60% had STEMI and IABP support)	Survival to hospital discharge	Survival rates at discharge: 47%. Vascular complications: 53%.
Nichol et al. [111]	1494 (84 studies)	Systematic review	VA-ECMO	Cardiogenic shock or cardiac arrest	Survival to hospital discharge	Survival to hospital discharge: 50%.
Sheu et al. [112]	Group 1: 115 Group 2: 219	Observational	Group 1: profound shock without ECMO versus group 2: profound shock with ECMO	AMI and profound cardiogenic shock (SBP <75 mmHg despite IABP and vasopressor support)	30-day survival	ECMO group had higher survival rates: 60.9% versus 28% in non-ECMO group.
Takayama et al. [113]	90	Observational	VA-ECMO	Refractory cardiac shock (AMI in 49%)	Survival to hospital discharge	Survival to hospital discharge: 49%. Bleeding and stroke rates: 26%; and LV distension and pulmonary edema: 18%.

Abbreviations: ACS, acute coronary syndrome; AMI, acute myocardial infarction; CI, cardiac index; IABP, intraaortic balloon pump; IMPRESS in Severe SHOCK, IMPella versus IABP Reduces mortality in STEMI patients treated with primary PCI in Severe cardiogenic SHOCK; ISAR-SHOCK, Impella LP 2.5 versus IABP in Cardiogenic SHOCK; LVEF, left ventricular ejection fraction; MCS, mechanical circulatory support; NRMI, National Registry of Myocardial Infarction; PCI, percutaneous coronary intervention; RCT, randomized controlled study; SBP, systolic blood pressure; STEMI, ST-elevation myocardial infarction; VA-ECMO, venoarterial extracorporeal membrane oxygenation.

Table 4. Main Clinical Studies of Percutaneous MCS devices in High-Risk PCI.

First Author/Study (Ref. #)	N	Study Type	Study Arms	Definition	Primary Endpoint	Salient Findings
IABP						
BCIS-1 [3]	301	RCT	Elective IABP versus no IABP before PCI	High-risk PCI without cardiogenic shock, LVEF < 30%, severe CAD (jeopardy score > 8)	MACE: Composite of death, AMI, stroke, revascularization at hospital discharge	No reduction in MACE. No difference in survival rates at 6 months. Decreased major procedural complications with planned IABP (mainly hypotension).
Extended BCIS-1 [70]	301	RCT	Elective IABP versus no IABP before PCI	High-risk PCI without cardiogenic shock, LVEF < 30%, severe CAD (jeopardy score > 8)	Long-term All-cause mortality	Elective IABP use was associated with a 34% relative reduction in all-cause mortality at 4 years post PCI.
CRISP-AMI [68]	337	RCT	Elective IABP prior to PCI until at least 12 h post versus no IABP	Acute anterior MI without cardiogenic shock	Infarct size measured by cardiac MRI at 3–5 days post PCI	No reduction in infarct size with IABP use. Survival at 6 months and procedural complications were similar between groups.
NCDR [69]	181,599	Observational	Elective IABP versus no IABP before PCI	LVEF < 30%, severe CAD, including patients with cardiogenic shock	In-hospital mortality	IABP use varied significantly across hospitals. No association with differences in in-hospital mortality.

Table 4. Cont.

First Author/Study (Ref. #)	N	Study Type	Study Arms	Definition	Primary Endpoint	Salient Findings
Impella						
Henriques et al. [77]	19	Observational	Impella 2.5	High-risk PCI (elderly, most with prior MI, poor surgical candidates, LVEF < 40%)	Safety and feasibility of Impella use	A 100% procedural success and no important device-related adverse events.
PROTECT I [78]	20	Prospective, nonrandomized	Impella 2.5	High-risk PCI (LVEF < 35%, UPLM disease or last patent vessel)	Safety and feasibility of Impella use	Impella is safe, easy to implant, and provides excellent hemodynamic support during high-risk PCI.
USPella [14]	175	Observational	Impella 2.5	High-risk PCI (severe three-vessel disease or UPLM, mean SYNTAX score 36, low LVEF)	MACE at 30 days	MACE: 8%. 30-day, 6-month, and 12-month survival: 96%, 91%, and 88%, respectively.
PROTECT II [4]	452	RCT	Impella 2.5 versus IABP	High-risk PCI (LVEF < 35%, UPLM, three-vessel or last patent vessel disease)	MACE (a composite of 11 adverse events) at 30 days	30-day MACE was similar between groups (ITT) and trend for lower MACE with Impella (PP). 90-day MACE was similar (ITT) and significantly lower with Impella (PP).
Ameelot et al. [8]	198	Observational	Impella CP, heartmate PHP, or PulseCath iVAC2L versus unprotected PCI	Prophylactic high-risk PCI	A composite of procedure-related adverse events	Lower rates of periprocedural adverse events with Impella devices. 30-day survival was significantly higher with Impella versus unsupported PCI.

Table 4. *Cont.*

First Author/Study (Ref. #)	N	Study Type	Study Arms	Definition	Primary Endpoint	Salient Findings
TandemHeart						
Alli et al. [82]	54	Observational	TandemHeart	Prophylactic high-risk PCI (STS score 13%, SYNTAX score 33, three-vessel and UPLM disease)	6-month survival	6-month survival: 87%. Major vascular complications: 13%.
Briasoulis et al. [83]	205	Meta-analysis (8 cohort studies)	TandemHeart	Prophylactic high-risk PCI	30-day all-cause mortality	30-day mortality: 8%. Major bleeding rates: 3.6%.
VA-ECMO						
Teirstein et al. [114]	389 (prophylactic support) 180 (standby support)	Observational	VA-ECMO	High-risk PCI (LVEF < 25%, culprit lesion supplying > 50% of the myocardium)	PCI success rates and major complications rates	Comparable results in the prophylactic compared with the standby VA-ECMO support groups. Patients with extremely low LVEF may benefit more from prophylactic support.
Schreiber et al. [115]	149	Observational	VA-ECMO versus IABP	High-risk PCI (low LVEF and multivessel PCI)	MACE: Composite of MI, stroke, death, CABG	No difference in MACE between VA-ECMO and IABP groups. Higher multivessel PCI success rates with VA-ECMO.

Abbreviations: AMI, acute myocardial infarction; BCIS-1, the Balloon pump-assisted Coronary Intervention Study; CRISP-AMI, the Counterpulsation to Reduce Infarct Size Pre-PCI Acute Myocardial Infarction; CABG, coronary artery bypass grafting; IABP, intraaortic balloon pump; ITT, intention to treat analysis; LVEF, left ventricular ejection fraction; MACE, major adverse cardiac events; MCS, mechanical circulatory support; MI, myocardial infarction; NCDR, National Cardiovascular Data Registry; PCI, percutaneous coronary intervention; PP, per protocol analysis; RCT, randomized controlled study; SYNTAX, Synergy between Percutaneous Coronary Intervention with TAXUS and Cardiac Surgery; UPLM, unprotected left main; VA-ECMO, venoarterial extracorporeal membrane oxygenation.

9. Conclusions

The use of MCS devices is expanding and several MCS devices are currently available and can provide varying magnitude of hemodynamic support during high-risk and complex PCIs. Small randomized controlled trials have provided conflicting results regarding survival benefit using these devices despite substantial hemodynamic and metabolic benefit. However, given the high morbidity and mortality burden among patients undergoing high-risk and complex PCI, detailed hemodynamic assessment and careful patient selection is mandatory to achieve incremental benefit over early revascularization and pharmacologic therapy with utilizing these devices. Furthermore, the optimal timing and magnitude of hemodynamic support during PCI as well as prevention of device-related complications are all important considerations in future research in this field. Until adequate data supporting MCS use in a broader patient population is available, MCS devices during PCI should be individualized based on multiple factors with a recommended use in patients with the greatest potential benefit and a relatively low risk of device-related complications.

Author Contributions: Conceptualization, R.A. and J.R.R.; methodology, R.A. and J.R.R.; formal analysis, R.A. and J.R.R.; data curation, R.A. and J.R.R.; writing—original draft preparation, R.A. and J.R.R.; writing—review and editing, R.A. and J.R.R.

Funding: This research received no external funding.

Conflicts of Interest: The authors have no conflict of interest to disclose.

References

1. Waldo, S.W.; Secemsky, E.A.; O'Brien, C.; Kennedy, K.F.; Pomerantsev, E.; Sundt, T.M., 3rd; McNulty, E.J.; Scirica, B.M.; Yeh, R.W. Surgical ineligibility and mortality among patients with unprotected left main or multivessel coronary artery disease undergoing percutaneous coronary intervention. *Circulation* **2014**, *130*, 2295–2301. [CrossRef] [PubMed]
2. Atkinson, T.M.; Ohman, E.M.; O'Neill, W.W.; Rab, T.; Cigarroa, J.E. A practical approach to mechanical circulatory support in patients undergoing percutaneous coronary intervention an interventional perspective. *JACC Cardiovasc. Interv.* **2016**, *9*, 871–883. [CrossRef] [PubMed]
3. Perera, D.; Stables, R.; Thomas, M.; Booth, J.; Pitt, M.; Blackman, D.; de Belder, A.; Redwood, S. BCSI-1 Investigators. Elective intra-aortic balloon counterpulsation during high-risk percutaneous coronary intervention: A randomized controlled trial. *JAMA* **2010**, *304*, 867–874. [CrossRef] [PubMed]
4. O'Neill, W.W.; Kleiman, N.S.; Moses, J.; Henriques, J.P.; Dixon, S.; Massaro, J.; Palacios, I.; Maini, B.; Mulukutla, S.; Dzavík, V. A prospective, randomized clinical trial of hemodynamic support with impella 2.5 versus intra-aortic balloon pump in patients undergoing high-risk percutaneous coronary intervention: The PROTECT II study. *Circulation* **2012**, *126*, 1717–1727. [CrossRef] [PubMed]
5. Thiele, H.; Zeymer, U.; Neumann, F.J.; Ferenc, M.; Olbrich, H.G.; Hausleiter, J.; Richardt, G.; Hennersdorf, M.; Empen, K.; Fuernau, G. Intraaortic balloon support for myocardial infarction with cardiogenic shock. *N. Engl. J. Med.* **2012**, *367*, 1287–1296. [CrossRef] [PubMed]
6. Ouweneel, D.M.; Eriksen, E.; Sjauw, K.D.; van Dongen, I.M.; Hirsch, A.; Packer, E.J.; Vis, M.M.; Wykrzykowska, J.J.; Koch, K.T.; Baan, J.; et al. Percutaneous mechanical circulatory support versus intra-aortic balloon pump in cardiogenic shock after acute myocardial infarction. *J. Am. Coll. Cardiol.* **2017**, *69*, 278–287. [CrossRef] [PubMed]
7. Basir, M.B.; Kapur, N.K.; Patel, K.; Salam, M.A.; Schreiber, T.; Kaki, A.; Hanson, I.; Almany, S.; Timmis, S.; Dixon, S.; et al. Improved outcomes associated with the use of shock protocols: Updates from the national cardiogenic shock initiative. *Catheter Cardiovasc. Interv.* **2019**, *93*, 1173–1183. [CrossRef] [PubMed]
8. Ameloot, K.; Bastos, M.B.; Daemen, J.; Schreuder, J.; Boersma, E.; Zijlstra, F.; Van Mieghem, N.M. New generation mechanical circulatory support during high-risk PCI: A cross sectional analysis. *EuroIntervention* **2019**. [CrossRef]
9. Damluji, A.A.; Bandeen-Roche, K.; Berkower, C.; Boyd, C.M.; Al-Damluji, M.S.; Cohen, M.G.; Forman, D.E.; Chaudhary, R.; Gerstenblith, G.; Walston, J.D.; et al. Percutaneous coronary intervention in older patients

with ST-segment elevation myocardial infarction and cardiogenic shock. *J. Am. Coll. Cardiol.* **2019**, *73*, 1890–1900. [CrossRef] [PubMed]

10. Ibanez, B.; James, S.; Agewall, S.; Antunes, M.J.; Bucciarelli-Ducci, C.; Bueno, H.; Caforio, A.L.P.; Crea, F.; Goudevenos, J.A.; Halvorsen, S.; et al. 2017 ESC Guidelines for the management of acute myocardial infarction in patients presenting with ST-segment elevation. *Eur. Heart J.* **2018**, *39*, 119–177. [CrossRef] [PubMed]

11. Rihal, C.S.; Naidu, S.S.; Givertz, M.M.; Szeto, W.Y.; Burke, J.A.; Kapur, N.K.; Kern, M.; Garratt, K.N.; Goldstein, J.A.; Dimas, V.; et al. 2015 SCAI/ACC/HFSA/STS clinical expert consensus statement on the use of percutaneous mechanical circulatory support devices in cardiovascular care. *J. Am. Coll. Cardiol.* **2015**, *65*, e7–e26. [CrossRef] [PubMed]

12. Levine, G.N.; Bates, E.R.; Blankenship, J.C.; Bailey, S.R.; Bittl, J.A.; Cercek, B.; Chambers, C.E.; Ellis, S.G.; Guyton, R.A.; Hollenberg, S.M.; et al. 2011 ACCF/AHA/SCAI guideline for percutaneous coronary intervention. *J. Am. Coll. Cardiol.* **2011**, *124*, e574–e651. [CrossRef]

13. Wallace, T.W.; Berger, J.S.; Wang, A.; Velazquez, E.J.; Brown, DL. Impact of left ventricular dysfunction on hospital mortality among patients undergoing elective percutaneous coronary intervention. *Am. J. Cardiol.* **2009**. [CrossRef] [PubMed]

14. Maini, B.; Naidu, S.S.; Mulukutla, S.; Kleiman, N.; Schreiber, T.; Wohns, D.; Dixon, S.; Rihal, C.; Dave, R.; O'Nell, W. Real-world use of the Impella 2.5 circulatory support system in complex high-risk percutaneous coronary intervention: The USpella registry. *Catheter Cardiovasc. Interv.* **2012**, *80*, 717–725. [CrossRef] [PubMed]

15. Krone, R.J.; Shaw, R.E.; Klein, L.W.; Block, P.C.; Anderson, H.V.; Weintraub, W.S.; Brindis, R.G.; McKay, C.R.; ACC-National Cardiovascular Data Registry. Evaluation of the American College of Cardiology/American Heart Association and the Society for Coronary Angiography and Interventions lesion classification system in the current "stent era" of coronary interventions (from the ACC-National Cardiovascular. *Am. J. Cardiol.* **2003**, *92*, 389–394. [CrossRef]

16. Sakakura, K.; Ako, J.; Wada, H.; Kubo, N.; Momomura, S.I. ACC/AHA classification of coronary lesions reflects medical resource use in current percutaneous coronary interventions. *Catheter Cardiovasc. Interv.* **2012**. [CrossRef] [PubMed]

17. Brennan, J.M.; Curtis, J.P.; Dai, D.; Fitzgerald, S.; Khandelwal, A.K.; Spertus, J.A.; Rao, S.V.; Singh, M.; Shaw, R.E.; Ho, K.K.; et al. Enhanced mortality risk prediction with a focus on high-risk percutaneous coronary intervention: Results from 1,208,137 procedures in the NCDR (national cardiovascular data registry). *JACC Cardiovasc. Interv.* **2013**, *6*, 790–799. [CrossRef] [PubMed]

18. Burkhoff, D.; Sayer, G.; Doshi, D.; Uriel, N. Hemodynamics of mechanical circulatory support. *J. Am. Coll. Cardiol.* **2015**. [CrossRef]

19. Van Diepen, S.; Katz, J.N.; Albert, N.M.; Henry, T.D.; Jacobs, A.K.; Kapur, N.K.; Kilic, A.; Menon, V.; Ohman, E.M.; Sweitzer, N.K.; et al. Contemporary management of cardiogenic shock: A scientific statement from the american heart association. *Circulation* **2017**, *136*, e232–e268. [CrossRef]

20. Reynolds, H.R.; Hochman, J.S. Cardiogenic shock current concepts and improving outcomes. *Circulation* **2008**. [CrossRef]

21. Miller, L. Cardiogenic shock in acute myocardial infarction the era of mechanical support. *J. Am. Coll. Cardiol.* **2016**. [CrossRef]

22. Masoudi, F.A.; Ponirakis, A.; de Lemos, J.A.; Jollis, J.G.; Kremers, M.; Messenger, J.C.; Moore, J.W.M.; Moussa, I.; Oetgen, W.J.; Varosy, P.D.; et al. Trends in U.S. cardiovascular care: 2016 report from 4 ACC national cardiovascular data registries. *J. Am. Coll. Cardiol.* **2017**, *69*, 1427–1450. [CrossRef] [PubMed]

23. Babaev, A.; Frederick, P.D.; Pasta, D.J.; Every, N.; Sichrovsky, T.; Hochman, J.S. Trends in management and outcomes of patients with acute myocardial infarction complicated by cardiogenic shock. *J. Am. Med. Assoc.* **2005**. [CrossRef] [PubMed]

24. Basir, M.B.; Schreiber, T.L.; Grines, C.L.; Dixon, S.R.; Moses, J.W.; Maini, B.J.; Khandelwal, A.K.; Ohman, E.M.; O'Nell, W.W. Effect of early initiation of mechanical circulatory support on survival in cardiogenic shock. *Am. J. Cardiol.* **2017**, *119*, 845–851. [CrossRef] [PubMed]

25. Remmelink, M.; Sjauw, K.D.; Henriques, J.P.S.; Vis, M.M.; van der Schaaf, R.J.; Koch, K.T.; Tijssen, J.G.; de Wintr, R.J.; Piek, J.J.; Baan, J., Jr. Acute left ventricular dynamic effects of primary percutaneous coronary intervention. From occlusion to reperfusion. *J. Am. Coll. Cardiol.* **2009**, *53*, 1498–1502. [CrossRef] [PubMed]

26. Borlaug, B.A.; Kass, D.A. Invasive hemodynamic assessment in heart failure. *Cardiol. Clin.* **2011**. [CrossRef] [PubMed]
27. Uriel, N.; Sayer, G.; Annamalai, S.; Kapur, N.K.; Burkhoff, D. Mechanical unloading in heart failure. *J. Am. Coll. Cardiol.* **2018**. [CrossRef] [PubMed]
28. Rab, T.; O'Neill, W. Mechanical circulatory support for patients with cardiogenic shock. *Trends Cardiovasc. Med.* **2018**. [CrossRef]
29. Thiele, H.; Ohman, E.M.; Desch, S.; Eitel, I.; De Waha, S. Management of cardiogenic shock. *Eur. Heart J.* **2015**. [CrossRef]
30. Csepe, T.A.; Kilic, A. Advancements in mechanical circulatory support for patients in acute and chronic heart failure. *J. Thorac. Dis.* **2017**. [CrossRef]
31. Tan, L.B. Cardiac pumping capability and prognosis in heart failure. *Lancet* **1986**. [CrossRef]
32. Lang, C.C.; Karlin, P.; Haythe, J.; Levy, W.; Lim, T.K.; Mancini, D.M. Peak cardiac power, measured non-invasively, is a powerful predictor of mortality in chronic heart failure. *Circulation* **2007**, *22*, 33–38.
33. WEBER, KT. Intra-aortic balloon pumping. *Ann. Intern. Med.* **2013**. [CrossRef]
34. Papaioannou, T.G.; Stefanadis, C. Basic principles of the intraaortic balloon pump and mechanisms affecting its performance. *ASAIO J.* **2005**. [CrossRef]
35. Rastan, A.J.; Tillmann, E.; Subramanian, S.; Lehmkuhl, L.; Funkat, A.K.; Leontyev, S.; Doenst, T.; Walther, T.; Gutberlet, M.; Mohr, F.W. Visceral arterial compromise during intra-aortic balloon counterpulsation therapy. *Circulation* **2010**. [CrossRef]
36. Herrera-Perez, D.; Haslam, A.; Crain, T.; Gill, J.; Livingston, C.; Kaestner, V.; Hayes, M.; Morgan, D.; Cifu, A.S.; Prasad, V. A comprehensive review of randomized clinical trials in three medical journals reveals 396 medical reversals. *Elife* **2019**. [CrossRef] [PubMed]
37. Basra, S.S.; Loyalka, P.; Kar, B. Current status of percutaneous ventricular assist devices for cardiogenic shock. *Curr. Opin. Cardiol.* **2011**. [CrossRef] [PubMed]
38. Möbius-Winkler, S.; Fritzenwanger, M.; Pfeifer, R.; Schulze, P.C. Percutaneous support of the failing left and right ventricle—Recommendations for the use of mechanical device therapy. *Heart Fail. Rev.* **2018**. [CrossRef]
39. Lauten, A.; Engström, A.E.; Jung, C.; Empen, K.; Erne, P.; Cook, S.; Windecker, S.; Bergmann, M.W.; Klingenberg, R.; Lüscher, T.F.; et al. Percutaneous left-ventricular support with the impella-2.5-assist device in acute cardiogenic shock results of the impella-EUROSHOCK-registry. *Circ. Hear Fail.* **2013**, *6*, 23–30. [CrossRef] [PubMed]
40. Remmelink, M.; Sjauw, K.D.; Henriques, J.P.; De Winter, R.J.; Vis, M.M.; Koch, K.T.; Paulus, W.J.; De Mol, B.A.; Tijssen, J.G.; Piek, J.J.; et al. Effects of mechanical left ventricular unloading by impella on left ventricular dynamics in high-risk and primary percutaneous coronary intervention patients. *Catheter Cardiovasc. Interv.* **2010**. [CrossRef]
41. Doshi, R.; Patel, K.; Decter, D.; Gupta, R.; Meraj, P. Trends in the utilisation and in-hospital mortality associated with short-term mechanical circulatory support for heart failure with reduced ejection fraction. *Hear Lung Circ.* **2019**. [CrossRef] [PubMed]
42. Martinez, C.A.; Singh, V.; Londoño, J.C.; Cohen, M.G.; Alfonso, C.E.; O'Neill, W.W.; Heldman, A.W. Percutaneous retrograde left ventricular assist support for patients with aortic stenosis and left ventricular dysfunction. *J. Am. Coll. Cardiol.* **2011**, *80*, 1201–1209. [CrossRef] [PubMed]
43. Kar, B.; Gregoric, I.D.; Basra, S.S.; Idelchik, G.M.; Loyalka, P. The percutaneous ventricular assist device in severe refractory cardiogenic shock. *J. Am. Coll. Cardiol.* **2010**. [CrossRef] [PubMed]
44. Burkhoff, D.; Naidu, S.S. The science behind percutaneous hemodynamic support: A review and comparison of support strategies. *Catheter Cardiovasc. Interv.* **2012**. [CrossRef] [PubMed]
45. Kono, S.; Nishimura, K.; Nishina, T.; Komeda, M.; Akamatsu, T. Auto-synchronized systolic unloading during left ventricular assist with centrifugal pump. *ASAIO J.* **1999**. [CrossRef]
46. Pham, D.T.; Al-Quthami, A.; Kapur, N.K. Percutaneous left ventricular support in cardiogenic shock and severe aortic regurgitation. *Catheter Cardiovasc. Interv.* **2013**. [CrossRef]
47. Ouweneel, D.M.; Schotborgh, J.V.; Limpens, J.; Sjauw, K.D.; Engström, A.E.; Lagrand, W.K.; Cherpanath, T.G.V.; Driessen, A.H.G.; De Mol, B.A.J.M.; Henriques, J.P.S. Extracorporeal life support during cardiac arrest and cardiogenic shock: A systematic review and meta-analysis. *Intensive Care Med.* **2016**. [CrossRef]
48. Thiagarajan, R.R.; Barbaro, R.P.; Rycus, P.T.; McMullan, D.M.; Conrad, S.A.; Fortenberry, J.D.; Paden, M.L. Extracorporeal life support organization registry international report 2016. *ASAIO J.* **2017**. [CrossRef]

49. Aghili, N.; Kang, S.; Kapur, N.K. The fundamentals of extra-corporeal membrane oxygenation. *Minerva Cardioangiol.* **2015**, *63*, 75–85.
50. MacLaren, G.; Combes, A.; Bartlett, R.H. Contemporary extracorporeal membrane oxygenation for adult respiratory failure: Life support in the new era. *Intensive Care Med.* **2012**. [CrossRef]
51. Russo, J.J.; Aleksova, N.; Pitcher, I.; Couture, E.; Parlow, S.; Faraz, M.; Visintini, S.; Simard, T.; Di Santo, P.; Mathew, R.; et al. Left ventricular unloading during extracorporeal membrane oxygenation in patients with cardiogenic shock. *J. Am. Coll. Cardiol.* **2019**. [CrossRef]
52. Koeckert, M.S.; Jorde, U.P.; Naka, Y.; Moses, J.W.; Takayama, H. Impella LP 2.5 for left ventricular unloading during venoarterial extracorporeal membrane oxygenation support. *J. Cardiol. Surg.* **2011**. [CrossRef]
53. Ostadal, P.; Mlcek, M.; Gorhan, H.; Simundic, I.; Strunina, S.; Hrachovina, M.; Krüger, A.; Vondrakova, D.; Janotka, M.; Hala, P.; et al. Electrocardiogram-synchronized pulsatile extracorporeal life support preserves left ventricular function and coronary flow in a porcine model of cardiogenic shock. *PLoS ONE* **2018**. [CrossRef]
54. Wang, S.; Izer, J.M.; Clark, J.B.; Patel, S.; Pauliks, L.; Kunselman, A.R.; Leach, D.; Cooper, T.K.; Wilson, R.P.; Ündar, A. In vivo hemodynamic performance evaluation of novel electrocardiogram-synchronized pulsatile and nonpulsatile extracorporeal life support systems in an adult swine model. *Artif. Organs* **2015**. [CrossRef]
55. Wolfe, R.; Strother, A.; Wang, S.; Kunselman, A.R.; Ündar, A. Impact of pulsatility and flow rates on hemodynamic energy transmission in an adult extracorporeal life support system. *Artif. Organs* **2015**. [CrossRef]
56. Pöss, J.; Kriechbaum, S.; Ewen, S.; Graf, J.; Hager, I.; Hennersdorf, M.; Petros, S.; Link, A.; Bohm, M.; Thiele, H.; et al. First-in-man analysis of the i-cor assist device in patients with cardiogenic shock. *Eur. Heart J. Acute Cardiovasc. Care* **2015**. [CrossRef]
57. Masyuk, M.; Abel, P.; Hug, M.; Wernly, B.; Haneya, A.; Sack, S.; Sideris, K.; Langwieser, N.; Graf, T.; Fuernau, G.; et al. Real-world clinical experience with the percutaneous extracorporeal life support system: Results from the German Lifebridge® Registry. *Clin. Res. Cardiol.* **2019**. [CrossRef]
58. Cheng, R.; Hachamovitch, R.; Kittleson, M.; Patel, J.; Arabia, F.; Moriguchi, J.; Esmailian, F.; Azarbal, B. Complications of extracorporeal membrane oxygenation for treatment of cardiogenic shock and cardiac arrest: A meta-analysis of 1,866 adult patients. *Ann. Thorac. Surg.* **2014**. [CrossRef]
59. Uil, C.D.; Daemen, J.; Lenzen, M.; Maugenest, A.-M.; Joziasse, L.; Van Geuns, R.; Van Mieghem, N. Pulsatile iVAC 2L circulatory support in high-risk percutaneous coronary intervention. *EuroIntervention* **2017**. [CrossRef]
60. McLaughlin, V.V.; Archer, S.L.; Badesch, D.B.; Barst, R.J.; Farber, H.W.; Lindner, J.R.; Mathier, M.A.; McGoon, M.D.; Park, M.H.; Rosenson, R.S.; et al. ACCF/AHA 2009 expert consensus document on pulmonary hypertension. A report of the American College of Cardiology Foundation task force on expert consensus documents and the American Heart Association Developed in Collaboration with the American College of Chest Physicians; American Thoracic Society, Inc.; and the Pulmonary Hypertension Association. *J. Am. Coll. Cardiol.* **2009**. [CrossRef]
61. Anderson, M.B.; Goldstein, J.; Milano, C.; Morris, L.D.; Kormos, R.L.; Bhama, J.; Kapur, N.K.; Bansal, A.; Garcia, J.; Baker, J.N.; et al. Benefits of a novel percutaneous ventricular assist device for right heart failure: The prospective RECOVER RIGHT study of the Impella RP device. *J. Heart Lung Transplant.* **2015**. [CrossRef]
62. Harris, S.; Tepper, D.; Ip, R. Comparison of hospital mortality with intra-aortic balloon counterpulsation insertion before vs after primary percutaneous coronary intervention for cardiogenic shock complicating acute myocardial infarction. *Congest. Heart Fail.* **2010**. [CrossRef]
63. Sjauw, K.D.; Engström, A.E.; Vis, M.M.; van der Schaaf, R.J.; Baan, J., Jr.; Koch, K.T.; de Winter, R.J.; Piek, J.J.; Tijssen, J.G.; Henriques, J.P. A systematic review and meta-analysis of intra-aortic balloon pump therapy in ST-elevation myocardial infarction: Should we change the guidelines? *Eur. Heart J.* **2009**. [CrossRef]

64. Hochman, J.S.; Sleeper, L.A.; Webb, J.G.; Sanborn, T.A.; White, H.D.; Talley, J.D.; Buller, C.E.; Jacobs, A.K.; Slater, J.N.; Col, J.; et al. Early revascularization in acute myocardial infarction complicated by cardiogenic shock. SHOCK Investigators. Should we emergently revascularize occluded coronaries for cardiogenic shock. *N. Engl. J. Med.* **1999**. [CrossRef]
65. Thiele, H.; Zeymer, U.; Neumann, F.-J.; Ferenc, M.; Olbrich, H.-G.; Hausleiter, J.; De Waha, A.; Richardt, G.; Hennersdorf, M.; Empen, K.; et al. Intra-aortic balloon counterpulsation in acute myocardial infarction complicated by cardiogenic shock (IABP-SHOCK II): Final 12 month results of a randomised, open-label trial. *Lancet* **2013**. [CrossRef]
66. Thiele, H.; Zeymer, U.; Thelemann, N.; Neumann, F.J.; Hausleiter, J.; Abdel-Wahab, M.; Meyer-Saraei, R.; Fuernau, G.; Eitel, I.; Hambrecht, R.; et al. Intraaortic balloon pump in cardiogenic shock complicating acute myocardial infarction: Long-term 6-year outcome of the randomized IABP-SHOCK II trial. *Circulation* **2018**. [CrossRef]
67. Dehmer, G.J.; Blankenship, J.C.; Cilingiroglu, M.; Dwyer, J.G.; Feldman, D.N.; Gardner, T.J.; Grines, C.L.; Singh, M. SCAI/ACC/AHA Expert consensus document: 2014 update on percutaneous coronary intervention without on-site surgical backup. *Catheter Cardiovasc. Interv.* **2014**. [CrossRef]
68. Patel, M.R.; Smalling, R.W.; Thiele, H.; Barnhart, H.X.; Zhou, Y.; Chandra, P.; Chew, D.; Choen, M.; French, J.; Perera, D.; et al. Intra-aortic balloon counterpulsation and infarct size in patients with acute anterior myocardial infarction without shock: The CRISP AMI randomized trial. *JAMA-J. Am. Med. Assoc.* **2011**. [CrossRef]
69. Curtis, J.P.; Rathore, S.S.; Wang, Y.; Chen, J.; Nallamothu, B.K.; Krumholz, H.M. Use and effectiveness of intra-Aortic balloon pumps among patients undergoing high risk percutaneous coronary intervention: Insights from the national cardiovascular data registry. *Circ. Cardiovasc. Qual. Outcomes* **2012**. [CrossRef]
70. Perera, D.; Stables, R.; Clayton, T.; De Silva, K.; Lumley, M.; Clack, L.; Thomas, M.; Redwood, S.; BCSI-1 Investigators. Long-term mortality data from the balloon pump–assisted coronary intervention study (BCIS-1). *Circulation* **2012**. [CrossRef]
71. O'Gara, P.T.; Kushner, F.G.; Ascheim, D.D.; E Casey, D.; Chung, M.K.; A De Lemos, J.; Ettinger, S.M.; Fang, J.C.; Fesmire, F.M.; A Franklin, B.; et al. 2013 ACCF/AHA guideline for the management of st-elevation myocardial infarction: Executive summary: A report of the American college of cardiology foundation/american heart association task force on practice guidelines. *J. Am. Coll. Cardiol.* **2013**. [CrossRef]
72. Seyfarth, M.; Sibbing, D.; Bauer, I.; Fröhlich, G.; Bott-Flügel, L.; Byrne, R.; Dirschinger, J.; Kastrati, A.; Schömig, A. A Randomized clinical trial to evaluate the safety and efficacy of a percutaneous left ventricular assist device versus intra-aortic balloon pumping for treatment of cardiogenic shock caused by myocardial infarction. *J. Am. Coll. Cardiol.* **2008**. [CrossRef]
73. Zeymer, U.; Thiele, H. Mechanical support for cardiogenic shock: Lost in translation? *J. Am. Coll. Cardiol.* **2017**. [CrossRef]
74. Karatolios, K.; Chatzis, G.; Markus, B.; Luesebrink, U.; Ahrens, H.; Dersch, W.; Betz, S.; Ploeger, B.; Boesl, E.; O'Neill, W.; et al. Impella support compared to medical treatment for post-cardiac arrest shock after out of hospital cardiac arrest. *Resuscitation* **2018**. [CrossRef]
75. Schrage, B.; Ibrahim, K.; Loehn, T.; Werner, N.; Sinning, J.-M.; Pappalardo, F.; Pieri, M.; Skurk, C.; Lauten, A.; Landmesser, U.; et al. Impella support for acute myocardial infarction complicated by cardiogenic shock. *Circulation* **2019**. [CrossRef]
76. Wernly, B.; Seelmaier, C.; Leistner, D.; Stähli, B.E.; Pretsch, I.; Lichtenauer, M.; Jung, C.; Hoppe, U.C.; Landmesser, U.; Thiele, H.; et al. Mechanical circulatory support with Impella versus intra-aortic balloon pump or medical treatment in cardiogenic shock—A critical appraisal of current data. *Clin. Res. Cardiol.* **2019**. [CrossRef]
77. Henriques, J.P.; Remmelink, M.; Baan, J.; Van Der Schaaf, R.J.; Vis, M.M.; Koch, K.T.; Scholten, E.W.; De Mol, B.A.; Tijssen, J.G.; Piek, J.J.; et al. Safety and feasibility of elective high-risk percutaneous coronary intervention procedures with left ventricular support of the impella recover LP 2.5. *Am. J. Cardiol.* **2006**. [CrossRef]
78. Dixon, S.R.; Henriques, J.P.; Mauri, L.; Sjauw, K.; Civitello, A.; Kar, B.; Loyalka, P.; Resnic, F.S.; Teirstein, P.; Makkar, R.; et al. A prospective feasibility trial investigating the use of the impella 2.5 system in patients undergoing high-risk percutaneous coronary intervention (The PROTECT I Trial). Initial U.S. Experience. *JACC Cardiovasc. Interv.* **2009**. [CrossRef]

79. Dangas, G.D.; Kini, A.S.; Sharma, S.K.; Henriques, J.P.; Claessen, B.E.; Dixon, S.R.; Massaro, J.M.; Palacios, I.; Popma, J.J.; Ohman, E.M.; et al. Impact of hemodynamic support with impella 2.5 versus intra-aortic balloon pump on prognostically important clinical outcomes in patients undergoing high-risk percutaneous coronary intervention (from the PROTECT II randomized trial). *Am. J. Cardiol.* **2014**. [CrossRef]
80. Thiele, H.; Sick, P.; Boudriot, E.; Diederich, K.-W.; Hambrecht, R.; Niebauer, J.; Schuler, G. Randomized comparison of intra-aortic balloon support with a percutaneous left ventricular assist device in patients with revascularized acute myocardial infarction complicated by cardiogenic shock. *Eur. Heart J.* **2005**. [CrossRef]
81. Burkhoff, D.; Cohen, H.; Brunckhorst, C.; O'Neill, W.W. A randomized multicenter clinical study to evaluate the safety and efficacy of the TandemHeart percutaneous ventricular assist device versus conventional therapy with intraaortic balloon pumping for treatment of cardiogenic shock. *Am. Heart J.* **2006**. [CrossRef]
82. Alli, O.O.; Singh, I.M.; Holmes, D.R.; Pulido, J.N.; Park, S.J.; Rihal, C.S. Percutaneous left ventricular assist device with TandemHeart for high-risk percutaneous coronary intervention: The Mayo Clinic experience. *Catheter Cardiovasc. Interv.* **2012**. [CrossRef]
83. Briasoulis, A.; Telila, T.; Palla, M.; Mercado, N.; Kondur, A.; Grines, C.; Schreiber, T. Meta-analysis of usefulness of percutaneous left ventricular assist devices for high-risk percutaneous coronary interventions. *Am. J. Cardiol.* **2016**. [CrossRef]
84. Bermudez, C.; Kormos, R.; Subramaniam, K.; Mulukutla, S.; Sappington, P.; Waters, J.; Khandhar, S.J.; Esper, S.A.; Dueweke, E.J. Extracorporeal Membrane oxygenation support in acute coronary syndromes complicated by cardiogenic shock. *Catheter Cardiovasc. Interv.* **2015**. [CrossRef]
85. Negi, S.I.; Sokolovic, M.; Koifman, E.; Kiramijyan, S.; Torguson, R.; Lindsay, J.; Ben-Dor, I.; Suddath, W.; Pichard, A.; Satler, L.; et al. Contemporary use of veno-arterial extracorporeal membrane oxygenation for refractory cardiogenic shock in acute coronary syndrome. *J. Invasive Cardiol.* **2016**, *28*, 52–57.
86. Chen, Y.-S.; Chao, A.; Yu, H.-Y.; Ko, W.-J.; Wu, I.-H.; Chen, R.J.-C.; Huang, S.-C.; Lin, F.-Y.; Wang, S.-S. Analysis and results of prolonged resuscitation in cardiac arrest patients rescued by extracorporeal membrane oxygenation. *J. Am. Coll. Cardiol.* **2003**. [CrossRef]
87. Schrage, B.; Burkhoff, D.; Rübsamen, N.; Becher, P.M.; Schwarzl, M.; Bernhardt, A.; Grahn, H.; Lubos, E.; Söffker, G.; Clemmensen, P.; et al. Unloading of the left ventricle during venoarterial extracorporeal membrane oxygenation therapy in cardiogenic shock. *JACC Heart Fail.* **2018**. [CrossRef]
88. Myat, A.; Patel, N.; Tehrani, S.; Banning, A.P.; Redwood, S.R.; Bhatt, D.L. Percutaneous circulatory assist devices for high-risk coronary intervention. *JACC Cardiovasc. Interv.* **2015**. [CrossRef]
89. Maini, B.; Gregory, D.; Scotti, D.J.; Buyantseva, L. Percutaneous cardiac assist devices compared with surgical hemodynamic support alternatives: Cost-effectiveness in the emergent setting. *Catheter Cardiovasc. Interv.* **2014**. [CrossRef]
90. Roos, J.B.; Doshi, S.N.; Konorza, T.; Palacios, I.; Schreiber, T.; Borisenko, O.V.; Henriques, J.P.S. The cost-effectiveness of a new percutaneous ventricular assist device for high-risk PCI patients: mid-stage evaluation from the European perspective. *J. Med. Econ.* **2013**. [CrossRef]
91. Udesen, N.J.; Møller, J.E.; Lindholm, M.G.; Eiskjær, H.; Schäfer, A.; Werner, N.; Holmvang, L.; Terkelsen, C.J.; Jensen, L.O.; Junker, A.; et al. Rationale and design of DanGer shock: Danish-German cardiogenic shock trial. *Am. Heart J.* **2019**. [CrossRef]
92. Jung, C.; Bueter, S.; Wernly, B.; Masyuk, M.; Saeed, D.; Albert, A.; Fuernau, G.; Kelm, M.; Westenfeld, R. Lactate clearance predicts good neurological outcomes in cardiac arrest patients treated with extracorporeal cardiopulmonary resuscitation. *J. Clin. Med.* **2019**. [CrossRef]
93. Slottosch, I.; Liakopoulos, O.; Kuhn, E.; Scherner, M.; Deppe, A.-C.; Sabashnikov, A.; Mader, N.; Choi, Y.-H.; Wippermann, J.; Wahlers, T. Lactate and lactate clearance as valuable tool to evaluate ECMO therapy in cardiogenic shock. *J. Crit. Care* **2017**. [CrossRef]
94. Fux, T.; Holm, M.; Corbascio, M.; van der Linden, J. cardiac arrest prior to venoarterial extracorporeal membrane oxygenation. *Crit. Care Med.* **2019**. [CrossRef]
95. Lee, W.-C.; Fang, C.-Y.; Chen, H.-C.; Chen, C.-J.; Yang, C.-H.; Hang, C.-L.; Yip, H.-K.; Fang, H.-Y.; Wu, C.-J. Associations with 30-day survival following extracorporeal membrane oxygenation in patients with acute ST segment elevation myocardial infarction and profound cardiogenic shock. *Heart Lung J. Acute Crit. Care* **2016**. [CrossRef]

96. Kapur, N.K.; Paruchuri, V.; Urbano-Morales, J.A.; Mackey, E.E.; Daly, G.H.; Qiao, X.; Pandian, N.; Perides, G.; Karas, R.H. Mechanically unloading the left ventricle before coronary reperfusion reduces left ventricular wall stress and myocardial infarct size. *Circulation* **2013**. [CrossRef]

97. Esposito, M.L.; Zhang, Y.; Qiao, X.; Reyelt, L.; Paruchuri, V.; Schnitzler, G.R.; Morine, K.J.; Annamalai, S.K.; Bogins, C.; Natov, P.S.; et al. Left ventricular unloading before reperfusion promotes functional recovery after acute myocardial infarction. *J. Am. Coll. Cardiol.* **2018**. [CrossRef]

98. Meyns, B.; Stolinski, J.; Leunens, V.; Verbeken, E.; Flameng, W. Left ventricular support by catheter-mounted axial flow pump reduces infarct size. *J. Am. Coll. Cardiol.* **2003**, *41*, 1087–1095. [CrossRef]

99. Kapur, N.K.; Qiao, X.; Paruchuri, V.; Morine, K.J.; Syed, W.; Dow, S.; Shah, N.; Pandian, N.; Karas, R.H. Mechanical pre-conditioning with acute circulatory support before reperfusion limits infarct size in acute myocardial infarction. *JACC Heart Fail.* **2015**. [CrossRef]

100. Kapur, N.K.; Alkhouli, M.A.; DeMartini, T.J.; Faraz, H.; George, Z.H.; Goodwin, M.J.; Hernandez-Montfort, J.A.; Iyer, V.S.; Josephy, N.; Kalra, S.; et al. Unloading the left ventricle before reperfusion in patients with anterior st-segment-elevation myocardial infarction: A pilot study using the impella CP. *Circulation* **2019**. [CrossRef]

101. O'Neill, W.W.; Grines, C.; Schreiber, T.; Moses, J.; Maini, B.; Dixon, S.R.; Ohman, E.M.; O'Neill, W.W. Analysis of outcomes for 15,259 US patients with acute myocardial infarction cardiogenic shock (AMICS) supported with the Impella device. *Am. Heart J.* **2018**. [CrossRef]

102. Flaherty, M.P.; Khan, A.R.; O'Neill, W.W. Early initiation of impella in acute myocardial infarction complicated by cardiogenic shock improves survival: A meta-analysis. *JACC Cardiovasc. Interv.* **2017**. [CrossRef]

103. Auffret, V.; Cottin, Y.; Leurent, G.; Gilard, M.; Beer, J.-C.; Zabalawi, A.; Chagué, F.; Filippi, E.; Brunet, D.; Hacot, J.-P.; et al. Predicting the development of in-hospital cardiogenic shock in patients with ST-segment elevation myocardial infarction treated by primary percutaneous coronary intervention: The ORBI risk score. *Eur. Heart J.* **2018**. [CrossRef]

104. Schrage, B.; Westermann, D. Reply: Does VA-ECMO plus impella work in refractory cardiogenic shock? *JACC Heatr Fail.* **2019**. [CrossRef]

105. Li, Y.; Yan, S.; Gao, S.; Liu, M.; Lou, S.; Liu, G.; Ji, B.; Gao, B. Effect of an intra-aortic balloon pump with venoarterial extracorporeal membrane oxygenation on mortality of patients with cardiogenic shock: A systematic review and meta-analysis. *Eur. J. Cardio-Thoracic Surg.* **2019**. [CrossRef]

106. Ohman, E.M.; Nanas, J.; Stomel, R.J.; Leesar, M.A.; Nielsen, D.W.T.; O'Dea, D.; Rogers, F.J.; Harber, D.; Hudson, M.P.; Fraulo, E.; et al. Thrombolysis and counterpulsation to improve survival in myocardial infarction complicated by hypotension and suspected cardiogenic shock or heart failure: Results of the TACTICS trial. *J. Thromb. Thrombolysis* **2005**. [CrossRef]

107. Waksman, R.; Weiss, A.T.; Gotsman, M.S.; Hasin, Y. Intra-aortic balloon counterpulsation improves survival in cardiogenic shock complicating acute myocardial infarction. *Eur. Heart J.* **1993**. [CrossRef]

108. Barron, H.V.; Every, N.R.; Parsons, L.S.; Angeja, B.; Goldberg, R.J.; Gore, J.M.; Chou, T.M. The use of intra-aortic balloon counterpulsation in patients with cardiogenic shock complicating acute myocardial infarction: Data from the national registry of myocardial infarction 2. *Am. Heart J.* **2001**. [CrossRef]

109. Cheng, J.M.; Uil, C.A.D.; Hoeks, S.E.; Van Der Ent, M.; Jewbali, L.S.; Van Domburg, R.T.; Serruys, P.W. Percutaneous left ventricular assist devices vs. intra-aortic balloon pump counterpulsation for treatment of cardiogenic shock: A meta-analysis of controlled trials. *Eur. Heart J.* **2009**. [CrossRef]

110. Alushi, B.; Douedari, A.; Froehlich, G.; Knie, W.; Leistner, D.; Staehli, B.; Mochmann, H.-C.; Pieske, B.; Landmesser, U.; Krackhardt, F.; et al. P2481Impella assist device or intraaortic balloon pump for treatment of cardiogenic shock due to acute coronary syndrome. *Eur. Heart J.* **2018**. [CrossRef]

111. Nichol, G.; Karmy-Jones, R.; Salerno, C.; Cantore, L.; Becker, L. Systematic review of percutaneous cardiopulmonary bypass for cardiac arrest or cardiogenic shock states. *Resuscitation* **2006**. [CrossRef]

112. Sheu, J.-J.; Tsai, T.-H.; Lee, F.-Y.; Fang, H.-Y.; Sun, C.-K.; Leu, S.; Yang, C.-H.; Chen, S.-M.; Hang, C.-L.; Hsieh, Y.-K.; et al. Early extracorporeal membrane oxygenator-assisted primary percutaneous coronary intervention improved 30-day clinical outcomes in patients with ST-segment elevation myocardial infarction complicated with profound cardiogenic shock. *Crit. Care Med.* **2010**. [CrossRef]

113. Takayama, H.; Truby, L.; Koekort, M.; Uriel, N.; Colombo, P.; Mancini, D.M.; Jorde, U.P.; Naka, Y. Clinical outcome of mechanical circulatory support for refractory cardiogenic shock in the current era. *J. Heart Lung Transplant* **2013**. [CrossRef]

114. Teirstein, P.S.; Vogel, R.A.; Dorros, G.; Stertzer, S.H.; Vandormael, M.; Smith, S.C.; Overlie, P.A.; O'Neill, W.W. Prophylactic versus standby cardiopulmonary support for high risk percutaneous transluminal coronary angioplasty. *J. Am. Coll. Cardiol.* **1993**. [CrossRef]
115. Schreiber, T.L.; Kodali, U.R.; O'Neill, W.W.; Gangadharan, V.; Puchrowicz-Ochocki, S.B.; Grines, C.L. Comparison of acute results of prophylactic intraaortic balloon pumping with cardiopulmonary support for percutaneous transluminal coronary angioplasty (PTCA). *Catheter Cardiovasc. Diagn.* **1998**. [CrossRef]

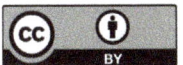

© 2019 by the authors. Licensee MDPI, Basel, Switzerland. This article is an open access article distributed under the terms and conditions of the Creative Commons Attribution (CC BY) license (http://creativecommons.org/licenses/by/4.0/).

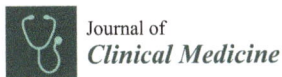

Review

Subclinical Atherosclerosis Imaging in People Living with HIV

Isabella C. Schoepf [1], Ronny R. Buechel [2], Helen Kovari [3], Dima A. Hammoud [4] and Philip E. Tarr [1],*

[1] University Department of Medicine and Infectious Diseases Service, Kantonsspital Baselland, University of Basel, 4101 Bruderholz, Switzerland
[2] Department of Nuclear Medicine, Cardiac Imaging, University Hospital Zurich, University of Zurich, 8091 Zurich, Switzerland
[3] Division of Infectious Diseases and Hospital Epidemiology, University of Zurich, 8091 Zurich, Switzerland
[4] Center for Infectious Disease Imaging, Radiology and Imaging Sciences, National Institutes of Health, Bethesda, MD 20892, USA
* Correspondence: philip.tarr@unibas.ch; Tel.: +41-61-436-2212; Fax: +41-61-436-3670

Received: 3 July 2019; Accepted: 26 July 2019; Published: 29 July 2019

Abstract: In many, but not all studies, people living with HIV (PLWH) have an increased risk of coronary artery disease (CAD) events compared to the general population. This has generated considerable interest in the early, non-invasive detection of asymptomatic (subclinical) atherosclerosis in PLWH. Ultrasound studies assessing carotid artery intima-media thickness (CIMT) have tended to show a somewhat greater thickness in HIV+ compared to HIV−, likely due to an increased prevalence of cardiovascular (CV) risk factors in PLWH. Coronary artery calcification (CAC) determination by non-contrast computed tomography (CT) seems promising to predict CV events but is limited to the detection of calcified plaque. Coronary CT angiography (CCTA) detects calcified and non-calcified plaque and predicts CAD better than either CAC or CIMT. A normal CCTA predicts survival free of CV events over a very long time-span. Research imaging techniques, including black-blood magnetic resonance imaging of the vessel wall and 18F-fluorodeoxyglucose positron emission tomography for the assessment of arterial inflammation have provided insights into the prevalence of HIV-vasculopathy and associated risk factors, but their clinical applicability remains limited. Therefore, CCTA currently appears as the most promising cardiac imaging modality in PLWH for the evaluation of suspected CAD, particularly in patients <50 years, in whom most atherosclerotic coronary lesions are non-calcified.

Keywords: subclinical coronary artery disease; accelerated atherosclerosis; HIV infection; carotid intima-media thickness; coronary calcium scoring; coronary CT angiography; magnetic resonance angiography; fluorodeoxyglucose positron emission tomography

1. Introduction

Cardiovascular disease (CVD) has become one of the leading causes of death in people living with HIV (PLWH) worldwide [1–4]. Reducing the burden of CVD, particularly coronary artery disease (CAD), is therefore emerging as a major public health goal in medical care for PLWH [5,6].

Data is inconsistent with respect to whether PLWH have an increased incidence of CAD events compared to the general population [2,7] or not [8–10]. Early reports have observed a 2- to almost 4-fold increased rate in CAD events as compared to HIV-negative patients [11,12], but traditional risk factors, particularly smoking, and socioeconomic factors were not always adjusted for in those studies [13]. Danish data suggest a 1.5- to 2-fold increase in CAD events in PLWH vs. controls [14]; a 2-fold CAD event increase in PLWH was also the conclusion of a recent systematic review and meta-analysis [2].

Other studies have reported smaller increases [15–17] in cardiovascular (CV) events in PLWH. In a large cohort study from California that evaluated the myocardial infarction (MI) risk from 1996 to 2011, a declining relative risk for MI was observed in PLWH vs. HIV-negative persons over time. Between 2010 and 2011, no increased risk of MI was seen in PLWH [17]. In a cohort of US veterans, a 50% increased risk in acute MI was recorded, after adjusting for Framingham risk score, comorbidities and substance use [16]. In another large North American analysis, HIV infection was associated with only a 21% increased incidence of CV events in comparison with a well-matched HIV-negative control group, and the risk increase was not statistically significant in the age group ≥60 years of age [15]. Moreover, in recent studies from Switzerland and Denmark, no increased risk of CAD events and, in Switzerland, no increased subclinical atherosclerosis prevalence was described, perhaps due to the prevalence of modern antiretroviral therapy (ART) regimens, reliably suppressive ART, decreased smoking prevalence, and access to regular medical follow-up [8,9,18]. Also, the data do not generally suggest that CV events occur earlier in PLWH, contradicting the widely held notion of "accelerated atherosclerosis" or even "accelerated aging". Some reports that CV events occur at a younger age seem to be related to the younger median age of many HIV+ populations compared to the general population [19].

The pathogenesis of CV events in HIV-positive individuals likely represents a complex interaction of different factors that contribute to the development of atherosclerosis [18,20–23]. Studies in multiple countries have consistently recorded an increased prevalence of smoking and drug use in PLWH [11,13]. A link between inflammation related to HIV infection and CAD in PLWH is well documented. Several serum biomarkers that are associated with CV risk or overall mortality may be elevated in PLWH compared to HIV-negative persons, including biomarkers of systemic inflammation (high sensitivity C-reactive protein, interleukin-6, soluble tumor necrosis factor-α receptor 1) [24–27], coagulation (D-dimer, fibrinogen) [24–27], monocyte activation (lipopolysaccharide, soluble CD14, CD163, CC-chemokine ligand 2) [24,28–31], and endothelial dysfunction (intercellular adhesion molecule 1) [24]. Although the exact mechanisms underlying the development of atherosclerosis in PLWH have not been conclusively determined, smooth muscle cell proliferation may play an important role [32]. Moreover, endothelial dysfunction due to adhesion molecules may lead to adhesion of circulating leukocytes, transmigration of monocytes/macrophages to the intima and subsequently to vascular inflammation [20,32,33]. In combination with procoagulatory mechanisms in the setting of increased concentrations of D-dimer and coagulation factors, and in the presence of other metabolic disorders (e.g., dyslipidemia), the progression of atherosclerosis might be enhanced in PLWH [20,32].

It is well accepted that viral suppression, in the setting of adequate ART, is associated with lower levels of inflammatory biomarkers and decreased CV risk [34,35]. Advanced immunosuppression has contributed to CV risk in PLWH in some [15,36,37] but not in other studies [38,39].

Also, certain ART agents have been associated with increased CV risk. This notion is most reliably based on findings from the large, multinational, observational D:A:D study [20,23,39]. Dyslipidemia was among the first described deleterious metabolic effects of ART, most notably in the setting of certain protease inhibitors, i.e., lopinavir, indinavir and darunavir [23,40,41]. Within the drug class of nucleoside reverse transcriptase inhibitors, abacavir and didanosine were found to increase CV risk [42].

The potentially increased CV event rate in PLWH has generated considerable interest in early detection of asymptomatic (subclinical) atherosclerosis, in order to improve CAD event prediction and to allow appropriate CVD prevention by early intervention [21]. Most published literature on noninvasive cardiac imaging for the detection of subclinical atherosclerosis in PLWH has focused on carotid artery intima-media thickness (CIMT), coronary artery calcification (CAC), coronary CT angiography (CCTA) [18,43,44] and, more recently, magnetic resonance imaging of the vessel wall (MRI) and 18F- fluorodeoxyglucose positron emission tomography (FDG-PET).

2. Carotid Artery Intima-Media Thickness (CIMT)

CIMT is an ultrasound technique to measure the thickness of the two layers of the carotid artery wall, the intima and the media [45]. CIMT is well recorded to predict future CV events in the general population [46–49]. According to the results of a 2009 meta-analysis that analyzed six cross-sectional, seven case-control and 13 cohort studies (5456 HIV positive and 3600 HIV negative patients) PLWH tend to show a greater thickness in CIMT (0.04 mm thicker; 95% confidence interval: 0.02–0.06 mm, $p < 0.001$) when compared to HIV-negative controls [50]. However, the findings are not concordant with some studies showing increased CIMT was increased in PLWH compared to HIV-negative controls [12,51–71] while other studies did not show a difference or showed only weakly increased CIMT in PLWH [12,45,50–59,61–68]. Those discordant findings may be attributable to differences in study design, participant characteristics, duration of follow-up, and different approaches of ultrasound measurement [45,50].

The largest differences in CIMT between HIV-positive and HIV-negative participants were noted in studies with the greatest demographic differences between the analyzed groups [45,50]. Moreover, small studies were more likely than larger studies to identify an increase in CIMT in PLWH vs. controls [45,50]. In addition, a large report of repeated CIMT measurements over a median of 7 years did not find accelerated CIMT progression in PLWH (747 women, 530 men) compared to HIV-negative controls (264 women, 284 men), but focal plaque prevalence was increased, after adjusting for traditional CV risk factors [70]. These findings are in accordance with another report that observed no different progression in CIMT over 144 weeks in 133 extensively matched HIV+ and HIV− participants [59].

CIMT has a number of limitations for the prediction of CV events, including a limited correlation with angiographically defined atherosclerosis [72,73], limited improvement in CV event prediction by the addition of CIMT to the Framingham risk score [46], and different results when CIMT findings at the common carotid artery level are compared with results obtained at the carotid bifurcation and/or the internal carotid artery level [45,61,65]. Finally, CIMT measurement is dependent on investigator experience, with the reproducibility of results generally being higher in research settings than in practitioner-based settings [74].

3. Coronary Artery Calcium (CAC) Scoring

CAC scoring using non-contrast enhanced CT is a well-established and easily applicable tool for detection and quantification of coronary calcifications [75–80] (Figure 1). Applying different scoring systems, most frequently the Agatston score, based on the landmark work of Arthur Agatston in the late 1980s [81], CAC scoring has emerged as a robust non-invasive atherosclerosis imaging modality characterized by high inter- and intra-observer reliability [74,80,82].

In the general population, there is a strong correlation between CAC score and future CV endpoints [74,80,83–86]. Persons with no detectable coronary calcium have a very low risk for CV events over the following years [87,88] and a ten-year survival of 99.4% [89]. Longitudinal CAC studies have suggested that annual CAC score change of ≥15% may constitute CVD progression [90]. CV event prediction by CAC and CIMT were similar in one report [91], but CAC was a more reliable CV event predictor than CIMT in several other reports [86,92–94]. CV event prediction may be improved when CAC is added to Framingham risk score [88,89].

Current evidence remains equivocal as to whether the presence of HIV is associated with an increased prevalence of coronary calcifications [18,71,95,96]. An increased vascular age was identified in Italian PLWH compared with age-specific CAC percentiles based on the MESA study done in a general US population [95]. However, these findings were not confirmed in a recent study assessing a large Swiss cohort [18]; other studies have also found similar CAC scores in HIV-positive and HIV-negative persons [18,50,96]. High pre-treatment HIV viremia levels were associated with a CAC score >0 [18]. In the US MACS study, CAC scores were elevated in those with metabolic syndrome but were not altered by HIV serostatus [57,96].

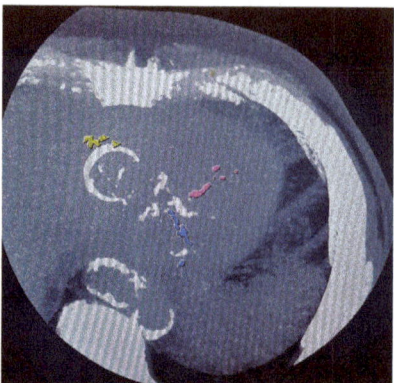

Figure 1. Coronary artery calcium scoring in an asymptomatic 43-year old HIV-positive male patient. Maximum intensity projection depicts extensive calcifications in the left anterior descending artery (purple), in the left circumflex artery (blue), and in the right coronary artery (yellow). The total Agatston score was 1031, classifying this patient as at high risk for future CV events and prompting lifestyle interventions and the initiation of a statin.

A major limitation of CAC is the inability to detect non-calcified plaque. This is of importance because a non-calcified or only partially calcified plaque is more likely to take on morphological features typical of high-risk plaque which is prone to adverse future CV events (e.g., plaque rupture or erosion potentially leading to MI) [97,98]. In addition, coronary artery plaque is predominantly non-calcified in patients <50 years of age [80,99,100]. This point may be particularly relevant to PLWH: as, in Western countries, even though HIV-positive populations are aging, their median age is still relatively low, e.g., 48 years in the Swiss HIV cohort study (www.shcs.ch and [101]). Their Framingham risk scores and CAD event rates have also been relatively low, and the median age at the time of the first CAD event in SHCS participants was 50 years [38].

4. Coronary CT Angiography (CCTA)

CCTA is a non-invasive imaging technique involving contrast-enhanced multi-slice CT for the accurate morphological assessment of the coronary arteries [102] (Figure 2).

Importantly, and in contrast to CIMT and CAC, CCTA can be used to detect calcified and non-calcified plaques, and due to its high spatial resolution also allows for the accurate assessment of plaque composition [74,103] (Figure 3).

CCTA has seen a tremendous development over the last two decades, both in terms of hardware advancements and improvements in image acquisition protocols. Among the latter, the introduction of prospectively electrocardiogram-triggered acquisition has contributed most substantially to lowering radiation dose exposure from 15–20 millisieverts (mSv) [104–106] down to 2–3 mSv [104,107–110]. The addition of sophisticated reconstruction algorithms and widespread use of latest-generation wide-coverage CT devices may now enable routine scanning in the sub-millisievert range [111]. Sensitivity of CCTA in the detection of relevant coronary stenosis is similar to standard invasive coronary angiography [112–114]. However, both modalities inherently lack the ability to predict hemodynamic relevance if a stenosis is found. This is of the utmost importance because the optimal treatment, i.e., the benefit of optimal medical therapy versus revascularization, depends heavily on the presence and extent of myocardial ischemia [115]. While, theoretically, measurement of pressure drops along a vessel and the derivation of the so-called fractional flow reserve constitutes an invasive technique to overcome this limitation, the application of hybrid imaging, that is, the combination and fusion of two non-invasive imaging modalities, has evolved into a robust and elegant technique for the assessment of both coronary anatomy and potential hemodynamical effects of any given lesion, hence providing the non-invasive grounds for optimized patient management decisions (Figure 4).

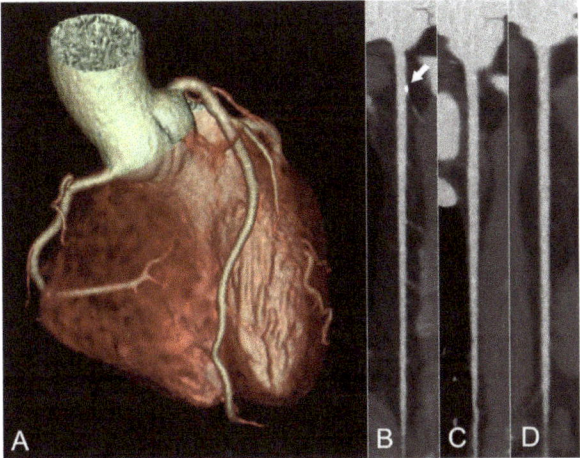

Figure 2. Coronary computed tomography angiography of a 48-year old HIV+ female patient with typical angina. The patient had a positive family history for cardiovascular events and was an active smoker, putting her at intermediate risk for having coronary artery disease. Volume rendering (**A**) of the image datasets depicts normal coronary anatomy, while the curved multiplanar reformats of the left anterior descending (**B**), the left circumflex (**C**), and the right coronary (**D**) arteries reveal only minimal and non-obstructive coronary atherosclerosis in the proximal left anterior descending (white arrow). Coronary artery disease was, therefore, excluded as a cause for her symptoms. BMI 24.2 kg/m^2. Radiation dose exposure 0.57 mSv. Contrast volume 40 mL.

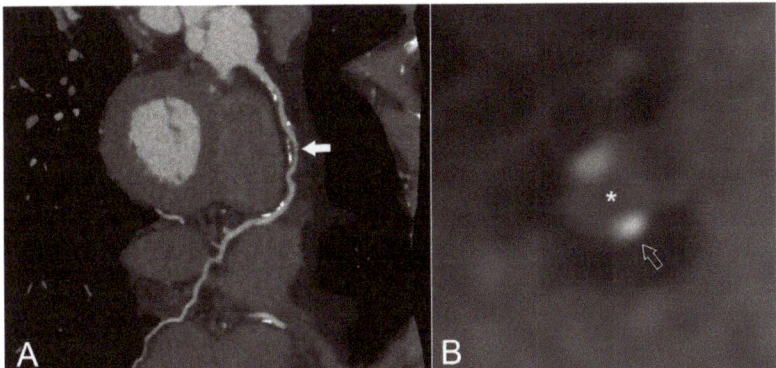

Figure 3. Non-invasive evaluation of an asymptomatic 65-year old HIV+ male patient. The patient had a history of treated arterial hypertension, was an active smoker and suffered from peripheral artery disease with the latter prompting further cardiovascular work-up despite a normal stress-electrocardiogram. Multiplanar curved reconstruction of the coronary computed tomography angiography dataset (**A**) reveals multiple calcified but non-obstructive lesions and 70–90% stenosis (white filled arrow) in the mid-right coronary artery. This obstructive lesion (**B**, cross sectional view) exhibits several morphological high-risk features typical for an event-prone lesion, such as positive remodeling and a low-attenuation core (*) with calcifications only at the edge of the lesion (white empty arrow), constituting the so-called napkin-ring sign.

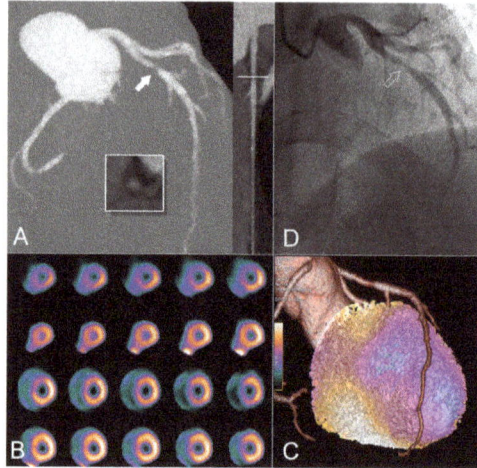

Figure 4. Evaluation of a 49-year old HIV+ male patient with typical angina. The patient had no cardiovascular risk factors and he was referred for exclusion of coronary artery disease with a calculated pre-test probability of 69%. Total cholesterol was 3.6 mmol/L (<5.0), HDL-cholesterol 1.45 mmol/L (>1.0), and LDL-cholesterol 1.8 mmol/L (<3.0). Maximum intensity projection and multiplanar curved reconstruction of the coronary computed tomography angiography (CCTA) datasets (**A**) depict a 70–90% stenosis (white filled arrow) in the proximal left anterior descending artery as shown in the cross-section (inlet). As per clinical routine and in accordance with current guidelines, lesions are primarily graded visually with regard to maximal percent diameter stenosis in our institution. In this particular patient, the qualitative evaluation was complemented by quantitative measurements (using version 2 of CardIQ Xpress/GE Healthcare), because the lesion in the LAD was non-calcified, allowing for more accurate lumen delineation due to the lack of blooming artifacts. The quantitative analysis resulted in a diameter stenosis of 75%. Myocardial perfusion single-photon-computed-emission-tomography (SPECT, (**B**)) confirmed hemodynamical relevance of the lesion, revealing a large perfusion defect during stress (top rows) with reversibility during rest (bottom rows), constituting ischemia in the anteroseptal wall of the left ventricular myocardium. Hybrid CCTA/SPECT imaging (**C**) clearly demonstrates a large area of ischemia in the myocardium subtended by the left anterior descending artery. Finally, obstructive coronary artery disease (white empty arrow) was confirmed during invasive coronary angiography (**D**), and the lesion was treated with a drug-eluting stent.

Compared to intravascular ultrasound, CCTA can precisely detect coronary plaque with a positive and negative predictive value >98% [18,107,116,117]. It is well recorded, however, that CCTA tends to overestimate the degree of coronary stenosis [118,119]. In the general population, among individuals without known CVD, the large scale CONFIRM study documented that the degree of non-obstructive and obstructive coronary artery stenosis and the number of vessels affected in CCTA are closely correlated with CV events and mortality rates over 3 years of follow-up [107]. CCTA improves prediction of future CV events compared to Framingham risk score [120], CAC [107,108,121] or CIMT [108,118].

In early studies, results regarding the presence of subclinical atherosclerosis in CCTA in HIV-positive relative to HIV-negative persons were not uniform. Some investigators recorded an increased [44,100,122–124] prevalence, while others noted a similar [18,43,125] or even lower prevalence in PLWH, compared to HIV-negative controls [18,103]. In a 2015 meta-analysis summarizing initial CCTA studies (1229 HIV-positive and 1029 HIV negative participants), a 3-fold higher prevalence of non-calcified coronary artery plaque on CCTA was recorded in asymptomatic HIV+ compared to HIV-negative subjects [100]. The analyzed studies typically included a small number of participants, that, in addition, were not always matched on CV risk factors [124].

Today, there are three published CCTA studies that enrolled large numbers of HIV+ and HIV-negative participants, with the following key findings: In men who had sex with men that were enrolled in the US-American multicenter AIDS cohort study (MACS), Post et al. [44] recorded a higher prevalence of any coronary plaque and non-calcified plaque in 618 HIV+ compared to 383 HIV-negative men in the baseline CCTA. In a follow-up report, with a median interval of 4.5 years between CCTAs, increased progression of coronary plaques was observed in HIV-positive compared to the HIV-negative MACS participants, but only in men with detectable HIV viremia and, thus, presumably, higher degrees of ongoing systemic inflammation, compared to persons with optimal virological control [44,126].

Lai et al. described the presence of subclinical atherosclerosis in CCTA of 953 HIV+ and 476 HIV-negative African American study participants from Baltimore/USA of whom more than 50% were frequent cocaine users [43]. In this study, there was a trend towards HIV infection being independently associated with non-calcified plaque, however, this association was largely explained by chronic cocaine use.

In addition to these two studies from the US [43,44,126], we recently assessed subclinical atherosclerosis in a cross-sectional study of 428 HIV-positive participants of the Swiss HIV Cohort Study (SHCS) and 276 HIV-negative control individuals with similar Framingham risk scores. HIV-positive participants had similar degrees of non-calcified/mixed plaque and high risk [97] plaque, and, indeed, had less calcified coronary plaque, and lower coronary atherosclerosis involvement and severity scores compared to their negative controls with similar Framingham risk score [18]. These Swiss CCTA results, together with Swiss data showing similar CV incidence rates in HIV+ and HIV-persons [8], attenuate concerns about accelerated atherosclerosis in HIV, and have prompted experts to ask the question whether the prevalent notion of increased CV risk in PLWH amounts to "much ado about nothing" [127].

The different CCTA results in these three large studies [18,43,44] might be related to a number of features. First, CAD rates are lower in southern/central Europe compared to the US [128,129]. Second, we speculate that the low subclinical atherosclerosis prevalence in Swiss PLWH might further be attributable to high rates of successful treatment in the setting of modern ART regimens, regular follow-up, and declining smoking rates in recent years [9,130].

As regards the duration of ART, the Swiss study did not find any association with any type of plaque. This was in line with findings from Lai et al. in the group of non-cocaine users and contrary to MACS [18,43,44]. Concerning the use of antiretroviral agents and subclinical atherosclerosis, the MACS investigators observed no clear association between different ART drugs and any form of coronary artery plaque on CCTA [131]. In contrast, the Swiss study identified an association with exposure to abacavir and an increased prevalence of non-calcified/mixed plaque [132]. This observation seems important, as it may afford a mechanism by which abacavir increases CV risk, i.e., the promotion of atherosclerosis, in addition to putative deleterious effects of abacavir on platelet reactivity [133,134].

Consistent with the MACS findings, the Swiss patients with a low nadir CD4+ cell count had more non-calcified plaque [18,44] and more coronary stenosis greater than 50% [44]. These findings suggest that advanced immunosuppression may contribute to subclinical atherosclerosis in PLWH [100].

In summary, coronary plaque in young persons typically is non-calcified [80,99,100]. CCTA (but not CAC) can detect non-calcified plaque [74] and predicts CVD better than CAC [107] or CIMT [118]. Therefore, and because the median age of most populations of PLWH remains below 50 years today, CCTA is emerging as the preferred research-setting imaging tool to detect subclinical atherosclerosis. There remains a need for additional studies to examine the exact role that CCTA may play in clinical HIV practice.

5. Magnetic Resonance Rmaging (MRI)

Based on CIMT being strongly predictive of CV events [135], multiple studies have reported the use of MRI rather than ultrasound in assessing CVD in PLWH [103,136–139]. Such studies mainly used black-blood MRI (BBMRI), an advanced imaging technique relying on nulling of the MR signal from the vascular lumen while retaining signal from the vascular wall, allowing better visualization of the wall thickness [140,141]. Multiple variations of the BBMRI technique have already been used in extracranial (e.g., aorta, carotid and coronary arteries) as well as intracranial vessel wall imaging [140–146].

In age-related atherosclerosis, BBMRI is generally used to assess the vulnerability characteristics of eccentric, lipid-rich plaques (e.g., lipid core, fibrous cap, hemorrhage). In HIV vasculopathy on the other hand, where intimal smooth muscle hypertrophy occurs in a symmetrical circumferential manner [32,33], BBMRI is more commonly used to assess diffuse wall thickening. This is why the majority of vessel wall imaging studies in HIV have concentrated on measuring the vessel wall thickness (VWT) akin to the measurement of CIMT using ultrasound [103,138,147,148]. In a group of treated HIV+ subjects with low measurable CVD risk, HIV-status was significantly associated with increased wall/outer-wall ratio (W/OW), an index of vascular thickening, after adjusting for age [139]. In another study, increased carotid artery wall thickness was noted in HIV+ subjects on chronic ART compared to controls with similar CVD risk, [137]. Interestingly, while in one study [139], no correlation of CVD with the type of ART was identified, another study [137] found that a longer duration of protease inhibitor therapy was associated with greater wall thickness. Using MRI to assess coronary rather than carotid arteries, subclinical CAD has been documented in ART-treated subjects, with HIV infection being independently associated with increased proximal right coronary artery wall thickness [103].

The connection between HIV-associated inflammation and atherosclerosis burden in HIV infection was also evaluated in a group of HIV+ subjects (treated and untreated) in comparison to a group of demographically similar controls. As expected, HIV-1 viral burden was found to be associated with higher serum levels of the chemokines monocyte chemoattractant protein-1/CC-chemokinligand 2 (MCP-1/CCL2). At the same time, HIV infection correlated with atherosclerosis burden, mainly detectable as increased vessel wall area and thickness in the thoracic aorta [148].

BBMRI has also been important in delineating that traditional CVD risk factors, which seem to disproportionately burden PLWH, need to be controlled. In one study evaluating asymptomatic, young-to-middle-aged African-Americans with and without HIV infection and cocaine use, only total cholesterol (and not HIV status) was significantly associated with the presence of a lipid core in carotid plaques [136]. In another more recent study, carotid VWT was increased in treated PLWH relative to controls with the 10-year ASCVD (atherosclerotic cardiovascular disease) risk score being the only variable significantly associated with VWT whereas HIV status was not. The authors concluded that traditional CVD risk factors in PLWH are adequately captured in the ASCVD risk score which was closely associated with subclinical carotid disease [138].

Over the last few years, there have been significant advances made in MR imaging of the vessel wall, with the ability nowadays of assessing atherosclerotic involvement of the intracranial arteries. To our knowledge, such high-resolution techniques have not yet been applied in the evaluation of PLWH [146,149–153]. At this point, BBMRI of the vessel wall remains a research application rather than a clinically used technique in assessing CVD in PLWH (Figure 5). Whether this would eventually change in the future, as PLWH get older, remains unclear.

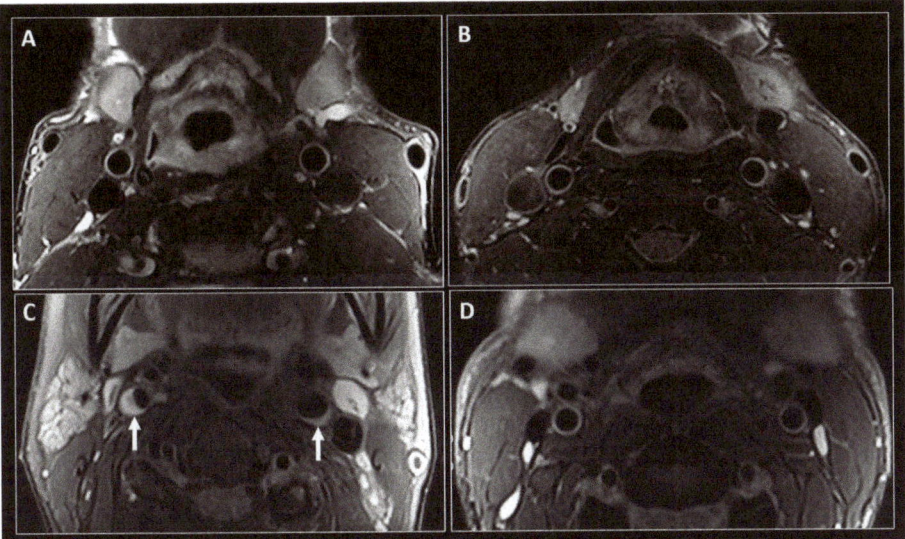

Figure 5. Black-blood MR imaging of the carotid arteries. Fat saturated T2-weighted black-blood MR images at the level of the common carotid arteries in a 56-year-old HIV+ man (**A**) and a 47-year-old HIV− man (**B**). Similar imaging technique at the level of the internal carotid arteries (ICAs) in a 56-year-old HIV+ woman (**C**) shows narrowing of the vascular lumen bilaterally by a plaque (small arrows), more significant on the right side. (**D**) shows similar imaging at the level of ICAs in a 47-year-old HIV negative man with no evidence of atherosclerosis.

6. 18F-Fluorodeoxyglucose Positron Emission Tomography (FDG PET)

The most common application of FDG PET imaging in the clinic is the baseline assessment and follow-up of neoplastic diseases. Applications in imaging infectious and inflammatory diseases using FDG PET, however, have been increasing in the last decade.

One such use is the assessment of vasculitis seen as increased glucose metabolism of the vessel wall, reflecting inflammatory changes [154] (Figure 6).

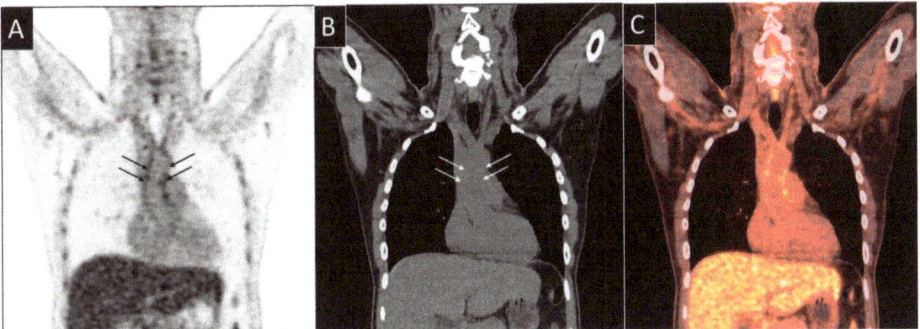

Figure 6. FDG-PET imaging of the major vessels. (**A**) Coronal FDG PET images, (**B**) coronal CT scan images and (**C**) fused PET CT scans show subtle FDG uptake in the vascular wall of the ascending aorta (arrows).

A similar approach has been used by multiple groups to assess HIV-vasculopathy using FDG PET [155–162]. A common presumption is that PLWH will demonstrate increased vessel wall FDG uptake reflecting premature aging and atherosclerotic changes. In fact, in one paper assessing only HIV+ patients, a relationship was found between arterial inflammation on FDG PET and features of high-risk coronary atherosclerotic disease including number of low attenuation plaques and plaque vulnerability characteristics [160].

The results from studies utilizing FDG PET to assess HIV-vasculopathy, however, have been rather inconsistent. In one paper [162], arterial inflammation in the aorta (measured as aortic target to background ratio (TBR)) was higher in the HIV+ group compared to the non-HIV control group matched for CVD, even after adjusting for traditional CV risk factors [162]. More recently, HIV was found to be associated with 0.16 higher aortic TBR compared to controls, independent of traditional risk factors [155]. On the other hand, in one paper assessing virologically controlled HIV+ persons with no known CVD, there was no evidence of increased arterial inflammation on FDG PET compared to healthy volunteers [159]. In a more recent paper looking at a larger group of patients, there was only a marginally higher TBR in PLWH, with significant overlap of TBR values with HIV-negative controls [156]. The discrepancy in the results of those studies could be related to variations in study populations, treatment status of patients and the presence or absence of co-morbid CVD. Another element of variability could also be related to the imaging technique and analysis methods.

Another use for FDG PET is in longitudinally assessing PLWH for changes in arterial inflammation over time. To our knowledge, only one such longitudinal study has been reported, with twelve ART naïve subjects imaged at baseline and again six months after ART initiation. Interestingly, there were no significant changes in TBR between baseline and follow-up scans [157]. This could be due to short interval imaging after ART initiation. Another paper assessing PLWH treated with statins versus placebo found no significant change in arterial inflammation as measured by FDG PET despite the fact that statin therapy reduced non-calcified plaque volume and high-risk coronary plaque features on CCTA [158].

At this point, using FDG PET in PLWH is more likely to be useful in evaluating co-morbidities, specific organ involvement or assessment of central nervous system involvement [163–167]. The role of FDG PET in assessing CVD in individual subjects on the other hand remains uncertain.

7. Outlook

Consistent with Swiss data [8], a nationwide cohort study in Denmark found that after the exclusion of participants with risk factors including illicit drug use or hepatitis B or C co-infections, the mortality rate was similar in HIV-positive and HIV-negative persons [168]. In general, persons with well-controlled HIV infection and a healthy lifestyle appear to have similar survival rates today as do HIV-negative persons, with potentially increased death rates mainly ascribed to traditional risk factors [168,169]. Thus, for efficient primary CAD prevention in PLWH, our aim should be the optimization of traditional risk factor management, early initiation of ART therapy, and regular patient follow-up.

Few studies have simultaneously applied more than one cardiac imaging modality (CIMT and CAC [170], CCTA and MRI [103]) in the same patients, but did not correlate CIMT results with CAC or MRI with CCTA results. Hsue and colleagues found that with or without detectable CAC, PLWH had higher CIMT than HIV-negative controls [171]. Interestingly, among those without detectable CAC, a third of PLWH but no controls had increased CIMT.

CCTA is emerging as an accurate and reliable non-invasive imaging modality for detection of subclinical atherosclerosis in PLWH, especially in persons <50 years who typically have non-calcified or partially calcified plaque. However, in asymptomatic PLWH today, cardiac imaging is not yet indicated to assess coronary atherosclerosis. The exception might be asymptomatic persons with diabetes [172]. Studies that compared coronary imaging to optimization of medical treatment in asymptomatic patients have not yet shown any clinical benefit, but a number of relevant studies are ongoing. Particularly in patients with atypical symptoms suggestive of myocardial ischemia, or in patients with suspected acute coronary syndrome but without ST-segment elevations on EKG, CCTA is now increasingly well established as a valuable diagnostic tool to rule out CAD in the emergency room [173–175], because of its non-invasiveness compared to coronary angiography and its extremely high negative predictive value [176].

Author Contributions: Literature review: I.C.S., D.A.H., P.E.T.; writing—original draft preparation, writing—critical insights during review and editing I.C.S., R.R.B., H.K., D.A.H., P.E.T. Preparation of cardiac imaging figures: R.R.B., D.A.H.

Funding: No external funding was obtained for preparation of this article.

Conflicts of Interest: P.E.T.'s institution has received research grants and advisory fees from ViiV and Gilead. The research of I.C.S., R.R.B., H.K., and P.E.T. supported by the Swiss National Science Foundation and the Swiss HIV Cohort Study. The other authors declare no conflicts of interest.

References

1. Mozaffarian, D.; Benjamin, E.J.; Go, A.S.; Arnett, D.K.; Blaha, M.J.; Cushman, M.; Das, S.R.; de Ferranti, S.; Després, J.; Fullerton, H.J.; et al. Heart Disease and Stroke Statistics-2016 Update: A Report From the American Heart Association. *Circulation* **2015**, *133*, 38–360. [CrossRef] [PubMed]
2. Shah, A.S.V.; Stelzle, D.; Lee, K.K.; Beck, E.J.; Alam, S.; Clifford, S.; Longenecker, C.T.; Strachan, F.; Bagchi, S.; Whiteley, W.; et al. Global Burden of Atherosclerotic Cardiovascular Disease in People Living With HIV. *Circulation* **2018**, *138*, 1100–1112. [CrossRef] [PubMed]
3. Weber, R.; Ruppik, M.; Rickenbach, M.; Spoerri, A.; Furrer, H.; Battegay, M.; Cavassini, M.; Calmy, A.; Bernasconi, E.; Schmid, P.; et al. Decreasing mortality and changing patterns of causes of death in the Swiss HIV Cohort Study. *HIV Med.* **2013**, *14*, 195–207. [CrossRef] [PubMed]
4. Smith, C.J.; Ryom, L.; Weber, R.; Morlat, P.; Pradier, C.; Reiss, P.; Kowalska, J.D.; de Wit, S.; Law, M.; el Sadr, W.; et al. Trends over time in underlying causes of death amongst HIV-positive individuals from 1999 to 2011. *Lancet* **2014**, *384*, 241–248. [CrossRef]
5. Frieden, T.R.; Jaffe, M.G. Saving 100 million lives by improving global treatment of hypertension and reducing cardiovascular disease risk factors. *J. Clin. Hypertens.* **2018**, *20*, 208–211. [CrossRef] [PubMed]
6. Patel, P.; Sabin, K.; Godfrey-Faussett, P. Approaches to Improve the Surveillance, Monitoring, and Management of Noncommunicable Diseases in HIV-Infected Persons: Viewpoint. *JMIR Public Heal. Surveill.* **2018**, *4*, e10989. [CrossRef] [PubMed]
7. Hsue, P.Y.; Waters, D.D. Time to Recognize HIV Infection as a Major Cardiovascular Risk Factor. *Circulation* **2018**, *138*, 1113–1115. [CrossRef]
8. Hasse, B.; Tarr, P.E.; Marques-Vidal, P.; Waeber, G.; Preisig, M.; Mooser, V.; Valeri, F.; Djalali, S.; Andri, R.; Bernasconie, E.; et al. Strong Impact of Smoking on Multimorbidity Immunodeficiency Virus-Infected Individuals in and Cardiovascular Risk Among Human Comparison With the General Population. *Open Forum Infect. Dis.* **2015**. [CrossRef]
9. Rasmussen, L.D.; Helleberg, M.; May, M.T.; Afzal, S.; Kronborg, G.; Larsen, C.S.; Pedersen, C.; Gerstoft, J.; Nordestgaard, B.G.; Obel, N. Myocardial infarction among danish HIV-infected individuals: Population-attributable fractions associated with smoking. *Clin. Infect. Dis.* **2015**, *60*, 1415–1423. [CrossRef]
10. Engel, T.; Raffenberg, M.; Marzolini, C.; Cavassini, M.; Kovari, H.; Hasse, B.; Tarr, P.E. HIV and Aging-Perhaps Not as Dramatic as We Feared? *Gerontology* **2018**, *64*, 446–456. [CrossRef]
11. Triant, V.A.; Lee, H.; Hadigan, C.; Grinspoon, S.K. Increased acute myocardial infarction rates and cardiovascular risk factors among patients with human immunodeficiency virus disease. *J. Clin. Endocrinol. Metab.* **2007**, *92*, 2506–2512. [CrossRef] [PubMed]
12. De Lima, L.R.; Petroski, E.L.; Moreno, Y.M.; Silva, D.A.; Trindade, E.B.; de Carvalho, A.P.; de Carlos Back, I. Dyslipidemia, chronic inflammation, and subclinical atherosclerosis in children and adolescents infected with HIV: The PositHIVe Health Study. *PLoS ONE* **2018**, *13*, 1–17.

13. Mallon, P.W.G. Getting to the Heart of HIV and Myocardial Infarction. *JAMA Intern. Med.* **2013**, *173*, 622. [CrossRef] [PubMed]
14. Rasmussen, L.D.; May, M.T.; Kronborg, G.; Larsen, C.S.; Pedersen, C.; Gerstoft, J.; Obel, N. Time trends for risk of severe age-related diseases in individuals with and without HIV infection in Denmark: A nationwide population-based cohort study. *Lancet HIV* **2015**, *2*, e288–e298. [CrossRef]
15. Drozd, D.R.; Kitahata, M.M.; Althoff, K.N.; Zhang, J.; Gange, S.J.; Napravnik, S.; Burkholder, G.A.; Mathews, W.C.; Silverberg, M.J.; Sterling, T.R.; et al. Increased Risk of Myocardial Infarction in HIV-Infected Individuals in North America Compared with the General Population. *J. Acquir. Immune Defic. Syndr.* **2017**, *75*, 568–576. [CrossRef] [PubMed]
16. Freiberg, M.S.; Chang, C.C.H.; Kuller, L.H.; Skanderson, M.; Lowy, E.; Kraemer, K.L.; Butt, A.A.; Goetz, M.B.; Leaf, D.; Oursler, K.A.; et al. HIV infection and the risk of acute myocardial infarction. *JAMA Intern. Med.* **2013**, *173*, 614–622. [CrossRef] [PubMed]
17. Klein, D.B.; Leyden, W.A.; Xu, L.; Chao, C.R.; Horberg, M.A.; Towner, W.J.; Hurley, L.B.; Marcus, J.L.; Quesenberry, C.P.; Silverberg, M.J. Declining relative risk for myocardial infarction among HIV-positive compared with HIV-negative individuals with access to care. *Clin. Infect. Dis.* **2015**, *60*, 1278–1280. [CrossRef] [PubMed]
18. Tarr, P.E.; Ledergerber, B.; Calmy, A.; Doco-Lecompte, T.; Marzel, A.; Weber, R.; Kaufmann, P.A.; Nkoulou, R.; Buechel, R.R.; Kovari, H. Subclinical coronary artery disease in Swiss HIV-positive and HIV-negative persons. *Eur. Heart J.* **2018**, *39*, 2147–2154. [CrossRef] [PubMed]
19. Lang, S.; Mary-Krausea, M.; Cotte, L.; Gilquind, J.; Partisanie, M.; Simonf, A.; Boccarag, F.; Binghamh, A.; Dominique, C.; for the French Hospital Database on HIV-ANRS CO4. Increased risk of myocardial infarction in HIV-infected patients in France, relative to the general population. *Res. Lett.* **2010**, *24*, 1228–1230. [CrossRef]
20. Boccara, F.; Lang, S.; Meuleman, C.; Ederhy, S.; Mary-Krause, M.; Costagliola, D.; Capeau, J.; Cohen, A. HIV and coronary heart disease: Time for a better understanding. *J. Am. Coll. Cardiol.* **2013**, *61*, 511–523. [CrossRef]
21. Vachiat, A.; McCutcheon, K.; Tsabedze, N.; Zachariah, D.; Manga, P. HIV and Ischemic Heart Disease. *J. Am. Coll. Cardiol.* **2017**, *69*, 73–82. [CrossRef]
22. Wang, X.; Chai, H.; Yao, Q.; Chen, C. Molecular Mechanisms of HIV Protease Inhibitor-Induced. *J. Acquir. Immune Defic. Syndr.* **2007**, *44*, 493–499. [CrossRef]
23. Worm, S.W.; Sabin, C.; Weber, R.; Reiss, P.; El-Sadr, W.; Dabis, F.; De Wit, S.; Law, M.; Monforte, A.D.; Friis-Møller, N.; et al. Risk of Myocardial Infarction in Patients with HIV Infection Exposed to Specific Individual Antiretroviral Drugs from the 3 Major Drug Classes: The Data Collection on Adverse Events of Anti-HIV Drugs (D:A:D) Study. *J. Infect. Dis.* **2009**, *201*, 318–330. [CrossRef]
24. Subramanya, V.; McKay, H.S.; Brusca, R.M.; Palella, F.J.; Kingsley, L.A.; Witt, M.D.; Hodis, H.N.; Tracy, R.P.; Post, W.S.; Haberlen, S.A. Inflammatory biomarkers and subclinical carotid atherosclerosis in HIV-infected and HIV-uninfected men in the Multicenter AIDS Cohort Study. *PLoS ONE* **2019**, *14*, e0214735. [CrossRef]
25. Tenorio, A.R.; Zheng, Y.; Bosch, R.J.; Krishnan, S.; Rodriguez, B.; Hunt, P.W.; Plants, J.; Seth, A.; Wilson, C.C.; Deeks, S.G.; et al. Soluble Markers of In flammation and Coagulation but Not T-Cell Activation Predict Non-AIDS-Defining Morbid Events During Suppressive Antiretroviral Treatment. *J. Infect. Dis.* **2014**, *210*, 1248–1259. [CrossRef]
26. Kuller, L.H.; Tracy, R.; Belloso, W.; De Wit, S.; Drummond, F.; Lane, H.C.; Ledergerber, B.; Lundgren, J.; Neuhaus, J.; Nixon, D.; et al. Inflammatory and Coagulation Biomarkers and Mortality in Patients with HIV Infection. *PLoS Med.* **2008**, *5*, e203. [CrossRef]
27. So-Armah, K.A.; Tate, J.P.; Chang, C.H.; Butt, A.A.; Gerschenson, M.; Gibert, C.L.; Leaf, D.; Rimland, D.; Rodriguez-barradas, M.C.; Budoff, M.J.; et al. Do Biomarkers of Inflammation, Monocyte Activation, and Altered Coagulation Explain Excess Mortality Between HIV Infected and Uninfected People? *J. Acquir. Immune Defic. Syndr.* **2016**, *72*, 206–213. [CrossRef]
28. Sandler, N.G.; Wand, H.; Roque, A.; Law, M.; Nason, M.C.; Nixon, D.E.; Pedersen, C.; Ruxrungtham, K.; Lewin, S.R.; Emery, S.; et al. Plasma Levels of Soluble CD14 Independently Predict Mortality in HIV Infection. 2011, 203, 780–790. *J. Infect. Dis.* **2011**, *203*, 780–790. [CrossRef]

29. Kelesidis, T.; Kendall, M.A.; Yang, O.O.; Hodis, H.N.; Currier, J.S. Biomarkers of Microbial Translocation and Macrophage Activation: Association with Progression of Subclinical Atherosclerosis in HIV-1 Infection. *J. Infect. Dis.* **2012**, *206*, 1558–1567. [CrossRef]
30. Hanna, D.B.; Lin, J.; Post, W.S.; Hodis, H.N.; Xue, X.; Anastos, K.; Cohen, M.H.; Gange, S.J.; Haberlen, S.A.; Heath, S.L.; et al. Association of Macrophage Inflammation Biomarkers With Progression of Subclinical Carotid Artery Atherosclerosis in HIV-Infected Women and Men. *J. Infect. Dis.* **2017**, *10461*, 1352–1361. [CrossRef]
31. Burdo, T.H.; Lo, J.; Abbara, S.; Wei, J.; Delelys, M.E.; Preffer, F.; Rosenberg, E.S.; Williams, K.C.; Grinspoon, S. Soluble CD163, a Novel Marker of Activated Macrophages, Is Elevated and Associated With Noncalcified Coronary Plaque in HIV-Infected Patients. *J. Infect. Dis.* **2011**, *204*, 1227–1236. [CrossRef]
32. Eugenin, E.A.; Morgello, S.; Klotman, M.E.; Mosoian, A.; Lento, P.A.; Berman, J.W.; Schecter, A.D. Human Immunodeficiency Virus (HIV) Infects Human Arterial Smooth Muscle Cells in Vivo and in Vitro Implications for the Pathogenesis of HIV-Mediated Vascular Disease. *Am. J. Pathol.* **2008**, *172*, 1100–1111. [CrossRef]
33. Tabib, A.; Mornex, C.; Leroux, J.-F.; Loire, R. Accelerated coronary atherosclerosis and arteriosclerosis in young human-immunodeficiency-virus-positive patients. *Coron. Artery Dis.* **2000**, *11*, 41–46. [CrossRef]
34. Zanni, M.V.; Schouten, J.; Grinspoon, S.K.; Reiss, P. Risk of coronary heart disease in patients with HIV infection. *Nat. Rev. Cardiol.* **2014**, *11*, 728. [CrossRef]
35. Wolf, K.; Tsakiris, D.A.; Weber, R.; Erb, P.; Battegay, M. Antiretroviral Therapy Reduces Markers of Endothelial and Coagulation Activation in Patients Infected with Human Immunodeficiency Virus Type 1. *J. Infect. Dis.* **2002**, *185*, 456–462. [CrossRef]
36. Lang, S.; Mary-Krause, M.; Simon, A.; Partisani, M.; Gilquin, J.; Cotte, L.; Boccara, F.; Costagliola, D. HIV Replication and Immune Status Are Independent Predictors of the Risk of Myocardial Infarction in HIV-Infected Individuals. *Clin. Infect. Dis.* **2012**, *55*, 600–607. [CrossRef]
37. Michael, S.; Leyden, W.A.; Xu, L.; Horberg, M.A.; Chao, C.R.; Towner, W.J.; Hurley, L.B.; Quesenberry, C.P.; Klein, D.B. Immunodeficiency and risk of myocardial infarction among HIV-positive individuals with access to care. *J. Acquir. Immune Defic. Syndr.* **2014**, *65*, 160–166.
38. Rotger, M.; Glass, T.R.; Junier, T.; Lundgren, J.; Neaton, J.D.; Poloni, E.S.; Van 'T Wout, A.B.; Lubomirov, R.; Colombo, S.; Martinez, R.; et al. Contribution of genetic background, traditional risk factors, and HIV-related factors to coronary artery disease events in HIV-positive persons. *Clin. Infect. Dis.* **2013**, *57*, 112–121. [CrossRef]
39. Sabin, C.A.; Ryom, L.; De Wit, S.; Mocroft, A.; Phillips, A.N.; Worm, S.W.; Weber, R.; Monforte, A.D.; Reiss, P.; Kamara, D.; et al. Associations between immune depression and cardiovascular events in HIV infection. *AIDS* **2013**, *27*, 2735–2748. [CrossRef]
40. Périard, D.; Telenti, A.; Sudre, P.; Cheseaux, J.J.; Halfon, P.; Reymond, M.J.; Marcovina, S.M.; Glauser, M.P.; Nicod, P.; Darioli, R.; et al. Atherogenic dyslipidemia in HIV-infected individuals treated with protease inhibitors. *Circulation* **1999**, *100*, 700–705. [CrossRef]
41. Ryom, L.; Lundgren, J.D.; El-Sadr, W.; Reiss, P.; Kirk, O.; Law, M.; Phillips, A.; Weber, R.; Fontas, E.; d'Arminio Monforte, A.; et al. Cardiovascular disease and use of contemporary protease inhibitors: The D:A:D international prospective multicohort study. *Lancet HIV* **2018**, *5*, e291–e300. [CrossRef]
42. Sabin, C.A.; Worm, S.W.; Weber, R.; Reiss, P.; El-Sadr, W.; Dabis, F.; De Wit, S.; Law, M.; D'Arminio Monforte, A.; Friis-Møller, N.; et al. Use of nucleoside reverse transcriptase inhibitors and risk of myocardial infarction in HIV-infected patients enrolled in the D:A:D study: A multi-cohort collaboration. *Lancet* **2008**, *371*, 1417–1426.
43. Lai, H.; Moore, R.; Celentano, D.D.; Gerstenblith, G.; Treisman, G.; Keruly, J.C.; Kickler, T.; Li, J.; Chen, S.; Lai, S.; et al. HIV infection itself may not be associated with subclinical coronary artery disease among African Americans without cardiovascular symptoms. *J. Am. Heart Assoc.* **2015**, *5*, 1–16. [CrossRef]
44. Post, W.S.; Budoff, M.; Kingsley, L.; Palella, F.J.; Witt, M.D.; Li, X.; George, R.T.; Brown, T.; Jacobson, L.P. Associations between HIV Infection and Subclinical Coronary Atherosclerosis: The Multicenter AIDS Cohort Study (MACS). *Ann. Intern. Med.* **2014**, *160*, 458–467. [CrossRef]
45. Stein, J.H.; Currier, J.S.; Hsue, P.Y. Arterial Disease in Patients With Human Immunodeficiency Virus Infection. *JACC Cardiovasc. Imaging* **2014**, *7*, 515–525. [CrossRef]
46. Inaba, Y.; Chen, J.A.; Bergmann, S.R. Carotid Intima-Media Thickness and Cardiovascular Events. *N. Engl. J. Med.* **2011**, *365*, 1640–1642.

47. Lorenz, M.W.; Polak, J.F.; Kavousi, M.; Mathiesen, E.B.; Völzke, H.; Tuomainen, T.P.; Sander, D.; Plichart, M.; Catapano, A.L.; Robertson, C.M.; et al. Carotid intima-media thickness progression to predict cardiovascular events in the general population (the PROG-IMT collaborative project): A meta-analysis of individual participant data. *Lancet* **2012**, *379*, 2053–2062. [CrossRef]
48. O'Leary, D.H.; Polak, J.F.; Kronmal, R.A.; Manolio, T.A.; Burke, G.L.; Wolfson, S.K. Carotid-Artery Intima and Media Thickness as a Risk Factor for Myocardial Infarction and Stroke in Older Adults. *N. Engl. J. Med.* **2002**, *340*, 14–22. [CrossRef]
49. Den Ruijter, H.M.; Peters, S.A.E.; Anderson, T.J.; Britton, A.R.; Dekker, J.M.; Eijkemans, M.J.; Engström, G.; Evans, G.W.; de Graaf, J.; Grobbee, D.E.; et al. Common carotid intima-media thickness measurements in cardiovascular risk prediction: A meta-analysis. *JAMA* **2012**, *308*, 796–803. [CrossRef]
50. Hulten, E.; Mitchell, J.; Scally, J.; Gibbs, B.; Villines, T.C. HIV positivity, protease inhibitor exposure and subclinical atherosclerosis: A systematic review and meta-analysis of observational studies. *Heart* **2009**, *95*, 1826–1835. [CrossRef]
51. Maggi, P.; Serio, G.; Epifani, G.; Fiorentino, G.; Saracino, A.; Fico, C.; Perilli, F.; Lillo, A.; Ferraro, S.; Gargiulo, M.; et al. Premature lesions of the carotid vessels in HIV-1-infected patients treated with protease inhibitors. *AIDS* **2000**, *14*, F123–F128. [CrossRef]
52. Maggi, P.; Lillo, A.; Perilli, F.; Maserati, R.; Chirianni, A.; Epifani, G.; Fiorentino, G.; Ladisa, N.; Pastore, G.; Angiletta, D.; et al. Colour-Doppler ultrasonography of carotid vessels in patients treated with antiretroviral therapy: A comparative study. *AIDS* **2004**, *18*, 1023–1028. [CrossRef]
53. Hsue, P.Y.; Lo, J.C.; Franklin, A.; Bolger, A.F.; Martin, J.N.; Deeks, S.G.; Waters, D.D. Progression of Atherosclerosis as Assessed by Carotid Intima-Media Thickness in Patients with HIV Infection. *Circulation* **2004**, *109*, 1603–1608. [CrossRef]
54. Mercié, P.; Thiébaut, R.; Aurillac-Lavignolle, V.; Pellegrin, J.L.; Yvorra-Vives, M.C.; Cipriano, C.; Neau, D.; Morlat, P.; Ragnaud, J.M.; Dupon, M.; et al. Carotid intima-media thickness is slightly increased over time in HIV-1-infected patients. *HIV Med.* **2005**, *6*, 380–387. [CrossRef]
55. Hsue, P.Y.; Hunt, P.W.; Sinclair, E.; Bredt, B.; Franklin, A.; Killian, M.; Hoh, R.; Martin, J.N.; McCune, J.M.; Waters, D.D.; et al. Increased carotid intima-media thickness in HIV patients is associated with increased cytomegalovirus-specific T-cell responses. *AIDS* **2006**, *20*, 2275–2283. [CrossRef]
56. Thiebaut, R.; Aurillac-Lavignolleb, V.; Bonnetb, F.; Ibrahimd, N.; Cipriancc, C.; Neauc, D.; Duponc, M.; Dabisb, F.; Mercie, P.; Groupe d'Epidemiologie Clinique du Sida en Aquitaine (GECSA). Change in atherosclerosis progression in HIV infected patients: ANRS Aquitaine Cohort, 1999–2004. *AIDS* **2005**, *19*, 729–731. [CrossRef]
57. Johnsen, S.; Dolan, S.E.; Fitch, K.V.; Kanter, J.R.; Hemphill, L.C.; Connelly, J.M.; Lees, R.S.; Lee, H.; Grinspoon, S. Carotid intimal medial thickness in human immunodeficiency virus-infected women: Effects of protease inhibitor use, cardiac risk factors, and the metabolic syndrome. *J. Clin. Endocrinol. Metab.* **2006**, *91*, 4916–4924. [CrossRef]
58. Van Wijk, J.P.H.; De Koning, E.J.P.; Cabezas, M.C.; Joven, J.; Op't Roodt, J.; Rabelink, T.J.; Hoepelman, A.M. Functional and structural markers of atherosclerosis in human immunodeficiency virus-infected patients. *J. Am. Coll. Cardiol.* **2006**, *47*, 1117–1123. [CrossRef]
59. Currier, J.S.; Kendall, M.A.; Henry, W.K.; Alston-Smith, B.; Torriani, F.J.; Tebas, P.; Li, Y.; Hodis, H.N. Progression of carotid artery intima-media thickening in HIV-infected and uninfected adults. *AIDS* **2007**, *21*, 1137–1145. [CrossRef]
60. Jericó, C.; Knobel, H.; Calvo, N.; Sorli, M.L.; Guelar, A.; Gimeno-Bayón, J.L.; Saballs, P.; López-Colomés, J.L.; Pedro-Botet, J. Subclinical carotid atherosclerosis in HIV-infected patients: Role of combination antiretroviral therapy. *Stroke* **2006**, *37*, 812–817. [CrossRef]
61. Lorenz, M.W.; Stephan, C.; Harmjanz, A.; Staszewski, S.; Buehler, A.; Bickel, M.; von Kegler, S.; Ruhkamp, D.; Steinmetz, H.; Sitzer, M. Both long-term HIV infection and highly active antiretroviral therapy are independent risk factors for early carotid atherosclerosis. *Atherosclerosis* **2008**, *196*, 720–726. [CrossRef]
62. Coll, B.; Parra, S.; Alonso-Villaverde, C.; Aragonés, G.; Montero, M.; Camps, J.; Joven, J.; Masana, L. The role of immunity and inflammation in the progression of atherosclerosis in patients with HIV infection. *Stroke* **2007**, *38*, 2477–2484. [CrossRef]

63. Depairon, M.; Chessex, S.; Sudre, P.; Rodondi, N.; Doser, N.; Chave, J.P.; Riesen, W.; Nicod, P.; Darioli, R.; Telenti, A.; et al. Premature atherosclerosis in hiv-infected individuals focus on protease inhibitor therapy. *AIDS* **2001**, *15*, 329–334. [CrossRef]
64. Maggi, P.; Perilli, F.; Lillo, A.; Gargiulo, M.; Ferraro, S.; Grisorio, B.; Ferrara, S.; Carito, V.; Bellacosa, C.; Pastore, G.; et al. Rapid progression of carotid lesions in HAART-treated HIV-1 patients. *Atherosclerosis* **2007**, *192*, 407–412. [CrossRef]
65. Grunfeld, C.; Delaney, J.A.; Wanke, C.; Currier, J.S.; Scherzer, R.; Biggs, M.L.; Tien, P.C.; Shlipak, M.G.; Sidney, S.; Polak, J.F.; et al. Preclinical atherosclerosis due to HIV infection: Carotid intima-medial thickness measurements from the FRAM study. *AIDS* **2009**, *23*, 1841–1849. [CrossRef]
66. Hsue, P.Y.; Hunt, P.W.; Schnell, A.; Kalapus, S.C.; Hoh, R.; Ganz, P.; Martin, J.N.; Deeks, S.G. Role of viral replication, antiretroviral therapy, and immunodeficiency in HIV-associated atherosclerosis. *AIDS* **2009**, *23*, 1059–1067. [CrossRef]
67. Cabello, C.M.; Bair, W.B.; Lamore, S.D.; Ley, S.; Alexandra, S.; Azimian, S.; Wondrak, G.T. Silencing of germline-expressed genes by DNA elimination in somatic cells. *Dev. Cell* **2010**, *46*, 220–231.
68. Kaplan, R.C.; Sinclair, E.; Landay, A.L.; Lurain, N.; Sharrett, A.R.; Gange, S.J.; Xue, X.; Hunt, P.; Karim, R.; Kern, D.M.; et al. T Cell Activation and Senescence Predict Subclinical Carotid Artery Disease in HIV-Infected Women. *J. Infect. Dis.* **2011**, *203*, 452–463. [CrossRef]
69. Sainz, T.; Álvarez-Fuente, M.; Navarro, M.L.; Díaz, L.; Rojo, P.; Blázquez, D.; De José, M.I.; Ramos, J.T.; Serrano-Villar, S.; Martínez, J.; et al. Subclinical atherosclerosis and markers of immune activation in hiv-infected children and adolescents: The carovih study. *J. Acquir. Immune Defic. Syndr.* **2014**, *65*, 42–49. [CrossRef]
70. Hanna, D.B.; Post, W.S.; Deal, J.A.; Hodis, H.N.; Jacobson, L.P.; Mack, W.J.; Anastos, K.; Gange, S.J.; Landay, A.L.; Lazar, J.M.; et al. HIV Infection Is Associated with Progression of Subclinical Carotid Atherosclerosis. *Clin. Infect. Dis.* **2015**, *61*, 640–650. [CrossRef]
71. Hsue, P.Y.; Scherzer, R.; Hunt, P.W.; Schnell, A.; Bolger, A.F.; Kalapus, S.C.; Maka, K.; Martin, J.N.; Ganz, P.; Deeks, S.G. Carotid Intima-Media Thickness Progression in HIV-Infected Adults Occurs Preferentially at the Carotid Bifurcation and Is Predicted by Inflammation. *J. Am. Heart Assoc.* **2012**, *1*, 1–12. [CrossRef]
72. Bots, M.L.; Baldassarre, D.; Simon, A.; De Groot, E.; O'Leary, D.H.; Riley, W.; Kastelein, J.J.; Grobbee, D.E. Carotid intima-media thickness and coronary atherosclerosis: Weak or strong relations? *Eur. Heart J.* **2007**, *28*, 398–406. [CrossRef]
73. Hodis, H.N.; Mack, W.J.; Labree, L.; Selzer, R.H. The Role of Carotid Arterial Intima-Media Thickness in Predicting Clinical Coronary Events Methods Study Design. *Annals Intern. Med.* **2006**, *128*, 262–269. [CrossRef]
74. Greenland, P.; Alpert, J.S.; Beller, G.; Benjamin, E.J.; Budoff, M.J.; Fayad, Z.A.; Foster, E.; Hlatky, M.A.; Hodgson, J.M.; Kushner, F.G.; et al. 2010 ACCF/AHA Guideline for Assessment of Cardiovascular Risk in Asymptomatic Adults. *J. Am. Coll. Cardiol.* **2010**, *56*, 50–103. [CrossRef]
75. Callister, T.Q.; Cooil, B.; Raya, S.; Lippolis, N.J.; Russo, D.J.; Raggi, P. Coronary artery disease: improved reproducibility of calcium scoring with an electron-beam CT volumetric method. *Radiology* **2014**, *208*, 807–814. [CrossRef]
76. Callister, T.Q.; Raggi, P.; Cooil, B.; Lippolis, N.J.; Russo, D.J. Effect of HMG-CoA Reductase Inhibitors on Coronary Artery Disease as Assessed by Electron-Beam Computed Tomography. *N. Engl. J. Med.* **2002**, *339*, 1972–1978. [CrossRef]
77. Raggi, P.; Callister, T.Q.; Shaw, L.J. Progression of coronary artery calcium and risk of first myocardial infarction in patients receiving cholesterol-lowering therapy. *Arterioscler. Thromb. Vasc. Biol.* **2004**, *24*, 1272–1277. [CrossRef]
78. Raggi, P.; Davidson, M.; Callister, T.Q.; Welty, F.K.; Bachmann, G.A.; Hecht, H.; Rumberger, J.A. Aggressive Versus Moderate Lipid-Lowering Therapy in Hypercholesterolemic Postmenopausal Women. *Circulation* **2005**, *112*, 563–571. [CrossRef]
79. Achenbach, S.; Ropers, D.; Pohle, K.; Leber, A.; Thilo, C.; Knez, A.; Menendez, T.; Maeffert, R.; Kusus, M.; Regenfus, M.; et al. Influence of lipid-lowering therapy on the progression of coronary artery calcification: A prospective evaluation. *Circulation* **2002**, *106*, 1077–1082. [CrossRef]
80. Bonow, R.O. Should Coronary Calcium Screening Be Used in Cardiovascular Prevention Strategies? *N. Engl. J. Med.* **2009**, *361*, 990–997. [CrossRef]

81. Hoffmann, U.; Brady, T.J.; Muller, J. Use of New Imaging Techniques to Screen for Coronary Artery Disease. *Circulation* **2003**, *108*, 1–4. [CrossRef]
82. Polonsky, T.S.; Mcclelland, R.L.; Jorgensen, N.W.; Bild, D.E.; Burke, G.L.; Guerci, A.D.; Greenland, P. Coronary artery calcium score and risk classification for coronary heart disease prediction. *JAMA* **2011**, *303*, 1610–1616. [CrossRef]
83. Schmermund, A.; Baumgart, D.; Möhlenkamp, S.; Kriener, P.; Pump, H.; Grönemeyer, D.; Seibel, R.; Erbel, R. Natural History and Topographic Pattern of Progression of Coronary Calcification in Symptomatic Patients. *Arterioscler. Thromb. Vasc. Biol.* **2011**, *21*, 421–426. [CrossRef]
84. Detrano, R.; Guerci, A.D.; Carr, J.J.; Bild, D.E.; Burke, G.; Folsom, A.R.; Liu, K.; Shea, S.; Szklo, M.; Bluemke, D.A.; et al. Coronary Calcium as a Predictor of Coronary Events in Four Racial or Ethnic Groups. *N. Engl. J. Med.* **2008**, *358*, 1336–1345. [CrossRef]
85. Pletcher, M.; Tice, J.; Pignone, M.; Browner, W. Using the Coronary Artery Calcium Score to Predict Coronary Heart Disease Events. *Arch. Intern. Med.* **2004**, *164*, 1285–1292. [CrossRef]
86. Folsam, A.; Kronmal, R.A.; Detrano, R.; O'Leary, D.; Bild, D.E.; Bluemke, D.A.; Budoff, M.J.; Liu, K.; Shea, S.; Szklo, M.; et al. Coronary Artery Calcification Compared With Carotid Intima-Media Thickness in the Prediction of Cardiovascular Disease Incidence. *Arch. Intern. Med.* **2008**, *168*, 1333–1339. [CrossRef]
87. Taylor, A.J.; Bindeman, J.; Feuerstein, I.; Cao, F.; Brazaitis, M.; O'Malley, P.G. Coronary Calcium Independently Predicts Incident Premature Coronary Heart Disease Over Measured Cardiovascular Risk Factors. *J. Am. Coll. Cardiol.* **2005**, *46*, 807–814. [CrossRef]
88. Arad, Y.; Goodman, K.J.; Roth, M.; Newstein, D.; Guerci, A.D. Coronary calcification, coronary disease risk factors, C-reactive protein, and atherosclerotic cardiovascular disease events: The St. Francis heart study. *J. Am. Coll. Cardiol.* **2005**, *46*, 158–165. [CrossRef]
89. Budoff, M.J.; Shaw, L.J.; Liu, S.T.; Weinstein, S.R.; Mosler, T.P.; Tseng, P.H.; Flores, F.R.; Callister, T.Q.; Raggi, P.; Berman, D.S. Long-Term Prognosis Associated With Coronary Calcification. Observations From a Registry of 25,253 Patients. *J. Am. Coll. Cardiol.* **2007**, *49*, 1860–1870. [CrossRef]
90. Raggi, P.; Cooil, B.; Shaw, L.J.; Aboulhson, J.; Takasu, J.; Budoff, M.; Callister, T.Q. Progression of coronary calcium on serial electron beam tomographic scanning is greater in patients with future myocardial infarction. *Am. J. Cardiol.* **2003**, *92*, 827–829. [CrossRef]
91. Newman, A.B.; Naydeck, B.; Ives, D.; Boudreau, R.; Sutton-Tyrrell, K.; O'Leary, D.H.; Kuller, L.H. Coronary Artery Calcium, Carotid Artery Wall Thickness and Cardiovascular Disease Outcomes in Adults 70 to 99 Years Old. *Am. J. Cardiol.* **2010**, *46*, 220–231. [CrossRef]
92. Vliegenthart, R.; Oudkerk, M.; Hofman, A.; Oei, H.-H.; van Dijck, W.; Van Rooij, F.J.A.; Witteman, J.C.M. Coronary Calcification Improves Cardiovascular Risk Prediction in the Elderly. *Circulation* **2005**, 572–577. [CrossRef]
93. Jain, A.; McClelland, R.L.; Polak, J.F.; Shea, S.; Burke, G.L.; Bild, D.E.; Watson, K.E.; Budoff, M.J.; Liu, K.; Post, W.S.; et al. Cardiovascular imaging for assessing cardiovascular risk in asymptomatic men versus women the Multi-Ethnic Study of Atherosclerosis (MESA). *Circ. Cardiovasc. Imaging* **2011**, *4*, 8–15. [CrossRef]
94. Yeboah, J.; Mcclelland, R.L.; Polonsky, T.S.; Burke, G.L.; Sibley, C.T.; O'Leary, D.H.; Carr, J.J.; Goff, D.C.; Greenland, P.; Herrington, D.M. Comparison of novel risk markers for improvement in cardiovascular risk assessment in intermediate-risk individuals. *JAMA* **2012**, *308*, 788–795. [CrossRef]
95. Guaraldi, G.; Zona, S.; Alexopoulos, N.; Orlando, G.; Carli, F.; Ligabue, G.; Fiocchi, F.; Lattanzi, A.; Rossi, R.; Modena, M.G.; et al. Coronary Aging in HIV-Infected Patients. *Clin. Infect. Dis.* **2009**, *49*, 1756–1762. [CrossRef]
96. Kingsley, L.A.; Cuervo-Rojas, J.; Muñoz, A.; Palella, F.J.; Post, W.; Witt, M.D.; Budoff, M.; Kuller, L. Subclinical coronary atherosclerosis, HIV infection and antiretroviral therapy: Multicenter AIDS Cohort Study. *AIDS* **2008**, *22*, 1589–1599. [CrossRef]
97. Motoyama, S.; Ito, H.; Sarai, M.; Kondo, T.; Kawai, H.; Nagahara, Y.; Harigaya, H.; Kan, S.; Anno, H.; Takahashi, H.; et al. Plaque characterization by coronary computed tomography angiography and the likelihood of acute coronary events in mid-term follow-up. *J. Am. Coll. Cardiol.* **2015**, *66*, 337–346. [CrossRef]
98. Giannopoulos, A.A.; Benz, D.C.; Gräni, C.; Buechel, R.R. Imaging the event-prone coronary artery plaque. *J. Nucl. Cardiol.* **2019**, *26*, 141–153. [CrossRef]

99. Monroe, A.K.; Haberlen, S.A.; Post, W.S.; Palella, F.; Kingsley, L.A.; Witts, M.D.; Budoff, M.; Jacobson, L.; Brown, T.T. Cardiovascular Disease Risk Scores' Relationship to Subclinical Cardiovascular Disease Among HIV-Infected and HIV-Uninfected Men. *AIDS* **2015**, *155*, 1683–1695. [CrossRef]
100. Ascenzo, F.D.; Cerrato, E.; Calcagno, A.; Grossomarra, W.; Montefusco, A.; Veglia, S.; Barbero, U.; Gili, S.; Cannillo, M.; Pianelli, M.; et al. High prevalence at computed coronary tomography of non-calcified plaques in asymptomatic HIV patients treated with HAART: A meta-analysis. *Atherosclerosis* **2015**, *240*, 197–204. [CrossRef]
101. Schoeni-Affolter, F.; Ledergerber, B.; Rickenbach, M.; Rudin, C.; Günthard, H.F.; Telenti, A.; Furrer, H.; Yerly, S.; Francioli, P. Cohort profile: The Swiss HIV cohort study. *Int. J. Epidemiol.* **2010**, *39*, 1179–1189.
102. Min, J.K.; Shaw, L.J.; Devereux, R.B.; Okin, P.M.; Weinsaft, J.W.; Russo, D.J.; Lippolis, N.J.; Berman, D.S.; Callister, T.Q. Prognostic Value of Multidetector Coronary Computed Tomographic Angiography for Prediction of All-Cause Mortality. *J. Am. Coll. Cardiol.* **2007**, *50*, 1161–1170. [CrossRef]
103. Abd-Elmoniem, K.Z.; Unsal, A.B.; Eshera, S.; Matta, J.R.; Muldoon, N.; McAreavey, D.; Purdy, J.B.; Hazra, R.; Hadigan, C.; Gharib, A.M. Increased coronary vessel wall thickness in HIV-infected young adults. *Clin. Infect. Dis.* **2014**, *59*, 1779–1786. [CrossRef]
104. Husmann, L.; Valenta, I.; Gaemperli, O.; Adda, O.; Treyer, V.; Wyss, C.A.; Veit-haibach, P.; Tatsugami, F.; Von Schulthess, G.K.; Kaufmann, P.A. Feasibility of low-dose coronary CT angiography: First experience with prospective. *Eur. Heart J.* **2008**, *29*, 191–197. [CrossRef]
105. Buechel, R.R.; Husmann, L.; Herzog, B.A.; Pazhenkottil, A.P.; Nkoulou, R.; Ghadri, J.R.; Treyer, V.; Von Schulthess, P.; Kaufmann, P.A. Low-dose computed tomography coronary angiography with prospective electrocardiogram triggering: Feasibility in a large population. *J. Am. Coll. Cardiol.* **2011**, *57*, 332–336. [CrossRef]
106. Kaufmann, P.A. Low-Dose Computed Tomography Coronary Angiography With Prospective Triggering. A Promise for the Future. *J. Am. Coll. Cardiol.* **2008**, *52*, 1456–1457. [CrossRef]
107. Min, J.K.; Dunning, A.; Lin, F.Y.; Achenbach, S.; Al-Mallah, M.; Budoff, M.J.; Cademartiri, F.; Callister, T.Q.; Chang, H.J.; Cheng, V.; et al. Age- and sex-related differences in all-cause mortality risk based on coronary computed tomography angiography findings: Results from the international multicenter CONFIRM (Coronary CT Angiography Evaluation for Clinical Outcomes: An International Multice. *J. Am. Coll. Cardiol.* **2011**, *58*, 849–860. [CrossRef]
108. Hadamitzky, M.; Freißmuth, B.; Meyer, T.; Hein, F.; Kastrati, A.; Martinoff, S.; Schömig, A.; Hausleiter, J. Prognostic Value of Coronary Computed Tomographic Angiography for Prediction of Cardiac Events in Patients With Suspected Coronary Artery Disease. *JACC Cardiovasc. Imaging* **2009**, *2*, 404–411. [CrossRef]
109. McEvoy, J.W.; Blaha, M.J.; Nasir, K.; Yoon, Y.E.; Choi, E.K.; Cho, I.S.; Chun, E.J.; Choi, S.I.; Rivera, J.J.; Blumenthal, R.S.; et al. Impact of coronary computed tomographic angiography results on patient and physician behavior in a low-risk population. *Arch. Intern. Med.* **2011**, *171*, 1260–1268. [CrossRef]
110. Herzog, B.A.; Wyss, C.A.; Husmann, L.; Gaemperli, O.; Valenta, I.; Treyer, V.; Landmesser, U.; Kaufmann, P.A. First head-to-head comparison of effective radiation dose from low-dose 64-slice CT with prospective ECG-triggering versus invasive coronary angiography. *Heart* **2009**, *95*, 1656–1661. [CrossRef]
111. Benz, D.C.; Gräni, C.; Hirt Moch, B.; Mikulicic, F.; Vontobel, J.; Fuchs, T.; Stehli, J.; Clerc, O.; Possner, M.; Pazhenkottil, A.; et al. A low-dose and an ultra-low-dose contrast agent protocol for coronary CT angiography in a clinical setting: Quantitative and qualitative comparison to a standard dose protocol. *Br. J. Radiolody* **2017**, *90*, 1–10. [CrossRef]
112. Litt, H.; Gatsonis, C.; Snyder, B.; Singh, H.; Miller, C.; Entrikin, D.; Leaming, J.; Gavin, L.; Pacella, C.; Hollander, J. CT Angiography for Safe Discharge of Patients with Possible Acute Coronary Syndromes. *N. Engl. J. Med.* **2012**, *366*, 1393–1403. [CrossRef]
113. Wyler von Ballmoos, M.; Haring, B.; Juillerat, P.; Alkadhi, H. Meta-analysis: Diagnostic Performance of Low-Radiation-Dose Coronary Computed Tomography Angiography. *Ann. Intern. Med.* **2011**, *154*, 413–420. [CrossRef]
114. Goldstein, J.A.; Chinnaiyan, K.M.; Abidov, A.; Achenbach, S.; Berman, D.S.; Hayes, S.W.; Hoffmann, U.; Lesser, J.R.; Mikati, I.A.; Neil, B.J.O.; et al. The CT-STAT (Coronary Computed Tomographic Angiography for Systematic Triage of Acute Chest Pain Patients to Treatment) Trial. *J. Am. Coll. Cardiol.* **2011**, *58*, 1414–1422. [CrossRef]

115. Hachamovitch, R.; Hayes, S.W.; Friedman, J.D.; Cohen, I.; Berman, D.S. Comparison of the short-term survival benefit associated with revascularization compared with medical therapy in patients with no prior coronary artery disease undergoing stress myocardial perfusion single photon emission computed tomography. *Circulation* **2003**, *107*, 2900–2906. [CrossRef]
116. Petoumenos, K.; Law, M. Comment HIV-infection and comorbidities: A complex mix. *Lancet HIV* **2015**, *2*, e265–e266. [CrossRef]
117. Gharib, A.M.; Abd-Elmoniem, K.Z.; Pettigrew, R.I.; Hadigan, C. Noninvasive Coronary Imaging for Atherosclerosis in Human Immunodeficiency Virus Infection. *Curr. Probl. Diagn. Radiol.* **2011**, *40*, 262–267. [CrossRef]
118. Van Velzen, J.E.; Schuijf, J.D.; De Graaf, F.R.; Boersma, E.; Pundziute, G.; Spanó, F.; Boogers, M.J.; Schalij, M.J.; Kroft, L.J.; De Roos, A.; et al. Diagnostic performance of non-invasive multidetector computed tomography coronary angiography to detect coronary artery disease using different endpoints: Detection of significant stenosis vs. detection of atherosclerosis. *Eur. Heart J.* **2011**, *32*, 637–645. [CrossRef]
119. Wijns, W.; Kolh, P.; Danchin, N.; Di Mario, C.; Falk, V.; Folliguet, T.; Garg, S.; Huber, K.; James, S.; Knuuti, J.; et al. Guidelines on myocardial revascularization: The Task Force on Myocardial Revascularization of the European Society of Cardiology (ESC) and the European Association for Cardio-Thoracic Surgery (EACTS). *Eur. Heart J.* **2010**, *31*, 2501–2555.
120. Lin, F.Y.; Shaw, L.J.; Dunning, A.M.; Labounty, T.M.; Choi, J.; Weinsaft, J.W.; Koduru, S.; Gomez, M.J.; Delago, A.J.; Callister, T.Q.; et al. Mortality Risk in Symptomatic Patients with Nonobstructive Coronary Artery Disease. *J. Am. Coll. Cardiol.* **2011**, *58*, 510–519. [CrossRef]
121. Kristensen, T.S.; Kofoed, K.F.; Khl, J.T.; Nielsen, W.B.; Nielsen, M.B.; Kelbæk, H. Prognostic implications of nonobstructive coronary plaques in patients with NonST-segment elevation myocardial infarction: A multidetector computed tomography study. *J. Am. Coll. Cardiol.* **2011**, *58*, 502–509. [CrossRef]
122. Fitch, K.V.; Lo, J.; Abbara, S.; Ghoshhajra, B.; Shturman, L.; Soni, A.; Sacks, R.; Wei, J.; Grinspoon, S. Increased coronary artery calcium score and noncalcified plaque among HIV-infected men: Relationship to metabolic syndrome and cardiac risk parameters. *J. Acquir. Immune Defic. Syndr.* **2010**, *55*, 495–499. [CrossRef]
123. Lai, S.; Bartlett, J.; Lai, H.; Moore, R.; Cofrancesco, J.; Pannu, H.; Tong, W.; Meng, W.; Sun, H.; Fishman, E.K. Long-Term Combination Antiretroviral Therapy Is Associated with the Risk of Coronary Plaques in African Americans with HIV Infection. *AIDS Patient Care STDS* **2009**, *23*, 815–824. [CrossRef]
124. Loa, J.; Abbarab, S.; Shturmanc, L.; Sonic, A.; Weia, J.; Rocha-Filhoc, J.; Nasirc, K.; Grinspoona, S.K. Increased prevalence of subclinical coronary atherosclerosis detected by coronary computed tomography angiography in HIV-infected men. *AIDS* **2010**, *24*, 243–253. [CrossRef]
125. Duarte, H.; Matta, J.R.; Muldoon, N.; Masur, H.; Hadigan, C.; Gharib, A.M. Non-calcified coronary plaque volume inversely related to CD4(+)T-cell count in HIV infection. *Antivir. Ther.* **2012**, *17*, 763–767. [CrossRef]
126. Post, W.S.; Haberlen, S.A.; Zhang, L. HIV infection is associated with progression of high risk coronary plaques in the MACS. In Proceedings of the Conference on Retroviruses and Opportunistic Infections, Boston, MA, USA, 4–7 March 2018.
127. Ma, G.S.; Cotter, B.R. HIV and cardiovascular disease: much ado about nothing? *Eur. Heart J.* **2018**, *39*, 2155–2157. [CrossRef]
128. Tunstall-Pedoe, H.; Kuulasmaa, K.; Amouyel, P.; Arveiler, D.; Rajakangas, A.M.; Pajak, A. Myocardial infarction and coronary deaths in the World Health Organization MONICA Project. Registration procedures, event rates, and case-fatality rates in 38 populations from 21 countries in four continents. *Circulation* **1994**, *90*, 583–612. [CrossRef]
129. Piepoli, M.; Hoes, A.; Agewall, S.; Albus, C.; Brotons, C.; Catapano, A.; Cooney, M.-T.; Corra, U.; Verschuren, W.M.M. New European guidelines for cardiovascular disease prevention in clinical practice. *Clin. Chem. Lab. Med.* **2009**, *47*, 2315–2381.
130. Huber, M.; Ledergerber, B.; Sauter, R.; Young, J.; Fehr, J.; Cusini, A.; Battegay, M.; Calmy, A.; Orasch, C.; Nicca, D.; et al. Outcome of smoking cessation counselling of HIV-positive persons by HIV care physicians. *HIV Med.* **2012**, *13*, 387–397. [CrossRef]
131. Guajira, T.P.; Xiuhong, L.; Post, W.S.; Jacobson, L.P.; Witt, M.D.; Brown, T.T.; Kingsley, L.A.; Phair, J.P.; Palella, F.J. Associations between antiretroviral use and subclinical coronary atherosclerosis. *AIDS* **2016**, *30*, 2477–2486.

132. Kovari, H.; Calmy, A.; Doco-Lecompte, T.; Nkoulou, R.; Marzel, A.; Weber, R.; Kaufmann, P.A.; Buechel, R.R.; Ledergerber, B.; Tarr, P.E. Antiretroviral Drugs Associated with Subclinical Coronary Artery Disease in the Swiss HIV Cohort Study. *Clin. Infect. Dis.* **2019**, *30*, 9.

133. Duprez, D.A.; Neuhaus, J.; Kuller, L.H.; Tracy, R.; Belloso, W.; De Wit, S.; Drummond, F.; Lane, H.C.; Ledergerber, B.; Lundgren, J.; et al. Inflammation, coagulation and cardiovascular disease in HIV-infected individuals. *PLoS ONE* **2012**, *7*, e44454. [CrossRef]

134. Calmy, A.; Gayet-Ageron, A.; Montecucco, F.; Nguyen, A.; Mach, F.; Burger, F.; Ubolyam, S.; Carr, A.; Ruxungtham, K.; Hirschel, B.; et al. HIV increases markers of cardiovascular risk: Results from a randomized, treatment interruption trial. *AIDS* **2009**, *23*, 929–939. [CrossRef]

135. Polak, J.F.; Leary, D.H.O. Carotid Intima-Media Thickness as Surrogate for and Predictor of CVD. *Glob. Heart* **2016**, *11*, 295–312. [CrossRef]

136. Du, J.; Wasserman, A.; Tong, W. Cholesterol Is Associated with the Presence of a Lipid Core in Carotid Plaque of Asymptomatic, Young-to-Middle-Aged African Americans with and without HIV Infection and Cocaine Use Residing in Inner-City Baltimore, Md., USA. *Cerebrovasc. Dis.* **2012**, *21287*, 295–301. [CrossRef]

137. Labounty, T.M.; Hardy, W.D.; Fan, Z.; Yumul, R.; Li, D.; Dharmakumar, R.; Conte, A.H. Carotid artery thickness is associated with chronic use of highly active antiretroviral therapy in patients infected with human immunode ficiency virus: A 3.0 Tesla magnetic resonance imaging study. *Br. HIV Assoc.* **2016**, *17*, 516–523.

138. Mee, T.C.; Aepfelbacher, J.; Krakora, R.; Chairez, C.; Kvaratskhelia, N.; Smith, B.; Sandfort, V.; Hadigan, C.; Morse, C.; Hammoud, D.A. Carotid magnetic resonance imaging in persons living with HIV and 10-year atherosclerotic cardiovascular disease risk score Short communication Carotid magnetic resonance imaging in persons living with HIV and 10-year atherosclerotic cardiovascular diseas. *Antivir. Ther.* **2018**, *23*, 695–698. [CrossRef]

139. Rose, K.A.M.; Vera, J.H.; Drivas, P.; Banya, W.; Pennell, D.J.; Winston, A. Europe PMC Funders Group Atherosclerosis is evident in treated HIV-infected subjects with low cardiovascular risk by carotid cardiovascular magnetic resonance. *J. Acquir. Immune Defic. Syndr.* **2016**, *71*, 514–521. [CrossRef]

140. Wasserman, B.A. Advanced Contrast-Enhanced MRI for Looking Beyond the Lumen to Predict Stroke Building a Risk Profile for Carotid Plaque. *Stroke* **2010**, *41*, 12–16. [CrossRef]

141. Wasserman, B.A.; Wityk, R.J.; Iii, H.H.T.; Virmani, R. Low-Grade Carotid Stenosis Looking Beyond the Lumen With MRI. *Stroke* **2005**, *36*, 2504–2513. [CrossRef]

142. Fayad, Z.A.; Fuster, V.; Fallon, J.T.; Jayasundera, T.; Worthley, S.G.; Helft, G.; Aguinaldo, J.G.; Badimon, J.J.; Sharma, S.K. Noninvasive In Vivo Human Coronary Artery Lumen and Wall Imaging Using Black-Blood Magnetic Resonance Imaging. *Circulation* **2000**, *102*, 506–510. [CrossRef]

143. U-king-im, J.M.; Trivedi, R.A.; Sala, E.; Graves, M.J.; Higgins, N.J.; Cross, J.C.; Hollingworth, W.; Coulden, R.A.; Kirkpatrick, P.J.; Antoun, N.M.; et al. Evaluation of carotid stenosis with axial high-resolution black-blood MR imaging. *Eur. Radiol.* **2004**, *14*, 1154–1161. [CrossRef]

144. Krishnamurthy, R.; Cheong, B.; Muthupillai, R. Tools for cardiovascular magnetic resonance imaging. *Cardiovasc. Dis. Ther.* **2014**, *4*, 104–125.

145. Saam, T.; Habs, M.; Buchholz, M.; Schindler, A.; Bayer-karpinska, A.; Cyran, C.C.; Yuan, C.; Reiser, M.; Helck, A. Expansive arterial remodeling of the carotid arteries and its effect on atherosclerotic plaque composition and vulnerability: An in-vivo black-blood 3T CMR study in symptomatic stroke patients. *J. Cardiovasc. Magn. Reson.* **2016**, *18*, 11. [CrossRef]

146. Al-Smadi, A.S.; Abdalla, R.N.; Elmokadem, A.H.; Shaibani, A.; Hurley, M.C.; Potts, M.B.; Jahromi, B.S.; Carroll, T.J.; Ansari, S.A. Diagnostic Accuracy of High-Resolution Black-Blood MRI in the Evaluation of Intracranial Large-Vessel Arterial Occlusions. *Am. J. Neuroradiol.* **2019**, *40*, 1–6. [CrossRef]

147. Ripa, R.S.; Knudsen, A.; Hag, A.M.F.; Lebech, A.; Loft, A.; Sune, H. Feasibility of simultaneous PET/MR of the carotid artery: first clinical experience and comparison to PET/CT. *Am. J. Nucl. Med. Mol. Imaging* **2013**, *3*, 361–371.

148. Floris-moore, M.A.; Fayad, Z.A.; Berman, J.W.; Schoenbaum, E.E.; Klein, R.S.; Weinshelbaum, K.B.; Fuster, V.; Howard, A.A.; Lo, Y.; Schecter, D. Association of HIV Viral Load with Monocyte Chemoattractant Protein-1 and Atherosclerosis Burden Measured by Magnetic Resonance Imaging. *AIDS* **2010**, *23*, 941–949. [CrossRef]

149. Bai, X.; Lv, P.; Liu, K.; Li, Q.; Ding, J.; Qu, J.; Lin, J. 3D Black-Blood Luminal Angiography Derived from High-Resolution MR Vessel Wall Imaging in Detecting MCA Stenosis: A Preliminary Study. *Am. J. Neuroradiol.* **2018**, *39*, 1827–1832. [CrossRef]

150. Eiden, S.; Beck, C.; Venhoff, N.; Elsheikh, S.; Id, G.I.; Urbach, H.; Id, S.M. High-resolution contrast-enhanced vessel wall imaging in patients with suspected cerebral vasculitis: Prospective comparison of whole-brain 3D T1 SPACE versus 2D T1 black blood MRI at 3 Tesla. *PLoS Med.* **2019**, *14*, 1–14. [CrossRef]

151. Takano, K.; Hida, K.; Iwaasa, M. Three-Dimensional Spin-Echo-Based Black-Blood MRA in the Detection of Vasospasm Following Subarachnoid Hemorrhage. *J. Magn. Reson. Imaging* **2018**, *49*, 800–887. [CrossRef]

152. Suri, M.; Qiao, Y.; Ma, X.; Guallar, E.; Zhou, J.; Zhang, Y.; Liu, L.; Chu, H.; Qureshi, A.I.; Alonso, A.; et al. Prevalence of Intracranial Atherosclerotic Stenosis Using High-Resolution Magnetic Resonance Angiography in the General Population The Atherosclerosis Risk in Communities Study. *Stroke* **2016**, *47*, 1187–1193. [CrossRef]

153. Dearborn, J.L.; Zhang, Y.; Qiao, Y.; Suri, M.F.; Liu, L.; Gottesman, R.F.; Rawlings, A.M.; Mosley, T.H.; Alonso, A.; Knopman, D.S.; et al. Intracranial atherosclerosis and dementia The Atherosclerosis Risk in Communities (ARIC) Study. *Neurology* **2017**, *88*, 1556–1563. [CrossRef]

154. Jiemy, F.W.; Heeringa, P.; Kamps, J.A.A.M.; van der Laken, C.J.; Slart, R.H.J.A.; Brouwer, E. Positron emission tomography (PET) and single photon emission computed tomography (SPECT) imaging of macrophages in large vessel vasculitis: Current status and future prospects. *Autoimmun. Rev.* **2018**, *17*, 715–726. [CrossRef]

155. Longenecker, C.T.; Sullivan, C.E.; Morrison, J.; Hileman, C.O.; Zidar, D.A.; Gilkeson, R.; O'Donnell, J.; Mc Comsey, G.A. The effects of HIV and smoking on aortic and splenic inflammation. *AIDS* **2019**, *32*, 89–94. [CrossRef]

156. Lawal, I.O.; Ankrah, A.O.; Popoola, G.O. Arterial inflammation in young patients with human immunodeficiency virus infection: A cross-sectional study using F-18 FDG PET/CT. *J. Nucl. Cardiol.* **2018**. [CrossRef]

157. Zanni, M.V.; Toribio, M.; Robbins, G.K.; Burdo, T.H.; Lu, M.T.; Ishai, A.E.; Feldpausch, M.N.; Martin, A.; Melbourne, K.; Triant, V.A.; et al. Effects of Antiretroviral Therapy on Immune Function and Arterial Inflammation in Treatment-Naive Patients With Human Immunodeficiency Virus Infection. *JAMA Cardiol.* **2016**, *1*, 474–480. [CrossRef]

158. Lo, J.; Lu, M.T.; Ihenachor, E.J.; Wei, J.; Looby, S.E.; Fitch, K.V.; Oh, J.; Zimmerman, C.O.; Hwang, J.; Abbara, S.; et al. Effects of Statin Therapy on Coronary Artery Plaque Volume and High Risk Plaque Morphology in HIV-Infected Patients with Subclinical Atherosclerosis: a Randomized Double-Blind Placebo-Controlled Trial. *Lancet HIV* **2016**, *2*, e52–e63. [CrossRef]

159. Knudsen, A.; Fisker, M.; Loft, A.; Lebech, A.; Ripa, S. HIV infection and arterial inflammation assessed by 18 F-fluorodeoxyglucose (FDG) positron emission tomography (PET): A prospective cross-sectional study. *J. Nucl. Cardiol.* **2015**, *22*, 372–380. [CrossRef]

160. Tawakol, A.; Lo, J.; Zanni, M.; Marmarelis, E.; Ihenachor, E.; MacNabb, M.; Wai, B.; Hoffmann, U.; Abbara, S.; Grinspoon, S. Increased Arterial Inflammation Relates to High-risk Coronary Plaque Morphology in HIV-Infected Patients. *J. Acquir. Immune Defic. Syndr.* **2015**, *66*, 164–171. [CrossRef]

161. Yarasheski, K.E.; Laciny, E.; Overton, E.T.; Reeds, D.N.; Harrod, M.; Baldwin, S.; Dávila-román, V.G. 18FDG PET-CT PET-CT imaging detects arterial inflammation and early atherosclerosis in HIV-infected adults with cardiovascular disease risk factors. *J. Inflamm.* **2012**, *9*, 1–9. [CrossRef]

162. Subramanian, S.; Tawakol, A.; Burdo, T.H.; Wei, J.; Corsini, E.; Hoffmann, U.; Williams, K.C.; Lo, J.; Grinspoon, S.K. Arterial Inflammation in Patients With HIV. *JAMA* **2012**, *308*, 379–386. [CrossRef]

163. Mhlanga, J.C.; Durand, D.; Tsai, H.-L.; Durand, C.M.; Leal, J.P.; Wang, H.; Moore, R.; Wahl, R.L. Differentiation of HIV-associated lymphoma from HIV-associated reactive adenopathy using quantitative FDG PET and symmetry. *Eur. J. Nucl. Med. Mol. Imaging* **2014**, *41*, 596–604. [CrossRef]

164. Esmail, H.; Lai, R.P.; Lesosky, M.; Wilkinson, K.A.; Graham, C.M.; Coussens, A.K.; Oni, T. Europe PMC Funders Group Characterization of progressive HIV-associated tuberculosis using 2-deoxy-2-[^{18}F] fluoro-D-glucose positron emission and computed tomography. *Nat. Med.* **2017**, *22*, 1090–1093. [CrossRef]

165. Hammoud, D.A.; Boulougoura, A.; Papadakis, G.Z.; Wang, J.; Dodd, L.E.; Rupert, A.; Higgins, J.; Roby, G.; Metzger, D.; Laidlaw, E.; et al. Increased Metabolic Activity on 18 F-Fluorodeoxyglucose Positron Emission Tomography-Computed Tomography in Human Immunodeficiency Virus-Associated Immune Reconstitution Inflammatory Syndrome. *Clin. Infect. Dis.* **2019**, *68*, 229–238. [CrossRef]

166. Hammoud, D.A.; Sinharay, S.; Steinbach, S.; Wakim, P.G. Global and regional brain hypometabolism on FDG-PET in treated HIV-infected individuals. *Neurology* **2018**, *91*, 1–12. [CrossRef]
167. Schreiber-stainthorp, W.; Sinharay, S.; Srinivasula, S.; Shah, S.; Wang, J.; Dodd, L.; Lane, H.C.; Di Mascio, M.; Hammoud, D.A. Brain ^{18}F-FDG PET of SIV-infected macaques after treatment interruption or initiation. *J. Neuroinflammation* **2018**, *15*, 1–9. [CrossRef]
168. Obel, N.; Omland, L.H.; Kronborg, G.; Larsen, C.S.; Pedersen, C.; Pedersen, G.; Sørensen, H.T.; Gerstoft, J. Impact of Non-HIV and HIV risk factors on survival in HIV-Infected patients on HAART: A Population-Based nationwide cohort study. *PLoS ONE* **2011**, *6*, 5–10. [CrossRef]
169. Gueler, A.; Moser, A.; Calmy, A.; Günthard, H.F.; Bernasconi, E.; Furrer, H.; Fux, C.A.; Battegay, M.; Cavassini, M.; Vernazza, P.; et al. Life expectancy in HIV-positive persons in Switzerland: Matched comparison with general population. *AIDS* **2017**, *31*, 427–436. [CrossRef]
170. Mangili, A.; Gerrior, J.; Tang, A.M.; Leary, D.H.O.; Polak, J.K.; Schaefer, E.J.; Gorbach, S.L.; Wanke, C.A. Risk of Cardiovascular Disease in a Cohort of HIV-Infected Adults: A Study Using Carotid Intima-Media Thickness and Coronary Artery Calcium Score. *Clin. Infect. Dis.* **2006**, *43*, 1482–1489. [CrossRef]
171. Hsue, P.Y.; Ordovas, K.; Lee, T.; Reddy, G.; Gotway, M.; Schnell, A.; Ho, J.E.; Selby, V.; Madden, E.; Martin, J.N.; et al. Carotid Intima-Media Thickness Among Human Immunodeficiency Virus-Infected Patients Without Coronary Calcium. *Am. J. Cardiol.* **2012**, *109*, 742–747. [CrossRef]
172. Andreini, D. Screening CT Angiography in Asymptomatic Diabetes Mellitus? *JACC Cardiovasc. Imaging* **2016**, *9*, 1301–1303. [CrossRef]
173. Roffi, M.; Patrono, C.; Collet, J.P.; Mueller, C.; Valgimigli, M.; Andreotti, F.; Bax, J.J.; Borger, M.A.; Brotons, C.; Chew, D.P.; et al. [2015 ESC Guidelines for the management of acute coronary syndromes in patients presenting without persistent ST-segment elevation. Task Force for the Management of Acute Coronary Syndromes in Patients Presenting without Persistent ST-Segment Elevation of the European Society of Cardiology (ESC)]. *Eur. Heart J.* **2016**, *37*, 267–315.
174. The SCOT Heart Investigators Coronary CT Angiography and 5-Year Risk of Myocardial Infarction. *N. Engl. J. Med.* **2018**, *379*, 924–933. [CrossRef]
175. Hoffmann, U.; Udelson, J.E. Imaging Coronary Anatomy and Reducing Myocardial Infarction. *N. Engl. J. Med.* **2018**, *379*, 977–978. [CrossRef]
176. Ryan, T.; Affandi, J.S.; Gahungu, N.; Dwivedi, G. Noninvasive Cardiovascular Imaging: Emergence of a Powerful Tool for Early Identification of Cardiovascular Risk in People Living With HIV. *Can. J. Cardiol.* **2019**, *35*, 260–269. [CrossRef]

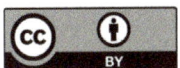

© 2019 by the authors. Licensee MDPI, Basel, Switzerland. This article is an open access article distributed under the terms and conditions of the Creative Commons Attribution (CC BY) license (http://creativecommons.org/licenses/by/4.0/).

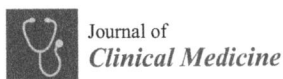

Review

Effect of Statin Therapy on Arterial Wall Inflammation Based on 18F-FDG PET/CT: A Systematic Review and Meta-Analysis of Interventional Studies

Matteo Pirro [1], Luis E. Simental-Mendía [2], Vanessa Bianconi [1], Gerald F. Watts [3,4], Maciej Banach [5,6] and Amirhossein Sahebkar [7,8,9,*]

1. Unit of Internal Medicine, Angiology and Arteriosclerosis Diseases, Department of Medicine, University of Perugia, 06129 Perugia, Italy; matteo.pirro@unipg.it (M.P.); v.bianconi.vb@gmail.com (V.B.)
2. Biomedical Research Unit, Mexican Social Security Institute, Durango 34067, Mexico; luis_simental81@hotmail.com
3. School of Medicine, Faculty of Health and Medical Sciences, University of Western Australia, Perth X2213, Australia; gerald.watts@uwa.edu.au
4. Lipid Disorders Clinic, Cardiometabolic Services, Department of Cardiology, Royal Perth Hospital, Perth X2213, Australia
5. Department of Hypertension, WAM University Hospital in Lodz, Medical University of Lodz, Zeromskiego 113, 93-338 Lodz, Poland; maciej.banach@umed.lodz.pl
6. Polish Mother's Memorial Hospital Research Institute (PMMHRI), 93-338 Lodz, Poland
7. Biotechnology Research Center, Pharmaceutical Technology Institute, Mashhad University of Medical Sciences, Mashhad 9177948564, Iran
8. Neurogenic Inflammation Research Center, Mashhad University of Medical Sciences, Mashhad 9177948564, Iran
9. School of Pharmacy, Mashhad University of Medical Sciences, Mashhad 9177948564, Iran
* Correspondence: sahebkara@mums.ac.ir; Tel.: +98-51-3800-2276

Received: 3 November 2018; Accepted: 14 January 2019; Published: 18 January 2019

Abstract: Aim. To evaluate by meta-analysis of interventional studies the effect of statin therapy on arterial wall inflammation. **Background.** Arterial exposure to low-density lipoprotein (LDL) cholesterol levels is responsible for initiation and progression of atherosclerosis and arterial wall inflammation. 18F-fluorodeoxyglucose Positron Emission Tomography-Computed Tomography (18F-FDG PET/CT) has been used to detect arterial wall inflammation and monitor the vascular anti-inflammatory effects of lipid-lowering therapy. Despite a number of statin-based interventional studies exploring 18F-FDG uptake, these trials have produced inconsistent results. **Methods.** Trials with at least one statin treatment arm were searched in PubMed-Medline, SCOPUS, ISI Web of Knowledge, and Google Scholar databases. Target-to-background ratio (TBR), an indicator of blood-corrected 18F-FDG uptake, was used as the target variable of the statin anti-inflammatory activity. Evaluation of studies biases, a random-effects model with generic inverse variance weighting, and sensitivity analysis were performed for qualitative and quantitative data assessment and synthesis. Subgroup and meta-regression analyses were also performed. **Results.** Meta-analysis of seven eligible studies, comprising 10 treatment arms with 287 subjects showed a significant reduction of TBR following statin treatment (Weighted Mean Difference (WMD): -0.104, $p = 0.002$), which was consistent both in high-intensity (WMD: -0.132, $p = 0.019$) and low-to-moderate intensity statin trials (WMD: -0.069, $p = 0.037$). Statin dose/duration, plasma cholesterol and C-reactive protein level changes, and baseline TBR did not affect the TBR treatment response to statins. **Conclusions.** Statins were effective in reducing arterial wall inflammation, as assessed by 18F-FDG PET/CT imaging. Larger clinical trials should clarify whether either cholesterol-lowering or other pleiotropic mechanisms were responsible for this effect.

Keywords: atherosclerosis; cholesterol; FDG; inflammation; PET; statins

1. Introduction

Atherosclerosis, the leading cause of cardiovascular (CV)-related deaths worldwide [1], is a disease process that is initiated, maintained and destabilized by an abnormal engagement of several cellular and molecular pathways of the inflammation cascade [2]. Exposure to elevated plasma low-density lipoprotein (LDL) cholesterol levels, either in the presence of or in the absence of additional CV risk factors, initiates and drives progressive lipid and inflammatory cell infiltration in the arterial wall [1,2], which may result in atherosclerotic plaque complications (e.g., erosion, rupture, etc.), ischemic-related organ injury and death [3,4].

Due to the recognized role of LDL cholesterol (LDL-C) in initiating and promoting atherosclerosis, followed by arterial wall inflammation [1,2], the anti-inflammatory effect of statins, as the most widely prescribed class of cholesterol-lowering drugs, has been largely explored [5–8]. Among a plethora of documented pleiotropic actions [9–14], there is accumulating evidence showing that statin therapy reduces inflammation in vitro, in experimental and clinical studies, though it is still debated whether it may depend on either cholesterol-lowering or pleiotropism [15]. Regardless of the mechanisms underlying the anti-inflammatory effects of statins, several circulating biomarkers of inflammation and acute phase reactants are down-regulated by statin treatment [7,15]. Despite low-grade systemic inflammation being frequently associated with atherosclerosis [16,17], the relationship with serum is sometimes contradictory [18–20], possibly suggesting that plasma biomarkers might not accurately reflect the degree of arterial wall inflammation. Hence, diagnostic tools that are more directly reflective of arterial inflammation have been sought.

One such method is 18F-fluorodeoxyglucose Positron Emission Tomography (18F-FDG PET) combined with computed tomography (CT), which has been used in both preclinical and clinical studies for the evaluation of inflammation in the arterial wall [18–22]. Over the last few years, significant technical progresses have been achieved in order to extend the CV applications of 18F-FDG PET/CT, which include improved image acquisition, measurements, and reconstruction protocols [23]. This has allowed a number of clinical trials to provide promising results of 18F-FDG PET/CT in detecting atherosclerotic plaque inflammation [18–20], discriminating stable from unstable plaques [24,25], predicting CV prognosis [26–29], and monitoring response to CV-related therapies [21,30,31].

In addition, 18F-FDG PET has been used to assess the impact of statin treatment on arterial wall inflammation in a few interventional studies [32–38]. In these studies [32–38], arterial 18F-FDG uptake was expressed as the Target-to-Background Ratio (TBR), that is a measure of the blood-normalized standardized uptake value (SUV). Since the reliability of TBR may be hampered by the low spatial resolution of PET, CT has been combined to improve 18F-FDG detection [21]. In these studies [32–38], the impact of different statins, at different doses, on inflammation of different arterial segments and in different clinical settings has been investigated. However, most of the studies have involved small numbers of patients, different clinical settings, varying statins with varying doses and treatment duration, different arterial segments, image acquisition/analysis, etc. Not surprisingly, the results of statin therapy on arterial wall inflammation using 18F-FDG PET/CT have been varied and inconclusive [32–38].

In order to overcome some of the inconsistencies, we carried out a systematic review and meta-analysis of previously reported trials with statins and 18F-FDG uptake, expressed as TBR.

2. Methods

2.1. Search Strategy

This study was designed according to the guidelines of the preferred reporting items for systematic reviews and meta-analysis (PRISMA) statement. PubMed-Medline, Scopus, ISI Web of Knowledge and Google Scholar databases were searched using the following search terms in titles and abstracts: (18F-fluorodeoxyglucose OR "18 F-fluorodeoxyglucose" OR FDG OR "18 F-FDG" OR "FDG-18 F" OR "18F-FDG" OR "FDG-18F" OR fluorodeoxyglucose OR "18 F FDG" OR "18F FDG" OR 18FDG OR "18 FDG") AND (atorvastatin OR simvastatin OR rosuvastatin OR lovastatin OR fluvastatin OR pravastatin OR pitavastatin). The wild-card term "*" was used to increase the sensitivity of the search strategy. The search was limited to articles published in English language. The literature was searched from inception to 19 January 2018.

2.2. Study Selection

Original studies were included if they met the following inclusion criteria: (i) being an interventional study with a statin treatment arm, (ii) investigating the impact of statin treatment on arterial wall inflammation based on the 18F-FDG PET/CT method, and (iii) presentation of arterial wall FDG uptake as TBR values (as a vein-normalized index) at baseline and after statin therapy or presenting the net change values. Exclusion criteria were: (i) non-clinical studies, (ii) non-interventional studies, e.g., observational studies with case-control, cross-sectional, or cohort designs, and (iii) lack of sufficient information on baseline or follow-up TBR values or presenting arterial wall FDG uptake as non-normalized indices.

2.3. Data Extraction

Eligible studies were reviewed and the following data were abstracted: (1) first author's name, (2) year of publication, (3) country where the study was performed, (4) study design, (5) number of treated subjects, (6) type of statin used, (7) statin dose, (8) duration of treatment, (9) age, gender and body mass index (BMI) of study participants, (10) baseline and follow-up TBR values, and (11) concentrations of plasma lipids, lipoproteins, and C-reactive protein (CRP).

2.4. Quality Assessment

The quality of involved studies in this meta-analysis was evaluated using the Cochrane criteria as previously described [39].

2.5. Quantitative Data Synthesis

Meta-analysis was conducted using Comprehensive Meta-Analysis (CMA) V2 software (Biostat, NJ, USA). A random-effects model (using DerSimonian-Laird method) and the generic inverse variance weighting method were used to compensate for the heterogeneity of studies in terms of study design, treatment protocol and the populations being studied [40]. Standard deviations (SDs) of the mean difference were calculated as follows: SD = square root $(SD_{post\text{-}treatment})^2 - (2R \times SD_{pre\text{-}treatment} \times SD_{post\text{-}treatment})$, assuming a correlation coefficient $(R) = 0.5$. Where standard error of the mean (SEM) was only reported, SD was estimated using the following formula: SD = SEM × sqrt (n), where n is the number of subjects. Heterogeneity was assessed quantitatively using Cochrane Q and I^2 statistic. Effect sizes were expressed as weighted mean difference (WMD) and 95% confidence interval (CI). If the outcome measures were reported in median and range (or 95% confidence interval [25]), mean and SD values were estimated using the method described by Wan et al. [41]. In order to evaluate the influence of each study on the overall effect size, a sensitivity analysis was conducted using the leave-one-out method (i.e., removing one study each time and repeating the analysis) [42,43]. Subgroup analyses were performed to evaluate the impact of treatment intensity on the estimated effect size and also to assess the effect size based on the TBR of most-diseased segment (MDS) of the index vessel.

2.6. Meta-Regression

As potential confounders of treatment response, duration of treatment, statin dose, mean changes in plasma levels of LDL-C and CRP, and baseline TBR were entered into a random-effects meta-regression model to explore their association with the estimated effect size on arterial wall inflammation.

2.7. Publication Bias

Evaluation of the funnel plot, Begg's rank correlation, and Egger's weighted regression tests were employed to assess the presence of publication bias in the meta-analysis. When there was an evidence of funnel plot asymmetry, potentially missing studies were imputed using the "trim and fill" method [44]. The number of potentially missing studies required to make the *p*-value non-significant was estimated using the "fail-safe N" method as another index of publication bias.

3. Results

Overall, 77 articles were found following the multi-database search. After screening of titles and abstracts, 16 articles were assessed in full text. Of these, nine were excluded because of a duplicate report ($n = 3$), not reporting TBR values ($n = 5$), and non-interventional study ($n = 1$). This left seven eligible articles for meta-analysis (Figure 1).

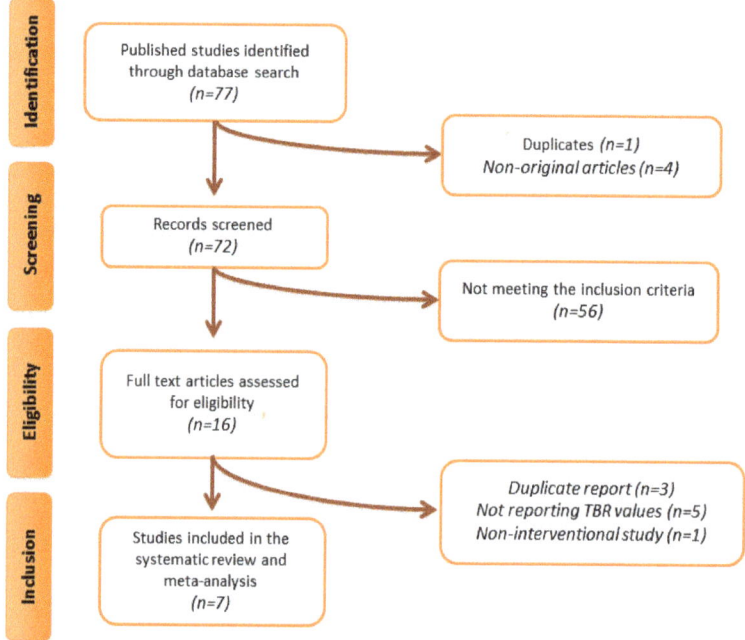

Figure 1. Flow chart of studies. Procedure of studies identification and inclusion into the meta-analysis.

3.1. Study Characteristics

Data were pooled from seven clinical trials comprising 10 treatment arms with 287 individuals. Of the selected studies, all reported whole vessel TBR of the index vessel. Aside from whole vessel TBR, three trials also reported TBR of the MDS of the index vessel. The included studies [32–38] used different types and doses of statins, and they were published between 2010 [33] and 2016 [36]. The range of treatment duration was from three months [32,35,36,38] to one year [34]. Study designs of included trials were open-label [32,33,36–38] and parallel group [34,35]. Selected studies enrolled subjects with atherosclerosis [32,38], hyperlipidemia [37], stable angina pectoris [33], HIV-infection [34], arterial inflammation [35], and ankylosing spondylitis [36]. The clinical and biochemical characteristics of the included clinical trials are presented in Table 1.

Table 1. Characteristics of studies included in the meta-analysis.

Author	Study Design	Target Population	Treatment Duration	n	Study Groups	Age (years)	Female (n, %)	BMI (kg/m²)	Total Cholesterol (mg/dL)	LDL Cholesterol (mg/dL) *	HDL Cholesterol (mg/dL)	Triglycerides (mg/dL)	C-reactive Protein (mg/L)	TBR in Index Vessel
Emami et al. (2015) [32]	Open-label trial	History of atherosclerosis	3 months	24 24	Atorvastatin 80 mg/day Placebo	62.1 ± 5.9 62.8 ± 7.1	8 (33.3) 6 (25)	ND ND	ND ND	92 ± 19 91 ± 24	53 ± 14 49 ± 11	ND ND	1.0 (2.4) * 1.6 (3.4) *	2.41 ± 0.33 2.50 ± 0.59
Ishii et al. (2010) [33]	Randomized, open-label trial	Japanese adults with stable angina pectoris	6 months	15 15	Atorvastatin 5 mg/day Atorvastatin 20 mg/day	55 ± 10 53 ± 11	7 (46.7) 5 (33.3)	ND ND	234 ± 36 244 ± 25	150 ± 28 162 ± 20	48 ± 14 47 ± 13	170 ± 121 189 ± 81	1.0 ± 0.6 1.4 ± 0.9	Ascending aorta 1.11 ± 0.10 1.15 ± 0.14 Femoral artery 1.10 ± 0.16 1.12 ± 0.11
Lo et al. (2015) [34]	Randomized, double-blind, placebo-controlled	HIV-infected patients	1 year	19 21	Atorvastatin 40 mg/day Placebo	52.2 ± 3.8 50.0 ± 5.6	4 (21) 4 (19)	25.6 ± 2.9 25.8 ± 4.8	198.8 ± 37.9 192.2 ± 27.1	123.7 ± 36.7 124.9 ± 32.1	51.8 ± 19.3 50.7 ± 15.1	120.5 (97.4–204.6) * 113.4 (92.1–135.5) *	0.8 (0.3–1.9) * 1.1 (0.4–2.4) *	Aorta 2.08 ± 0.32 2.20 ± 0.37 Segment of aorta 2.18 ± 0.33 2.26 ± 0.37
Tawakol et al. (2013) [35]	Randomized, double-blind trial	Individuals with arterial inflammation	3 months	34 34	Atorvastatin 10 mg/day Atorvastatin 80 mg/day	61 (53–68) * 58.5 (53–68) *	8 (23.5) 8 (23.5)	31.1 (26.9–32.5) * 32 (26.7–35.5) *	176.5 (161–192) * 178 (154–203) *	104 (86–118) * 107.5 (85–129) *	49 (43–60) * 44 (39–48) *	114.5 (78–182) * 129 (87–179) *	ND ND	MDS 2.34 (2.01–2.93) * 2.48 (2.23–2.81) * WV 2.21 (2.02–2.49) * 2.28 (2.06–2.52) *
van der Valk et al. (2016) [36]	Open-label trial	Patients with ankylosing spondylitis	3 months	18 20	Atorvastatin 40 mg/day Control	46 ± 9 48 ± 7	6 (33.3) 8 (40.0)	26 ± 4 26 ± 3	212.7 ± 48.7 207.3 ± 38.7	137.3 ± 44.5 124.1 ± 39.4	50.7 ± 15.5 65.7 ± 13.5	95.7 (70.9–167.4) * 78.8 (41.6–128.4) *	5.0 (1.5–9.3) * 1.1 (0.7–1.5) *	1.50 ± 0.14 1.37 ± 0.15
Watanabe et al. (2015) [37]	Randomized, open-label trial	Patients with hyperlipidemia	6 months	10 10	Pitavastatin 2 mg/day Pravastatin 10 mg/day	68 ± 5 64 ± 11	2 (20) 3 (30)	ND ND	202 ± 67 225 ± 21	150 ± 21 142 ± 24	52 ± 12 54 ± 15	134 ± 35 167 ± 63	2.8 ± 4.1 1.7 ± 2.2	1.29 ± 0.22 1.19 ± 0.16
Wu et al. (2012) [38]	Open-label trial	Subjects with atherosclerosis	3 months	43	Atorvastatin 40 mg/day	54 ± 10	19 (44.1)	24.5 ± 3.2	199 ± 42	108 ± 36	45 ± 12	154 ± 70	1.2 ± 1.4	1.31 ± 0.21

Values are expressed as mean ± SD. * Mean (interquartile range). Abbreviations: ND, no data; BMI, body mass index; MDS, most-diseased segment; WV, whole vessel.

3.2. F18-FDG PET/CT Procedure

FDG-PET and contrast-enhanced CT imaging of the arteries was performed in different vessels. In this regard, Emami et al. [32] assessed the arterial FDG in the right carotid, left carotid, and aorta. Ishii et al. [33] evaluated the ascending aorta and the right and left femoral arteries. Lo et al. [34] measured FDG-PET of the aorta. Two studies [35,37] performed FDG-PET/CT imaging of the thoracic aorta and carotid arteries. Van der Valk et al. [36] assessed arterial wall inflammation in carotid arteries. Finally, Wu et al. [38] determined FDG uptake in several arterial segments, including the ascending aorta, arch, thoracic descending aorta, abdominal aorta, and bilaterial iliofemoral arteries.

3.3. Risk of Bias Assessment

With respect to the random sequence generation and allocation concealment, two trials exhibited high risk of bias [36,38]. Additionally, several studies had risk of bias for blinding of participants, personnel, and outcome assessors [32,33,36–38]. Nonetheless, all selected studies showed low risk of bias for incomplete outcome data and selective outcome reporting. Details of the risk of bias assessment are shown in Table 2.

Table 2. Quality of bias assessment of the included studies, according to the Cochrane guidelines.

Study	Sequence Generation	Allocation Concealment	Blinding of Participants, Personnel and Outcome Assessors	Incomplete Outcome Data	Selective Outcome Reporting	Other Sources of Bias
Emami et al. (2015) [32]	U	U	H	L	L	U
Ishii et al. (2010) [33]	U	L	H	L	L	U
Lo et al. (2015) [34]	L	L	L	L	L	L
Tawakol et al. (2013) [35]	U	U	U	L	L	U
van der Valk et al. (2016) [36]	H	H	H	L	L	U
Watanabe et al. (2015) [37]	U	U	H	L	L	U
Wu et al. (2012) [38]	H	H	H	L	L	U

L, low risk of bias; H, high risk of bias; U, unclear risk of bias.

3.4. Quantitative Data Synthesis

Meta-analysis of data from seven studies comprising 10 treatment arms suggested a significant reduction of arterial wall FDG uptake based on TBR index following treatment with statins (WMD: −0.104, 95% CI: −0.171, −0.038, $p = 0.002$; I^2: 89.32%) (Figure 2A). The effect size was robust in the leave-one-out sensitivity analysis (Figure 2B) and not mainly driven by any single study. Four studies comprising five treatment arms reported arterial MDS TBR, which showed a significant reduction by statin therapy (WMD: −0.186, 95% CI: −0.272, −0.100, $p < 0.001$; I^2: 61.71%) (Figure 3A). Subgroup analysis showed a significant reduction of arterial wall TBR with both high-intensity (WMD: −0.132, 95% CI: −0.242, −0.021, $p = 0.019$; I^2: 93.44%) and low-to-moderate-intensity (WMD: −0.069, 95% CI: −0.134, −0.004, $p = 0.037$; I^2: 64.93%) statin therapy (Figure 3B); however, there was no significant difference between the two subgroups ($p = 0.340$).

3.5. Meta-Regression

Random-effects meta-regression was performed to assess the impact of potential confounders on the effects of statin therapy on arterial wall inflammation. The results did not suggest a significant association between the impact of statins on TBR and treatment duration (slope: 0.005; 95% CI: −0.002, 0.01; $p = 0.138$), atorvastatin dose (slope: −0.001; 95% CI: −0.004, 0.002; $p = 0.512$), LDL-C change (slope: 0.004; 95% CI: −0.0002, 0.01; $p = 0.062$), CRP change (slope: 0.05; 95% CI: −0.01, 0.11; $p = 0.087$), and baseline TBR (slope: 0.023; 95% CI: −0.136, 0.181; $p = 0.779$) (Figure 4).

A

Study name	Difference in means	Standard error	Variance	Lower limit	Upper limit	Z-Value	p-Value
			Statistics for each study				
Wu et al., 2012	-0.330	0.029	0.001	-0.387	-0.273	-11.342	0.000
van der Valk et al., 2016	-0.100	0.029	0.001	-0.156	-0.044	-3.499	0.000
Watanabe et al., 2015a	-0.250	0.071	0.005	-0.390	-0.110	-3.511	0.000
Watanabe et al., 2015b	0.000	0.054	0.003	-0.106	0.106	0.000	1.000
Tawakol et al., 2013a	0.000	0.062	0.004	-0.121	0.121	0.000	1.000
Tawakol et al., 2013b	-0.150	0.062	0.004	-0.271	-0.029	-2.430	0.015
Emami et al., 2015	-0.090	0.016	0.000	-0.122	-0.058	-5.511	0.000
Ishii et al., 2010a	-0.040	0.024	0.001	-0.086	0.006	-1.690	0.091
Ishii et al., 2010b	-0.100	0.034	0.001	-0.166	-0.034	-2.953	0.003
Lo et al., 2015	0.040	0.066	0.004	-0.090	0.170	0.602	0.547
	-0.104	0.034	0.001	-0.171	-0.038	-3.071	0.002

B

Study name	Point	Standard error	Variance	Lower limit	Upper limit	Z-Value	p-Value
			Statistics with study removed				
Wu et al., 2012	-0.076	0.019	0.000	-0.113	-0.038	-3.981	0.000
van der Valk et al., 2016	-0.104	0.039	0.002	-0.181	-0.028	-2.669	0.008
Watanabe et al., 2015a	-0.092	0.035	0.001	-0.161	-0.023	-2.605	0.009
Watanabe et al., 2015b	-0.115	0.036	0.001	-0.185	-0.045	-3.212	0.001
Tawakol et al., 2013a	-0.114	0.036	0.001	-0.184	-0.044	-3.199	0.001
Tawakol et al., 2013b	-0.100	0.036	0.001	-0.171	-0.029	-2.753	0.006
Emami et al., 2015	-0.105	0.043	0.002	-0.190	-0.021	-2.445	0.014
Ishii et al., 2010a	-0.112	0.038	0.001	-0.187	-0.037	-2.938	0.003
Ishii et al., 2010b	-0.104	0.038	0.001	-0.179	-0.030	-2.735	0.006
Lo et al., 2015	-0.117	0.035	0.001	-0.186	-0.049	-3.340	0.001
	-0.104	0.034	0.001	-0.171	-0.038	-3.071	0.002

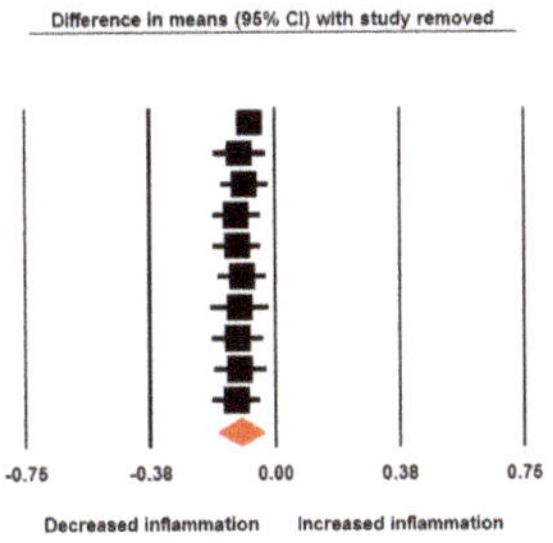

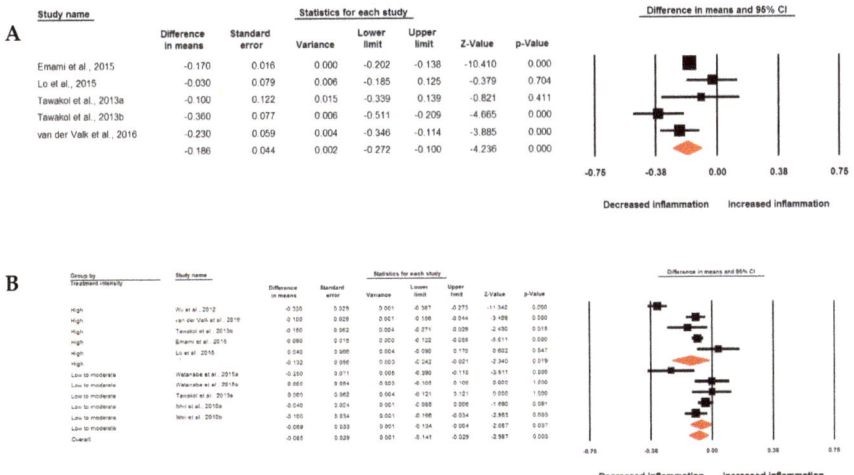

Figure 2. Impact of statin treatment on arterial wall fluorodeoxyglucose (FDG) uptake. Forest plot displaying weighted mean difference and 95% confidence intervals for the impact of statin therapy on arterial wall FDG uptake based on whole vessel target-to-background ratio (TBR) index (**A**). (**B**) shows the results of leave-one-out sensitivity analysis.

A

Study name	Difference in means	Standard error	Variance	Lower limit	Upper limit	Z-Value	p-Value
			Statistics for each study				
Emami et al., 2015	-0.170	0.016	0.000	-0.202	-0.138	-10.410	0.000
Lo et al., 2015	-0.030	0.079	0.006	-0.185	0.125	-0.379	0.704
Tawakol et al., 2013a	-0.100	0.122	0.015	-0.339	0.139	-0.821	0.411
Tawakol et al., 2013b	-0.360	0.077	0.006	-0.511	-0.209	-4.665	0.000
van der Valk et al., 2016	-0.230	0.059	0.004	-0.346	-0.114	-3.885	0.000
	-0.186	0.044	0.002	-0.272	-0.100	-4.236	0.000

B

Group by Treatment intensity	Study name	Difference in means	Standard error	Variance	Lower limit	Upper limit	Z-Value	p-Value
				Statistics for each study				
High	Wu et al., 2012	-0.330	0.029	0.001	-0.387	-0.273	-11.342	0.000
High	van der Valk et al., 2016	-0.100	0.029	0.001	-0.156	-0.044	-3.499	0.000
High	Tawakol et al., 2013b	-0.150	0.062	0.004	-0.271	-0.029	-2.430	0.015
High	Emami et al., 2015	-0.090	0.016	0.000	-0.122	-0.058	-5.511	0.000
High	Lo et al., 2015	0.040	0.066	0.004	-0.090	0.170	0.602	0.547
High		-0.132	0.056	0.003	-0.242	-0.021	-2.340	0.019
Low to moderate	Watanabe et al., 2015a	-0.250	0.071	0.005	-0.390	-0.110	-3.511	0.000
Low to moderate	Watanabe et al., 2015b	0.000	0.054	0.003	-0.106	0.106	0.000	1.000
Low to moderate	Tawakol et al., 2013a	0.000	0.062	0.004	-0.121	0.121	0.000	1.000
Low to moderate	Ishii et al., 2010a	-0.040	0.024	0.001	-0.086	0.006	-1.690	0.091
Low to moderate	Ishii et al., 2010b	-0.100	0.034	0.001	-0.166	-0.034	-2.953	0.003
Low to moderate		-0.069	0.033	0.001	-0.134	-0.004	-2.087	0.037
Overall		-0.085	0.029	0.001	-0.141	-0.029	-2.987	0.003

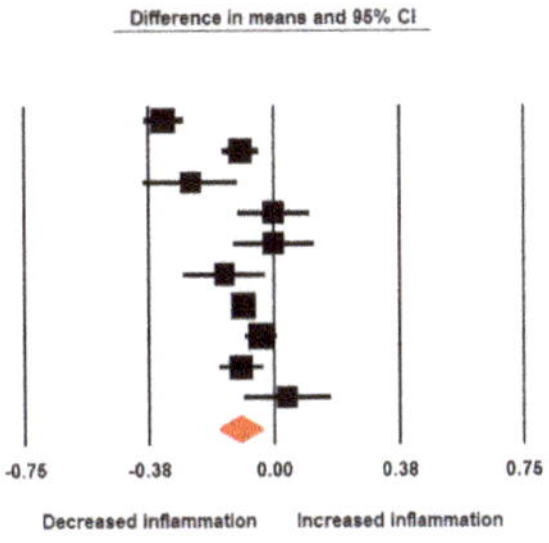

Figure 3. Impact of statin treatment on FDG uptake of the most diseased arterial segment. Forest plot displaying weighted mean difference and 95% confidence intervals for the impact of statin therapy on arterial wall FDG uptake based on the most diseased segment of vessel TBR (**A**). (**B**) shows the results of meta-analysis stratified according to the intensity (high versus low-to-moderate) of statin therapy.

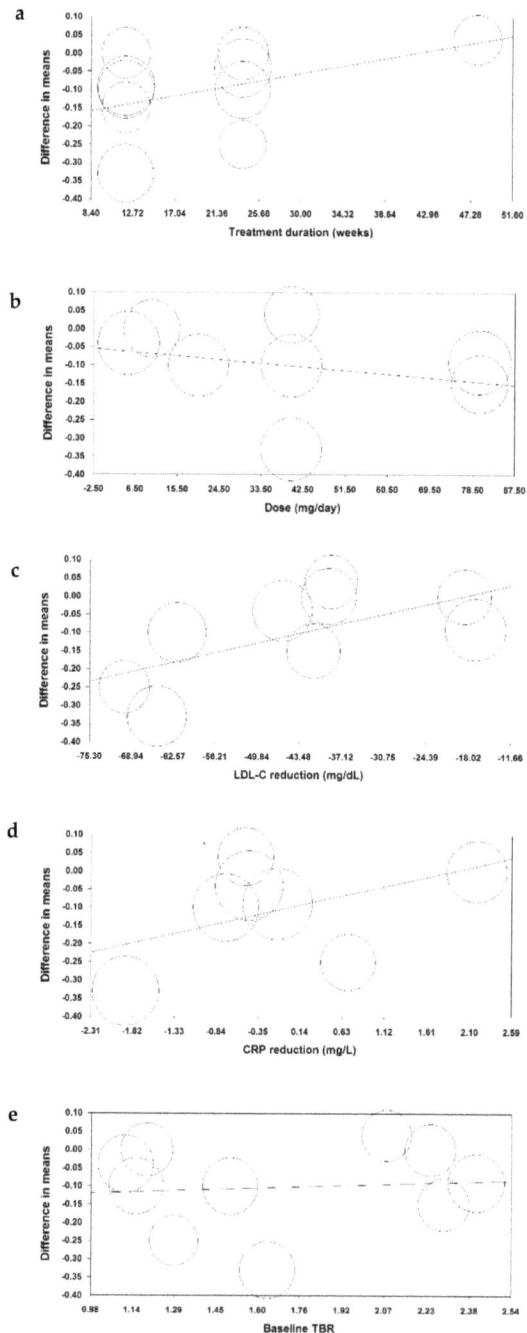

Figure 4. Associations of potential confounders with changes in arterial wall TBR. Meta-regression bubble plots of the association between mean changes in arterial wall TBR index with treatment duration (**a**), atorvastatin dose (**b**) and mean changes in plasma LDL-cholesterol (**c**), C-reactive protein (**d**), and baseline TBR (**e**). The size of each circle is inversely proportional to the variance of change.

3.6. Publication Bias

Visual inspection of Begg's funnel plots showed a slight asymmetry in the meta-analyses of statins' effects on arterial wall inflammation. This asymmetry was corrected by imputing one potentially missing study using "trim and fill" method, yielding a corrected effect size of −0.12 (95% CI: −0.18, −0.05) (Figure 5). Begg's rank correlation (tau = −0.11, z = 0.45, p = 0.655) and Egger's regression test (t = 0.02, df = 8, p = 0.988) did not suggest the presence of publication bias. The results of "fail-safe N" test suggested that 230 missing studies would be required to make the observed significant result non-significant. Given that for this meta-analysis we were able to identify seven eligible studies (with 10 treatment arms), it is far too unlikely that 230 studies were missed, thereby implying the lack of any significant publication bias.

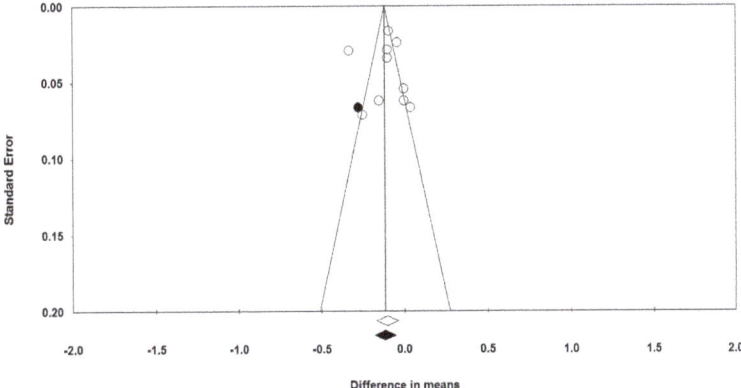

Figure 5. Publication biases. Funnel plot detailing publication bias in the studies reporting statin therapy on arterial wall FDG uptake based on whole vessel TBR index. Open and closed circles represent reported studies and potentially missing studies imputed using "trim and fill" method.

4. Discussion

In this meta-analysis, statin treatment resulted in a significant reduction of arterial wall inflammation, based on TBR measurement by 18F-FDG PET/CT imaging. Although the included clinical trials recruited only a limited number of patients for larger subgroup analyses and estimate of confounders, we did not find any significant influence of statin doses, duration of treatment, and cholesterol-lowering efficacy on TBR changes.

The pro-inflammatory role of increased LDL cholesterol levels has been documented by in vitro, experimental and clinical studies [1,2,45–47]. Additionally, statin-related cholesterol-lowering has been accompanied by the down-regulation of multiple pro-inflammatory pathways in atherogenesis [48]. Intriguingly, early anti-inflammatory effects of statins have often been described even before the reduction of plasma cholesterol levels occurs, thus suggesting that the anti-inflammatory effects of statins might be, at least in part, independent of their cholesterol-lowering action [15]. Irrespective of the mechanisms explaining the recognized ability of statin therapy to suppress inflammation, statin-related reduction of plasma CRP levels has been prospectively associated with atherosclerotic plaque regression [49] and reduction of several clinical meaningful CV end-points [50], though this has not been always confirmed [51].

Measurement of some plasma biomarkers may be useful to detect atherosclerosis-related systemic inflammation [52–55]; however, the same biomarkers may not accurately reflect the degree of the inflammatory burden within the arterial wall and, more specifically, in the atherosclerotic plaques. In this regard, the association between inflammation at the plasma and arterial wall levels was not always confirmed across the different studies [18–20]. Based on this background, several techniques have been proposed with the aim of detecting inflammation within the arterial wall and atherosclerotic plaques [23]. 18F-FDG PET/CT has been used for this purpose both in preclinical and clinical studies, with the progressive attempt to improve and standardize image acquisition and reconstruction protocols, as well as measurement of 18F-FDG uptake [18–31]. Overall, these studies have consistently demonstrated that 18F-FDG is taken up mostly by macrophages within the atherosclerotic plaques, albeit other cells (i.e., endothelial cells, vascular smooth muscle cells, neutrophils, lymphocytes) may participate in tracer uptake [21,22]. TBR, as a measure of SUV, demonstrated to be a reproducible index for quantification of 18F-FDG uptake in the inflamed arterial wall [21]. However, although TBR represents a useful tool for detecting arterial inflammation, it must be underlined that arterial 18F-FDG uptake is not necessarily atherosclerosis-related, but may be associated with other less frequent disease processes (e.g., giant cell arteritis, Takayasu arteritis, arterial grafts and aortic aneurysm infections, periaortitis, chemotherapy- or radiation-induced arterial inflammation, etc.) in the absence of atherosclerosis [56]. Regardless of this limitation, TBR was able to discriminate stable from unstable plaques (i.e., culprit lesions), as well as patients with stable angina from those with unstable angina [24,25]. In a retrospective study of 309 older subjects without history of cancer and coronary heart disease at baseline, ascending aorta TBR has been associated with coronary heart disease events [27]. Also, a few studies have revealed that arterial 18F-FDG uptake was prospectively associated with an unfavorable CV prognosis [26,28,29]. Hence, 18F-FDG PET/CT has been increasingly considered as a promising diagnostic and prognostic tool in the atherosclerosis-mediated CV disease field.

An additional use of 18F-FDG PET/CT is the monitoring of vascular wall inflammation during treatment of CV risk factors [21,30–38]. Few interventional studies in humans have reported the impact of statin treatment on arterial TBR values extracted from 18F-FDG PET/CT analysis [32–38]. In particular, seven studies (including 10 treatment arms) fulfilled the inclusion/exclusion criteria of this meta-analysis. Arterial TBR improved in 6 out of 10 arms [32,33,35–38], with the remaining four [33–35,37] showing unaltered TBR after statin treatment. Specifically, TBR of the thoracic aorta and carotid atherosclerotic plaques did not improve in one arm, including hyperlipidemic patients taking low-dose (10 mg/daily) pravastatin therapy [37]; in this study, not including a placebo-controlled arm, a modest 27% reduction of plasma LDL cholesterol level was observed along with a 2.29-fold increase in plasma CRP level. Two additional studies not including a placebo-controlled arm did not observe a significant arterial TBR change after low-dose atorvastatin treatment [33,35]. Specifically, only 5 mg/daily of atorvastatin has been used by Ishii et al [33]. Also, in the 10 mg/daily atorvastatin arm of the study by Tawakol et al. [35], 65% of patients received a statin before randomization to atorvastatin, thus limiting the ability of the low-dose atorvastatin 10 mg/daily to improve a baseline statin-influenced TBR value. This limitation was overcome, however, by atorvastatin 80 mg/daily in the second arm of the study by Tawakol et al. [35]. Finally, 40 mg/daily of atorvastatin was administered for one year in the study by Lo et al [34], but this was not sufficient to improve aortic TBR in HIV-infected patients receiving antiretroviral therapy, despite a significant 31% LDL cholesterol reduction and a three-fold decrease of plasma CRP level. However, as stated in Reference [34], technical issues compromised the possibility of reaching adequate statistical power to detect changes in the arterial wall inflammation. Regardless of the possible reasons explaining the failure of statin therapy in 4 out of 10 arms, it must be pointed out that: (1) overall, statin therapy significantly reduced arterial wall TBR, (2) neither duration/dose of statin treatment nor statin-related changes in plasma LDL cholesterol and CRP levels had a significant influence on the association between statin treatment and TBR improvement, and (3) unmeasured confounding variables or combinations of confounders might have interfered with the latter association, which was not tested in this meta-analysis.

There were some limitations for this meta-analysis. The overall sample size was relatively small, and populations differed in health status at baseline, statin preparations, doses, and duration of therapy, which limited the ability to draw direct conclusions, as well as the statistical power for additional subgroup and meta-regression analyses. However, it is worth noting that the present meta-analysis could provide a total population size that is considerably higher than the numbers recruited in each individual study, thus providing a more reliable conclusion. We also reported the presence of biases with respect to random sequence generation, allocation concealment, and blinding procedures in some studies, which may have reduced the quality of the results. Finally, heterogeneity of clinical settings and arterial segments examined by 18F-FDG PET/CT, in the absence of a larger sample size, have precluded the possibility to explore the impact of statin treatment in specific populations and arterial regions. Despite these potential limitations, statistical compensation for heterogeneity was performed, and the overall result of this meta-analysis was robust in sensitivity analysis.

In conclusion, our meta-analysis showed the significant anti-inflammatory effect of statin treatment at the arterial wall level; however, unresolved issues remain regarding the presumptive factors that either mediate or confound such an effect. Larger clinical trials are warranted to resolve this uncertainty and to verify whether the local anti-inflammatory effects of satins, as detected by arterial 18F-FDG PET/CT, might translate into favorable clinical outcomes. Moreover, given that most of the studies included in this analysis had a relatively short duration of follow-up, it remains to be established if the anti-inflammatory effects of statins, as assessed by 18F-FDG PET/CT, are enhanced over time and following prolonged exposure of arteries to low concentrations of LDL. It also remains to be investigated if the findings of 18F-FDG PET/CT are correlated with alterations of biomarkers of vascular inflammation, as well as circulating levels of pro-inflammatory cytokines in statin-treated subjects. Finally, biomimetic nanoparticles have recently emerged as potential tools for targeting and imaging of inflammation, e.g., through mimicking the interactions between cell adhesion molecules and selectins in the inflamed vascular site [57,58]. The use of these nanoparticles, with modalities like radioisotope imaging, magnetic resonance imaging, and ultrasound, could allow efficient monitoring of the anti-inflammatory action of statins and other lipid-lowering therapies on the arterial wall and could be confirmatory to 18F-FDG PET/CT findings as detailed in this study.

Funding: No funding was received for this study.

Acknowledgments: The authors thank Evan A. Stein for his valuable help in improving the manuscript.

Conflicts of Interest: This meta-analysis was written independently; no company or institution supported it financially. Gerald F. Watts has received honoraria for advisory boards and lectures from Amgen, Sanofi, Regeneron, Kowa and MSD. Maciej Banach: speakers bureau: Abbott/Mylan, Abbott Vascular, Actavis, Akcea, Amgen, Biofarm, KRKA, MSD, Sanofi-Aventis, Servier and Valeant; consultant to Abbott Vascular, Akcea, Amgen, Daichii Sankyo, Esperion, Lilly, MSD, Resverlogix, Sanofi-Aventis; Grants from Sanofi and Valeant.

References

1. Roth, G.A.; Johnson, C.; Abajobir, A.; Abd-Allah, F.; Abera, S.F.; Abyu, G.; Ahmed, M.; Aksut, B.; Alam, T.; Alam, K.; et al. Global, Regional, and National Burden of Cardiovascular Diseases for 10 Causes, 1990 to 2015. *J. Am. Coll. Cardiol.* **2017**, *70*, 1–25. [CrossRef]
2. Hansson, G.K. Inflammation and Atherosclerosis: The End of a Controversy. *Circulation* **2017**, *136*, 1875–1877. [CrossRef]
3. Catapano, A.L.; Graham, I.; De Backer, G.; Wiklund, O.; Chapman, M.J.; Drexel, H.; Hoes, A.W.; Jennings, C.S.; Landmesser, U.; Pedersen, T.R.; et al. ESC Scientific Document Group. 2016 ESC/EAS Guidelines for the Management of Dyslipidaemias. *Eur. Heart J.* **2016**, *37*, 2999–3058. [CrossRef] [PubMed]
4. Ference, B.A.; Ginsberg, H.N.; Graham, I.; Ray, K.K.; Packard, C.J.; Bruckert, E.; Hegele, R.A.; Krauss, R.M.; Raal, F.J.; Schunkert, H.; et al. Low-density lipoproteins cause atherosclerotic cardiovascular disease. 1. Evidence from genetic, epidemiologic, and clinical studies. A consensus statement from the European Atherosclerosis Society Consensus Panel. *Eur Heart J.* **2017**, *38*, 2459–2472. [CrossRef] [PubMed]
5. Deshmukh, H.; Chasman, D.; Trompet, S.; Li, X.; Sun, F.; Hitman, G.; Colhoun, H. Meta-analysis of genome-wide association studies to assess C-reactive protein response to statin therapy. *Lancet* **2016**, *387*, S37. [CrossRef]
6. Ridker, P.M.; Danielson, E.; Fonseca, F.A.; Genest, J.; Gotto, A.M., Jr.; Kastelein, J.J.; Koenig, W.; Libby, P.; Lorenzatti, A.J.; MacFadyen, J.G.; et al. Rosuvastatin to prevent vascular events in men and women with elevated C-reactive protein. *N. Engl. J. Med.* **2008**, *359*, 2195–2207. [CrossRef] [PubMed]

7. Zhang, L.; Zhang, S.; Jiang, H.; Sun, A.; Wang, Y.; Zou, Y.; Ge, J.; Chen, H. Effects of statin therapy on inflammatory markers in chronic heart failure: A meta-analysis of randomized controlled trials. *Arch. Med. Res.* **2010**, *41*, 464–471. [CrossRef]
8. Bielecka-Dabrowa, A.; Mikhailidis, D.P.; Rizzo, M.; von Haehling, S.; Rysz, J.; Banach, M. The influence of atorvastatin on parameters of inflammation left ventricular function, hospitalizations and mortality in patients with dilated cardiomyopathy—5-year follow-up. *Lipids Health Dis.* **2013**, *12*, 47. [CrossRef] [PubMed]
9. Mohajeri, M.; Banach, M.; Atkin, S.L.; Butler, A.E.; Ruscica, M.; Watts, G.F.; Sahebkar, A. MicroRNAs: Novel Molecular Targets and Response Modulators of Statin Therapy. *Trends Pharmacol. Sci.* **2018**, *39*, 967–981. [CrossRef]
10. Bahrami, A.; Parsamanesh, N.; Atkin, S.L.; Banach, M.; Sahebkar, A. Effect of statins on toll-like receptors: A new insight to pleiotropic effects. *Pharmacol. Res.* **2018**, *135*, 230–238. [CrossRef]
11. Sahebkar, A.; Kotani, K.; Serban, C.; Ursoniu, S.; Mikhailidis, D.P.; Jones, S.R.; Ray, K.K.; Blaha, M.J.; Rysz, J.; Toth, P.P.; et al. Statin therapy reduces plasma endothelin-1 concentrations: A meta-analysis of 15 randomized controlled trials. *Atherosclerosis* **2015**, *241*, 433–442. [CrossRef] [PubMed]
12. Parizadeh, S.M.R.; Azarpazhooh, M.R.; Moohebati, M.; Nematy, M.; Ghayour-Mobarhan, M.; Tavallaie, S.; Rahsepar, A.A.; Amini, M.; Sahebkar, A.; Mohammadi, M.; et al. Simvastatin therapy reduces prooxidant-antioxidant balance: Results of a placebo-controlled cross-over trial. *Lipids* **2011**, *46*, 333–340. [CrossRef] [PubMed]
13. Serban, C.; Sahebkar, A.; Ursoniu, S.; Mikhailidis, D.P.; Rizzo, M.; Lip, G.Y.H.; Kees Hovingh, G.; Kastelein, J.J.P.; Kalinowski, L.; Rysz, J.; et al. A systematic review and meta-analysis of the effect of statins on plasma asymmetric dimethylarginine concentrations. *Sci. Rep.* **2015**, *5*, 9902. [CrossRef]
14. Sahebkar, A.; Serban, C.; Mikhailidis, D.P.; Undas, A.; Lip, G.Y.H.; Muntner, P.; Bittner, V.; Ray, K.K.; Watts, G.F.; Hovingh, G.K.; et al. Association between statin use and plasma d-dimer levels: A systematic review and meta-analysis of randomised controlled trials. *Thromb. Haemost.* **2015**, *114*, 546–557. [CrossRef] [PubMed]
15. Diamantis, E.; Kyriakos, G.; Quiles-Sanchez, L.V.; Farmaki, P.; Troupis, T. The Anti-Inflammatory Effects of Statins on Coronary Artery Disease: An Updated Review of the Literature. *Curr. Cardiol. Rev.* **2017**, *13*, 209–216. [CrossRef] [PubMed]
16. Buffon, A.; Biasucci, L.M.; Liuzzo, G.; D'Onofrio, G.; Crea, F.; Maseri, A. Widespread coronary inflammation in unstable angina. *N. Engl. J. Med.* **2002**, *347*, 5–12. [CrossRef] [PubMed]
17. Libby, P.; Ridker, P.M.; Hansson, G.K. Progress and challenges in translating the biology of atherosclerosis. *Nature* **2011**, *473*, 317–325. [CrossRef] [PubMed]
18. Duivenvoorden, R.; Mani, V.; Woodward, M.; Kallend, D.; Suchankova, G.; Fuster, V.; Rudd, J.H.; Tawakol, A.; Farkouh, M.E.; Fayad, Z.A. Relationship of serum inflammatory biomarkers with plaque inflammation assessed by FDG PET/CT: The dal-PLAQUE study. *JACC Cardiovasc. Imaging* **2013**, *6*, 1087–1094. [CrossRef] [PubMed]
19. Rudd, J.H.; Bansilal, S.; Machac, J.; Woodward, M.; Fuster, V. Relationships among regional arterial inflammation, calcification, risk factors, and biomarkers: A prospective fluorodeoxyglucose positron-emission tomography/computed tomography imaging study. *Circ. Cardiovasc. Imaging* **2009**, *2*, 107–115. [CrossRef] [PubMed]
20. Yang, S.J.; Kim, S.; Choi, H.Y.; Kim, T.N.; Yoo, H.J.; Seo, J.A.; Kim, S.G.; Kim, N.H.; Baik, S.H.; Choi, D.S.; et al. High-sensitivity C-reactive protein in the low- and intermediate-Framingham risk score groups: Analysis with 18F-fluorodeoxyglucose positron emission tomography. *Int. J. Cardiol.* **2013**, *163*, 277–281. [CrossRef] [PubMed]
21. Rosenbaum, D.; Millon, A.; Fayad, Z.A. Molecular imaging in atherosclerosis: FDG PET. *Curr. Atheroscler. Rep.* **2012**, *14*, 429–437. [CrossRef] [PubMed]
22. Tarkin, J.M.; Joshi, F.R.; Rajani, N.K.; Rudd, J.H. PET imaging of atherosclerosis. *Future Cardiol.* **2015**, *11*, 115–131. [CrossRef] [PubMed]
23. Huet, P.; Burg, S.; Le Guludec, D.; Hyafil, F.; Buvat, I. Variability and uncertainty of 18F-FDG PET imaging protocols for assessing inflammation in atherosclerosis: Suggestions for improvement. *J. Nucl. Med.* **2015**, *56*, 552–559. [CrossRef]

24. Dilsizian, V.; Jadvar, H. Science to Practice: Does FDG Differentiate Morphologically Unstable from Stable Atherosclerotic Plaque? *Radiolog* **2017**, *283*, 1–3. [CrossRef]
25. Rogers, I.S.; Nasir, K.; Figueroa, A.L.; Cury, R.C.; Hoffmann, U.; Vermylen, D.A.; Brady, T.J.; Tawakol, A. Feasibility of FDG imaging of the coronary arteries: Comparison between acute coronary syndrome and stable angina. *JACC Cardiovasc. Imaging* **2010**, *3*, 388–397. [CrossRef] [PubMed]
26. Figueroa, A.L.; Abdelbaky, A.; Truong, Q.A.; Corsini, E.; MacNabb, M.H.; Lavender, Z.R.; Lawler, M.A.; Grinspoon, S.K.; Brady, T.J.; Nasir, K.; et al. Measurement of arterial activity on routine FDG PET/CT images improves prediction of risk of future CV events. *JACC Cardiovasc. Imaging* **2013**, *6*, 1250–1259. [CrossRef] [PubMed]
27. Iwatsuka, R.; Matsue, Y.; Yonetsu, T.; O'uchi, T.; Matsumura, A.; Hashimoto, Y.; Hirao, K. Arterial inflammation measured by 18F-FDG-PET-CT to predict coronary events in older subjects. *Atherosclerosis* **2018**, *268*, 49–54. [CrossRef]
28. Marnane, M.; Merwick, A.; Sheehan, O.C.; Hannon, N.; Foran, P.; Grant, T.; Dolan, E.; Moroney, J.; Murphy, S.; O'rourke, K.; et al. Carotid plaque inflammation on 18F-fluorodeoxyglucose positron emission tomography predicts early stroke recurrence. *Ann. Neurol.* **2012**, *71*, 709–718. [CrossRef]
29. Rominger, A.; Saam, T.; Wolpers, S.; Cyran, C.C.; Schmidt, M.; Foerster, S.; Nikolaou, K.; Reiser, M.F.; Bartenstein, P.; Hacker, M. 18F-FDG PET/CT identifies patients at risk for future vascular events in an otherwise asymptomatic cohort with neoplastic disease. *J. Nucl. Med.* **2009**, *50*, 1611–1620. [CrossRef] [PubMed]
30. Van Wijk, D.F.; Sjouke, B.; Figueroa, A.; Emami, H.; van der Valk, F.M.; MacNabb, M.H.; Hemphill, L.C.; Schulte, D.M.; Koopman, M.G.; Lobatto, M.E.; et al. Nonpharmacological lipoprotein apheresis reduces arterial inflammation in familial hypercholesterolemia. *J. Am. Coll. Cardiol.* **2014**, *64*, 1418–1426. [CrossRef]
31. Xu, J.; Nie, M.; Li, J.; Xu, Z.; Zhang, M.; Yan, Y.; Feng, T.; Zhao, X.; Zhao, Q. Effect of pioglitazone on inflammation and calcification in atherosclerotic rabbits: An 18F-FDG-PET/CT in vivo imaging study. *Herz* **2017**, *43*, 733–740. [CrossRef]
32. Emami, H.; Vucic, E.; Subramanian, S.; Abdelbaky, A.; Fayad, Z.A.; Du, S.; Roth, E.; Ballantyne, C.M.; Mohler, E.R.; Farkouh, M.E.; et al. The effect of BMS-582949, a P38 mitogen-activated protein kinase (P38 MAPK) inhibitor on arterial inflammation: A multicenter FDG-PET trial. *Atherosclerosis* **2015**, *240*, 490–496. [CrossRef] [PubMed]
33. Ishii, H.; Nishio, M.; Takahashi, H.; Aoyama, T.; Tanaka, M.; Toriyama, T.; Tamaki, T.; Yoshikawa, D.; Hayashi, M.; Amano, T.; et al. Comparison of atorvastatin 5 and 20 mg/d for reducing F-18 fluorodeoxyglucose uptake in atherosclerotic plaques on positron emission tomography/computed tomography: A randomized, investigator-blinded, open-label, 6-month study in Japanese adults scheduled for percutaneous coronary intervention. *Clin. Ther.* **2010**, *32*, 2337–2347. [CrossRef] [PubMed]
34. Lo, J.; Lu, M.T.; Ihenachor, E.J.; Wei, J.; Looby, S.E.; Fitch, K.V.; Oh, J.; Zimmerman, C.O.; Hwang, J.; Abbara, S.; et al. Effects of statin therapy on coronary artery plaque volume and high-risk plaque morphology in HIV-infected patients with subclinical atherosclerosis: A randomised, double-blind, placebo-controlled trial. *Lancet HIV* **2015**, *2*, e52–e63. [CrossRef]
35. Tawakol, A.; Fayad, Z.A.; Mogg, R.; Alon, A.; Klimas, M.T.; Dansky, H.; Subramanian, S.S.; Abdelbaky, A.; Rudd, J.H.; Farkouh, M.E.; et al. Intensification of statin therapy results in a rapid reduction in atherosclerotic inflammation: Results of a multicenter fluorodeoxyglucose-positron emission tomography/computed tomography feasibility study. *J. Am. Coll. Cardiol.* **2013**, *62*, 909–917. [CrossRef] [PubMed]
36. Van der Valk, F.M.; Moens, S.J.; Verweij, S.L.; Strang, A.C.; Nederveen, A.J.; Verberne, H.J.; Nurmohamed, M.T.; Baeten, D.L.; Stroes, E.S. Increased arterial wall inflammation in patients with ankylosing spondylitis is reduced by statin therapy. *Ann. Rheum. Dis.* **2016**, *75*, 1848–1851. [CrossRef]
37. Watanabe, T.; Kawasaki, M.; Tanaka, R.; Ono, K.; Kako, N.; Saeki, M.; Onishi, N.; Nagaya, M.; Sato, N.; Miwa, H.; et al. Anti-inflammatory and morphologic effects of pitavastatin on carotid arteries and thoracic aorta evaluated by integrated backscatter trans-esophageal ultrasound and PET/CT: A prospective randomized comparative study with pravastatin (EPICENTRE study). *Cardiovasc. Ultrasound* **2015**, *13*. [CrossRef]
38. Wu, Y.W.; Kao, H.L.; Huang, C.L.; Chen, M.F.; Lin, L.Y.; Wang, Y.C.; Lin, Y.H.; Lin, H.J.; Tzen, K.Y.; Yen, R.F.; et al. The effects of 3-month atorvastatin therapy on arterial inflammation, calcification, abdominal adipose tissue and circulating biomarkers. *Eur. J. Nucl. Med. Mol. Imaging* **2012**, *39*, 399–407. [CrossRef]

39. Green, S.; Higgins, J. (Eds.) *Cochrane Handbook for Systematic Reviews of Interventions*; Version 5.0.2; The Cochrane Collaboration: London, UK, 2009.
40. Sutton, A.J.; Abrams, K.R.; Jones, D.R.; Jones, D.R.; Sheldon, T.A.; Song, F. *Methods for Meta-Analysis in Medical Research*; J. Wiley: Hoboken, NJ, USA, 2000.
41. Wan, X.; Wang, W.; Liu, J.; Tong, T. Estimating the sample mean and standard deviation from the sample size, median, range and/or interquartile range. *BMC Med. Res. Methodol.* **2014**, *14*, 135. [CrossRef]
42. Sahebkar, A.; Simental-Mendía, L.E.; Watts, G.F.; Serban, M.C.; Banach, M. Comparison of the effects of fibrates versus statins on plasma lipoprotein(a) concentrations: A systematic review and meta-analysis of head-to-head randomized controlled trials. *BMC Med.* **2017**, *15*, 22. [CrossRef]
43. Sahebkar, A. Does PPARγ2 gene Pro12Ala polymorphism affect nonalcoholic fatty liver disease risk? Evidence from a meta-analysis. *DNA Cell Biol.* **2013**, *32*, 188–198. [CrossRef] [PubMed]
44. Duval, S.; Tweedie, R. Trim and fill: A simple funnel-plot-based method of testing and adjusting for publication bias in meta-analysis. *Biometrics* **2000**, *56*, 455–463. [CrossRef] [PubMed]
45. Paciullo, F.; Fallarino, F.; Bianconi, V.; Mannarino, M.R.; Sahebkar, A.; Pirro, M. PCSK9 at the crossroad of cholesterol metabolism and immune function during infections. *J. Cell. Physiol.* **2017**, *232*, 2330–2338. [CrossRef] [PubMed]
46. Pirro, M.; Bianconi, V.; Paciullo, F.; Mannarino, M.R.; Bagaglia, F.; Sahebkar, A. Lipoprotein(a) and inflammation: A dangerous duet leading to endothelial loss of integrity. *Pharm. Res.* **2017**, *119*, 178–187. [CrossRef] [PubMed]
47. Pirro, M.; Schillaci, G.; Savarese, G.; Gemelli, F.; Mannarino, M.R.; Siepi, D.; Bagaglia, F.; Mannarino, E. Attenuation of inflammation with short-term dietary intervention is associated with a reduction of arterial stiffness in subjects with hypercholesterolaemia. *Eur. J. Cardiovasc. Prev. Rehabil.* **2004**, *11*, 497–502. [CrossRef] [PubMed]
48. Montecucco, F.; Mach, F. Update on statin-mediated anti-inflammatory activities in atherosclerosis. *Semin. Immunopathol.* **2009**, *31*, 127–142. [CrossRef]
49. Nissen, S.E.; Tuzcu, E.M.; Schoenhagen, P.; Crowe, T.; Sasiela, W.J.; Tsai, J.; Orazem, J.; Magorien, R.D.; O'shaughnessy, C.; Ganz, P. Statin therapy, LDL cholesterol, C-reactive protein, and coronary artery disease. *N. Engl. J. Med.* **2005**, *352*, 29–38. [CrossRef] [PubMed]
50. Ridker, P.M.; Cannon, C.P.; Morrow, D.; Rifai, N.; Rose, L.M.; McCabe, C.H.; Pfeffer, M.A.; Braunwald, E. C-reactive protein levels and outcomes after statin therapy. *N. Engl. J. Med.* **2005**, *352*, 20–28. [CrossRef]
51. Yousuf, O.; Mohanty, B.D.; Martin, S.S.; Joshi, P.H.; Blaha, M.J.; Nasir, K.; Blumenthal, R.S.; Budoff, M.J. High-sensitivity C-reactive protein and cardiovascular disease: A resolute belief or an elusive link? *J. Am. Coll. Cardiol.* **2013**, *62*, 397–408. [CrossRef]
52. Krintus, M.; Kozinski, M.; Kubica, J.; Sypniewska, G. Critical appraisal of inflammatory markers in cardiovascular risk stratification. *Crit. Rev. Clin. Lab. Sci.* **2014**, *51*, 263–279. [CrossRef]
53. Mannarino, E.; Pirro, M. Endothelial injury and repair: A novel theory for atherosclerosis. *Angiology* **2008**, *59*, 69S–72S. [CrossRef] [PubMed]
54. St-Pierre, A.C.; Bergeron, J.; Pirro, M.; Cantin, B.; Dagenais, G.R.; Després, J.P.; Lamarche, B. Effect of plasma C-reactive protein levels in modulating the risk of coronary heart disease associated with small, dense, low-density lipoproteins in men (The Quebec Cardiovascular Study). *Am. J. Cardiol.* **2003**, *91*, 555–558. [CrossRef]
55. Wang, J.; Tan, G.J.; Han, L.N.; Bai, Y.Y.; He, M.; Liu, H.B. Novel biomarkers for cardiovascular risk prediction. *J. Geriatr. Cardiol.* **2017**, *14*, 135–150. [PubMed]
56. Chrapko, B.E.; Chrapko, M.; Nocuń, A.; Stefaniak, B.; Zubilewicz, T.; Drop, A. Role of 18F-FDG PET/CT in the diagnosis of inflammatory and infectious vascular disease. *Nucl. Med. Rev.* **2016**, *19*, 28–36. [CrossRef] [PubMed]
57. Chacko, A.M.; Hood, E.D.; Zern, B.J.; Muzykantov, V.R. Targeted Nanocarriers for Imaging and Therapy of Vascular Inflammation. *Curr. Opin. Colloid Interface Sci.* **2011**, *16*, 215–227. [CrossRef] [PubMed]
58. Jin, K.; Luo, Z.; Zhang, B.; Pang, Z. Biomimetic nanoparticles for inflammation targeting. *Acta Pharm. Sin. B* **2018**, *8*, 23–33. [CrossRef] [PubMed]

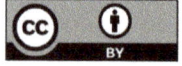

© 2019 by the authors. Licensee MDPI, Basel, Switzerland. This article is an open access article distributed under the terms and conditions of the Creative Commons Attribution (CC BY) license (http://creativecommons.org/licenses/by/4.0/).

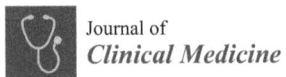

Review

Accuracy of Commonly-Used Imaging Modalities in Assessing Left Atrial Appendage for Interventional Closure: Review Article

Ramez Morcos [1], Haider Al Taii [2], Priya Bansal [2], Joel Casale [1], Rupesh Manam [1], Vikram Patel [1], Anthony Cioci [3], Michael Kucharik [3], Arjun Malhotra [4] and Brijeshwar Maini [5,*]

1. Department of Internal Medicine, Florida Atlantic University, Boca Raton, FL 33431, USA; morcos.ramez@gmail.com (R.M.); jcasale3@health.fau.edu (J.C.); rmanam@health.fau.edu (R.M.); patelv@health.fau.edu (V.P.)
2. Department of Cardiovascular Diseases, Florida Atlantic University, Boca Raton, FL 33431, USA; haltaii@health.fau.edu (H.A.T.); Pbansal@health.fau.edu (P.B.)
3. College of Medicine, Florida Atlantic University, Boca Raton, FL 33431, USA; acioci@health.fau.edu (A.C.); mkucharik2016@health.fau.edu (M.K.)
4. University of Miami, Coral Gables, FL 33124, USA; a.malhotra2@umiami.edu
5. Tenet Florida & Department of Cardiovascular Diseases, Florida Atlantic University, Boca Raton, FL 33431, USA
* Correspondence: brijmaini1@gmail.com; Tel.: +1-561-498-2249

Received: 16 October 2018; Accepted: 10 November 2018; Published: 14 November 2018

Abstract: Periprocedural imaging assessment for percutaneous Left Atrial Appendage (LAA) transcatheter occlusion can be obtained by utilizing different imaging modalities including fluoroscopy, magnetic resonance imaging (MRI), computed tomography (CT), and ultrasound imaging. Given the complex and variable morphology of the left atrial appendage, it is crucial to obtain the most accurate LAA dimensions to prevent intra-procedural device changes, recapture maneuvers, and prolonged procedure time. We therefore sought to examine the accuracy of the most commonly utilized imaging modalities in LAA occlusion. Institutional Review Board (IRB) approval was waived as we only reviewed published data. By utilizing PUBMED which is an integrated online website to list the published literature based on its relevance, we retrieved thirty-two articles on the accuracy of most commonly used imaging modalities for pre-procedural assessment of the left atrial appendage morphology, namely, two-dimensional transesophageal echocardiography, three-dimensional transesophageal echocardiography, computed tomography, and three-dimensional printing. There is strong evidence that real-time three-dimensional transesophageal echocardiography is more accurate than two-dimensional transesophageal echocardiography. Three-dimensional computed tomography has recently emerged as an imaging modality and it showed exceptional accuracy when merged with three-dimensional printing technology. However, real time three-dimensional transesophageal echocardiography may be considered the preferred imaging modality as it can provide accurate measurements without requiring radiation exposure or contrast administration. We will present the most common imaging modality used for LAA assessment and will provide an algorithmic approach including preprocedural, periprocedural, intraprocedural, and postprocedural.

Keywords: left atrial appendage; WATCHMAN occlusive device; 2D transesophageal echocardiography; 3D transesophageal echocardiography; computerized tomography

1. Introduction

Atrial Fibrillation (AF) is a major burden on public health, it is estimated to be the cause of ≥15% of all strokes in the United States, and >100,000–125,000 embolic strokes per year, of which >20% are fatal [1]. AF risk factors, pathogenesis, prevention, and treatment are beyond the scope of this review. We will focus on the classification when patients may or may not have valvular heart disease. The distinction still an area of debate. Valvular AF is the terminology used in those patients who have heart valve disorder or a prosthetic heart valve. Nonvalvular AF is generally referred in those patients who have other etiology causing the AF. The rapid and chaotic heartbeats restrict the left atrium from pumping the blood properly, which may cause it to pool and form a clot. More than 90% of thrombi in AF is formed in the left atrial appendage (LAA) [2]. The standard treatment for AF is heart rate or rhythm control and stroke prevention. Prophylactic anticoagulation is the gold standard to prevent embolic strokes in AF patients with CHADS-VASC score greater than or equal to two. For many years there has been no alternative treatment available to prevent strokes in AF patients who have high risk of bleeding and only 50–60% are therapeutically anticoagulated which make the effective long-term anticoagulation very challenging [3].

In 2001 a successful percutaneous implantation of a device to occlude the LAA cavity was done in a patient with non-valvular AF to prevent embolism [4]. Interventional closure of the LAA employing the Watchman device (Boston Scientific) was shown to be non-inferior to Oral anticoagulation (OAC) in randomized trials and has since been approved in the United States and Europe [5]. The LAA exhibits complex anatomy that commonly varies morphologically among different individuals. Post-mortem analysis of 100 left atrial appendages has demonstrated significant variability in appendage shape, dimensions, and the number of lobes presents [6]. Therefore, accurate visualization of the LAA and appreciation of its morphological considerations is an essential step in occlusion procedures. Specifically, accurately measuring the dimensions of the LAA ostium, landing zone, and maximum length of the main anchoring lobe is necessary for selecting an adequately sized occlusion device successful device placement [4]. Choosing a device that is too small increases the risk of device instability and peri-device leakage, whereas selecting a device that is too large increases the risk of LAA perforation and cardiac tamponade [7,8]. Additionally, improper device selection can result in intra-procedural device changes and recapture maneuvers and increasing length of the procedure [9].

We present a review on the most commonly used imaging modality for pre-procedural planning and assessment of the LAA morphology, which include 2D Transesophageal echocardiography (2D TEE), 3D Transesophageal echocardiography (3D TEE), Computed tomography (CT), and 3D Printing (3DP).

1.1. 3D TEE Modality Is Superior to 2D TEE

2D TEE has been the most commonly used imaging modality for pre-procedural planning. However, three-dimensional multiplanar transesophageal electrocardiography is a more accurate alternative to 2D TEE in the assessment of the LAA morphology. Advantages of 3D TEE vs. 2D TEE are illustrated in (Table 1), and comparative studies using 3D TEE are illustrated in (Table 2).

Zhou et al. found 3D TEE to be more accurate than 2D TEE for measuring the LAA Landing zone, LAA depth, and LAA ostial dimensions, LAA morphology after the occlusion device deployment, and visualizing any residual shunts around the entire device in one more view. In the Zhou et al. study, a residual shunt of less than 1mm was identified in three cases by 3D TEE and only once by 2D TEE [7]. Salzman et al. determined that area-derived diameter (ADD) and perimeter-derived diameter (PDD) measurements obtained via 3D TEE correlated well with the occlusion device size chosen in the procedure. Furthermore, the 3D landing zone measurements demonstrated a higher reproducibility relative to 2D TEE [8].

Yosefi et al. found that RT3DTEE provides more accurate measurements of the maximal LAA orifice than 2D TEE. 2D TEE significantly undersized the diameter of the LAA orifice relative to RT3DTEE, when compared to CT [10]. Nucifora et al. found that RT3DTEE is in more significant agreement with the dimensions obtained from CT as demonstrated by smaller bias and narrower limits of agreement with CT. Therefore, these authors believe that RT3DTEE may be the preferred imaging modality to assess LAA dimensions as it can provide accurate measurements of the LAA without requiring radiation exposure or contrast administration [11].

The real-time 3DTEE method is a feasible, fast way to assess the LAA number of lobes, the area of the orifice, maximal LAA diameter, minimum LAA diameter, and LAA depth with similar accuracy to RT3DTEE and CT according to a study published by Yosefy et al. Real-time 3DTEE consists of converting a 3DTEE image into three 2D planes (X,Y,Z), at which time a 360 degree rotational in the sagittal plane creates a single "stop shop" image that displays all aspects of the LAA morphology including number of lobes, orifice area, and maximal and minimal diameter [12]. Nakajima et al. determined that 3D TEE could accurately visualize LAA morphological variations. They studied 55 patients in normal sinus rhythm and 52 patients with atrial fibrillation. 3D TEE provides adequate 3D full volume images of all patients in NSR, whereas sufficient images were obtained in 94.6% of patients with AF using zoom mode. Excellent correlation was found between full volume mode and zoom mode [13].

Table 1. Advantages of 3D TEE vs. 2D TEE.

Author	Advantages of 3D TEE vs. 2D TEE	Study
Zhou et al.	-More accurate measuring of Landing zone and depth -More significant association between the closure device -Displaying cross-sectional images from any angle using Flexi Slice mode -Useful in displaying the LAA morphology after the occlusion device deployed -Visualizing any residual shunts around the entire device in one more view	[7]
Salzman et al.	-Producing (ADD) and (PDD) measurements of the LAA ostium -3D landing zone measurements demonstrated a higher reproducibility	[8]
Yosefi et al.	-3DTEE is a feasible, fast way to assess LAA morphology with similar accuracy to RT3DTEE and CT	[10]
Nucifora et al.	-RT3DTEE more significant agreement with the dimensions obtained from CT -RT3DTEE Provide accurate measurements without radiation exposure or contrast	[11]
Yosefi et al.	-RT3DTEE provides more accurate measurements of the maximal LAA orifice	[12]
Nakajima et al.	-Accurately visualize LAA morphological variations -Excellent correlation was found between full volume mode and zoom mode	[13]

Table 2. Literature review summary table for 3D TEE vs. 2D TEE in the preprocedural assessment of the left atrial appendage.

Ref	Author	Country	Date (mm/dd)	Objective	Study	Result/Outcome	Conclusion
[7]	Zhou et al.	China	01/17	To determine the clinical values of RT-3D TEE in the peri-procedure of LAA closure.	Observational study, of 38 patients conducted real-time 3D TEE (3D TEE) of the LAA for all subjects	-The landing zone dimension of LAA revealed by 2D TEE, showed statistical difference compared with the dimensions obtained from the 3D TEE -No statistical difference was noticed in the landing zone values of 3D TEE compared with that of X-ray -No statistical difference was noticed in the landing zone values of 3D TEE compared with that of X-ray	RT-3D TEE has better visualization of the LAA compared with 2D TEE.
[8]	Salzman et al.	Germany	07/17	To establish measurements based on 3D TEE imaging that would be most helpful in achieving successful cardiovascular intervention	Retrospective study analyzed 55 patient who underwent LAA occlusion using Watchman	ADD) and perimeter-derived diameter (PDD) from 3D TEE can reduce intra-procedural recapture maneuvers, peridevice leakage, and device size changes compared with two-dimensional (2D) measurements.	3D ADD and PDD may help with reducing intraprocedural recapture maneuvers, device size changes, and peridevice leakage.
[10]	Yosefi et al.	Israel	01/16	Compared RT3DTEE and 2DTEE versus CT when measuring LAA dimensions	Prospective study of 30 patients compared RT 3D TEE and 2D TEE versus 64 slice CT for measuring LAA dimensions	No difference was found between LAA depth using RT 3D TEE (19.5 ± 2.3 mm) vs. CT (19.6 ± 2.3, P = NS) and 2D TEE (19.4 ± 2.2 mm) vs. CT (P = NS). However, RT 3D TEE (24.5 ± 4.7 mm) vs. CT (24.6 ± 5, P = NS) was more accurate in measuring maximal LAA diameter compared to 2D TEE (23.5 ± 3.9 mm) vs. CT ($P < 0.01$).	RT3DTEE provides more accurate measurements of the maximal LAA orifice than 2D TEE.
[11]	Nucifora et al.	Switzerland	09/11	The accuracy of the measurements obtained via 2DTEE and RT3DTEE were subsequently compared against measurements obtained via CT.	Prospective study of 137 patients who underwent 2DTEE, RT3DTEE, and CT to measure the dimensions of the LAA orifice	-Compared to CT, both 2DTEE and RT3DTEE underestimated LAA dimensions. -RT3DTEE was found to be in greater agreement with the dimensions obtained from CT as demonstrated by smaller bias and narrower limits of agreement with CT	RT3DTEE may be the preferable imaging modality to assess LAA dimensions.

Table 2. *Cont.*

Ref	Author	Country	Date (mm/dd)	Objective	Study	Result/Outcome	Conclusion
[12]	Yosefi et al.	Israel	09/16	To validate the accuracy of Rotational 3DTEE versus RT3DTEE when assessing LAA	Prospective study of 41 patients who underwent a rotational 3D TEE	Rotational 3D TEE measurements of LAA were not statistically different from RT3DTEE and from 64-slice CT regarding Rotational 3D TEE is achieved by rotating the sagittal plane (in the green box, x-plane) 360° and allows for a faster method of achieving necessary LAA measurements.	Choosing the appropriate device size for LAA closure can be achieved by Rotational 3DTEE ("Yosefy rotation").
[13]	Nakajima et al.	Japan	09/10	To determined if 3D TEE could accurately visualize LAA morphological variations	Prospective od 107 patients, 55 were in SR in whom 3DTEE images were obtained from full-volume mode imaging, and 52 were in Afib, zoom-mode imaging was used.	3D TEE proviced adequate 3D full volume images of all patients in NSR, whereas adequate images were obtained in 94.6% of patients with AF using zoom mode. Excellent correlation was found between full volume mode and zoom mode.	3D TEE is a reliable modality when evaluating LAA geometry and LAA characteristics.

1.2. CT Is More Accurate Than TEE

CT has been considered the gold standard for visualizing the LAA for its ability to acquire 3D volumetric data of the LAA at various points in the cardiac cycle [4]. However, it has only recently emerged as an imaging modality for sizing the LAA before occlusion and for post-procedural evaluation of residual peri-device shunts. Although TEE remains the most commonly used imaging modality for sizing the LAA, CT may be the most accurate imaging modality. Yosefy et al. compared 2D TEE to CT and found 2D TEE to be non-inferior to CT for determining LAA area and volume. Additionally, Yosefy et al. found that of 30 patients who underwent routine TEE examination and CT in the workup of PE, RT3DTEE was found to yield measurements not significantly different than CT for the number of LAA lobes, LAA depth, LAA internal area, and LAA maximal and minimal diameter. They concluded that 3DTEE might be more practical for sizing the LAA due to its accuracy, lack of radiation, and bedside capabilities [10]. In contrast, other studies have demonstrated that measurements obtained via TEE and CT are not interchangeable and may result in clinically significant consequences. One such study by Sievert et al. showed that LAA sizing by 2D TEE alone might result in the selection of a closure device that is undersized by 20–40% [2]. Advantages of CT are illustrated in (Table 3), and comparative studies using CT are illustrated in (Table 4).

MSCT is a more accurate tool in selecting proper LAA closure device size than the conventionally used TEE according to the study by Chow et al. [14] 2D-TEE measurements of orifice size are not interchangeable with those obtained via CT according to a study by Rawjani et al. The researchers concluded that due to the irregular and eccentric nature of the LAA orifice, obtaining mean orifice diameter measurements may be more accurate than planar maximal diameters for sizing circular occluder devices [15].

In the study by Wang et al. patients who underwent advanced CT imaging at this site required 1.245 devices per implantation attempt with 100% success rate, compared to patients in the first half of the PROTECT AF study who averaged 1.8 devices used per implantation attempt with an 82% success rate. Accurate sizing of the LAA landing zone is critical in successful implantation of the WATCHMAN, and this study suggests high-resolution volumetric imaging with CT should be preferred over TEE [9].

Budge et al. determined that measurements obtained via CTsb, CTp, and TEE are not interchangeable. CTsb was found to yield larger mean orifice diameters than both TEE and CTp, which produced similar mean orifice diameters. It was speculated that this was due to foreshortening associated with 2D modalities. Furthermore, when compared to TEE, both CT modalities yielded larger ostial measurements for small LAA orifices and smaller ostial measurements for larger LAA orifices within this cohort [16].

Table 3. Advantages of CT when assessing the left atrial appendage.

Author	Advantages of CT	Study
Chow et al.	-Allows more accurate assessment of the LAA ostium and landing zone. -Allows higher appreciation for the morphology of the LAA and surrounding structures	[14]
Rawjani et al.	-device sizing by CT-derived mean diameter was in most agreement with the actual device implanted -Better in detection and avoidance of sizing error by 2D TOE	[15]
Wang et al.	-WATCHMAN device selection was 100% accurate when selected by CT imaging -Provides a comprehensive assessment for LAA which is accurate	[9]
Budge et al.	-Provides accurate sizing of LAA occlusion devices	[16]

Table 4. Literature review summary table of CT imaging in the preprocedural assessment of the left atrial appendage.

Ref	Author	Country	Date (mm/dd)	Objective	Study	Result/Outcome	Conclusion
[14]	Chow et al.	Denmark	06/17	To compare available LAA imaging and sizing modalities which lead to successful LAA closure	Retrospective, 67 patients who underwent preprocedural MSCT and 2D TEE for LAA closure device sizing from 2014 to 2016	MSCT resulted in correct LAA sizing in 83% of patients, whereas 2D TEE would have produced in only 57% proper sizing	CT derived PD mean diameter may be the optimal measurement for sizing 'closed-ended' devices (Amulet and WATCHMANFLX) whereas CT derived maximal diameter is more accurate for sizing 'open-ended' devices (WATCHMAN)
[15]	Rawjani et al.	Australia	12/17	To evaluate the use of CT, procedural safety, and outcomes for percutaneous LAA closure	A registry between July 2010 and December 2015 was prospectively established for individuals undergoing LAA closure	2D TEE sizing resulted in gross sizing errors in 3.4% of cases. 2D-TEE measurements resulted in device selection that was 3mm smaller than those from CT measurements	CT has excellent outcomes for procedural safety with absence of major residual leak
[9]	Wang et al.	USA	11/16	To determine the role of 3DCT guided planning for LAA occlusion on the early operator WATCHMAN learning curve	Prospective study studied 53 patients who underwent 2D TEE, 3D TEE, and 3D CT for Watchman device qualification and sizing	53 patients underwent successful device implantation. Compared with 2D and 3D TEE sizing, 3D CT maximal width of the LAA landing zone was larger ($p \leq 0.0001$). Pearson correlation coefficient showed a significant difference when sizing by CT against TEE ($r < 0.001$)	3D CT is an excellent tool in advanced case planning for precise WATCHMAN device size selection in LAA closure procedures compared to standard 2D TEE
[16]	Budge et al.	USA	11/08	To compare multiple different imaging modalities to assess the morphology of the LAA in AF patients	Prospective study of 66 patients where measurement relationships of TEE to planar CT (CTp), CTp to 3D cardiac segmented CT (CTsg), and CTsg to TEE were compared	Similar to CTp, CTsg orifice values were usually slightly smaller than TEE for large orifices, and larger than TEE for smaller orifices. LAA orifice measurements among CTsg, CTp, and TEE are not interchangeable which is clinically significant because of the need of accurate sizing of LAA occlusion devices	CTsg, either alone or in conjunction with TEE measurements, could allow for more accurate initial device sizing

1.3. The Use of 3D Printing Can Facilitate LAA Occlusion

As more LAA occlusion procedures have been conducted, physicians have recognized the unique and diverse morphology of the LAA [17]. This anatomical intricacy may be deceptively portrayed in standardized diagnostic modalities such as 2D and 3D transesophageal echocardiography (TEE), which are the conventional pre-procedural image technique. 3D CT characterization may provide exceptional accuracy when merged with 3D printing technology. By creating a model customized to each patient's anatomy, a physical Watchman device (Boston Scientific, Marlborough, MA, USA) can be implanted ex vivo so that spatial navigation and geographic accuracy of the left atrium may be established before the cardiac catheterization procedure commences. The following findings show this modality technology applied and successively replicated. They also suggest 3D CT as the best imaging technique when establishing device size. Hell et al. [18] and Li et al. [19] supported the use of 3D printing while, Goiten et al. did not support it [20] (Table 5).

Hell et al. and Li et al. in prospective studies both found that 3D printing of LAA was a feasible mechanism of predicting correct Watchman devices. In the study conducted by Hell et al. Mean LAA ostium diameter based on TEE was 22 ± 4 mm and based on CT 25 ± 3 mm (p = 0.014) [18]. Similarly, Li et al. performed successful Watchman implantation in 21 patients based on 3D model printing (3DP). In this study, although all patients in both groups underwent successful device implantation, significant differences did occur. After the occlusion, TOE showed that three patients in the control group had mild residual shunting (two patients with a 2 mm residual shunt, one patient with a 4 mm residual shunt). No residual shunt was observed in the 3DP group. The procedure times, contrast agent volumes, and costs were 96.4 ± 12.5 vs. 101.2 ± 13.6 min, 22.6 ± 3.0 vs. 26.9 ± 6.2 mL, and 12,676.1 vs. 12,088.6 USD for the 3DP and control groups, respectively. Compared with the control group, the radiographic exposure was significantly reduced in the 3DP group (561.4 ± 25.3 vs. 651.6 ± 32.1 mGy, p = 0.05) [19].

Goiten et al. found that LAA printed 3D models were accurate for prediction of LAA device size for the Amulet device but not for the Watchman device. Two procedures were aborted due to mismatch between LAA and any Watchman device dimensions in which all three interventional cardiology physicians that were involved in the study predicted the failures using the printed 3D model. Although 3D prints were found to be more accurate for Amulet compared to Watchman, strong agreement among physicians was demonstrated for both devices (average intra-class correlation of 0.915 for Amulet and 0.816 for Watchman) [20].

Table 5. Literature review summary table of CT 3D printing in the preprocedural assessment of the left atrial appendage.

Ref	Author	Country	Date (mm/dd)	Objective	Study	Result/Outcome	Conclusion
[17]	Hell et al.	Europe	11/17	To determine if using 3D-printed LAA models based on CT will permit accurate device sizing	Prospective study of 22 patients who underwent pre-procedure TEE and CT examinations in which a 3D printed model was created based on the CT images and CT measurements recorded.	-Implantation was successful in all patients -In 95% of the patients (21/22), predicted device size based on simulated implantation in the 3D model was equal to the device ultimately implanted. TEE would have undersized the device in 45% of the patients (10/22) and device compression determined in the 3D-CT model corresponded closely with compression upon implantation of Watchman device ($r = 0.622$, $p = 0.003$).	CT 3D-printing models may assist with device selection and the prediction of device compression.
[18]	Li et al.	China	03/17	To assess 3DP feasibility using CT for LAA closure	Prospective study for 42 patients were randomly split into 2 groups, one that had 3D LAA model printing and a control group. For the control group, device size was based on TEE, cardiac CT angiogram, and intraoperative LAA angiography only	The diameter of the occlusion devices used in the 3DP group and control group were 27.6 ± 2.4 mm (21–33 mm) and 26.3 ± 3.4 mm (21–33 mm), respectively. TOE showed that the compression ratios of the occlusion devices were $19.7\% \pm 0.8\%$ and $19.3 \pm 1.0\%$ ($p = 0.05$), respectively.	3DP enhance the work efficiency for LAA closure which is valuable for clinical application.
[19]	Goiten et al.	Israel	10/17	To determine the feasibility of MDCT when predicting the accurate size of device for LAA closure	Prospective study including 29 patients compared 3D LAA model printing for predicting occlusion device size based on pre-procedure CT scan Amplatzer Amulet (St. Jude Medical/Abbott) was deployed in 12 patients and the other 17 received the Watchman device	Two procedures were aborted due to mismatch between LAA and any Watchman device dimensions in which all three interventional cardiology physicians that were involved in the study predicted the failures using the printed 3D model According to Bland-Altman analysis, the average difference between the predicted Amulet size using the 3D LAA printed model and the inserted Amulet was 0.848 mm (95% limit of agreement (LOA): −4.215, 5.912). The average difference between the predicted Watchman size using the 3D print and the inserted Watchman was 0.956 mm (95% LOA: −6.534, 8.445)	LAA 3DP model is not accurate for prediction of LAA using WATCHMAN devi.

2. Algorithmic Approach for the WATCHMAN Procedural

Here, we will provide an algorithmic approach including preprocedural, periprocedural, intraprocedural, and postprocedural. (Figures 1 and 2) [21].

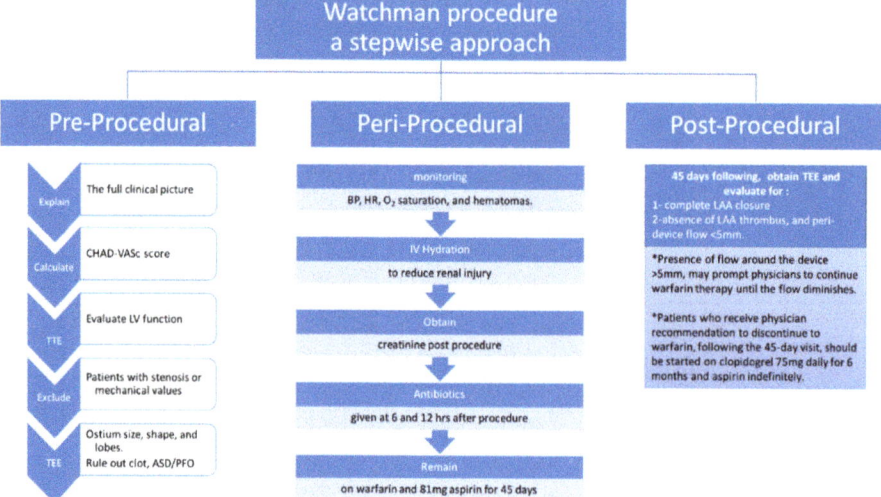

Figure 1. A stepwise approach for pre-, peri-, and post-procedure for the successful implantation of WATCHMAN device.

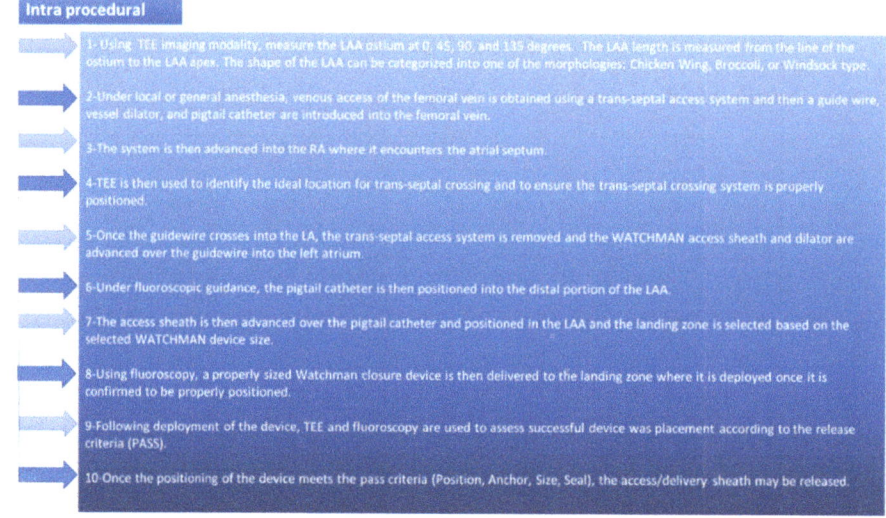

Figure 2. The WATCHMAN implant intra-procedural steps.

3. Pre-Procedural Assessment of the LAA

Here, we will provide the pre-procedural assessment of the LAA on 2D TEE, 3D TEE, and MDCT (Figure 3).

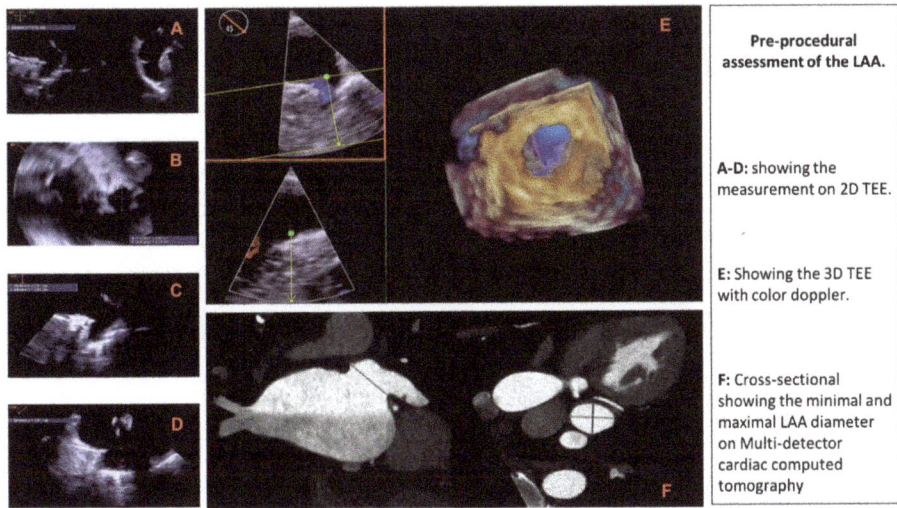

Figure 3. Pre-procedural assessment of the LAA using different imaging modalities.

4. Conclusions

Rotational three-dimensional transesophageal echocardiography is a more accurate alternative to two-dimensional transesophageal echocardiography in the assessment of the left atrial appendage morphology and has been the most commonly used imaging modality for sizing the left atrial appendage. Three-dimensional computed tomography has recently emerged as an imaging modality and it has showed exceptional accuracy when merged with three-dimensional printing technology. However, real-time three-dimensional transesophageal echocardiography may be considered the preferred imaging modality to assess left atrial appendage dimensions as it can provide accurate measurements without requiring radiation exposure or contrast administration (Table 6).

Table 6. Preprocedural imaging impact on predicting the correct size of the WATCHMAN device.

Imaging Modality	Impact on Implantation Success
2D TEE	Less accurate
3D TEE	Accurate without requiring radiation exposure or contrast administration
3D CT	Exceptional accuracy when merged with three-dimensional printing technology

Author Contributions: All authors contributed extensively to the work presented in this literature review. R.M. (Ramez Morcos) did the literature search, created the tables & the figures, and drafted the manuscript. H.T. & P.B. drafted the manuscript and provided revision. J.C., R.M. (Rupesh Manam) & V.P. drafted the manuscript. A.C., M.K. & A.M. collected the data, drafted the manuscript, and provided revisions. B.M. reviewed the manuscript and provided critical Revision.

Funding: This research received no external funding.

Conflicts of Interest: The authors declare no conflict of interest.

References

1. Reiffel, J.A. Atrial fibrillation and stroke: Epidemiology. *Am. J. Med.* **2014**, *127*, e15–e16. [CrossRef] [PubMed]
2. Sievert, H.; Lesh, M.D.; Trepels, T.; Omran, H.; Bartorelli, A.; Della Bella, P.; Nakai, T.; Reisman, M.; DiMario, C.; Block, P.; et al. Percutaneous left atrial appendage transcatheter occlusion to prevent stroke in high-risk patients with atrial fibrillation: Early clinical experience. *Circulation* **2002**, *105*, 1887–1889. [CrossRef] [PubMed]

3. Go, A.S.; Hylek, E.M.; Borowsky, L.H.; Phillips, K.A.; Selby, J.V.; Singer, D.E. Warfarin use among ambulatory patients with nonvalvular atrial fibrillation: The anticoagulation and risk factors in atrial fibrillation (ATRIA) study. *Ann. Intern. Med.* **1999**, *131*, 927–934. [CrossRef] [PubMed]
4. Wunderlich, N.C.; Beigel, R.; Swaans, M.J.; Ho, S.Y.; Siegel, R.J. Percutaneous interventions for left atrial appendage exclusion: Options, assessment, and imaging using 2D and 3D echocardiography. *JACC Cardiovasc. Imaging* **2015**, *8*, 472–488. [CrossRef] [PubMed]
5. Holmes, D.R.; Reddy, V.Y.; Turi, Z.G.; Doshi, S.K.; Sievert, H.; Buchbinder, M.; Mulli, M.; Sick, P. Percutaneous closure of the left atrial appendage versus warfarin therapy for prevention of stroke in patients with atrial fibrillation: A randomised non-inferiority trial. *Lancet* **2009**, *374*, 534–542. [CrossRef]
6. Kamiński, R.; Kosiński, A.; Brala, M.; Piwko, G.; Lewicka, E.; Dąbrowska-Kugacka, A.; Raczak, G.; Kozłowski, D.; Grzybiak, M. Variability of the Left Atrial Appendage in Human Hearts. *PLoS ONE* **2015**, *10*, e0141901. [CrossRef] [PubMed]
7. Zhou, Q.; Song, H.; Zhang, L.; Deng, Q.; Chen, J.; Hu, B.; Wang, Y.; Guo, R. Roles of real-time three-dimensional transesophageal echocardiography in peri-operation of transcatheter left atrial appendage closure. *Medicine* **2017**, *96*, e5637. [CrossRef] [PubMed]
8. Schmidt-Salzmann, M.; Meincke, F.; Kreidel, F.; Spangenberg, T.; Ghanem, A.; Kuck, K.H.; Bergmann, M.W. Improved Algorithm for Ostium Size Assessment in Watchman Left Atrial Appendage Occlusion Using Three-Dimensional Echocardiography. *J. Invasive Cardiol.* **2017**, *29*, 232–238. [PubMed]
9. Wang, D.D.; Eng, M.; Kupsky, D.; Myers, E.; Forbes, M.; Rahman, M.; Zaidan, M.; Parikh, S.; Wyman, J.; Pantelic, M.; et al. Application of 3-Dimensional Computed Tomographic Image Guidance to WATCHMAN Implantation and Impact on Early Operator Learning Curve: Single-Center Experience. *JACC Cardiovasc. Interv.* **2016**, *9*, 2329–2340. [CrossRef] [PubMed]
10. Yosefy, C.; Laish-Farkash, A.; Azhibekov, Y.; Khalameizer, V.; Brodkin, B.; Katz, A. A New Method for Direct Three-Dimensional Measurement of Left Atrial Appendage Dimensions during Transesophageal Echocardiography. *Echocardiography* **2016**, *33*, 69–76. [CrossRef] [PubMed]
11. Nucifora, G.; Faletra, F.F.; Regoli, F.; Pasotti, E.; Pedrazzini, G.; Moccetti, T.; Auricchio, A. Evaluation of the left atrial appendage with real-time 3-dimensional transesophageal echocardiography: Implications for catheter-based left atrial appendage closure. *Circ. Cardiovasc. Imaging* **2011**, *4*, 514–523. [CrossRef] [PubMed]
12. Yosefy, C.; Azhibekov, Y.; Brodkin, B.; Khalameizer, V.; Katz, A.; Laish-Farkash, A. Rotational method simplifies 3-dimensional measurement of left atrial appendage dimensions during transesophageal echocardiography. *Cardiovasc. Ultrasound* **2016**, *14*, 36. [CrossRef] [PubMed]
13. Nakajima, H.; Seo, Y.; Ishizu, T.; Yamamoto, M.; Machino, T.; Harimura, Y.; RyoKawamura, R.; Sekiguchi, Y.; Tada, H.; Aonuma, K. Analysis of the left atrial appendage by three-dimensional transesophageal echocardiography. *Am. J. Cardiol.* **2010**, *106*, 885–892. [CrossRef] [PubMed]
14. Chow, D.H.; Bieliauskas, G.; Sawaya, F.J.; Millan-Iturbe, O.; Kofoed, K.F.; Søndergaard, L.; De Backer, O. A comparative study of different imaging modalities for successful percutaneous left atrial appendage closure. *Open Heart* **2017**, *4*, e000627. [CrossRef] [PubMed]
15. Rajwani, A.; Nelson, A.J.; Shirazi, M.G.; Disney, P.J.; Teo, K.S.; Wong, D.T.; Young, G.D.; Worthley, S.G. CT sizing for left atrial appendage closure is associated with favourable outcomes for procedural safety. *Eur. Heart J. Cardiovasc. Imaging* **2017**, *18*, 1361–1368. [CrossRef] [PubMed]
16. Budge, L.P.; Shaffer, K.M.; Moorman, J.R.; Lake, D.E.; Ferguson, J.D.; Mangrum, J.M. Analysis of in vivo left atrial appendage morphology in patients with atrial fibrillation: A direct comparison of transesophageal echocardiography, planar cardiac CT, and segmented three-dimensional cardiac CT. *J. Interv. Card. Electrophysiol.* **2008**, *23*, 87–93. [CrossRef] [PubMed]
17. Wang, Y.A.N.; Di Biase, L.; Horton, R.P.; Nguyen, T.; Morhanty, P.; Natale, A. Left atrial appendage studied by computed tomography to help planning for appendage closure device placement. *J. Cardiovasc. Electrophysiol.* **2010**, *21*, 973–982. [CrossRef] [PubMed]
18. Hell, M.M.; Achenbach, S.; Yoo, I.S.; Franke, J.; Blachutzik, F.; Roether, J.; Graf, V.; Raaz-Schrauder, D.; Marwan, D.; Schlundt, C. 3D printing for sizing left atrial appendage closure device: Head-to-head comparison with computed tomography and transoesophageal echocardiography. *EuroIntervention* **2017**, *13*, 1234–1241. [CrossRef] [PubMed]
19. Li, H.; Shu, M.; Wang, X.; Song, Z. Application of 3D printing technology to left atrial appendage occlusion. *Int. J. Cardiol.* **2017**, *231*, 258–263. [CrossRef] [PubMed]

20. Goitein, O.; Fink, N.; Guetta, V.; Beinart, R.; Brodov, Y.; Konen, E.; Goitein, D.; Di Segni, E.; Grupper, A.; Glikson, M. Printed MDCT 3D models for prediction of left atrial appendage (LAA) occluder device size: A feasibility study. *EuroIntervention* **2017**, *13*, e1076–e1079. [CrossRef] [PubMed]
21. Möbius-Winkler, S.; Sandri, M.; Mangner, N.; Lurz, P.; Dähnert, I.; Schuler, G. The WATCHMAN left atrial appendage closure device for atrial fibrillation. *J. Vis. Exp.* **2012**. [CrossRef] [PubMed]

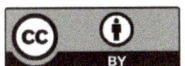

© 2018 by the authors. Licensee MDPI, Basel, Switzerland. This article is an open access article distributed under the terms and conditions of the Creative Commons Attribution (CC BY) license (http://creativecommons.org/licenses/by/4.0/).

MDPI
St. Alban-Anlage 66
4052 Basel
Switzerland
Tel. +41 61 683 77 34
Fax +41 61 302 89 18
www.mdpi.com

Journal of Clinical Medicine Editorial Office
E-mail: jcm@mdpi.com
www.mdpi.com/journal/jcm

www.ingramcontent.com/pod-product-compliance
Lightning Source LLC
LaVergne TN
LVHW070227100526
838202LV00015B/2102